Electrophysiological Foundations of Cardiac Arrhythmias

A Bridge Between Basic Mechanisms and Clinical Electrophysiology

Second Edition

ONLINE ACCESS

The purchase of a new copy of this book entitles the first retail purchaser to free personal online access to a digital version of this edition.

Please send a copy of your purchase receipt to info@cardiotext.com with subject EP FOUNDATIONS, 2ED, and we will email you a redemption code along with instructions on how to access the digital file.

Electrophysiological Foundations of Cardiac Arrhythmias

A Bridge Between Basic Mechanisms and Clinical Electrophysiology

Second Edition

Andrew L. Wit, PhD
Penelope A. Boyden, PhD
Mark E. Josephson, MD
Hein J. Wellens, MD, PhD

cardiotext PUBLISHING

Second Edition

Cardiotext Publishing, LLC
3405 W. 44th Street
Minneapolis, Minnesota 55410
USA

www.cardiotextpublishing.com

Any updates to this book may be found at:
www.cardiotextpublishing.com/electrophysiological-foundations-of-cardiac-arrhythmias-2ed

Comments, inquiries, and requests for bulk sales can be directed to the publisher at: info@cardiotextpublishing.com.

Library of Congress Control Number: 2020934194

ISBN: 978-1-942909-42-2

eISBN: 978-1-942909-48-4

20 21 22 23 24 25 26 10 9 8 7 6 5 4 3 2

Dedication

This book is dedicated to all our teachers who have inspired us to pursue the fascinating study of cardiac arrhythmias and to our families who have traveled with us on this journey.

In Memoriam

Mark E. Josephson passed away on January 11, 2017 as the first edition of this book went to press. His contributions remain a centerpiece of this second edition. His death is an enormous personal and professional loss to his co-authors and the cardiology community.

Acknowledgments

The authors would like to thank the following colleagues who reviewed parts of the manuscript of the first edition. However, any errors are entirely our own responsibility.

Penelope A. Boyden, PhD
Candido Cabo, PhD
Edward Ciaccio, PhD
Nicholas Peters, MD
Richard Robinson, PhD
Dan Roden, MD
Michael Rosen, MD
Albert Waldo, MD

We would also like to express our gratitude to Katharine Swenson, MD, for her excellent editorial assistance, which transformed our manuscript into the first edition of this book. Her work has infuenced the second edition as well.

Table of Contents

About the Authors

Andrew L. Wit, PhD, FACC
Emeritus Professor of Pharmacology, Department of Pharmacology
College of Physicians and Surgeons of Columbia University
New York, New York

Penelope A. Boyden, PhD
Emerita Professor of Pharmacology, Department of Pharmacology
College of Physicians and Surgeons of Columbia University
New York, New York

Mark E. Josephson, MD, FACC, FHRS, FAHA
Director, Harvard-Thorndike Electrophysiology Institute and Arrhythmia Service
Chief Emeritus, Division of Cardiovascular Medicine
Beth Israel Deaconess Medical Center
Herman C. Dana Professor of Medicine
Harvard Medical School
Boston, Massachusetts

Hein J. Wellens, MD, PhD, FACC, FAHA, FESC
Emeritus Professor of Cardiology, University of Maastricht
Maastricht, The Netherlands

PREFACE

Why Is Basic Cardiac Electrophysiology Important?

Approximately 55 years ago, the introduction of programmed electrical stimulation of the heart together with the recording of intracardiac electrograms, including that of the bundle of His, opened the door for better understanding of the underlying mechanisms of different types of cardiac arrhythmias. This initial diagnostic phase led to new therapeutic possibilities, such as arrhythmia surgery, better selection of antiarrhythmic drugs, antitachycardia pacing, and catheter ablation. In those 55 years, the number of cardiologists involved in cardiac arrhythmia management and the complexity of diagnosis and treatment options increased remarkably.

Of great importance has been a parallel increase in knowledge of the basic electrophysiology of the heart that has been essential for understanding the mechanisms of arrhythmogenesis and their clinical expression. A major factor was the introduction of the microelectrode technique for recording transmembrane action potentials from heart cells. This has led the authors of this book to the firm belief that practitioners of clinical cardiac electrophysiology should have a solid foundation in the basic electrophysiology responsible for the rhythm abnormalities that they are treating. This reasoning is two-fold.

First, understanding the electrophysiologic mechanism of an arrhythmia can help in selecting the appropriate treatment. Initially, the mechanism may not always be evident, but requires some probing to discover it. Appropriate reasoning and interpretations of test results to successfully identify the mechanism is based on knowledge of the electrophysiological properties of the different mechanisms.

Second, the development of modern clinical cardiac electrophysiology has been built on a foundation of the basic science of cardiac electrophysiology, without which the discipline would have stagnated. Discoveries that have moved the field forward and enabled it to accomplish previously unimaginable goals have been based on the interactions of laboratory and clinical research on basic mechanisms. For expert clinical practice and to make new discoveries in the field, current practitioners of clinical cardiac electrophysiology must have a solid basic knowledge foundation of basic electrophysiology.

This book is designed to lead the reader through the pathway from basic cardiac electrophysiology over the bridge to clinical cardiac electrophysiology. Basic cellular electrophysiology of the three main categories of arrhythmogenesis (automaticity, triggered activity, and reentry—see the Introduction and Table i-1) is described in sufficient detail to understand how alterations in cellular electrophysiology cause an arrhythmia. Then, these cellular electrophysiological mechanisms are related to the ECG appearance of that arrhythmia and how the arrhythmia responds to interventions such as programmed electrical stimulation and selected pharmacological agents that are mechanism-specific. Therapy for arrhythmias is not part of this curriculum.

In writing this book, it has not been our intent to provide a complete review or description of either the basic or the clinical electrophysiology of the heart. These fields are now so extensive that a complete review of both would be impossible undertakings for the authors and would require a number of contributors who are expert in all aspects of both basic and clinical cardiac electrophysiology. Rather, it is our purpose to provide the basic foundations of both cellular electrophysiology and the electrophysiology of selected arrhythmias, so that readers will be able to advance their education with additional texts written by experts. These texts typically assume the fundamental knowledge of basic and clinical electrophysiology found in this book.

This is the second edition of the book originally published in 2017. We have tried to make it more user-friendly by eliminating details that may not have been necessary for the understanding of basic concepts, shortening the book by about a third.

Andrew L. Wit, PhD
Penelope A. Boyden, PhD
Mark E. Josephson, MD
Hein J. Wellens, MD, PhD

INTRODUCTION

How This Book Is Organized

Although there are many kinds of clinical arrhythmias with many different pathological causes, in the final analysis, they all are the result of critical alterations in cardiac cellular electrophysiology. Since cellular electrophysiology is so important, it is the foundation for the description of mechanisms causing arrhythmias in this book. It is presented in the context of an arrhythmia mechanism and examples of the clinical arrhythmias that this mechanism causes.

The different cellular mechanisms that form the organization of the book are presented in **Table i-1**.

Table i-1 Electrophysiological Mechanisms of Cardiac Arrhythmias

I. Abnormal Impulse Initiation
A. Automaticity • normal automaticity • abnormal automaticity
B. Triggered Activity • delayed afterdepolarizations • early afterdepolarizations
II. Altered (Abnormal) Impulse Conduction
A. Conduction block leading to ectopic pacemaker "escape"
B. Unidirectional block and reentry • anatomical reentry • functional reentry

(Modified from Hoffman, BF, Rosen MR. Cellular mechanisms of cardiac arrhythmias. *Circ Res.* 1981;49:1–15.)

ABNORMAL IMPULSE INITIATION

This topic constitutes Chapters 1–8 of this book. The term "impulse initiation" is used to describe an electrical signal (impulse) that arises in a single cell or group of closely coupled cells through depolarization (decrease in negativity) of the cell membrane potential to a threshold that initiates an action potential. Once initiated, the action potential(s) form an electrical impulse that spreads to other regions of the heart.

Table i-1 subdivides the causes for impulse initiation into two categories: (A) automaticity and (B) triggered activity. Each has its own unique cellular mechanism resulting in the membrane depolarization that initiates impulses.

Automaticity

Automaticity is the result of spontaneous (diastolic) depolarization (SDD). **Chapters 1–4** describe the cellular mechanisms of automaticity and provide examples of the clinical arrhythmias that it causes. Automaticity is divided into two kinds, normal (**Chapters 1–3**) and abnormal (**Chapter 4**). Normal automaticity is found in the primary pacemaker of the heart—the sinus node (**Chapter 2**)—as well as in subsidiary or latent pacemakers found in certain regions of the atria, A-V junction, and ventricular specialized conducting system (**Chapter 3**). Impulse initiation is a normal property of these latent pacemakers.

On the other hand, abnormal automaticity (**Chapter 4**) occurs in cardiac cells when major (abnormal) changes occur in their transmembrane potentials due to pathology. Working atrial and ventricular myocardial cells do not normally have spontaneous diastolic depolarization and do not normally initiate spontaneous impulses. However, when their resting potentials are reduced sufficiently by disease, spontaneous diastolic depolarization may occur and cause repetitive impulse initiation, a phenomenon called depolarization-induced abnormal automaticity. Atrial and ventricular tachycardias occurring in a number of different diseases can be caused by abnormal automaticity.

Triggered Activity

Triggered activity (Table i-1 B), is a form of impulse initiation caused by afterdepolarizations. Afterdepolarizations are abnormal oscillations in membrane potential that occur after the rapid depolarization (Phase 0) of an action potential. Chapters 5–8 describe the electrophysiological mechanisms for afterdepolarizations and provides examples of the clinical arrhythmias that they cause. There are two types of afterdepolarizations that cause triggered activity. One type is delayed until repolarization is complete or nearly complete (delayed afterdepolarizations [DADs]) (**Chapters 5** and **6**). The other type is early, occurring before repolarization is complete (early after depolarizations [EADs]) (**Chapters 7** and **8**).

ALTERED (ABNORMAL) IMPULSE CONDUCTION

Altered (abnormal) impulse conduction (heading II in Table i-1) includes both arrhythmias due to conduction block leading to ectopic pacemaker escape and arrhythmias due to unidirectional block and reentry.

Conduction Block Leading to Ectopic Pacemaker "Escape"

Conduction block leading to ectopic pacemaker "escape" (subheading II, A) is described in **Chapters 1–4** as a mechanism for occurrence of some arrhythmias caused by normal and abnormal automaticity.

Unidirectional Block and Reentry

Unidirectional block and reentry are the subjects of **Chapters 9–12**. **Chapter 9** describes the basic cellular electrophysiology of impulse conduction in the heart and how this process is altered by disease to slow it or to cause it to fail (conduction block). These basic cellular concepts are then applied to the different mechanisms that cause reentrant excitation, a process whereby the propagating impulse can circulate and return to re-excite regions that it has already excited without the requirement for new impulse initiation. Reentrant circuits are described that are dependent on anatomical structures as well as functional properties of cardiac muscle and the characteristic responses to electrical stimulation and some pharmacological agents.

Chapters 10–12 describe the process of reentry in different regions of the heart (atria, A-V junction, ventricles). Each chapter also provides example arrhythmias that are caused by this mechanism.

THE BRIDGE BETWEEN BASIC MECHANISMS AND CLINICAL ELECTROPHYSIOLOGY

The purpose of this book is to explain how basic cardiac electrophysiology can elucidate mechanisms causing cardiac arrhythmias, that is, to provide a bridge between basic mechanisms and clinical electrophysiology. Concepts from basic electrophysiology are interwoven with the arrhythmia mechanisms and examples of clinical arrhythmias in order to show the close interrelationships between basic and clinical electrophysiology. With the appropriate background from medical school physiology, we hope these basic concepts are understandable as encountered while progressing through the book.

This same bridge is also a pathway from clinical arrhythmias to basic mechanisms. It is our belief that as the student becomes more familiar with the mechanisms of arrhythmogenesis, the information obtained from clinical electrophysiology will become easier to assimilate and to utilize for improved diagnosis and treatment of real-world arrhythmias.

SOURCES

Josephson ME. *Josephson's Clinical Cardiac Electrophysiology: Techniques and Interpretations* (5th ed.). Philadelphia, PA: Wolters Kluwer; 2016.

Wellens HJJ, Conover M. *The ECG in Emergency Decision Making*. St. Louis, MO: Saunders Elsevier; 2006.

Abbreviations and Ionic Currents Involved in Arrhythmogenesis

ABBREVIATIONS

ACh	acetylcholine
AF	atrial fibrillation
A-H	time interval from atrial deflection (A) to His bundle deflection (H) in the His bundle electrogram (HBE)
AIVR	accelerated idioventricular rhythm
AN	atrial to A-V nodal transitional region
ANS	autonomic nervous system
APD	action potential duration
APD	atrial premature depolarization
ARVC	arrhythmogenic right ventricular cardiomyopathy
ATP	adenosine triphosphate
A-V	atrioventricular
AVN	atrioventricular node
AVNRT	A-V nodal reentrant tachycardia
BBR	bundle branch reentry
BCL	basic cycle length
bpm	beats/min
cAMP	cyclic adenosine monophosphate
Casq2	calsequestrin 2
CL	cycle length
CMT	circus movement tachycardia
CN	compact region of the A-V node
CPVT	catecholaminergic polymorphic ventricular tachycardia
CSM	carotid sinus massage
CSO	coronary sinus ostium
CSRT	corrected sinus node recovery time
CT	crista terminalis
Cx	connexin
DAD	delayed afterdepolarization
DCM	dilated cardiomyopathy
EAD	early afterdepolarization
EG	electrogram
ERP	effective refractory period
HBE	His bundle electrogram comprised of atrial electrogram (A), His bundle electrogram (H), and ventricular electrogram (V)
HCM	hypertrophic cardiomyopathy
H-V	time interval from His bundle electrogram (H) to ventricular electrogram (V) in the His bundle electrogram
ID	intercalated disk
IVC	inferior vena cava
JET	junctional ectopic tachycardia
LBB	left bundle branch
LBBB	left bundle branch block
LCR	local calcium release
LE	left extension of A-V node
LP	left pathway
LQT	long QT interval
LQTS	long QT interval syndromes
LVOT	left ventricular outflow tract
MDP	maximum diastolic potential
mV	millivolts
NH	nodal to His bundle transitional region
NSR	normal sinus rhythm
PCL	paced cycle length
PE	posterior extension of A-V node
PES	programmed electrical stimulation
PF	Purkinje fiber
PN	perinodal
RBB	right bundle branch
RBBB	right bundle branch block
RC	return cycle
RCL	return cycle length
RE	right (posterior) extension of A-V node
RP	right pathway
RVOT	right ventricular outflow tract
RyR2	Ryanodine receptor in cardiac muscle
S-A	sino atrial
SACT	sinoatrial conduction time
SAN	sinoatrial node
SCL	sinus cycle length
SDD	spontaneous diastolic depolarization
SERCA	sarcoplasmic reticulum Ca^{2+} ATPase (SR Ca^{2+} pump)
SR	sarcoplasmic reticulum
SRT	sinus node recovery time
SVC	superior vena cava
SVT	supraventricular tachycardia
TP	threshold potential
VF	ventricular fibrillation
VPD	ventricular premature depolarization
VT	ventricular tachycardia
WPW	Wolff-Parkinson-White syndrome

IONIC CURRENTS INVOLVED IN ARRHYTHMOGENESIS

I_{CaL}	L-type (long lasting) inward calcium current that contributes to the plateau phase of muscle and Purkinje cells. Responsible for phase 0 of sinus node and compact A-V node cells.
I_{CaT}	T-type (transient) inward calcium current, may contribute to pacemaker activity in some cells.
I_{Cl}	Current carried by chloride ions. Physiological role in heart uncertain but may be involved in cell swelling and DAD formation.
I_f	Inward current that contributes to the pacemaker potential ("funny current"). This is also called I_h.
I_K	Outward potassium current, also called the delayed rectifier current, that contributes to repolarization.
I_{K1}	Outward potassium current called the inward rectifier, that is responsible for the resting potential and terminal phase of repolarization.
I_{KACh}	Outward potassium current that is increased by acetylcholine.
I_{KAdo}	Outward adenosine activated potassium current, probably through same channel as I_{KACh}, sometimes designated as $I_{KACh/Ado}$.
I_{KATP}	Outward potassium current activated by a decrease in adenosine triphosphate.
I_{Kr}	Outward potassium current that is the rapidly activating component of the delayed rectifier current (I_K), contributing to repolarization.
I_{Ks}	Outward potassium current that is the slowly activating component of the delayed rectifier current (I_K) contributing to repolarization.
I_{Kur}	Ultra rapid activating outward potassium current in atrial muscle contributing to repolarization.
I_{Na}	Fast inward sodium current responsible for phase 0 depolarization in working atrial and ventricular myocardial cells and Purkinje cells.
I_{NCX}	Current generated by sodium–calcium exchanger.
I_P	Current generated by sodium–potassium pump (pump current).
I_{st}	Sustained inward current carried by sodium ions that may contribute to pacemaking in sinus node.
I_{TI}	Transient inward current that causes delayed afterdepolarizations.
I_{to}	Transient outward potassium current contributing to early phase (1) repolarization.

CHAPTER

1

Basic Principles of Normal Automaticity

Automaticity is the term used to indicate the mechanism for the initiation of an electrical signal in a single cell or group of closely interacting (coupled) cells. This signal, in the form of an action potential, arises from spontaneous depolarization of the membrane potential. The action potential is the electrical signal or impulse that excites the heart, and the cell(s) that generate this signal are called "pacemakers."

"Normal automaticity" is found in the primary pacemaker of the heart, the sinus node, as well as in certain subsidiary or latent pacemakers that can become the pacemaker under special conditions (hence the term, latent). Impulse initiation is an intrinsic property of these latent pacemakers, as it is in the sinus node. ("Abnormal automaticity," described in Chapter 4, is related to pathological changes in a region of the heart, often where the cells do not have intrinsic pacemaker properties, although there are exceptions.) The recording of the transmembrane resting potential (often referred to here as simply the membrane potential) and action potentials as well as the membrane currents of individual myocardial cells has provided much of the information necessary for understanding the mechanism by which certain myocardial cells can generate impulses spontaneously by normal automaticity.

The cause of normal automaticity in the sinus node and latent pacemakers is a spontaneous decline (becoming less negative) in the membrane potential during diastole or phase 4. This decline in membrane potential is referred to as either the "pacemaker potential," "phase 4 depolarization," or "spontaneous diastolic depolarization" (SDD). **Figure 1-1** illustrates an action potential with a pacemaker potential in a myocardial cell with the property of normal automaticity and compares the automatic cell with a cell without normal automaticity (nonautomatic cell).

Panel A shows a nonautomatic cell with a steady level of resting (diastolic) potential during phase 4 (the resting potential [RP]) between action potentials (purple arrow). This type of cell must be excited from an external source (green arrow), either another connected cell or an applied electrical stimulus, to initiate an action potential. The action potential is comprised of phase 0 (rapid depolarization phase or "upstroke") and phases 1, 2, and 3 (repolarization phases).

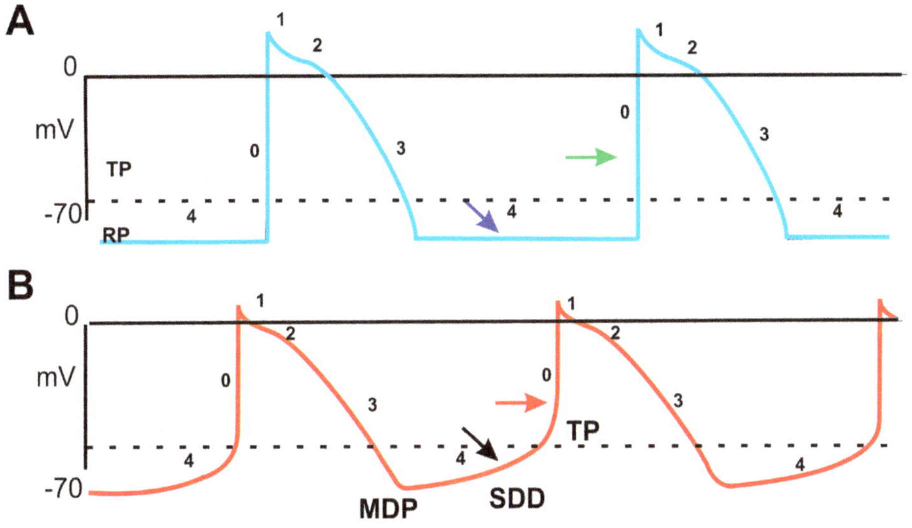

Figure 1-1 Diagrams of transmembrane action potentials characteristic of a nonautomatic cell (**Panel A**) and a normal automatic cell (**Panel B**). In each panel, the horizontal black line indicates "0" potential and the horizontal dashed line is the threshold potential (TP).

Electrophysiological Foundations of Cardiac Arrhythmias: A Bridge Between Basic Mechanisms and Clinical Electrophysiology, Second Edition.

Panel B shows a cell with normal automaticity. Spontaneous diastolic depolarization (the pacemaker potential) is that part of the membrane potential labeled "SDD" (black arrow) coinciding with phase 4 of the membrane potential. In Panel B, the membrane potential moves spontaneously in a positive direction from the maximum potential during diastole (maximum diastolic potential [MDP]) with a negative value of –70 mV until it reaches the threshold potential (TP), which is less negative at –60 mV. At this point, the inward depolarizing current (phase 0, red arrow) is activated, and this in turn causes the cell to generate an action potential. Phase 0 is responsible for conduction of the action potential from the pacemaker cell to surrounding cells. Depolarization of membrane potential during SDD represents the summation of a number of inward and outward transmembrane currents with depolarization resulting because inward current dominates.

In later chapters, we describe the specific ion channels and membrane currents that are involved in the genesis of the pacemaker depolarization, but these details are not necessary at this point for understanding the role of automaticity in causing arrhythmias.

General Principles of Normal Automaticity

1. Control of rate of automatic impulse initiation
2. Relationship between sinus node and latent pacemakers
3. Electrophysiological causes of ectopic automatic arrhythmias
4. General ECG characteristics of automatic arrhythmias
5. Effects of electrical stimulation and pharmacological agents on normal automaticity

CONTROL OF RATE OF AUTOMATIC IMPULSE INITIATION

The rate of automatic impulse initiation is determined by two major factors: the characteristics of the transmembrane potential and electrical coupling between pacemaker and nonpacemaker cells.

Transmembrane Potential

The intrinsic rate at which pacemaker cells initiate impulses is determined by the amount of time it takes for the membrane potential to move from its maximal negativity (maximum diastolic potential, MDP) after repolarization to the threshold potential to generate an action potential or impulse. Time to threshold potential is in turn dependent on the interplay of several factors (**Figure 1-2**), including:

- The level of the "maximum diastolic potential" (MDP), which is the maximum negativity attained after repolarization of the action potential. This term is used instead of resting potential (RP) since the membrane potential in a pacemaker cell does not have a period of rest as it does in a nonpacemaker cell (Figure 1-1, Panel B).
- The level of the "threshold potential" (TP) for initiation of phase 0 of the action potential. The threshold potential is the membrane potential at which the inward current causing phase 0 becomes regenerative to cause a conducted action potential.
- The slope of "spontaneous diastolic depolarization" (SDD), which is the rate of change of phase 4, also referred to as the pacemaker potential. This slope is dependent on the speed of activation and the magnitude of net inward current. Sometimes there may be two different slopes if the rate of change is not constant.
- The "action potential duration" (APD) is the time from depolarization phase 0 to complete repolarization at the end of phase 3.

These features of the transmembrane potential are under the control of the ion channels, pumps, and exchangers involved in the genesis of the pacemaker potential and action potential, which will be described in detail later in this chapter and in Chapters 2 and 3. A change in any one of the above parameters caused by changes in the membrane currents will alter the time required for SDD to move the membrane potential from its MDP to the TP, and thereby alter the rate of impulse initiation. Understanding the interplay of these factors is necessary for understanding how automatic arrhythmias occur.

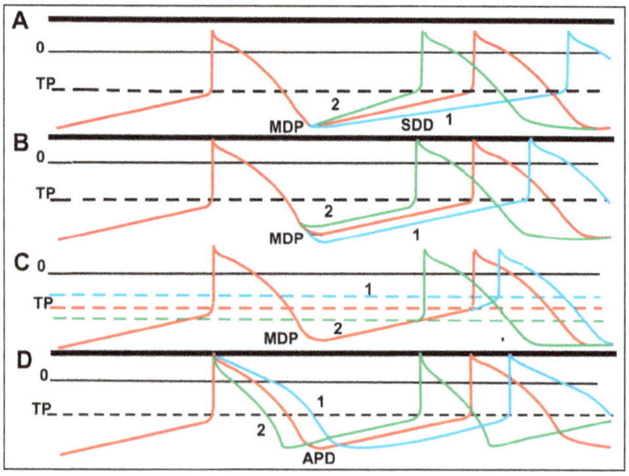

Figure 1-2 Factors that control intrinsic rate. **Panel A** shows effects of changes in slope of spontaneous diastolic depolarization (SDD). **Panel B** shows effects of changes in maximum diastolic potential (MDP). **Panel C** shows effects of changes in threshold potential (TP). **Panel D** shows effects of changes in action potential duration (APD).

Figure 1-2 illustrates how these parameters control the spontaneous rate. Panel A shows how changes in the slope of SDD can change the rate of automatic impulse initiation. The red trace shows action potentials with the initial intrinsic or automatic rate of the pacemaker cell, that is determined by the time required for SDD caused by the pacemaker current(s), to move the membrane potential from the MDP to TP. The blue trace (labeled 1) shows the effect of a decrease in the slope of SDD. This would be caused by a decrease in net inward pacemaker current, resulting in a longer interval between action potentials and a decrease in heart rate because of the longer time required for membrane potential to reach the threshold potential. Modest parasympathetic (vagal) activation is one condition that results in a decreased slope of SDD of sinus node pacemaker cells to slow the heart rate. Some antiarrhythmic drugs also have this effect on latent pacemakers. The green trace (labeled 2) shows the effect of an increase in the slope of SDD that increases heart rate. This would be caused by an increase in the net inward pacemaker current, which reduces the time to reach threshold potential and decreases the time between action potentials. Sympathetic activation, which accelerates the heart rate, is an example of this condition.

Figure 1-2, Panel B illustrates how a change in the MDP can change the rate of automatic impulse initiation. If the MDP increases (becomes more negative), going from the nadir of the solid red trace (initial intrinsic value) to the blue trace (labeled 1), then the SDD (or pacemaker potential) takes longer to reach threshold potential and the rate of impulse initiation slows. This occurs even if the slope of the SDD is not altered as shown in the figure. An increase in MDP results from a net increase in outward current during diastole which usually is also accompanied by a decrease in slope of SDD. Strong vagal activation causes an increase in MDP of sinus pacemaker cells in addition to the decreased slope of SDD, both of which slow sinus rate. Conversely, a decrease in the MDP (going from red to green trace, labeled 2), decreases the time it takes to go from MDP to TP and increases the rate of impulse initiation even if the slope of SDD is not altered as shown in the figure. However, a decrease in outward current during diastole that decreases MDP, often increases the slope of SDD. A simultaneous increase in sympathetic activity and decrease in vagal activity can produce this change and increase the sinus rate.

Figure 1-2, Panel C illustrates the effect of changes in TP on the rate of impulse initiation. The TP (dashed lines) is the membrane potential required for initiation of the upstroke (phase 0) of the action potential. When the TP is decreased from the initial level indicated by the red dashed line (associated with the solid red line action potential) to the less negative TP (blue dashed line, labeled 1), then the SDD must proceed for a longer time before an impulse is finally initiated (rapid upstroke, solid blue trace). Thus the heart rate is slower. Conversely, an increase in TP (from red to more negative green dashed line, labeled 2) accelerates the heart rate because SDD must proceed for a shorter time before an impulse is initiated, shown by the earlier green action potential.

Don't be confused by this terminology corresponding to negative values in which an *increase* in "potential"—the difference between the measured value and 0—is actually more negative, while a *decrease* in potential is less negative. On the other hand, when the term "threshold" is used by itself, an increase in threshold means "more difficult to excite" while a decrease in threshold means "more excitable."

Figure 1-2, Panel D, shows how changes in the APD can alter the rate of impulse initiation. The APD is controlled in part by the membrane currents that determine the time course for repolarization (phases 1, 2, and 3). SDD begins after completion of action potential repolarization. If APD lengthens (increases), as illustrated by the change from the red action potential at the left to the blue action potential (labeled 1) at the left, and the diastolic time remains constant, the rate of impulse initiation decreases (compare onset of the second red action potential with the later second blue action potential). A decrease in action potential duration shown by the green action potential (labeled 2) at the left compared with the red action potential, accelerates the rate (compare the earlier onset of the second green action potential with the later onset of the second red action potential) when diastolic time remains constant. Changes in APD do not normally apply to the physiological control of rate, but may be instrumental in the rate effect of drugs that alter repolarization.

Electrical Coupling Between Pacemaker and Nonpacemaker Cells

In addition to the changes discussed in Figure 1-2, electrical coupling between pacemaker and nonpacemaker cells provided by gap junctions, reduces the slope of SDD and slows or inhibits pacemaker cell impulse initiation by electrotonic current flow. The way this effect is exerted is diagrammed in **Figure 1-3**.

The lower part of the figure diagrams two adjacent cells, P and NP (yellow cylinder). Cell P is a pacemaker cell (action potential is above it) with SDD (black trace) and cell NP is a nonpacemaker cell (action potential is above it) with a more negative membrane potential during phase 4 (black trace). The broken double black lines between the two cells represents the adjacent cell membranes (sarcolemmae) of each cell, which abut to form the intercalated disk. In the disks are structures called "gap junctions," specialized regions of close interaction between the sarcolemmae of neighboring myocytes in which clusters of channels, formed by proteins called connexins, bridge the paired plasma membranes to connect the intracellular spaces of cell P and cell NP. Because gap-junctional membrane is several orders of magnitude more permeable than nonjunctional plasma membrane, it provides low resistance pathways for "electrotonic current flow" between myocardial cells (represented by the curved black arrows), which is important for impulse propagation. (The mechanism for impulse propagation is described in detail in, Chapter 9, Figure 9-4). Electrotonic current flow in the absence of propagation also influences impulse initiation by automaticity.

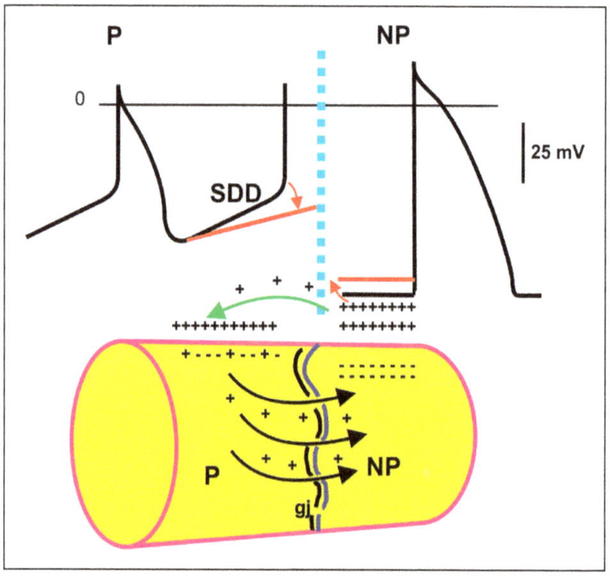

Figure 1-3 Influence of electrical coupling of pacemaker cell (P) to nonpacemaker cell (NP) on spontaneous diastolic depolarization (SDD).

During SDD, the membrane potential in the pacemaker cell (black trace in P) becomes much less negative than the membrane potential in the adjacent well coupled nonpacemaker cell (black trace in NP). As a result of this potential difference, current (positive charges) flows intracellularly from the pacemaker cell (P) towards the nonpacemaker cell (NP) through the gap junction channels (curved black arrows and + signs). It also flows in extracellular space from the nonpacemaker cell (NP) to the pacemaker cell (P), also down the potential gradient (curved green arrow and + signs). The addition of positive charges outside the membrane of P and removal of + charges from the inside of the membrane caused by the current flow push the membrane potential of the pacemaker cell in a negative direction and retards SDD (red arrow shows shift in slope of SDD from black to red trace) in the pacemaker cell. It also decreases the membrane potential of the nonpacemaker cell (red arrow in NP, from black to red trace).

The efficacy of this inhibitory effect of electrotonic current flow on SDD is dependent on the magnitude of the electrotonic current, which in turn is influenced by the conductance (ability to pass current) of the gap junctions. One determinant of conductance is the isoform of the connexin protein that forms the gap junction. There are five connexin isoforms that form gap junctions in the human heart. The conventional nomenclature for a connexin (Cx) includes a suffix referring to its molecular weight. Some connexin proteins (Cx40 and Cx43) have high conductance, and others (Cx45) have low conductance. Different types of connexins are located in different regions of the heart. In the sinus node region, where pacemaker cells are coupled to nonpacemaker atrial cells with a more negative membrane potential, it is important that the gap junctions between the two cell types have low conductance, or sinus node pacemaker activity might be silenced. However, the conductance must still be sufficient to allow impulse propagation. More details on gap junction function are described in Chapters 2–4, since a decrease in coupling between cells caused by changes in gap junctions can enhance automaticity and cause arrhythmias.

RELATIONSHIP BETWEEN SINUS NODE AND LATENT PACEMAKERS

Cells with normal pacemaker properties occur throughout the heart. There is a hierarchy of pacemaker impulse initiation such that the sinus node is normally the primary pacemaker. With the sinus node functioning normally, other pacemaker sites are effectively "silent." Why does impulse initiation in the normal heart reside in the sinus node and not at one of the ectopic sites, since they also have the property of normal automaticity? Two factors are involved: the hierarchy of pacemakers and overdrive suppression.

Sinus Node as the Primary Pacemaker in the Hierarchy of Pacemakers

The sinus node is the prototype of normal automaticity and the dominant pacemaker in the normal heart. In addition, there are other special regions throughout the heart where myocardial cells have the normal, intrinsic ability to initiate impulses by automaticity. Myocardial cells at these ectopic sites are called latent or subsidiary pacemakers (**Figure 1-4**).

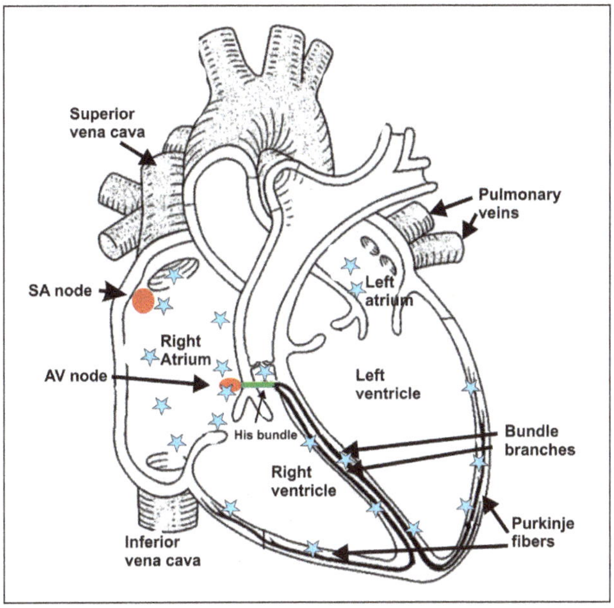

Figure 1-4 Location of pacemakers with normal automaticity (**blue stars**).

They include multiple sites in the right and left atria, the atrioventricular (AV) junction (AV node and His bundle), and the specialized conducting system of the ventricles (Purkinje system). Pacemaker cells at some of these sites such as the AV junction and Purkinje system can be identified by a specific histological structure while most pacemaker cells in the atria usually appear the same as the working myocardial cells with typical contractile structure and function.

The latent pacemakers have membrane currents causing SDD similar in many aspects to the mechanism described for the sinus node in Chapter 2 (Figure 2-6). In general, latent pacemaker sites with normal automaticity, like the sinus node, have cells with an isoform of a specific gene called the *HCN* gene (HCN stands for Hyperpolarization-activated Cyclic Nucleotide-gated). This gene controls the expression of a membrane channel that is involved in the genesis of the pacemaker current. Myocardial cells in atria and ventricles classified as "working," i.e., performing the contractile function, do not normally express pacemaker ability, although under pathological conditions, they may express abnormal automaticity (see Chapter 4).

Hierarchy of Pacemakers

Under normal conditions there is a difference in intrinsic rates among different pacemaker cells in various regions of the heart, which is called the hierarchy of pacemakers. The intrinsic rate is the rate at which a cell initiates automatic impulses in the absence of external inhibitory or stimulatory factors such as the autonomic nervous system. The sinus node pacemakers have the fastest intrinsic rates, followed by atrial pacemakers, AV nodal pacemakers, His bundle pacemakers, and then the Purkinje pacemakers in the distal ventricular conducting system. Because the sinus node has the fastest intrinsic rate, the latent pacemakers are excited by propagated impulses from the sinus node and discharge an action potential before sufficient time passes to allow them to depolarize spontaneously to threshold potential and initiate an impulse.

Overdrive Suppression of Latent Pacemakers by the Sinus Node

Not only are latent pacemakers prevented from initiating an impulse because they are depolarized by propagating electrical activity originating in the sinus node, but also, the SDD of latent pacemaker cells is actually inhibited when the cells are repeatedly depolarized by the impulses from the sinus node—a phenomenon called "overdrive suppression." The effect of overdrive suppression can be seen when there is sudden failure of the sinus node pacemaker to initiate impulses or failure of the impulses to conduct into the location of the latent pacemaker. Latent pacemaker impulse initiation does not arise immediately but is generally preceded by a period of quiescence. Overdrive suppression is exemplified by this period of quiescence after sudden inhibition of the sinus node pacemaker by vagal activity.

Figure 1-5 shows the ECG during vagal activation by carotid sinus massage beginning at the "R" in the top tracing, in a normal human subject. The quiescent period prior to the appearance of a junctional beat (first impulse in the second tracing) reflects the suppressive influence of overdrive suppression exerted on the latent pacemakers, including this junctional pacemaker, by the dominant sinus node pacemaker. Several more junctional beats occur prior to reappearance of sinus rhythm after carotid message is terminated at the x in the third tracing. The junctional pacemaker is not suppressed by the vagal activation (as are atrial pacemakers and mid AV nodal pacemakers), perhaps because it is in the lower AV node or His bundle where the vagus exerts little effect (see Chapter 3). In humans, ventricular pacemaker escape is rare after vagal activation, the usual site of escape being in the AV junction.

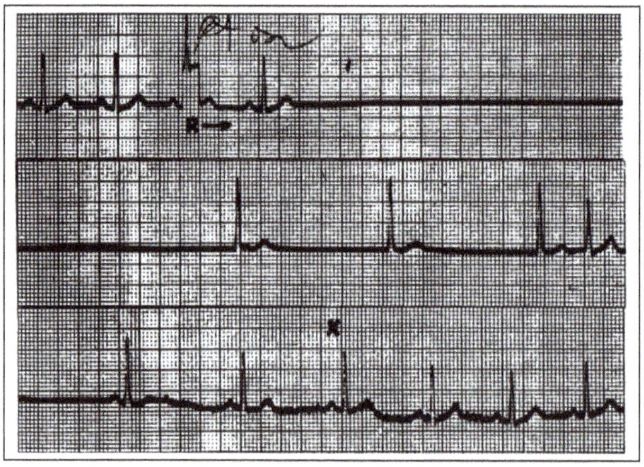

FFigure 1-5 Effects of carotid massage beginning at "R" in the **top trace**. (Reproduced from Heidorn DH, McNamara AP. Effect of carotid sinus stimulation on the electrocardiograms of clinically normal individuals. *Circulation*. 1956;14:1104–1113.)

Parenthetically, the sinus node pacemaker can also be overdrive-suppressed if there is a faster site of impulse initiation, such as during an ectopic tachycardia caused by any arrhythmogenic mechanism or by electrical stimulation (Chapter 2).

Role of the Na^+–K^+ Exchange Pump

In order to describe the mechanism for overdrive suppression, one of the membrane currents that influences SDD must be identified at this time. Recall that the pacemaker depolarization reflects both inward and outward currents, but depolarization occurs because there is a net inward current. One of the outward currents is generated by the activity of the Na^+–K^+ exchange pump. The Na^+–K^+ exchange pump resides in the cell membrane (sarcolemma) and transports 3 Na^+ out of the cell in exchange for 2 K^+, which are transported simultaneously into the cell. Both these ion movements occur against a concentration gradient (e.g., Na^+ concentration in the extracellular space is greater than in the intracellular space, K^+ concentration in the intracellular space is greater than in the extracellular space). Transporting ions against their concentration gradients requires energy derived from splitting adenosine triphosphate (ATP) by the enzyme ATPase. A primary role of the exchange pump is to prevent the cell from filling up with Na^+ and losing K^+ during electrical activity, since Na^+ enters most cardiac cells during each action potential upstroke while cells lose K^+, which exits the cell during action potential repolarization. The net outward movement of positive charges (more outward positively charged 3 Na^+ than inward positively charged 2 K^+) results in an outward membrane current designated I_P for pump current that occurs throughout the action potential and the diastolic interval (phase 4).

The Pump Current, I_P

During phase 4 in pacemaker cells, the outward directed I_P opposes the inward currents that cause SDD. It also has a hyperpolarizing effect on the MDP (making it more negative). Both effects serve to slow the rate of impulse initiation. Outward I_P reduces the slope of pacemaker depolarization (SDD) and slows the rate of impulse initiation (see Figure 1-2, Panel A: blue trace). The outward I_P also drives the MDP (normally determined by the K^+ current (I_{K1})) to more negative levels which slows the rate, as illustrated in Figure 1-2 Panel B. Other electrophysiological effects of I_P, such as effects on action potential duration that are involved in generation of arrhythmias, are described in Chapter 7. Overdrive suppression of latent pacemakers is mostly mediated by activity of the Na^+–K^+ exchange pump that is responsible for the I_P outward current, although other currents may sometimes contribute.

Role of I_P in Overdrive Suppression of Automaticity

Figure 1-6 is a schematic summarizing the mechanism for overdrive suppression of a pacemaker cell with a Na^+ dependent action potential phase 0 and the effects of increased rate of the driving impulses. Panel A shows transmembrane potentials of a latent pacemaker cell initiating impulses at its intrinsic rate (at the top).

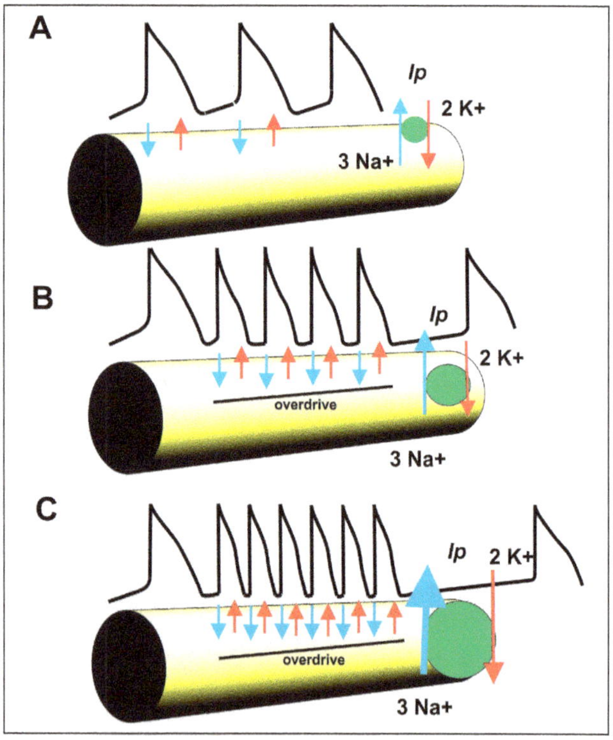

Figure 1-6 Mechanism for effects of overdrive suppression on automaticity.

The blue arrows under each action potential designates movement of Na^+ into a pacemaker cell (yellow cylinder) during phase 0 of the action potential, the red arrows indicate movement of K^+ out of the cell during repolarization. At the right, the green circle represents the Na^+–K^+ exchange pump moving 3 Na^+ out of the cell (blue arrow) in exchange for 2 K^+ into the cell (red arrow) generating the outward directed current, I_p. Panel B illustrates overdrive suppression. After the initial action potential, the spontaneous activity of the pacemaker is overdriven at a more rapid rate by an impulse arising elsewhere, such as the natural overdrive of a latent pacemaker during normal sinus rhythm or, alternatively, by electrical stimulation. During the overdrive period, more Na^+ enters (blue arrows) because of the increased number of action potentials, and the activity of the pump generating I_p increases (green circle at the right). The magnitude of I_p is directly related to the activity of the Na^+–K^+ exchange pump, which in turn is controlled by the amount of intracellular Na^+. I_p opposes SDD. At the right of Panel B, overdrive stimulation ceases, but the pump keeps generating increased I_p to remove excess Na^+; thus, pacemaker depolarization is suppressed, resulting in the long cycle length before a spontaneous action potential can occur (overdrive suppression). The rate of latent pacemaker activity gradually increases as Na^+ and I_p are progressively reduced to their basal level (not shown in the diagram). Panel C shows the effect of a period of a still faster overdrive rate on this cell. Since more action potential upstrokes occur per unit time, there is a further increase in Na^+ entering the cell (blue arrows) that increases the magnitude of I_p even further (green circle at right). After the termination of overdrive action potentials, the subsequent quiescent period is even longer than in Panel B. The enhanced I_p decreases net inward current during the pacemaker potential and suppresses SDD even more. The continued inhibition of SDD by the outward I_p (generated by the Na^+–K^+ pump), which is directly related to the previous rate of overdrive, is responsible for the period of quiescence. This quiescence lasts until the intracellular Na^+ concentration, and hence I_p, becomes small enough to allow the pacemaker potential of the latent pacemaker cells to depolarize spontaneously to threshold.

Figure 1-7, Panel A shows an example of overdrive suppression of an automatic Purkinje cell in a laboratory experiment, with SDD indicated by the small arrows at the left.

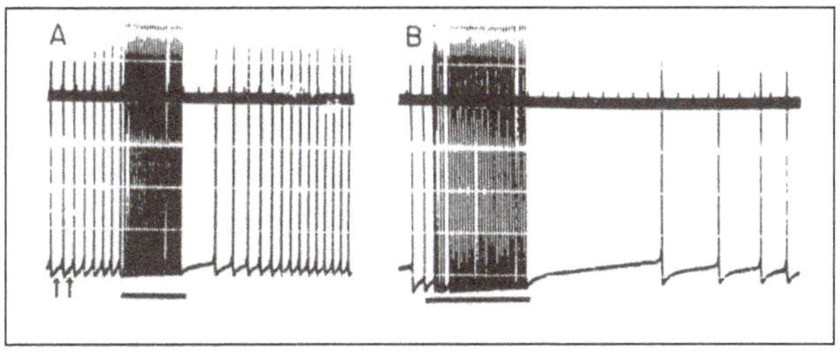

Figure 1-7 Transmembrane potential recordings showing overdrive suppression of an automatic canine Purkinje cell. Time marks on thick horizontal trace at the top are at 5-second intervals.

A period of rapid overdrive stimulation is applied during the time period indicated by the horizontal line under the recording. This is followed by a long cycle length indicating overdrive suppression, with reoccurrence of automatic activity at a rate gradually increasing to the pre-overdrive rate (warm up). Rate gradually speeds up to the intrinsic rate as intracellular Na^+ concentration is progressively decreased and I_p is reduced. In Figure 1-7, Panel B, overdrive suppression is enhanced when the period of overdrive at the same rate is prolonged (horizontal line under the recording). (The same effect occurs when the rate of overdrive is increased which was described in Figure 1-6). Both cause increased Na^+ to enter the pacemaker cell and thus stimulate I_p. Purkinje cells have a large inward I_{Na} that controls inward Na^+ movement, and a Na^+-K^+ pump that generates a strong pump current (I_p), accounting for the strong overdrive suppression.

Overdrive Electrical Stimulation Does Not Terminate Automatic Activity

A specific feature of overdrive suppression should be emphasized: automatic activity is not terminated by overdrive electrical stimulation. Although automaticity may be suppressed for many seconds, automatic impulse initiation returns after I_p has been reduced sufficiently by continuous pump activity to reduce intracellular Na^+. This characteristic response can be utilized in clinical electrophysiological studies to identify automaticity as a mechanism of arrhythmias since other arrhythmogenc mechanisms respond differently to overdrive.

ELECTROPHYSIOLOGICAL CAUSES OF ECTOPIC AUTOMATIC ARRHYTHMIAS

Enhanced or depressed automatic impulse initiation in the sinus node can lead to arrhythmias of sinus node origin caused by normal automaticity; sinus tachycardia and sinus bradycardia; Chapter 2. A shift in the site of impulse initiation from the sinus node to one of the regions where latent pacemakers with normal automaticity are located results in ectopic arrhythmias caused by normal automaticity. This happens when any of the following changes occur.

Decreased Effective Sinus Node Rate

The rate at which the sinus node activates latent pacemakers is decreased in a number of situations resulting in "escape" of a latent pacemaker (an escape rhythm) (Figure 1-5). As explained above, there is a natural hierarchy of intrinsic rates of latent pacemakers. Once overdrive suppression is decreased or removed by decreased sinus node impulse initiation or blocked conduction of the sinus impulse, the latent pacemaker with the fastest rate becomes the site of impulse origin. For example, impulse initiation by the sinus node is slowed or inhibited by heightened activity of the parasympathetic nervous system or by damage to the sinus node or its arterial supply. Degenerative structural changes in the node, caused by aging or sinus node disease such as the sick sinus syndrome, also may result in decreased rate of impulse initiation. Alternatively, any of the above can cause block of impulse conduction from the sinus node to the atria or block of conduction from the atria to the ventricles, both of which effectively decrease the rate at which the sinus node overdrives latent pacemakers distal to the region of block. Localized entrance block into an ectopic pacemaker site also shields the pacemaker from sinus activation and permits the pacemaker to initiate impulses at its intrinsic rate to cause arrhythmias as a parasystolic focus in the absence of exit block from the focus.

Figure 1-8 depicts these mechanisms for shifts of the dominant pacemaker from the sinus node to an ectopic site.

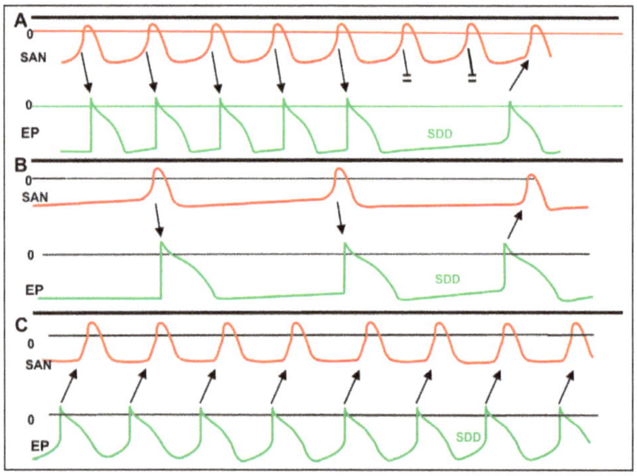

Figure 1-8 Mechanisms for emergence of ectopic automatic rhythms. The top trace in each panel shows action potentials of a sinus node pacemaker cell (**red, SAN**). The second trace shows action potentials of an ectopic pacemaker cell (**green, EP**). **Panels A** and **B** show decreased overdrive by sinus node; **Panel C** shows enhanced ectopic pacemaker firing.

In Panel A, black arrows indicate conduction from the sinus node (SAN, red action potentials) to activate the ectopic pacemaker (EP, green action potentials) before SDD of the ectopic pacemaker can reach threshold potential (first five action potentials). The next two sinus node action potentials block before reaching the ectopic pacemaker (indicated by short horizontal lines). This allows the SDD of this ectopic pacemaker to reach threshold to initiate an ectopic impulse that then propagates back to activate the sinus node (last action potential at the right; upward arrow). The period of time between the last latent pacemaker action potential activated by an impulse from the sinus node by normal conduction (downward arrow) and the first spontaneous action potential from the ectopic (latent) pacemaker is an indication of overdrive suppression of the latent pacemaker.

In Panel B, slowing of the sinus rate (red SAN action potentials) decreases overdrive suppression of the ectopic pacemaker resulting in an increase in slope of the SDD and an impulse is initiated from the latent pacemaker (last green action potential at the right, upward arrow). Pacemaker escape as shown in Panel B may be facilitated by a decrease in gap junction coupling (called "uncoupling") between latent pacemaker cells and surrounding nonpacemaker cells if there is an inhibitory influence of electrotonic current flow through gap junctions on the latent pacemakers (see Figure 1-3). Uncoupling removes the inhibitory influence and increases SDD to allow the latent pacemaker to fire closer to its intrinsic rate. Sinus node slowing is still required for such sites to become the dominant pacemaker, since the intrinsic rate is slower than the sinus rate. Gap junction coupling can be reduced by age related fibrosis, that can separate myocardial fibers and disrupt gap junction connections. Other factors that can decrease the ability of current to flow through gap junction channels (decreased conductance leading to uncoupling) are a decrease in intracellular pH as occurs in ischemia or an increase in intracellular Ca^{2+} that might result from digitalis.

Increased Rate of Ectopic Pacemakers

Enhancement of impulse initiation in latent pacemakers causes automatic ectopic tachycardias. Figure 1-8, Panel C diagrams an increase of the intrinsic rate of latent pacemaker cells, as may be the case with sympathetic stimulation. In this situation, the membrane potential of an ectopic pacemaker reaches threshold (bottom trace, EP, green action potentials) before it is activated by an impulse from the sinus node (top trace, SAN, red action potentials), resulting in impulse initiation from the ectopic site (upward-pointing arrows). The ectopic pacemaker can then suppress the sinus node by overdrive suppression. Enhancement of latent pacemaker impulse initiation can also occur in combination with decreased sinus node impulse initiation or conduction block.

An important cause of enhanced normal automaticity is sympathetic nerve activity. Norepinephrine released locally in the heart from sympathetic nerves acts on β_1-adrenergic receptors to increase net inward current in both latent pacemaker cells and sinus node cells. The slope of SDD is increased in both types of cell. Norepinephrine also decreases the inhibitory effects of overdrive because the enhanced pacemaker current is less easily suppressed. Localized enhancement of latent pacemaker rate can occur in the absence of sinus node stimulation, either when increased sympathetic activity is confined to localized regions of the heart or when sinus node rate is prevented from increasing by simultaneous vagal activation that is greater in this region than elsewhere. A decrease in sinus node pacemaker cells due to factors such as degenerative disease or aging might also reduce the ability of the sinus node to increase its rate in response to increased sympathetic activity. Circulating epinephrine may also have some of these effects. The upper limit for automatic rates generated by latent pacemakers in the atria in laboratory experiments is close to 200/min and in the Purkinje fibers of the ventricles is around 120/min.

Automatic tachycardias are not always dependent on sympathetic activity. Ion channel remodeling (e.g., change in ion channel properties caused by pathology) might increase inward current(s) involved in pacemaker activity or decrease outward currents. Stretch can also induce rapid automatic rates by increasing inward current through special stretch-activated channels.

GENERAL ECG CHARACTERISTICS OF AUTOMATIC ARRHYTHMIAS

Several characteristics of the ECG at the onset or termination of arrhythmias can help identify an automatic mechanism.

ECG Features of Automatic Arrhythmias Caused by Slowing of Sinus Rate

The onset of automatic arrhythmias with rates slower than sinus rhythm occurs after slowing of the effective sinus rate has allowed sufficient time for SDD of an ectopic pacemaker to reach threshold to generate an action potential. This "pacemaker escape" is facilitated by decreased overdrive suppression of the ectopic pacemaker. A single long sinus cycle length may allow the ectopic pacemaker to fire only once. More persistent sinus slowing or block can result in an escape rhythm. The first impulse of the escape rhythm occurs after a longer cycle length then the normal sinus cycle length reflecting the time required for the pacemaker potential to reach threshold.

Warm up, another characteristic of an automatic arrhythmia, refers to the gradual decrease in cycle length after onset, as the ectopic pacemaker continues to fire. This reflects the progressive decrease in pump current, until a steady cycle length is established. Warm-up does not always occur if most of the pump effect has been dissipated during the initial escape cycle. The rate of pacemaker firing may or may not be the expected intrinsic rate of firing of the ectopic site, depending on the influence of disease or the autonomic nervous system on the pacemaker. Rarely is there complete absence of autonomic effects on the pacemaker.

Termination of escape rhythms occurs when the sinus cycle length decreases and the sinus node again activates the region where the ectopic focus is located, at a rate faster than the ectopic pacemaker rate. During the ectopic rhythm, there may be transient activation (capture) of the heart by a sinus impulse, when it is initiated with appropriate timing prior to impulse initiation by the ectopic pacemaker and is able to reach the pacemaker before it fires.

ECG Features of Automatic Arrhythmias Caused by Increased Rate of Ectopic Pacemakers

The first impulse of ectopic automatic tachycardias caused by acceleration of ectopic pacemaker activity does not require sinus slowing and may or may not occur late in the diastolic interval (late coupled to the preceding sinus impulse). Since the time of appearance of the first ectopic impulse reflects the time that is required for the SDD to reach the threshold potential, it is unlikely that the first tachycardia impulse will appear very early in the cycle, as may occur with other arrhythmogenic mechanisms such as reentry or triggered activity. The tachycardia rate might speed up gradually after the first impulse (warm up) or if the pacemaker is markedly enhanced such as by sympathetic activity, maximum rate might be quickly established without the gradual warm up. There is no relationship between the rate of tachycardia and the prior sinus rate, such as may occur with triggered activity caused by delayed afterdepolarizations (Chapters 5 and 6).

In the case of ventricular automatic tachycardias, the presence of "AV dissociation" is usually indicative of an ectopic ventricular pacemaker, since the atrial pacemaker cannot capture the ventricle because of its slower automatic rate. Thus, the ventricles and atria are activated independently. AV dissociation may also occur with other mechanisms causing ventricular arrhythmias such as triggered activity (Chapters 5 and 6), but rarely occurs with reentrant arrhythmias. AV dissociation does not occur during an automatic ventricular tachycardia with 1:1 retrograde conduction from a ventricular pacemaker to the atria through the AV junction.

When automatic tachycardia terminates, its rate must be slower than the sinus allowing the sinus node to recapture the site of tachycardia origin, either through slowing of the ectopic pacemaker rate, acceleration of the sinus rate or a combination of the two. Automatic arrhythmias may sometimes be incessant, and onset and termination are not observable.

EFFECTS OF ELECTRICAL STIMULATION ON NORMAL AUTOMATICITY

Electrical stimulation of the heart through an electrode catheter is a valuable tool to identify mechanisms causing clinical arrhythmias. Programmed electrical stimulation (PES) refers to incremental pacing—that is, stimulation of the heart at faster rates (we use "overdrive stimulation" and "overdrive pacing" interchangeably)—and programmed premature stimulation, which is the application of single or multiple stimuli throughout the cycle of a regular rhythm. In general, automaticity responds to these patterns of electrical stimulation differently than the other arrhythmogenic mechanisms, triggered activity and reentrant excitation, enabling automaticity to be identified as an arrhythmogenic mechanism in a clinical electrophysiological study.

Overdrive Stimulation

Clinical overdrive stimulation protocols entail stimulating the heart at a rate more rapid than the rate of the spontaneous rhythm (overdrive) for a period of time and then observing the effects on the spontaneous rhythm immediately after stimulation is stopped. (We often express the rate in terms of its cycle length, particularly when referring to a short period of time.) Overdrive stimulation can be implemented during sinus rhythm either to investigate properties of sinus node automaticity such as sinus node recovery time or to determine whether a period of stimulation can induce an ectopic arrhythmia that has spontaneously appeared previously. Overdrive stimulation can also be implemented during an arrhythmia to determine whether overdrive can terminate it, or if it does not, to determine the effect of overdrive on characteristics of the arrhythmia, most important of which is the cycle length. The overdrive stimuli should be applied as close as possible to the arrhythmia origin that can often be deduced from the ECG characteristics, to insure that the stimulated impulses reach that site. In general, there are two variables in the overdrive protocol: the number of stimuli in the overdrive train and the cycle length at which the stimuli are delivered.

Figure 1-9 illustrates overdrive protocols and expected effects on a rhythm caused by normal automaticity (sinus or ectopic arrhythmia). An automatic rhythm with a cycle length of 400 ms is indicated by the vertical red bars at the left of each panel. The overdrive period is indicated by the vertical green bars and the horizontal green bar below them. Following overdrive (in green), a horizontal arrow indicates the time period to the reappearance of the spontaneous rhythm (vertical red bars to the right). In Panel A, overdrive of the spontaneous rhythm at a stimulus cycle length of 300 ms for 30 sec is followed by a post-overdrive cycle length of 500 ms. Subsequent cycle lengths shorten until the original cycle length of 400 ms is attained. The number of cycle lengths required to reach the pre-overdrive cycle length is variable depending on the properties of the automatic pacemaker. In carrying out the complete protocol, subsequent periods of stimulation at the same cycle length are progressively lengthened (Panel B for example) until maximum overdrive suppression occurs. In Panel B, the increase in overdrive duration to 60 sec (green bars) is followed by an increase in time period before reappearance of the spontaneous rhythm (horizontal arrow; post-overdrive cycle length is 600 ms) followed by gradual shortening of the spontaneous cycle length to the pre-overdrive rate.

Panels C and D illustrate an alternative protocol. Here, stimulation duration is fixed, (usually 30–60 sec), but the overdrive cycle length is decreased for each stimulation period. In Panels C and D, the effects of a decrease in cycle length of overdrive (vertical green bars, 250 and 200 ms) for 30 sec can be compared to Panel A, which uses the same time period. The decreased overdrive cycle length is followed by progressively longer overdrive suppression (horizontal arrows, 750 and 800 ms), after which there is a gradual decrease in cycle length to the pre-overdrive cycle length.

In summary, as shown in Figure 1-9:

- The overdrive suppression (prolongation of the first cycle length after stimulation), is increased with increased duration or rate of overdrive to a maximum that is determined by the properties of the pacemaker and accessibility of the site of pacemaker location to the rapidly stimulated impulses.

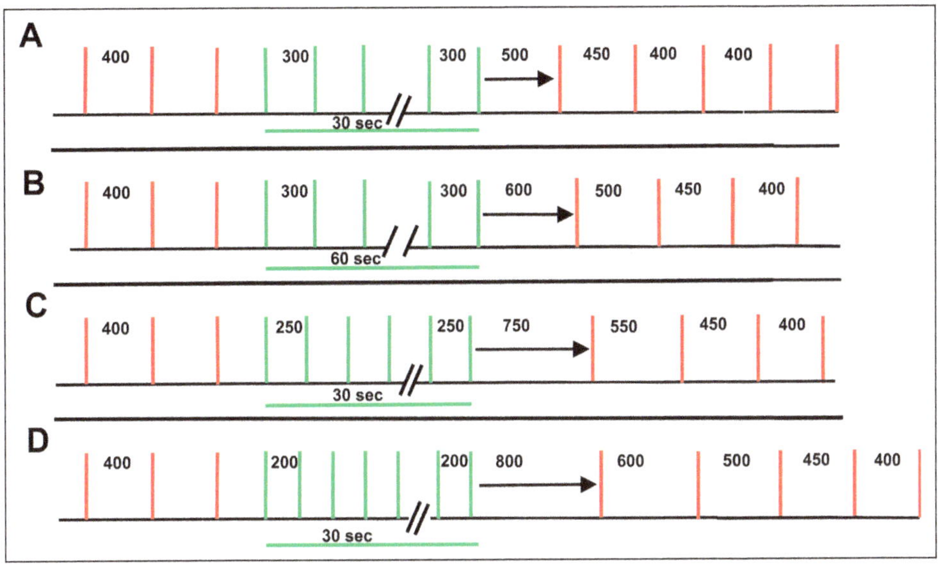

Figure 1-9 Overdrive stimulation protocol and effects on normal automaticity.

- The overdrive suppression is caused by increased activity of the Na^+–K^+ pump (I_P) as described in Figure 1-6. At fast rates of overdrive, if the stimulated impulses fail to conduct into the site where the pacemaker cells are located, the post-overdrive cycle length will suddenly shorten (not shown in Figure 1-9) due to a decrease in effects of overdrive at the pacemaker site, because blocked impulses did not reach the site.
- It is important to remember that overdrive stimulation does not terminate impulse initiation caused by normal automaticity (nor can it initiate this type of arrhythmia). The pre-over drive rhythm (sinus or ectopic in origin) resumes after the suppression by overdrive has worn off, as activity of the Na^+–K^+ pump returns to pre-overdrive levels.

Programmed Premature Stimulation

Programmed premature stimulation refers to the application of premature stimuli during the dominant rhythm. The term premature stimulus means that a stimulus is applied and a response is elicited that occurs earlier than the next expected spontaneously occurring impulse. To determine the mechanism of an arrhythmia, premature stimuli are applied at decreasing coupling intervals to the previous arrhythmic impulse, and the type of response that occurs is observed. The response to the application of controlled premature stimuli provides information for distinguishing an automatic pacemaker mechanism from the other arrhythmogenic mechanisms.

In the absence of an ongoing arrhythmia, premature stimuli can be used during sinus rhythm to evaluate the function of the sinus node pacemaker (Chapter 2) or to determine if an arrhythmia, sinus or ectopic, can be induced by the stimuli. A key feature of these protocols is that each premature stimulus is delivered at decreasing coupling intervals to the previous sinus impulse after allowing for a period of stabilization of the rhythm before the next (earlier) premature stimulus is delivered.

In attempting to induce an arrhythmia, the heart rate may also be controlled by a regular stimulus cycle length called the "basic cycle length," and premature stimuli are applied at progressively decreasing coupling intervals to the previous basic cycle stimulus.

Figure 1-10 shows an example protocol and illustrates the response of a rhythm caused by normal automaticity. The response to premature stimuli can be subdivided into four zones that are illustrated in the different panels in the figure. Not all zones necessarily occur during a single protocol.

- **Zone 1:** Compensatory pause (Panel A)
- **Zone 2:** Resetting (Panels B, C, and D)
- **Zone 3:** Interpolation (Panel E)
- **Zone 4:** Reentry (not shown here; will be described in Chapter 9)

In Figure 1-10, a stable automatic rhythm is diagrammed in each panel at the left (black downward arrows) with each spontaneous depolarization indicated by "A" (automatic impulse), occurring at a cycle length of 500 ms.

The pacemaker is located in region 1 and the automatic impulse propagates to region 2 (blue downward arrows) without significant delay. For now, we will not distinguish between sinus and ectopic pacemakers, although there may be some differences in their responses. In particular, the imposition of conduction delay between

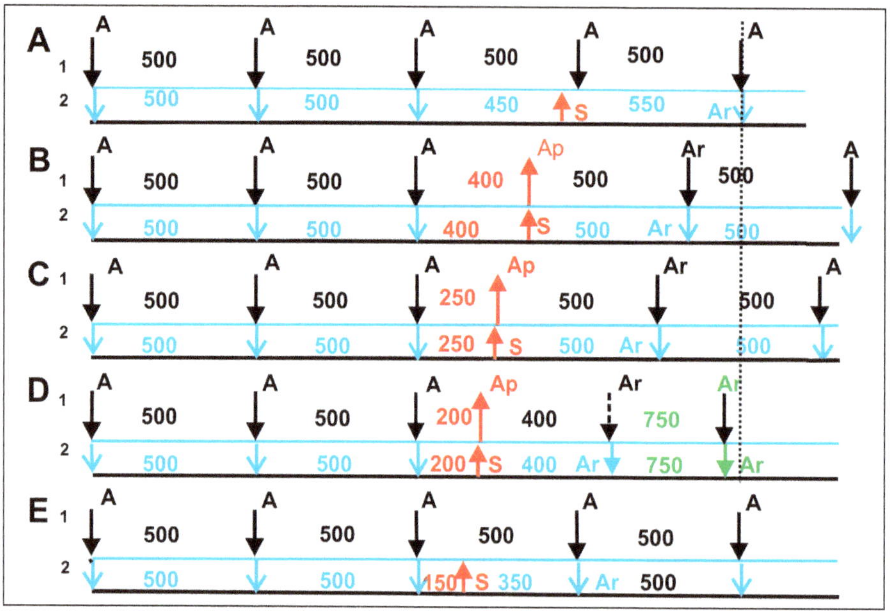

Figure 1-10 Effects of programmed premature stimulation on normal automaticity. In each panel, automatic impulse initiation in region 1 is indicated by the **downward, black arrows** (**A**). This impulse activates region 2 (**downward, blue arrow**). **Red S** and **upward arrows** indicate premature stimulation impulses in region 2. **Panel A:** compensatory pause; **vertical dashed black line. Panels B, C,** and **D:** reset; and **Panel E:** interpolation.

the stimulus site and the pacemaker can alter the perceived response. In Panel A (Zone 1; compensatory pause), a premature stimulus is applied in region 2, near the pacemaker site to initiate a premature impulse (red S and upward red arrow) at a coupling interval of 450 ms to the prior spontaneous depolarization (A). The A-to-S interval is the premature cycle length (450 ms). The spontaneous impulse (A) that occurs 50 ms after S cannot conduct to region 2; the next spontaneous depolarization in region 1 (A) was not affected by the premature stimulus and conducts to region 2 (blue arrow) at a cycle length of 550 ms after the premature impulse. This response in region 2 (the impulse that follows the premature impulse) is designated as the "return automatic impulse" (Ar) and the S-to-Ar interval is the "return cycle length" (550 ms).

A compensatory pause is demonstrated by observing that the sum total of the coupling interval of the premature impulse (premature cycle length = 450 ms) and the time required for the appearance of the first spontaneous impulse after the premature depolarization in region 2 (return cycle length = 550 ms) is 1000 ms. This is equal to two spontaneous cycle lengths. In other words, the spontaneous depolarization (blue Ar) in region 2 following the premature depolarization occurs exactly when expected, as if no premature impulse had been initiated. This type of response, a compensatory pause, is expected to occur when the premature depolarization has no effect on the spontaneous rhythm. As shown in the diagram in Figure 1-10, Panel A, the premature stimulation (S) has no effect other than depolarizing region 2 and making region 2 refractory, thus preventing the manifestation of the spontaneous impulse that was expected 50 ms later. There was no influence on the appearance of the next automatic (A) impulse in region 1, which occurred when expected. When a compensatory pause occurs, it can be assumed that conduction of S never reached the pacemaker site.

In this illustration, the premature stimuli are applied close to the pacemaker site, and as a result, the range of premature impulses over which there is a compensatory pause is small (as plotted in **Figure 1-11**). When a zone of conduction delay is interposed between the stimulus and pacemaker sites, this zone widens, since the possibility that the stimulated impulse does not reach the pacemaker is increased, as is described for the sinus node in Figure 2-14.

Figure 1-10, Panel B shows how the automatic rhythm is reset (Zone 2) in response to a premature stimulus. Just as in panel A, the premature impulse (red S and upward red arrow) is initiated at a shorter coupling interval to the preceding spontaneous impulse (A) (premature cycle length = 400 ms). This time, however, the premature impulse conducts to region 1 to prematurely excite the pacemaker (red upward arrow; Ap). The next spontaneous depolarization (Ar) in region 2 occurs at 500 ms after the premature impulse, and thus the sum of the premature cycle (400 ms) and the return cycle (500 ms) is 900 ms, which is less than two spontaneous cycle lengths (1000 ms). In other words, as shown in the diagram, the premature impulse (red S) caused the next depolarization of the pacemaker (red Ap in region 1) to occur earlier than it would have occurred without the premature impulse. This is the result of the premature impulse reaching the pacemaker to depolarize it early (upward red arrow, Ap), after which the pacemaker initiates an impulse. The diagram shows that the return cycle (S-Ar interval) in regions 1 and 2 was 500 ms, which is the same cycle as the unperturbed, spontaneous cycle length. Therefore, premature activation of the pacemaker did not influence the pacemaker current or the cycle length of automaticity.

In Figure 1-10, Panel C, at a shorter premature coupling interval (A-S = 250 ms), the cycle length between the premature impulse and the next spontaneous impulse in region 2 (return cycle length S-Ar) is still 500 ms. The pacemaker is still reset (Zone 2) since the premature coupling interval AS of 250 ms plus return cycle length (S-Ar) of 500 ms is still less than two spontaneous cycle lengths (1000 ms). The diagram shows that the stimulated impulse (red S) depolarized the pacemaker (upward red arrow) early and that the early pacemaker depolarization (Ap) is followed by appearance of the next spontaneous impulse (Ar) at a (return) cycle length of 500 ms, showing that the pacemaker mechanism has not been affected. However, this is not always the case, as diagrammed in Panel D.

In Figure 1-10, Panel D, the premature stimulus (red S) is applied after 200 ms (A-S = 200 ms) in region 2 and causes early depolarization of the pacemaker in region 1 (upward red arrow, Ap). Two possible responses are diagrammed, both of which indicate resetting (still Zone 2) according to the definition above. One is indicated by a shortened return response (S-Ar) of 400 ms (blue downward arrow). This would occur if the pacemaker mechanism was somehow enhanced (Ar with black dashed arrow) and less than the pre-stimulus pacemaker cycle length of 500 ms. The other possible response is a reset mechanism that prolongs the automatic pacemaker cycle indicated by a return response (S-Ar) of 750 ms (green downward arrow). This would occur if the pacemaker mechanism was somehow depressed, since it is longer than 500 ms. Changes in the return cycle length from the pre-stimulus automatic rate may sometimes occur. However, the reset pacemaker cycle length may also remain constant over a wide range of premature coupling intervals. Mechanisms for alterations in the pacemaker mechanism and related arrhythmias are described in Chapters 2 and 3.

Figure 1-10, Panel E, illustrates interpolation (Zone 3). The premature stimulus is initiated still earlier after a spontaneous depolarization (A-S = 150 ms). The return cycle length following S in region 2 (S-Ar) is 350 ms. The sum of A-S (150 ms) and S-Ar (350 ms) is equal to the spontaneous cycle length of the automatic rhythm (500 ms). In this situation, the premature impulse has no effect on the pacemaker and also has no effect on the ability of the pacemaker to express itself in region 2. That is, the following spontaneous depolarization occurs exactly when expected in region 2, as if no premature stimulus had been applied. This might occur if the premature impulse was confined to a small region and did not reach the pacemaker site or affect the exit of the spontaneous impulse from the pacemaker site.

Response Patterns in Clinical Studies

Effects of conduction delay. In actual clinical studies, the response to premature stimulation may vary due to conduction delay between the site where the premature stimulus is applied (region 2) and the site where the pacemaker is located (region 1). To reiterate, the description in Figure 1-10 of the effects of programmed premature stimulation assumes that there is no significant conduction delay. Conduction properties of intervening tissue between the stimulus site and the pacemaker site can alter the characteristic response measured near the stimulus site, as discussed in Chapter 2 on resetting of the sinus node pacemaker.

Failure to initiate or terminate arrhythmias. It should be noted here that programmed stimulation of automatic arrhythmias, like overdrive stimulation, will not terminate the arrhythmia as it might do to some forms of triggered activity or reentrant excitation, thus distinguishing automaticity from these other mechanisms. Based on the supposition that electrical stimulation does not terminate normal automaticity, failure of cardioversion is also evidence for automaticity although it sometimes may fail to terminate other mechanisms. To reiterate, programmed stimulation, overdrive or premature, will not initiate an ectopic automatic arrhythmia if applied during sinus rhythm—in contrast to some forms of triggered activity or reentrant excitation.

Specificity of response pattern. The response pattern in Figure 1-10 is not only diagnostic for an automatic rhythm but it can also occur in response to premature stimulation of a reentrant tachycardia, particularly during circus movement tachycardia using an accessory pathway (described in Chapter 10). Depending upon the timing and distance between the reentry circuit and the stimulus site, a compensatory pause or reset can occur. The significant difference is that a premature stimulus can start and terminate reentrant tachycardia but, as described above, not automatic tachycardia. The mechanisms are described in Chapter 10.

Graphing clinical study data. Figure 1-11 is a typical graphic display used in clinical studies of the responses of a normal automatic pacemaker to programmed premature stimuli (using data from Figure 1-10). The premature coupling interval is on the abscissa (A-S); it can also be expressed as a percent of the spontaneous cycle length, A-S/A-A. The cycle length following the premature interval (return cycle length, S-Ar) is on the ordinate; it can also be expressed as a percent of the spontaneous cycle length, S-Ar/A-A. The horizontal dashed line on the graph indicates the spontaneous cycle length (500 ms in Figure 1-10).

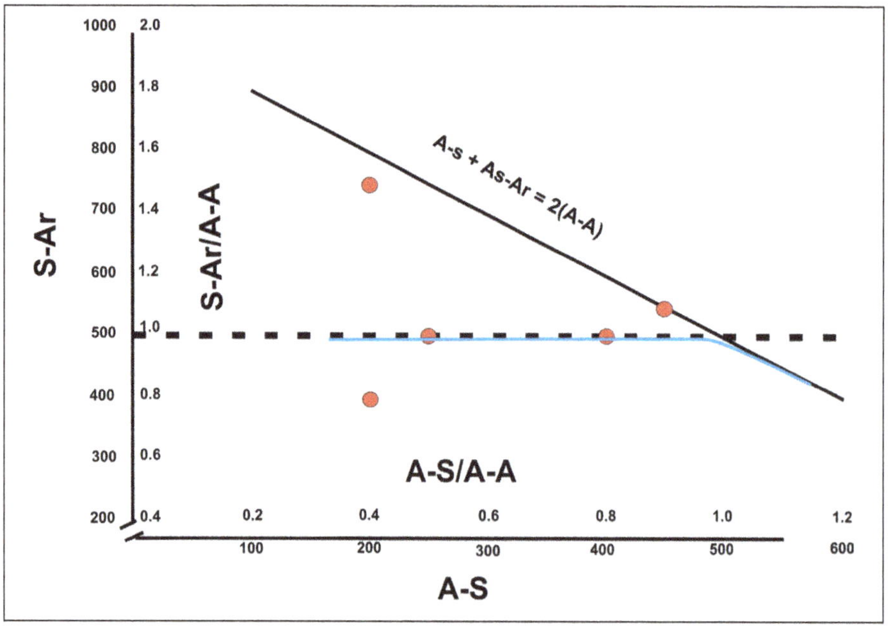

Figure 1-11 Graphic display of data from the resetting response of the automatic pacemaker in Figure 1-10.

The diagonal solid line in Figure 1-11 indicates where the response would occur due to a compensatory pause; the sum of A-S and S-Ar of each point falling on the line is equal to twice the spontaneous cycle length. At a coupling interval of 450 ms in Figure 1-10, a compensatory response occurred (red circle on the diagonal line in Figure 1-11). As explained above, the zone of compensatory responses is small when the stimulus is applied close to the pacemaker. In Figure 1-10, resetting occurred at coupling intervals less than 450 ms and down to 200 ms. Thus, all points during this resetting zone fall below the line of compensatory pause (are less than compensatory). When the return cycle length (S-Ar) equals the spontaneous cycle length, they fall along the dashed line (blue line). When the return cycle is more than the spontaneous cycle, the points are above the dashed line, and when the return cycle is less than the spontaneous cycle, they fall below the dashed line, as shown by two separate red circles at A-S of 200 ms. Nevertheless, they are still less than compensatory and indicate resetting. A short return cycle may also indicate reentry of the premature impulse, a completely different mechanism (Chapter 9).

PHARMACOLOGIC AGENTS

Pharmacologic agents that have characteristic effects on automatic arrhythmias, enabling them to be distinguished from arrhythmias caused by other mechanisms, are described Chapters 2 and 3.

SUMMARY

Normal automaticity is a normal property of sinus node and latent pacemaker cells in the atria, AV conducting system, and Purkinje cells of the ventricular specialized conducting system. It is characterized by spontaneous diastolic depolarization (SDD) caused by net inward pacemaker current. The control of rate of automatic impulse initiation is affected by properties of the transmembrane potential and electrical coupling between cells. The sinus node is the primary pacemaker with the fastest intrinsic rate compared to latent pacemakers (hierarchy of pacemakers). The sinus node inhibits activity of latent pacemakers located throughout the heart by the mechanism of overdrive suppression related to enhanced activity of the Na^{+}–K^{+} pump. Ectopic automatic arrhythmias can arise due to decreased effective sinus node rate, increased rate of ectopic pacemakers, or a combination of both. Certain ECG features suggest arrhythmias due to automatic impulse initiation. Electrophysiology testing protocols including overdrive stimulation or programmed premature stimulation are useful for identifying arrhythmias due to automaticity.

SOURCES

Carmeliet E. Cardiac ionic currents and acute ischemia: From channels to arrhythmias. *Physiol Rev.* 1999;79:917–987.

Carmeliet E, Vereecke J. *Cardiac Cellular Electrophysiology.* Dordrecht: Kluwer Academic Publ.; 2002.

Kerzner J, Marshal W, Kosowsky BD, Lown B. Ventricular ectopic rhythms following vagal stimulation in dogs with acute myocardial infarction. *Circulation.* 1973;47:44–50.

Mangoni MM, Nargeoy JL. Genesis and regulation of the heart automaticity. *Physiol Rev.* 2008;88: 919–982.

Vassalle M.The relationship among cardiac pacemakers; Overdrive suppression. *Circ. Res.* 1977;41:269–277.

Vassalle M, Caress DL, Slovin AJ, Stuckey JH. On the cause of ventricular asystole during vagal stimulation. *Circ Res.*1967;20: 228–241.

CHAPTER 2

Sinus Node Normal Automaticity and Automatic Arrhythmias

The sinus node is the prototype for normal automaticity. It is the location of the primary pacemaker. In addition to controlling the heart's normal rhythm, it can also be a cause of automatic arrhythmias.

To understand mechanisms for arrhythmias caused by normal automaticity, it is important to begin with the electrophysiological properties that enable impulses to be initiated by sinus node automaticity. As explained in Figure 1-4, other regions of the heart have the property of normal automaticity as well. The principles that are described in this chapter also apply to automaticity at the other (ectopic) sites that cause arrhythmias by the normal automatic mechanism (Chapter 3).

Basic Electrophysiological Mechanisms

SINUS NODE ANATOMY

Figure 2-1, left panel, shows the sinus node (dense greenish-blue staining region labeled SN) located subepicardially at the lateral junction of the superior vena cava (SVC) within the right atrium. It is an oval structure, usually arranged around a prominent nodal artery that is a branch of either the right coronary or circumflex artery. Sinus nodal cells, which are generally smaller and have fewer myofibrils than atrial myocardial cells, are embedded in a matrix of connective tissue. These structural features are among those that distinguish the "anatomical" node from the surrounding atrium. The node has extensions (right panel) both toward the superior vena cava and toward the orifice of the inferior vena cava in the intercaval region, which is adjacent to the thick muscular terminal crest (TC).

The anatomical sinus node is surrounded by connective tissue that forms a barrier between the node and the crista terminalis (endocardial manifestation of the terminal crest). This barrier electrically isolates the node from the surrounding atrial myocardium, except in several regions where exit pathways from the node permeate the barrier to connect to the crista (**Figure 2-2**). These exit pathways are composed of sinus nodal-like cells and transitional cells that have a structure intermediate between nodal and atrial cells.

In Figure 2-2, which shows the location of exit pathways, the anatomical node is indicated by the yellow oval region with the dark red-brown oval at its center, indicating the pacemaker location. The thick red lines indicate coronary arteries that also form barriers to electrical propagation. The exit pathways are indicated by the arrows pointing away from the sinus node: a pathway exits the node superiorly (upward arrow), other pathways exit laterally (leftward) toward the crista terminalis (CT) permeating the connective tissue barrier (dashed line), and still other pathways exit inferiorly (downward arrows). Except for exit pathways, the remaining margin of the node at the left is isolated from the crista by connective tissue (dashed line). An anatomical (and electrical) barrier at the septal margin of the node (dashed line at the right) is composed of connective tissue, fat, and coronary arteries. The number of exit pathways varies in different hearts and determines the earliest atrial activation sites under different physiological and pathological conditions.

Electrophysiological Foundations of Cardiac Arrhythmias: A Bridge Between Basic Mechanisms and Clinical Electrophysiology, Second Edition.

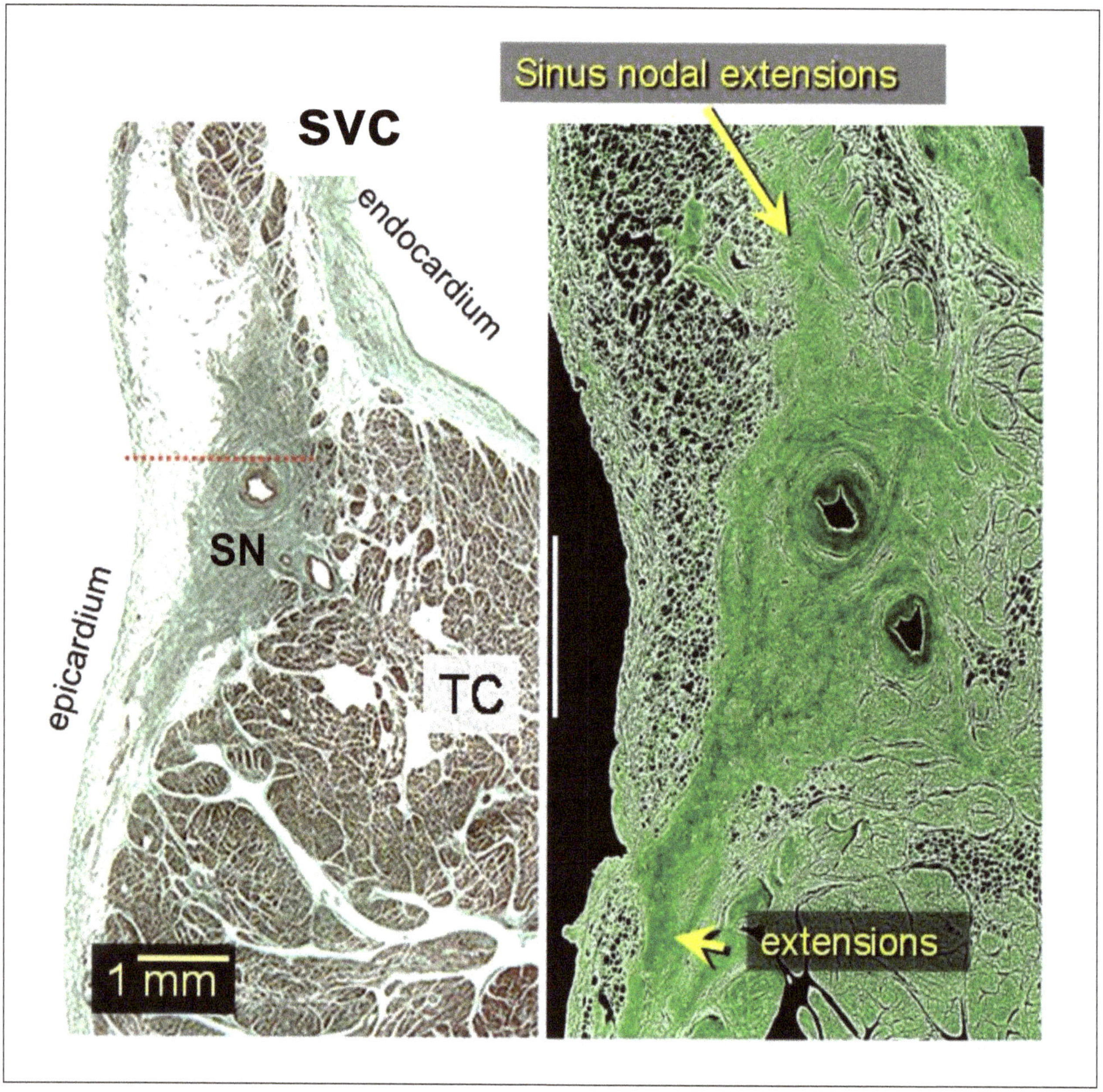

Figure 2-1 Histological sections of human sinus node. The **left panel** features the sinus nodal structure (SN), terminal crest (TC), and superior vena cava (SVC). The **right panel** shows extensions of the node in **dark green**. (Figure kindly provided by Jose Angel Cabrera and Damian Sanchez-Quintana.)

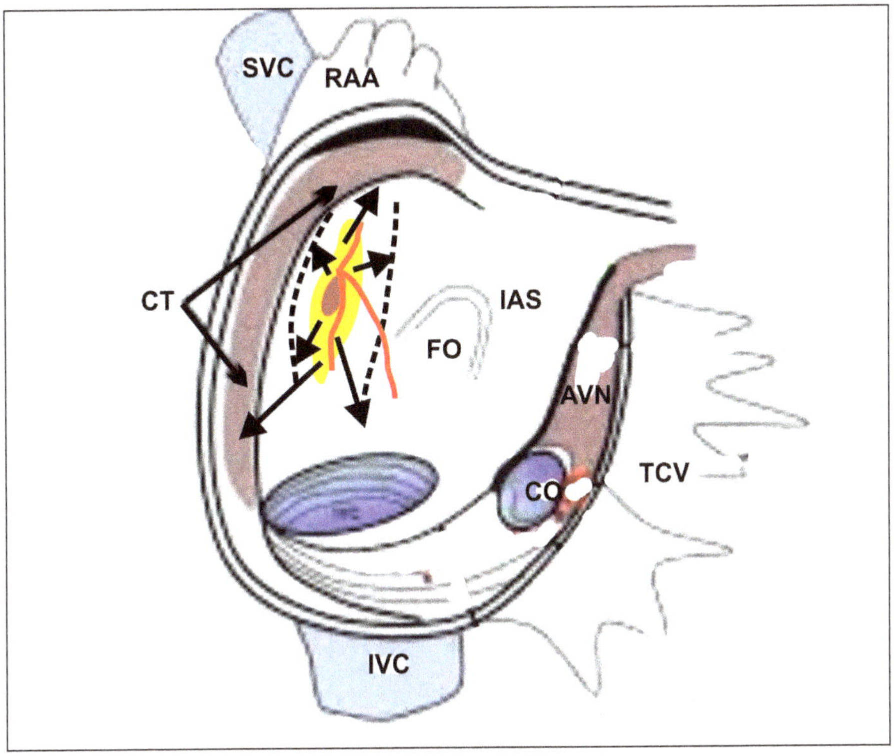

Figure 2-2 Endocardial view of right atrium. AVN, AV node; CO, ostium of coronary sinus; CT, crista terminalis; FO, fossa ovale; IAS, interatrial septum; IVC, inferior vena cava; RAA, right atrial appendage; SVC, superior vena cava, TCV, tricuspid valve. (Figure is based on data in publication of Fedorov VV, Glukhov AV, Chang R, et al. Optical mapping of the isolated coronary-perfused human sinus node. *J Am Coll Cardiol.* 2010;56:1386–1394.)

Earliest Atrial Activation

Normal pacemaker activity at typical sinus rates of around 60–100 impulses/min originates in the central region of the body of the anatomical node (red-brown oval in Figure 2-2) where the sinus node pacemaker cells are located. Sinus impulses propagate out of the node into atrial muscle of the terminal crest and crista terminalis through the exit pathways (arrows to the left and downward in Figure 2-2).

The earliest atrial activation may occur as late as 80 ms after earliest sinus node impulse initiation and may be at a distance of several mm from the anatomical node. Activation then spreads rapidly in the right atrium along the parallel oriented muscle bundles of the crista terminalis and towards the left atrium in the interatrial bundle (Bachmann's bundle). An example of atrial activation during sinus rhythm is shown in **Figure 2-3**.

In Figure 2-3, the first region of atrial myocardium to be activated during sinus rhythm is displayed in the light pinkish region in Panels A, B, and C (activated during the 0–5 ms isochrone on the color-coded time scale). Electrical activity of the sinus node itself is not represented for several reasons: (1) because of the small number of cells and their location deep to the epicardial surface, and (2) because these cells have low-amplitude action potentials that generate only a small extracellular signal that cannot be detected with standard methodology. The wavefront from this site of earliest atrial activation spreads sequentially to the regions represented by the dark red, orange, brown, yellow, green, and blue isochrones.

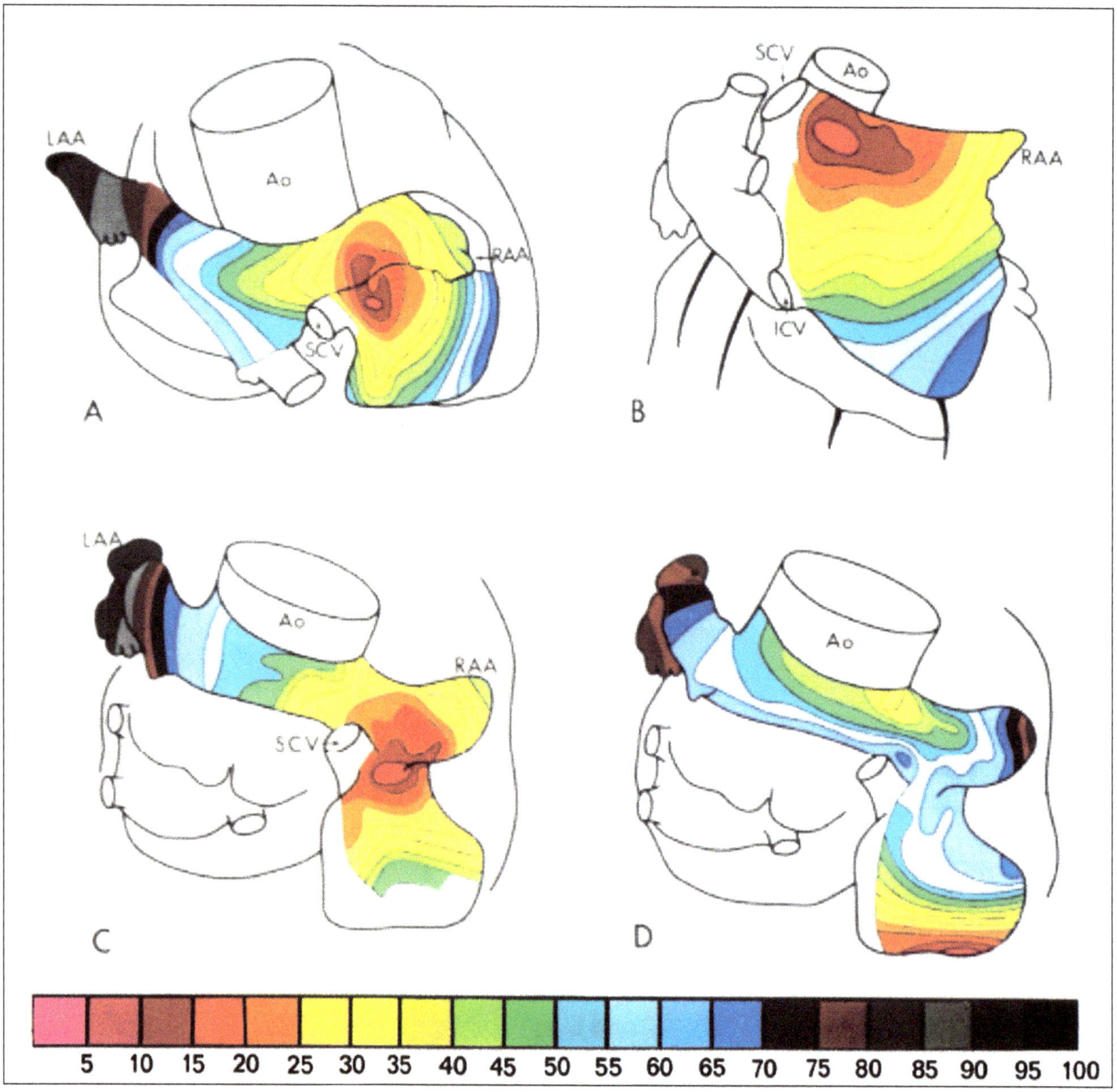

Figure 2-3 Isochronic representation of the activation of two human hearts. Color scheme is below, earliest activity on the atrial surface (with respect to a fixed reference electrode on the right atrial appendage) was taken as 0 time. **Panels A** and **B** show different aspects of the same heart during sinus rhythm. **Panel A** is a superior view of part of the right atrium and the musculature connecting right and left atria (interatrial band zone); the right atrial appendage is folded outward. **Panel B** is a posterior view of the right atrium. **Panels C** and **D** show the activation pattern of the interatrial band zone and right atrial surface of another heart during sinus rhythm (**Panel C**) and retrograde (V-A) conduction when stimulating the ventricles (**Panel D**). Ao, root of the aorta; ICV, inferior caval vein; LAA, left atrial appendage; RAA, right atrial appendage; SCV, superior caval vein. (Reproduced from Durrer D, van Dam R, et al. Total excitation of the isolated human heart. *Circulation*. 1970;41:899–912.)

SINUS NODE ELECTROPHYSIOLOGY

The special characteristics of the sinus node action potentials influence its normal automaticity and conduction properties and its role in the genesis of certain supraventricular arrhythmias.

The Sinus Node Action Potential

Many of the features of the sinus node action potential responsible for automatic impulse initiation conform to the prototype of automaticity described in Figure 1-1. These features are illustrated in **Figure 2-4**.

The prominent feature of the sinus node action potential (green tracing in Figure 2-4) is the spontaneous movement of membrane potential during diastole (phase 4, black arrow) in a positive direction from its maximum negativity (maximum diastolic potential, MDP) toward the threshold potential (TP). This is known as spontaneous diastolic depolarization (SDD), sometimes referred to as phase 4 depolarization or the pacemaker potential. The MDP of the pacemaker cell is between −70 and −50 mV. Note that phase 4 of the nonpacemaker atrial myocardial cell (in red) is more negative and has a stable value.

Once the SDD reaches the TP, the upstroke of the action potential (green, phase 0) occurs caused by activation of inward currents that moves the membrane potential to 0 or slightly into positive values. As shown in Figure 2-4, the rate of membrane potential change during phase 0 is relatively slow in the sinus node compared to phase 0 of the atrial cell (the reasons are discussed below). Following the upstroke, inactivation of the inward currents causing phase 0 occurs, and outward currents repolarize the cell back to its MDP (green, phases 2 and 3), from which the process begins again. (Phase 1, which is an initial rapid phase of repolarization found in ventricular muscle and Purkinje cells, is not evident in the sinus node and some atrial cell action potentials.)

Heterogeneous Sinus Node Action Potential Properties

Figure 2-5 shows an activation map and heterogeneous action potentials in different regions of the sinus node. The "true" pacemaker cells in the center of the node (lower left action potential at the origin of activation, time 0), in addition to the prominent SDD have low MDP (−50 to −70 mV) attributed to reduced I_{K1}, the outwardly directed K^+ current that is responsible for the high resting potential (more negative) in working atrial cells (Figure 2-4, red tracing) and ventricular myocardial cells. The slow depolarization during the upstroke (phase 0) of the action potential of the pacemaker cell (~20 V/sec) is a result of slow inward Ca^{2+} current mostly through L-type calcium channels (I_{CaL}) (T-type Ca^{2+} channels may play a minor role) with little or no contribution from the cardiac Na^+ current (I_{Na}), which is responsible for the upstroke of the action potential in working atrial myocardium. Moving toward the periphery of the node (action potentials at activation times 10, 20, 25 ms), MDP becomes more negative due to increasing I_{K1}, and phase 0 upstroke velocity becomes faster with a higher-amplitude phase 0 because of increasing I_{Na}.

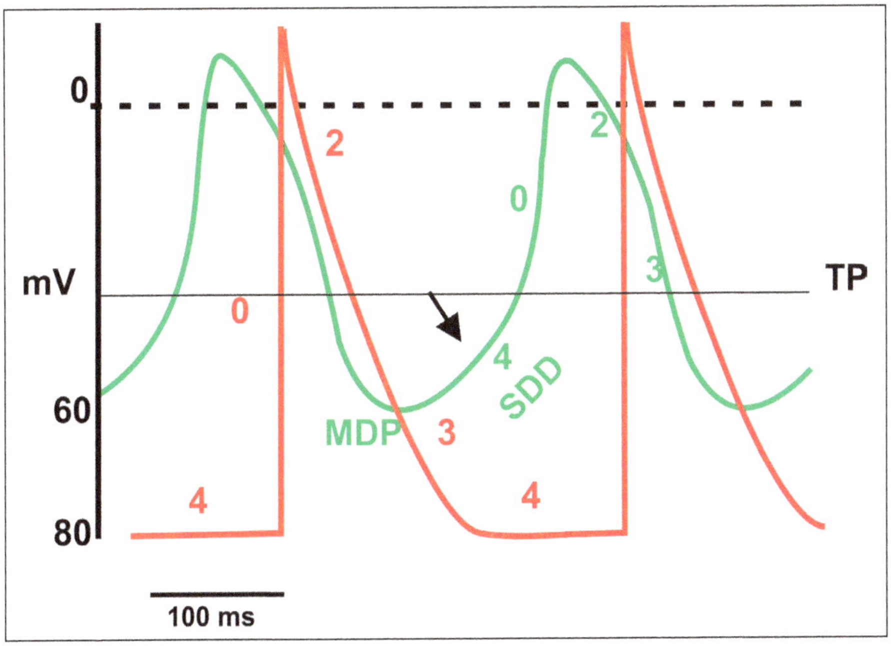

Figure 2-4 Diagrams of transmembrane action potentials of a pacemaker cell in the sinus node (**green**) and an atrial myocardial cell (**red**), which is not a pacemaker. The phases of the atrial action potential are indicated by **red numbers**, while phases of the sinus node action potential are indicated by **green numbers**.

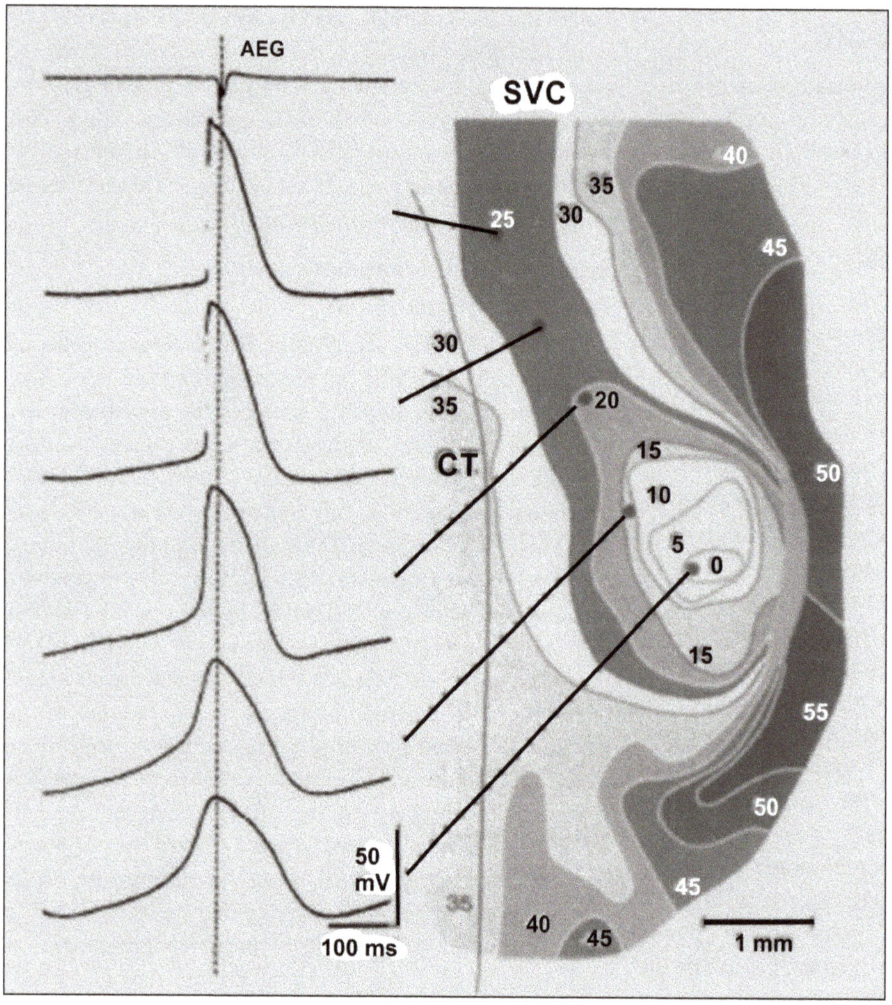

Figure 2-5 Action potentials recorded in the sinus node of the rabbit heart. The **right side** of the figure is a diagram of the sinus node region with the superior vena cava (SVC) at the top and the crista terminalis (CT) at the left. The isochrones show the spread of activation (numbers on map are in ms). The **left side** of the figure are action potentials recorded from sites shown by the lines. Vertical dashed line through action potentials indicates the time of atrial activation indicated by the atrial electrogram (AEG) in the top trace. (Reproduced from Bleeker WK, Mackaay AJC, et al. Functional and morphological organization of the rabbit sinus node. *Circ Res.* 1980;46:11–22.

The peripheral region of the node is sometimes referred to as the perinodal or paranodal region that determines conduction characteristics of impulses leaving and entering the node. Although there is some SDD here, it is less evident than in the central sinus node pacemaker. In fact, peripheral nodal cells are latent pacemakers that might become the dominant pacemaker under special conditions. Repolarization of both pacemaker and peripheral nodal cells is generally caused by inactivation of the inward currents causing phase 0 (I_{CaL} and/or I_{Na}) and by an outward K^+ current, the delayed rectifier current (I_K).

Ionic Currents and the Pacemaker Potential in the Sinus Node

The inward current that causes SDD and normal automaticity in the sinus node is the sum of a number of different currents with different properties flowing through ion channels in the cell membrane. Some of these currents flow inward (from extracellular space to intracellular space) in the depolarizing direction, and some flow outward (from intracellular space to extracellular space) in the repolarizing direction. However, the net current is inward, giving rise to the pacemaker potential or SDD. In **Figure 2-6**, these currents are represented schematically below the sinus node (SAN) action potentials that are displayed in the top trace. Inward currents are downward and outward currents upward. Although there are both inward and outward currents, the sum of all of them is a net inward depolarizing current causing SDD.

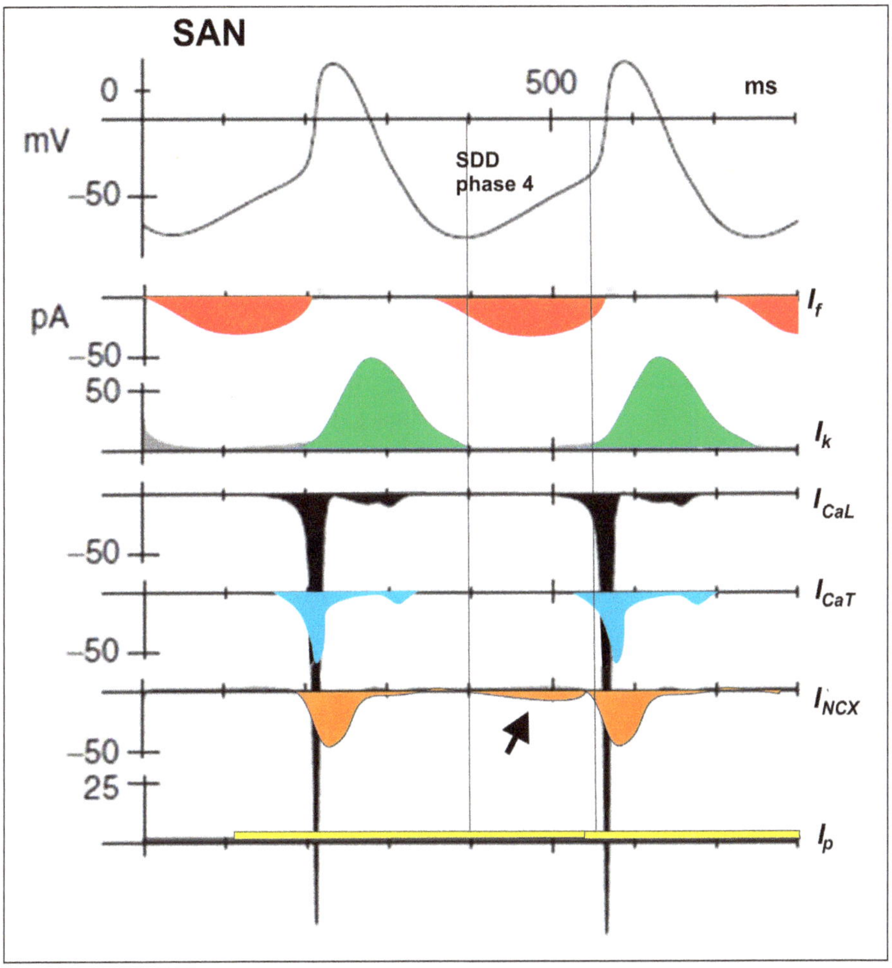

Figure 2-6 Schematic of ionic currents in a sinus node pacemaker cell. The top tracing is the sinus node (**SAN**) action potential in mV, with the time scale at the top in ms. Lower tracings are displays of membrane currents; timing is coordinated with the phases of the SAN action potential. Inward currents are downward and outward currents upward. Relative magnitudes are indicated by the magnitude of the vertical deflections although the drawing is not quantitatively exact. (Modified from Robinson RB, DiFrancesco DA. SA node and impulse initiation. In: *Foundations of Cardiac Arrhythmias*. PM Spooner and MR Rosen (eds). New York: Marcel Dekker; 2000;151–170.)

Inward Current Components of the Pacemaker Potential (SDD)

The I_f pacemaker channel/current. (Figure 2-6, red display). The I_f pacemaker current is a progressively increasing inward current during diastole. The "f" stands for "funny," since its properties were considered to be unusual when the current was first discovered. This channel is also called "I_h" because it is activated by hyperpolarization (h) rather than depolarization (activation by depolarization to a threshold value is a common feature of many voltage gated cardiac ion channels, e.g., I_{Na}, I_{CaL}). The channels for this current begin to open during repolarization of the previous action potential and are activated (open to the inward flow of ions) by the time the terminal segment of repolarization occurs; activation during movement of membrane potential in the repolarizing direction is the basis for the term "hyperpolarization." The threshold for activation is around –50 to –60 mV. Upon activation, an inward (depolarizing) membrane current flows. It is a mixed-cation current carried by Na^+ and K^+, but mostly by Na^+ under physiologic conditions. This current increases with time during pacemaker depolarization, causing the membrane depolarization during early phase 4 (the pacemaker potential, spontaneous phase 4 depolarization or SDD (shown in Figure 2-6) until the channels deactivate (close) late in diastole.

Expression of the I_f current in the sarcolemma of sinus node cells is primarily under the control of the gene *HCN4*, one of four gene isoforms of the hyperpolarization-activated cyclic nucleotide-gated channel. *HCN* was given that name to describe the activation of the current by hyperpolarization (repolarization) and its sensitivity to cyclic nucleotides, which are involved in the autonomic regulation of sinus rate. Modulation of I_f in SAN cells is independent of PKA phosphorylation. Rather, intracellular cAMP binds directly to the HCN protein to modulate its activity and hence modulate I_f. There is some controversy concerning the relative importance of this current in the sinus node relative to the other pacemaker currents.

Calcium channels/currents. The two major calcium channels, the L-type channel (I_{CaL}) and T-type calcium channel (I_{CaT}), both participate in the generation of the pacemaker potential.

I_{CaL} (Figure 2-6, black) in the sinus node activates when the membrane potential is depolarized by I_f to −50 to −30 mV, and therefore I_{CaL} flows during the latter segment of the pacemaker potential. It is represented by two L-type Ca^{2+} channel isoforms, Cav1.2 and Cav1.3 (products of *CACNA21C* and *CACNA1D* genes). Inward I_{CaL} is also the primary current responsible for the depolarization phase (upstroke, phase 0) of the sinus node action potential, particularly in the central part of the node—hence the large downward spike in Figure 2-6. I_{CaL} channels deactivate (close) during repolarization.

I_{CaT} (Figure 2-6, blue) is activated at more negative voltages than I_{CaL} and also may be a source of some of the inward current during the late part of the pacemaker potential. The proteins involved in channel formation are gene products of the *CACNA1G* gene.

Sustained inward current (I_{st}). A third inward current, of uncertain importance, results from a neuronal isoform of the Na^+ channel, Nav1.1, encoded by *SCNA1A*. It is designated I_{st} for sustained inward current (not shown in Figure 2-6). It is activated at around −70 mV and increases when membrane potential decreases to −50 mV. Although current is carried by Na^+, this channel is distinct from the one that carries inward current during phase 0 of the action potential in peripheral nodal cells.

Na^+/Ca^{2+} exchanger current (I_{NCX}). Another inward current carried by inward-moving positive charges is called the Na^+/Ca^{2+} exchanger current (I_{NCX}, Figure 2-6, orange). The Na^+/Ca^{2+} exchanger is an integral membrane protein and not a channel, that moves Ca^{2+} out of the cell against an electrochemical gradient, after its release from the sarcoplasmic reticulum (SR) that initiates contraction. SR Ca^{2+} release is triggered by Ca^{2+} entering the cell through the L-type Ca^{2+} channels and possibly the T-type Ca^{2+} channels during the action potential, acting on ryanodine receptor (RyR) channels in the SR (a process called Ca^{2+}-induced Ca^{2+} release). The extrusion of Ca^{2+} from the cell is in exchange for Na^+ that the exchanger moves into the cell. This process is sensitive to ryanodine, which blocks release of intracellular Ca^{2+}. The inward movement of Na^+ down its electrochemical gradient provides the energy required for the Ca^{2+} extrusion. There is a net inward movement of positive charge because 3 Na^+ ions (3 positive charges) are exchanged for 1 Ca^{2+} ion (2 positive charges). The inward current carried by the inward moving positive charges is called the Na^+/Ca^{2+} exchanger current, I_{NCX}. It occurs primarily during repolarization of the action potential. (It may be confusing, but earlier during initial repolarization, the current may be outward, as described in Chapter 5). Later during SDD, there is also a small Ca^{2+} release beneath the sarcolemma (termed "local calcium release" or LCR; small black arrow on I_{NCX} tracing in Figure 2-6) through the same ryanodine receptor-operated channels. The elevated subsarcolemmal Ca^{2+} from the LCR activates the inward I_{NCX} that contributes to the latter part of SDD. The magnitude of the Ca^{2+} release, which controls the magnitude of I_{NCX}, is related to the amount of Ca^{2+} in the SR and the threshold for opening the ryanodine receptor-operated channels. The greater the Ca^{2+} release, the steeper the slope of the terminal part of the pacemaker potential, which increases the sinus node firing rate. There is some controversy concerning the relative importance of I_f and I_{NCX} in the generation of the pacemaker potential in the sinus node.

Outward Current Components of the Pacemaker Potential (SDD)

I_K channels/current. Outward current components are primarily through several potassium channels serving to repolarize the cell after the upstroke of the action potential (Figure 2-6, green). I_{Kr} (a component of I_K) is probably the dominant repolarizing K^+ current in sinus node, although there are species differences. It reaches a maximum outward flow during repolarization at around −25 mV and then diminishes (channel deactivation) into diastole. By continuing to decrease during diastole, it increases net inward current, contributing to the initial phase of pacemaker depolarization.

I_{K1} channel/current (not shown in Figure 2-6). The low density of I_{K1}, an outward current (inward rectifying) that sets the resting potential or MDP, in sinus node cells facilitates depolarization during the pacemaker potential, since it contributes little or no outward current in opposition to the inward currents. I_{K1} becomes more of a factor in latent pacemaker cells toward the periphery and outside the node with higher negative levels of membrane potential, where it offsets the increased I_f in these cells.

Na^+/K^+ sarcolemmal pump current, I_p. The Na^+/K^+ pump is described in Figure 1-6. In Figure 2-6, it is displayed as I_p (yellow). Three Na^+ ions are extruded in exchange for two K^+ ions, generating a net outward movement of positive charges, e.g., a net outward current, designated as the pump current, I_p. In the sinus node I_p is present throughout the action potential and SDD, contributing to the maximum diastolic potential and the pacemaker potential (an outward current that opposes inward currents). I_p current may fluctuate during the sinus node action potential, although fluctuations are not represented in the diagram.

The magnitude of I_p is controlled by the level of intracellular Na^+. It may be quite small in pacemaker cells in the center of the node because of low Na^+ entry during the action potential, but increases toward the periphery of the node where there is increased Na^+ influx.

Effects of Cell Coupling on Sinus Node Pacemakers

The electrotonic coupling between pacemaker cells and nonpacemaker cells, whereby current flow between the two cell types through gap junctions can inhibit spontaneous diastolic depolarization, is described in Figure 1-3. In the central region of the sinus node the pacemaker cells are weakly coupled to surrounding (latent pacemaker) peripheral nodal cells. There is only weak inhibitory current flow because of the presence of low-conductance gap junctions formed by connexin (Cx) 45 and the paucity of high-conductance gap junctions formed by Cx40 and Cx43. This protects the central nodal pacemaker cells from the hyperpolarizing effects of more peripheral sinus node cells with higher membrane potentials that would serve to inhibit SDD (see Figure 1-3). Coupling among sinus node cells becomes stronger towards the periphery of the node, owing to an increased number of high-conductance Cx43 and Cx40 gap junctions. These gap junctions also provide connections with atrial myocardium that allow conduction from the node into the atria to begin atrial activation. However, the coupling between peripheral nodal cells and atrial myocardium is still weaker than between atrial myocardial cells with each other, thus protecting the node from stronger effects of electrotonic current flow between atrium and node that would inhibit pacemaker activity. Connective tissue barriers that isolate much of the node from atrial myocardium (see Figure 2-2) also protect sinus node pacemakers by decreasing cell-to-cell connections and electrotonic current flow between atrium and node. Nevertheless, there is some inhibition of pacemaker activity in the peripheral nodal cells through their coupling to atrial myocardium, thereby favoring the normal location of the pacemaker in the center of the node.

Sinus Node Conduction Properties

As described in Figures 2-3 and 2-5, during normal sinus impulse initiation, there is delay in the exit of the sinus node impulse into the atrium. This delay is caused by slow conduction in the node and perinodal region. The exact anatomical location of the perinodal region has not been precisely defined. It is likely located in the periphery of the anatomical node, particularly on the margin towards the crista terminalis (Figure 2-5), possibly extending into the exit pathways (Figure 2-2) and outside the node into adjacent atrium.

Slow Anisotropic Conduction

Conduction in the sinus node is slow and anisotropic. Conduction in the node is slow because of the low amplitude, slowly rising phase 0 of the action potentials and the weak electrical coupling between cells. The anisotropy (described in Chapter 9) is characterized by more rapid conduction in the superior and inferior directions (~6 to 8 cm/sec), slower conduction in the lateral direction towards the crista (~6 cm/sec), and even slower in the medial direction towards the atrial septum (~3 cm/sec). In contrast, atrial muscle has a velocity of around 30 cm/sec. In the periphery of the node and perinodal region, conduction is faster than in the central node because the cells have: an increased maximum diastolic potential (MDP) due to increased I_{K1}, and an increased phase 0 upstroke velocity due to increased I_{Na} (Figure 2-5). Cells are also better coupled to each other through an increased number of high-conductance (Cx43) gap junctions.

Time-Dependent Recovery of Excitability

Sinus node and perinodal cells have a time-dependent recovery of excitability shown in **Figure 2-7**.

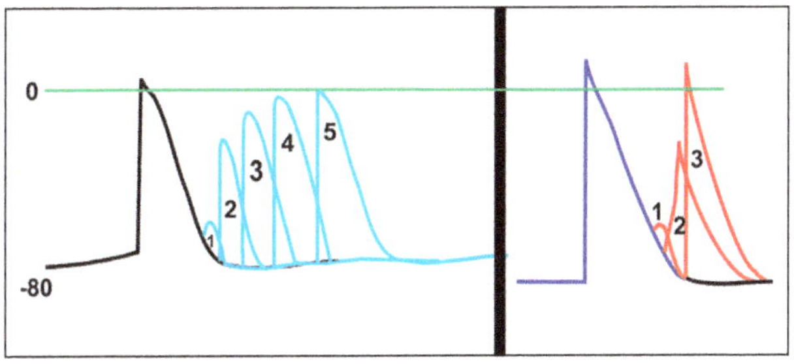

Figure 2-7 Diagrams of action potentials of perinodal cell (**left**) and atrial cell (**right**) and their response to premature activation (**blue, left panel and red, right panel**).

On the left side, a diagram of a perinodal cell action potential is shown in black. The light blue traces (numbers 1–5) represent premature action potentials initiated just before complete repolarization and later in diastole. Prior to complete repolarization, only a small response (1) occurs, which is not conducted. Responses (2–5) occurring later in diastole after complete repolarization, have still not returned to normal because of the time-dependent recovery of excitability, and therefore are slowly conducting.

On the other hand, in atrial cells, recovery of excitability is voltage-dependent, so normal action potentials can be elicited as soon as action potential repolarization is complete. The right side of the figure shows an atrial cell action potential (purple trace) and premature action potentials in red. Premature response 1 is not conducted because the cell is still refractory; response 2 during the latter part of repolarization has a reduced phase 0 and conducts slowly, but response 3, elicited at complete repolarization, has a normal phase 0 and rapid conduction.

The functional significance of the (time-dependent) delay in recovery of excitability in the perinodal cell is that it contributes to conduction slowing and delay of rapid repetitive and premature impulses into and out of the node. This is particularly significant when the origin of the impulses is outside the node and affects the invasion of the node by ectopic impulses, for example during atrial tachycardia or fibrillation. This functional significance is described in more detail in Figure 2-10, later in this chapter.

Control of the Rate of Sinus Node Impulse Initiation

The transmembrane potential characteristic that control the rate of automatic impulse initiation are defined and explained in Figure 1-2. These same factors—rate (slope) of SDD, level of MDP, level of TP, and action potential duration (APD)— apply to sinus node impulse initiation.

Control of Sinus Node Automaticity by the Autonomic Nervous System (ANS)

Sinus node automaticity is under control of the ANS, which, in addition to regulation of heart rate under normal physiological conditions, is responsible for arrhythmias originating in the node. Normal sinus rate and response to the ANS are dependent on age. Sympathetic activation increases net inward pacemaker current thereby increasing the rate of impulse initiation by increasing the slope of spontaneous diastolic depolarization (SDD) (Figure 1-2, Panel A). Parasympathetic activation decreases net inward pacemaker current and decreases the rate of impulse initiation by decreasing the slope of SDD. It also increases the maximum diastolic potential (MDP) (Figure 1-2, Panel B). In the basal state in humans, parasympathetic effects dominate, maintaining the sinus rate between approximately 60–90 impulses/min (normal sinus rhythm). During exercise or other forms of exertion, the sinus rate normally increases to 120–140 impulses/min caused by a decreased parasympathetic activity and an increased sympathetic activity. The site of impulse origin remains in the sinus node although the pacemaker or exit route may shift more cranially (see Figure 2-8). Atrial rates above 150 impulses/min during sympathetic activation may indicate a shift in the pacemaker to an ectopic atrial site where the maximum rate is faster than the sinus node.

Sympathetic nervous system. Sympathetic stimulation via the β_1 receptor affects several of the components of the pacemaker potential to increase the rate of automatic impulse initiation. β_1-adrenergic activation through a G protein-coupled pathway increases I_f by increasing adenyl cyclase activity, which converts adenosine triphoshpate (ATP) to cyclic adenosine monophosphate (cAMP). Elevated cAMP facilitates channel opening, increasing inward I_f pacemaker current and the speed (slope) of pacemaker depolarization (SDD). Elevated cAMP also activates protein kinase A, which phosphorylates L-type calcium channels, increasing I_{CaL} that may be involved in the increased pacemaker current (currents diagrammed in Figure 2-6). Calcium release from the SR is also under sympathetic control since phosphorylation of L-type calcium channels increases Ca^{2+} influx and augments the amount of Ca^{2+} pumped into the SR. The availability of the RyR2-operated channels is also increased by phosphorylation, all of which combine to increase the amount of calcium released during the pacemaker potential, thereby increasing inward I_{NCX}.

Parasympathetic nervous system. Parasympathetic stimulation slows the heart rate by binding of released acetylcholine (ACh) to muscarinic receptors (M_2 subtype) and activating a G protein-dependent pathway that inhibits cAMP formation. This G protein-dependent inhibition of cAMP has several different effects. One is through an inhibitory effect on the I_f pacemaker current, which decreases the rate of SDD. A second is activation of an outward K^+ current (I_{KACh}) through a channel specifically sensitive to ACh, which hyperpolarizes the MDP (Figure 1-2, Panel B). I_{KACh} is a membrane ion channel that is present in high density in SA nodal, atrial, and A-V nodal cells. The proteins that form the channel are encoded by the *Girk4* (*Kir3.4*) gene. Adenosine, a naturally occurring transmitter, although not considered to be part of the parasympathetic system, also activates this pathway to slow sinus rate by binding to adenosine receptors coupled to G protein. This activity makes adenosine useful to help identify arrhythmogenic mechanisms in clinical electrophysiological studies. One final mechanism for parasympathetic slowing of sinus rate may occur mainly when sinus node activity has been enhanced by β_1-adrenergic stimulation. Parasympathetic antagonism of this enhanced sympathetic effect is called "accentuated antagonism."

Age-Dependent Changes

Age is an important regulator of heart rate. The number of functionally active sinus node pacemaker cells decreases with increasing age, being markedly reduced by age 75. Concomitantly, there may be reduction in the density of several of the membrane channels (I_f and I_{CaL}) that give rise to the pacemaker current. There also may be a reduction of HCN_4 gene product causing a reduction of I_f. Connective tissue also increases within the node, disrupting the connections among sinus node cells. Conduction out of the node may become more tenuous owing to connective tissue barriers or decreased gap junctions. The net effect of all these changes is a decrease in both the intrinsic sinus rate as well as the maximal rate that can be attained during autonomic activation. During exercise testing, the maximum age-adjusted heart rate is reduced.

Rate-Dependent Shifts in Earliest Right Atrial Activation

The earliest site(s) of right atrial activation, which indicates the exit route from the sinus node to atrium, changes depending on the ANS effects on the heart rate. **Figure 2-8** shows this "multicentric" origin of atrial activation at different heart rates.

The pattern of activation is indicated by the different shaded isochrones according to the scale. The sites of earliest activation of the right atrium are at the "0" isochrone. In Panel A, during rapid sinus rate when sympathetic effects are predominant, the earliest site is superior to the SVC. In Panels C and D, the earliest site is shifted inferiorly when sinus rate is slowed during vagal domination. In Panel B, at an intermediate rate, there are two early sites activated simultaneously, one inferiorly and one superiorly. The shifts in site of earliest activation alter the pattern of atrial activation and the P-wave morphology changes (above each Panel). Atrial activation reaches the region around the IVC more rapidly when early activation is inferior to the SVC. Superior early activation (A) is associated with an upright P wave in leads I, II, and III. During inferior early activation (C, D), the P-wave axis moves leftward resulting in less positivity in lead III. The P wave in lead III may become isoelectric or even slightly negative, leading to some difficulty in distinguishing a sinus pacemaker from an inferior ectopic atrial pacemaker.

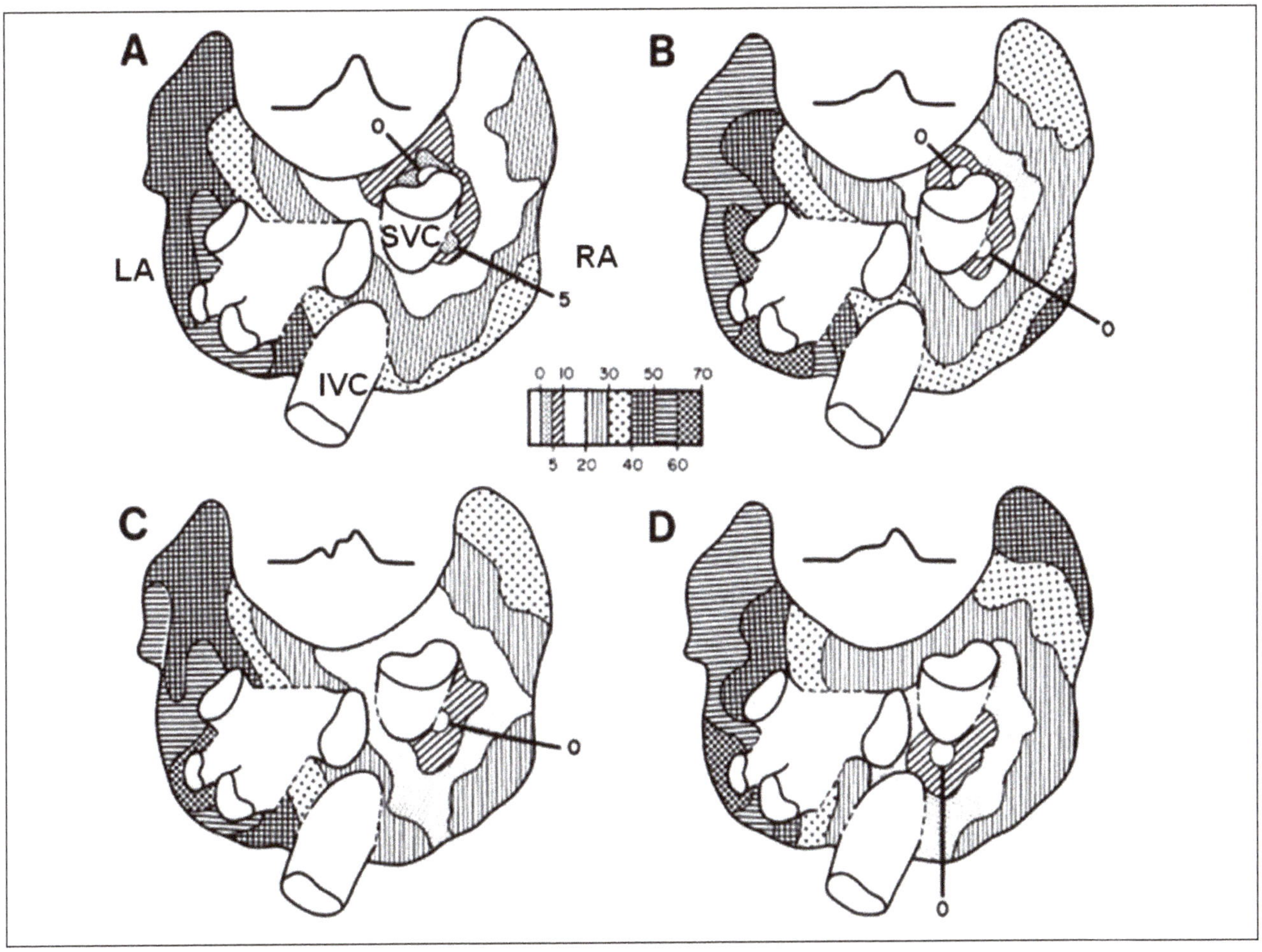

Figure 2-8 Activation maps showing changes in earliest activation with changes in sinus rate in the canine atria. IVC, inferior vena cava; LA, left atrium; RA, right atrium; SVC, superior vena cava. (Reproduced from Boineau JP, Schuessler RB, et al. Multicentric origin of the atrial depolarization wave: The pacemaker complex relation to dynamics of atrial conduction, P-wave changes, and heart rate control. *Circulation*. 1978;58;1036–1048.)

Possible mechanisms for shifts in earliest activation. The association of earliest superior right atrial activation with rapid sinus rates and earliest inferior activation with slow sinus rates has several possible explanations. There may be a relatively stationary, dominant pacemaker region within the compact sinus node that changes its automatic rate due to ANS influence without significantly changing its location. However, the exit routes from that pacemaker region may change depending on autonomic influences. In this model, sympathetic activity favors the superior exit pathway, while parasympathetic activity favors the inferior pathway. During intermediate rates, exit may occur through several pathways simultaneously, including the lateral ones. The mechanisms by which these effects might occur are speculative. The change in exit routes may depend on different densities of sympathetic and parasympathetic nerve endings in different regions of the node, favoring a sympathetic acceleration of conduction out of the superior exit pathway, and parasympathetic inhibition of the superior pathway leading to exit out of the inferior pathway. Other as yet undefined mechanisms are also feasible for differential effects on the different exit pathways.

Another possible mechanism for the change in earliest atrial activation is a shift in the pacemaker site within the sinus node, resulting in a change in the dominant exit route. Cells throughout the sinus node and adjacent perinodal region have pacemaking ability although their intrinsic rates vary. The site within the node that controls the sinus rate at any one time is the site that is initiating the highest frequency of action potentials that conduct to the atria. Other potential pacemaker cells within the node are activated by the high-frequency site before SDD in those cells reaches threshold potential. A pacemaker shift to the superior aspect of the node as would occur if there is a greater effect of the sympathetics to accelerate pacemaker activity in this region, would favor a superior exit route to the atrium. Increased inhibition of superior nodal pacemakers by the parasympathetics would favor the inferior exit route.

A change in pacemaker location to a region outside of the sinus node, such as in the adjacent crista terminalis, can also cause changes in the heart rate. The differential distribution of sympathetic and parasympathetic nerve endings or receptors within the node or different regional sensitivities of pacemaker currents to ANS mediators can also contribute to changes in pacemaker location.

ELECTRICAL STIMULATION OF THE SINUS NODE

Sinus Node Overdrive Stimulation: Basic Electrophysiology

The basic principles of overdrive suppression of automaticity by rapid stimulation (also called "overdrive pacing" in the clinical literature) are illustrated in Chapter 1, Figure 1-6.

Sinus Node Is Comparatively Resistant to Overdrive Suppression

Sinus node pacemaker cells can be overdrive suppressed but are more resistant to suppression than latent pacemakers. Resistance may ensure that the sinus node is not easily displaced from its normal role as dominant pacemaker. For example, during transient shifts of rhythm origin to ectopic sites during a paroxysmal tachycardia, the sinus node can rapidly regain control of the rhythm without a long period of depressed activity once the tachycardia ceases if nodal function is normal; however, the node becomes more susceptible to overdrive suppression in some pathological conditions.

Figure 2-9 shows the effects of overdrive stimulation on a rabbit sinus node pacemaker cell in a tissue chamber. The sinus node was stimulated directly to avoid conduction disturbances that can happen in the *in situ* node that make the response characteristics to overdrive more complicated.

In Panel A at the left, the sinus node pacemaker cell has an automatic rate of 198 impulses/min (cycle length (CL) of 300 ms indicated by the horizontal arrow). It is stimulated at a rate of 375 per min (CL = 160 ms) during the 30-sec period labeled "drive" (the complete 30-sec period is not displayed; also, the sinus rate of the rabbit heart is significantly more rapid than the human heart, so the overdrive stimulation rates are also more rapid than what would be used in a clinical study). After stimulation ends, there is a prolonged CL of 340 ms (horizontal arrow) until the first post overdrive spontaneous action potential due to overdrive suppression. The intrinsic CL of 300 ms is rapidly reestablished within several cycles.

In Panel B, the rate of overdrive is increased to 462 per min (CL = 130 ms) during the 30-sec drive period. Overdrive suppression after stimulation ends is lengthened to 375 ms, showing the rate related enhancement of overdrive suppression previously described in Figure 1-6. Again, there is rapid reestablishment of the pre-stimulus spontaneous rate.

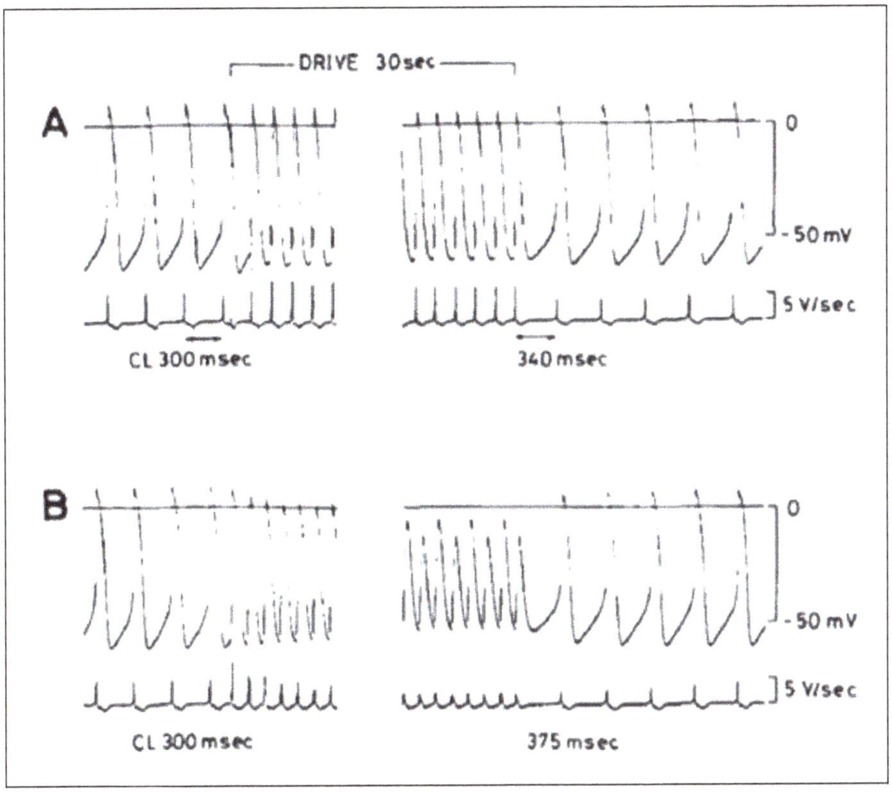

Figure 2-9 Effects of overdrive stimulation on rabbit sinus node cell. Below the action potential recording is its first time derivative that is used as an indicator of the rate of sinus node firing. (Reproduced from Kodama I, Goto J, et al. Effects of Rapid stimulation on the transmembrane action potentials of rabbit sinus node pacemaker cells. *Circ Res.* 1980;46:90–99.)

The overdrive suppression shown in this experiment is much less than suppression of ectopic pacemakers using the same experimental paradigm (see Figure 1-7 which shows the response to overdrive of a ventricular Purkinje cell). Another important point to emphasize is that automatic impulse initiation is not terminated by overdrive stimulation, as are other mechanisms for arrhythmias, DAD-triggered activity (Chapter 5), and reentry (Chapter 9).

Overdrive Results in Less I_p in the Sinus Node

Overdrive suppression of ectopic pacemakers is primarily caused by increased activity of the electrogenic Na^+–K^+ pump and the generation of outwardly directed pump current, I_p, that suppresses the pacemaker potential and hyperpolarizes the membrane potential (see Figure 1-6). The upstroke (phase 0) of the sinus node action potential is mainly due to inward L-type calcium current (I_{CaL}), rather than the sodium current (I_{Na}) that underlies phase 0 depolarization in some latent pacemakers (exceptions are A-V node and A-V valves). Therefore, the increment in internal Na^+ during overdrive is much less in sinus node pacemakers than in latent pacemakers, resulting in less of a stimulant to the pump and a smaller increase in I_p with pacing. (Some Na^+ does enter sinus node cells during the action potential but does not contribute significantly to phase 0 depolarization).

Other mechanisms might also be involved in sinus node overdrive suppression. One hypothesis attributes some of the overdrive suppression of sinus node pacemakers to an increase in Ca^{2+} that enters during the action potential upstroke owing to the increase in number of action potentials that occurs during overdrive. This increased Ca^{2+} at the internal surface of the membrane can in turn lead to a reduction in the Ca^{2+} current (I_{CaL}) by acting on the inside of the Ca^{2+} channel to potentiate inactivation of the channel (referred to as calcium-dependent inactivation). Since I_{CaL} likely contributes to the inward component of the pacemaker current in the sinus node (Figure 2-6), this decrease in the inward current that results would lead to some overdrive suppression.

I_p is likely to play a greater role for overdrive suppression of pacemakers in the more peripheral aspect of the node, which may control the rhythm under certain abnormal circumstances. I_{Na} contributes more to the depolarization phase (0) of these action potentials (see Figure 2-5), and therefore, internal Na^+ increases more during overdrive to provide a stronger activation of the pump.

Overdrive Stimulation of the Sinus Node *In Situ*

In clinical electrophysiology studies, overdrive stimulation (pacing) of the sinus node *in situ* usually does not involve its direct stimulation. The site of overdrive stimulation is in the atrium outside the node, and the effects of overdrive are also measured in the atrium. Therefore, the exact events occurring within the sinus node are not detected and must be deduced from the atrial response.

Influence of conduction delay and block on overdrive suppression. An important factor influencing the measured overdrive response is conduction delay and possible block of atrial stimulated impulses before they reach the pacemaker region of the node and/or conduction delay of the pacemaker impulse out of the node to the atrium. Conduction delay and block can occur either in the node, because of its low-amplitude action potentials with slow phase 0 and time-dependent recovery of excitability or in the perinodal region with time-dependent recovery of excitability (see Figure 2-7).

During normal sinus impulse initiation, there is delay in the exit of the sinus impulse into the atrium (antegrade direction) through the perinodal region. During atrial stimulation, the delay in the other (retrograde) direction, from atrium into sinus node, is greater because the safety factor for conduction decreases in this direction (while increasing from sinus pacemaker to atrium). The decrease in safety factor results from the progressive decrease in action potential upstroke velocity and amplitude going from the atrium into the node, resulting in each action potential in this direction of conduction being a weaker stimulus to the next action potential (Figure 2-5). (A more detailed description of safety factor for conduction is presented in Chapter 9, Figure 9-4.

Sinus Node Recovery Time (SRT)

Figure 2-10 shows how conduction properties of the perinodal region can influence the measured overdrive suppression response, which in clinical studies is called the "sinus node recovery time" (SRT). In these studies, the stimulation and recording sites are in the right atrium. (Compare the response to Figure 1-9 in which there is no region of conduction delay surrounding the pacemaker.) Figure 2-10 shows a standard ladder diagram depicting conduction (black downward arrows) of the automatic impulse (AI) arising in the sinus node (SAN), through the perinodal region (PN) into the adjacent atrium (ATR) to elicit an atrial response (A). The CL of AI initiation is 500 ms (at the left in each panel). Conduction delay in the perinodal region of 60 ms is indicated by the slanted segment of the arrows. In each panel, a 60-sec period of overdrive stimulation is applied to the atrium (S to AS, red upward arrows). Only the last three stimuli of the overdrive are shown in Panels A–D and the last four stimuli in Panel E. The stimulated impulses must pass through the perinodal region to reach and stimulate the nodal pacemaker (AS). As shown in the diagram, there is conduction delay (slanted red arrows).

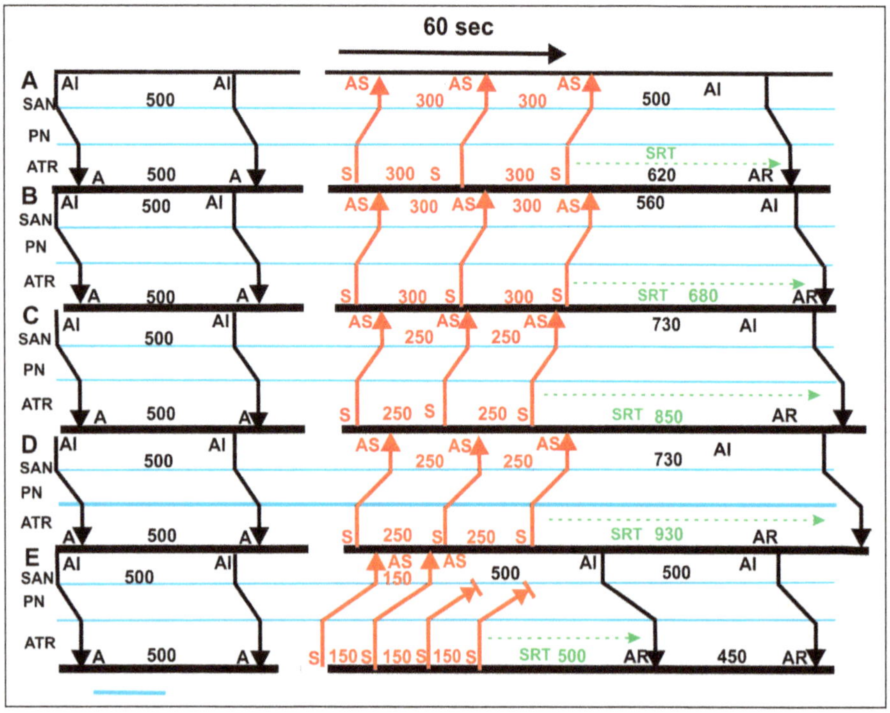

Figure 2-10 Ladder diagram describing how conduction of atrial stimulated impulses influences the measured overdrive response of the sinus node.

Panel A shows how overdrive suppression might be measured at the atrial recording site due to conduction delay, even though there is actually no suppression of the SAN. After stimulation at a CL of 300 ms, the first CL after overdrive (AS-AI) is 500 ms in the SAN, which is the same as the spontaneous CL. The measured SRT (dashed green arrow) at the atrial site is 620 ms because of the 60-ms delay in conduction of the last stimulated impulse through the perinodal region to the sinus node (red upward-slanted arrow) and the 60-ms conduction delay of the first sinus impulse after overdrive to the atrium back through the perinodal region to the atrial response (AR)—e.g., add these conduction delays totaling 120 ms to the SCL of 500 ms.

In Panel B, at the same overdrive CL of 300 ms, overdrive suppression of the sinus node pacemaker is depicted; AS-AI = 560 ms. Because of the same conduction delay into and out of the node through the perinodal region (60 ms in each direction) as in Panel A, the measured SRT in the atrium is 680 ms (dashed green arrow), 120 ms greater than the actual overdrive suppression of the node.

In Panel C, at a more rapid stimulation rate (S-S = 250), overdrive suppression of the sinus pacemaker (AS-AI) is increased to 730 ms and SRT measured at 850 ms in the atrium because of the same perinodal conduction delays.

Panel D shows another response in which perinodal conduction delay increases to 100 ms in each direction because of its time-dependent refractoriness (the stimulation CL stays the same at 250 ms). The measured SRT at the atrium (S-AR) would be even longer (730 + 200 = 930 ms) than in Panel C.

Panel E shows block of overdrive impulses in the perinodal region at a shorter overdrive CL of 150 ms (red arrow and horizontal bar). In this panel, the sinus node pacemaker is not effectively overdriven and no overdrive suppression is evident in the atrium (and even some overdrive acceleration) at the rapid stimulation CL.

In summary, Figure 2-10 diagrams the mechanism for SRT in clinical studies. The diagram illustrates the conduction delay in the perinodal region that contributes to the overdrive suppression measured from the last stimulated impulse to the appearance of the first spontaneous impulse in the atrium (AR).

Other Factors Affect Overdrive SRT

Change in pacemaker location. In some instances, suppression of the dominant pacemaker by overdrive may result in a shift of the pacemaker to another site within the node and shifts of the exit route. For example, shortening of the exit route because of a shift in the pacemaker toward the periphery of the node may decrease conduction time out of the node. Shifts in pacemaker site or exit routes can often be detected by a change in the P wave after the period of overdrive.

ANS - Acetylcholine (ACh). Electrical stimulation of atrial myocardium near the node during overdrive can release ACh from parasympathetic nerve endings. This ANS neurotransmitter can influence the response of *in situ* sinus node pacemakers to overdrive stimulation in multiple ways. ACh enhances overdrive suppression of sinus node pacemakers by increasing outward current components of the pacemaker potential (I_K, I_{K1}) and activating I_{KACh}, which is a specific K^+-channel outward current in the node. ACh also decreases inward I_f (Figure 2-6). It can also cause shifts in the pacemaker site and slow conduction or cause conduction block in some regions of the node by decreasing I_{CaL}, an important component of the depolarization phase (0) of sinus node cells. ACh can also slow conduction in the perinodal region by decreasing action potential amplitude and increasing time-dependent recovery of excitability related to a decrease in I_{CaL}. The possible effects of ACh release likely depend on the location of the stimulating electrodes. If ACh is released at a distance from the node during atrial stimulation, effective amounts are not likely to reach the sinus node pacemaker due to its rapid inactivation by cholinesterases in the blood. Clinical overdrive testing of sinus node function sometimes has poor reproducibility. One explanation for this may be changes in the amount and effect of ACh release on nodal pacemakers due to different locations of the atrial stimulating electrodes from one test to the next.

ANS—Sympathetic activity. A decrease in blood pressure during overdrive stimulation *in situ* might enhance reflex sympathetic nerve activity affecting the overdrive response of the sinus node. Norepinephrine from sympathetic nerve endings decreases overdrive suppression, likely related to norepinephrine enhancement of both I_f and I_{CaL} (Figure 2-6). Norepinephrine might also increase retrograde and antegrade conduction velocity and decrease block in the perinodal region by enhancing I_{CaL}, thereby decreasing the component of SRT attributable to perinodal conduction delay.

Finally, even the baseline autonomic tone influences overdrive suppression through the effects of ACh and/or norepinephrine as described above. Therefore, *in situ*, the intrinsic properties of the conduction and pacemaker properties in and surrounding the node can only be determined by removing these autonomic influences by muscarinic and β_1-receptor blockade.

Sinus Node Overdrive Stimulation (Pacing); Clinical Electrophysiology

Clinical Context

In clinical studies, the effects of overdrive stimulation on sinus rhythm provides specific information on the response of a rhythm that by definition is caused by normal automaticity. This provides a template for studying and interpreting the effects of overdrive on ectopic arrhythmias where the mechanism is uncertain and overdrive is used to determine if the cause is automaticity. The response of the sinus node to overdrive has also been used to evaluate whether it is functioning normally or has been altered by disease. However, because of the difficulties in interpreting the response as discussed above, it is not usually used as a diagnostic procedure to evaluate the properties of the sinus node.

A Normal Sinus Node Response

Figure 2-11 shows an example of the effects of overdrive on sinus rhythm in a heart with a normal sinus node. The spontaneous CL in normal sinus rhythm (NSR) is 720 ms, shown in the top recording. The bottom recording shows, at the left, the last 5 stimulated impulses of a period of 30 sec of overdrive pacing at a CL of 400 ms. The SRT is the interval from the last paced impulse (arrow) to the first sinus impulse (1120 ms). The time to resumption of the prestimulation CL (720 ms) is the total recovery time. This occurs after 3 impulses with gradual shortening CLs (warm up); total recovery time in this example is 4.4 sec.

In the normal sinus node response, the SRT increases as the overdrive rate is increased (decreased CL). **Figure 2-12** shows the overdrive (paced) CL (PCL) on the abscissa, plotted against the SRT (unfilled circles) on the ordinate. There is a progressive increase in SRT at shorter PCLs as expected of an automatic pacemaker, reaching a peak SRT (1100 ms) at an overdrive CL of 400 ms. Further shortening of the PCL results in a decrease in recovery time.

Interpreting the SRT

There are important factors that must be considered in interpreting the measured response of the sinus node *in situ* to overdrive stimulation, in addition to the effects of the overdrive on automaticity of the sinus node pacemaker cells. Two of these factors are conduction time and sinus node CL. The sinus node CL is used to calculate the corrected sinus node recovery time (CSRT) (see below).

Conduction time and block. The measured SRT is influenced by the conduction time from the site of atrial stimulation to the sinus node pacemaker and the conduction time from the pacemaker back to the site of measurement (see Figure 2-10). As the rate of stimulation increases, an increase in the measured SRT can occur due to both overdrive suppression of automaticity and increased conduction time into and out of the node (Figure 2-10, Panels C and D).

At a critically rapid overdrive rate, the SRT may decrease (Figure 2-12) for at least two reasons: (1) even if all the stimulated impulses succeed in entering the node, the sinus nodal pacemaker cells may not respond 1:1 to each stimulated impulse because of the long time-dependent refractory period of sinus nodal cells, and (2) conduction block of some of the stimulated impulses in the perinodal region or in the peripheral node itself may decrease the actual number of overdrive impulses reaching the pacemaker cells (Figure 2-10, Panel E). The decreased SRT in Figure 2-12 at the shorter overdrive CLs is likely caused by such block of overdrive impulses. Unfortunately, it is not possible to precisely quantify how much of the overdrive suppression response is caused by suppression of sinus node automaticity and how much by conduction changes. A rough estimate based on experimental laboratory studies is that conduction time into and out of the node may be as much as 120 ms, which must be subtracted from the SRT. Thus, measurements of SRT tend to overestimate the actual depression of sinus node pacemaker function. The only way of accurately evaluating the contribution of pacemaker suppression and conduction time *in situ* is by recording directly from the sinus node (called a sinus node electrogram). These recordings show the pacemaker depolarization in the node itself. This is not usually done in clinical studies owing to the difficulty in obtaining a satisfactory recording that is free of artifacts.

Sinus node CL and corrected sinus node recovery time (CSRT). The measurement of the SRT is also affected by the sinus node cycle length (SCL). To account for this property, the CSRT, calculated as SRT-SCL (triangles in Figure 2-12), is often used as a measurement of overdrive suppression. In **Figure 2-13**, the normal relationship of SRT to SCL is shown by the diagonal line. At shorter SCLs, the SRT is decreased.

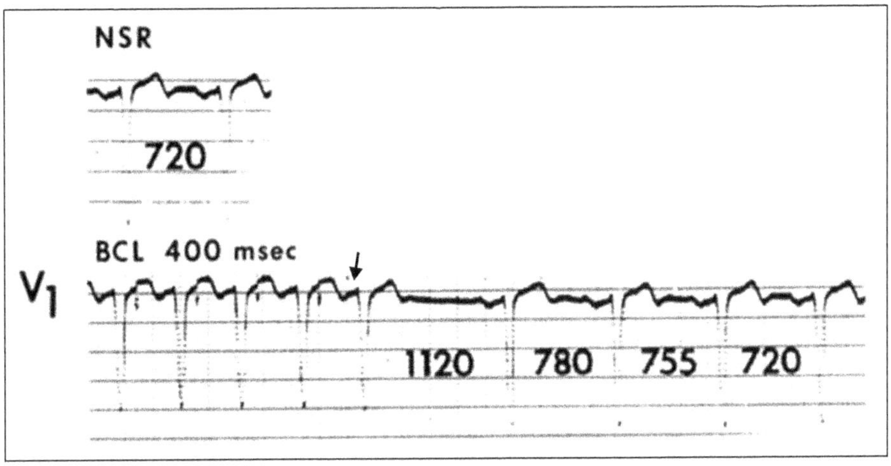

Figure 2-11 Normal sinus node response, to overdrive atrial pacing measured in ECG lead V_1. (Reproduced from Josephson ME. *Josephson's Clinical Cardiac Electrophysiology: Techniques and Interpretations* (5th ed.). Philadelphia, PA: Wolters Kluwer; 2016.)

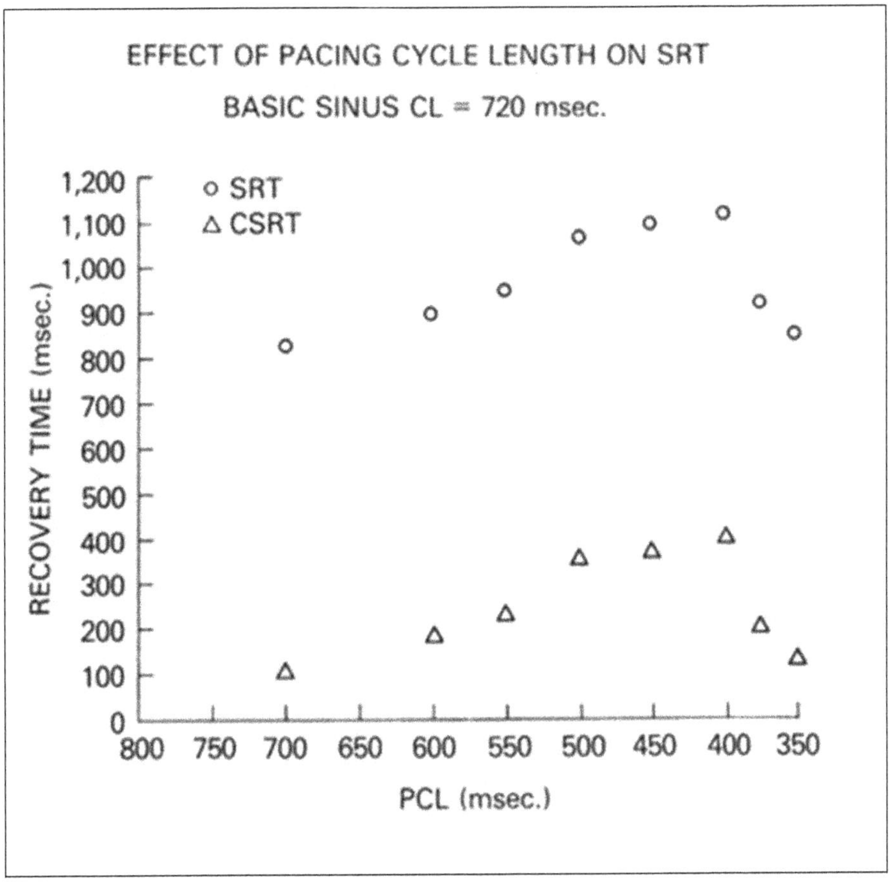

Figure 2-12 Typical relationship of sinus node recovery time (SRT) to paced cycle length (PCL) in a normal heart is shown by the circles. The corrected sinus node recovery (CSRT) time is shown by the **triangles**. (Reproduced from Josephson ME. *Josephson's Clinical Cardiac Electrophysiology: Techniques and Interpretations* (5th ed.). Philadelphia, PA: Wolters Kluwer; 2016.)

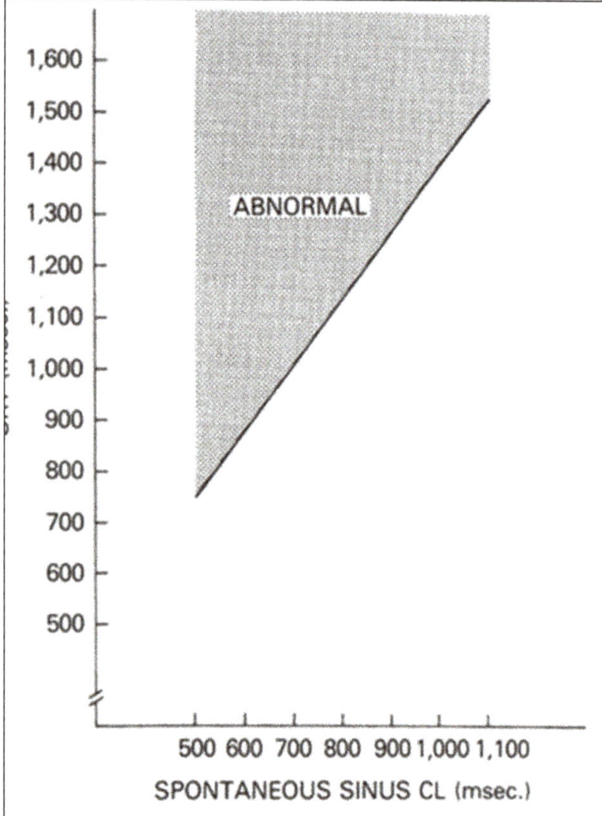

Figure 2-13 Relationship of maximum SRT (ordinate) to spontaneous SCL (abscissa). At any spontaneous SCL, the normal SRT ± 2 SD should fall to the **right of the diagonal line and stippled area**. (Reproduced from Mandel W, Hayakawa H, et al. Evaluation of sinoatrial node function in man by overdrive suppression. *Circulation.* 1971;44;59–66.)

The mechanism responsible for a decrease in SRT with a decrease in SCL is uncertain but may reflect the state of the ANS (decreased vagus and increased sympathetic activity at faster sinus rates), which can influence overdrive suppression. In general, the normal SRT and CSRT are decreased if vagal influences on the node are blocked by atropine. SRT is increased if sympathetic influences are blocked by propranolol.

Programmed Premature Stimulation—Basic Electrophysiology

Arrhythmias caused by automaticity in some respects respond differently to premature stimuli compared with the responses of other arrhythmogenic mechanisms. These differences may sometimes help in the identification of an automatic mechanism. The basic responses of automaticity are *compensatory pause*, *resetting*, and *interpolation*, as described in Figure 1-10 and Figure 1-11. This pattern is exemplified by the sinus node pacemaker when it is stimulated directly in experimental laboratory studies, providing a template for understanding the effects of premature excitation on ectopic pacemakers and the arrhythmias that they cause. The response of the sinus node to premature stimulation also provides information on normal and abnormal sinus node function. It should be emphasized again that automaticity is neither initiated nor terminated by premature stimulation as are other mechanisms that cause arrhythmias, DAD-triggered activity (Chapter 5) and reentry (Chapter 9).

Importance of Conduction Delay

The sinus node is not stimulated directly in clinical studies but rather, atrial stimulation is used. Therefore, of primary importance in interpreting the resetting response of the sinus node, when the premature stimuli are applied in the atrium and the sinus node response is measured in the atrium, is the conduction delay of the prematurely stimulated impulses into the node and conduction delay of the reset sinus node impulse out of the node to the atrial site where it is measured. **Figure 2-14** diagrams several possible effects of conduction on the resetting response.

The ladder diagram in Figure 2-14 (similar format as Figure 2-10) describes automatic impulse initiation (AI) in the sinus node (SAN) at a CL of 500 ms (black numbers), and propagation of the sinus impulse through the perinodal region (PN) with conduction delay (slanted black line) to the atrium (ATR) (black downward arrows) (blue A).

In Panel A, a late premature impulse (S) stimulated in the atrium with a coupling interval of 400 ms (upward red arrow, S), does not prematurely excite the sinus node at 400 ms but rather, because of conduction delay in the PN (slanted red arrow) collides with the automatic impulse (AI) (asterisks) before it reaches the pacemaker. The pacemaker continues to fire at the 500-ms cycle length. A compensatory pause of 600 ms from S to AR (atrial response; also called the return cycle (RCL) results in the atrium (vertical dashed line at far right indicates compensatory pause in the atrium based on the calculation: A-S (400 ms) + S-Ar (600 ms) = 2 × AI-AI (1000 ms)). Note that there is a 50-ms conduction delay from SAN to AR.

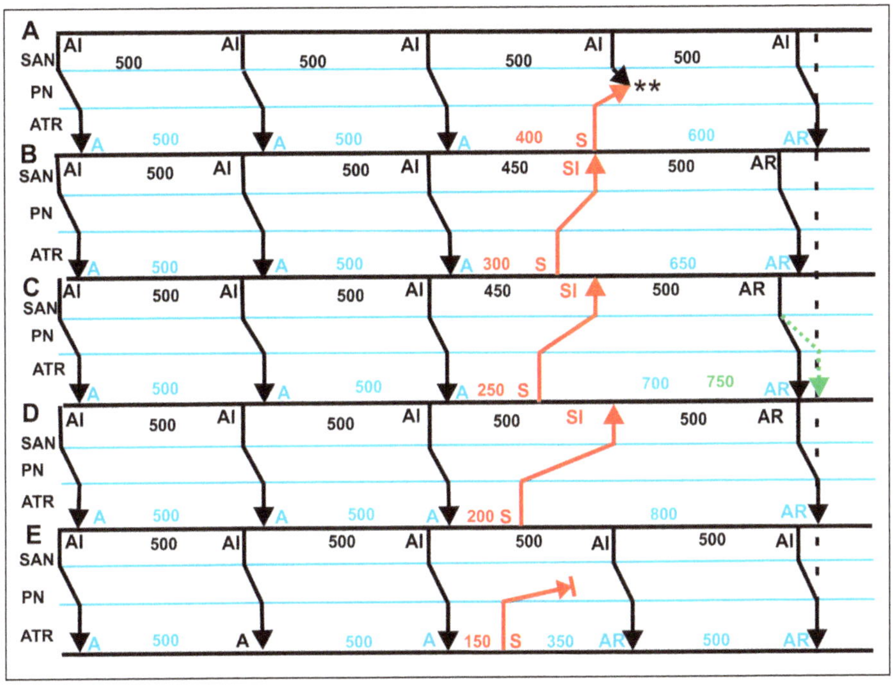

Figure 2-14 Ladder diagram describing how conduction of prematurely stimulated impulses (**S, red arrow**) in the atrium (ATR) influences the measured atrial response (**AR, blue**). In each panel (**Panels A–E**), automatic impulse initiation (AI) in the sinus node (SAN) is indicated by the downward pointing **black arrows**. The prematurely stimulated impulse in the ATR (S) and conduction through the PN region to the SAN (SI) are indicated by the **upward pointing red arrow**.

In Panel B, an earlier premature impulse (S) with a coupling interval of 300 ms, does conduct to the sinus node pacemaker and activates it earlier (stimulation impulse SI in red) than its spontaneous CL. Notice that additional conduction delay of 150 ms of the premature impulse in the perinodal region (slanted red line) results in a longer premature coupling interval in the SAN (450 ms) than at the atrial site of stimulation (300 ms). The SAN cycle length following premature activation (red SI) is still 500 ms (RCL), unchanged from the control since premature activation does not affect the pacemaker potential as previously explained in the description of Figure 1-10. The pacemaker response measured in the atrium (AR) has a RCL of 650 ms (blue), indicated by the downward black arrow, demonstrating resetting since A-S (300 ms) + S-AR (650 ms) is less than 2 × (AI-AI) (1000 ms). The atrial cycle length, however, is longer than the SAN cycle length because of conduction delay of the premature impulse into and out of the node.

Panels C and D show that earlier premature impulses (red S; 250 and 200 ms) conduct more slowly (compare to Panel B with the 300-ms coupling interval), since they are conducting in more refractory perinodal tissue. As a result, the coupling interval at the pacemaker site in the SAN does not decrease as expected. In Panel C, the premature coupling interval at the pacemaker site stays at the same 450 ms as in Panel B, despite increased prematurity at the site of stimulation to 250 ms. Resetting still occurs in the atrium (black arrow and blue AR at 700 ms CL). However, if there is some additional conduction delay from the SAN to ATR as diagrammed by the dashed green arrow, a compensatory response would be measured in the ATR (CL = green 750 ms). In extreme cases when there is marked delay of the stimulated premature impulse as diagrammed in Panel D, the SAN may not be excited prematurely at all; the coupling interval in SAN after premature atrial activation, S-AR = 200 ms is 500 ms because of a 300 ms conduction delay in the PN, which is the same as the spontaneous CL in Panel D. As a result, there is a compensatory pause in the atrium (black arrow and blue AR at CL = 800 ms).

Panel E shows that conduction block of an earlier premature impulse (red S, 150 ms A-S coupling) may also occur, resulting in failure to reach and reset the pacemaker and failure to affect conduction of the pacemaker impulse to the ATR. The AR following the premature impulse is at a cycle length of 350 ms, the exact time expected of the next sinus impulse if the SAN were not affected. This response indicates interpolation of the premature impulse, S.

Variable conduction delays. As previously described, the measured CL in the atrium following premature stimulation of the atrium (S-AR) (atrial return cycle, RCL) does not accurately reflect effects on the SAN pacemaker. It always includes the time it takes the stimulated impulse to reach the pacemaker site plus the time it takes the impulse to conduct from this site back to where the return cycle (AR) is measured. For example, in Panel B, the RCL following the premature impulse is 500 ms in the SAN (SI-AR), which is the same as the unperturbed pacemaker cycle length, but the RCL following the premature impulse at the site of stimulation in the atrium (AR) is 650 ms. As discussed previously, the retrograde conduction time from stimulated impulse to nodal cell may differ from the antegrade conduction time from nodal pacemaker to atrium. Although in Figure 2-14 Panels C and D, the prematurely stimulated atrial impulse entering the node conducts more slowly than the sinus impulse exiting the node because it encounters increasingly refractory perinodal tissue, this might not always be the case. In either case, the RCL (S-AR in Figure 2-14) is a measurement of the RCL of impulse initiation by the pacemaker plus conduction to and from the pacemaker site. One or all of these components can change, sometimes in opposite directions making the interpretation of the response pattern difficult. For example, the S-AR response may be compensatory even when the pacemaker is reset if there is sufficient conduction slowing (Figure 2-14, Panel C, green dashed arrow at 750 ms = AR).

In addition to the conduction delay in the sinus node and perinodal region described above, there can also be conduction delay in the atrium itself, between the atrial stimulation site and the SAN, which depends on the distance of the stimulating electrode from the SAN (not shown in Figure 2-14). The added atrial delay causes a shift in the resetting curve, which possibly results in measured compensatory responses over a wider range of premature coupling intervals.

Shifts in pacemaker site to the perinodal margins. After early premature impulses, antegrade conduction time from the pacemaker to the atrium may sometimes shorten because of a shift in the pacemaker site toward the peripheral margins of the node. As the early premature impulse enters the node, it first depolarizes latent pacemakers at the margin. As it slowly conducts toward the more centrally located dominant pacemaker, these peripheral pacemakers can recover. Since the true pacemaker is subsequently excited by the premature impulse after recovery of the peripheral latent pacemakers has taken place, there is sufficient time for the pacemaker potential of the latent pacemaker at the margin of the node to depolarize to threshold and initiate the next impulse closer to the margin with the atrium. The early premature impulse may also activate only part of the node where the dominant pacemaker resides, allowing a peripheral latent pacemaker that is not excited by the premature impulse, sufficient time to initiate impulses. This pacemaker may initiate the subsequent one or two impulses as well; before the original sinus node pacemaker regains control of the rhythm. A clue to pacemaker shift may be a change in the P wave if the shift causes a change in the exit route from the node.

Programmed Premature Stimulation: Clinical Electrophysiology

Based on the description above, it is apparent that interpretation of the responses of the *in situ* sinus node to premature stimulation during clinical electrophysiology studies is complicated. For this reason, this testing procedure is not often used to elucidate sinus node function for clinical care. The contribution of each of the features of conduction, pacemaker shift, and properties of automaticity that underlie the response are difficult to sort out without direct recordings from the sinus node pacemaker and its surrounding regions, which are not readily feasible in clinical studies. Nevertheless, the results of clinical studies show the relationship of basic electrophysiological properties of the sinus node to clinical function and offer a useful template for studies using these methods to determine the mechanism of impulse origin for the ectopic arrhythmias that are described in Chapter 3.

Clinical Studies of Sinus Node Reset Properties

Figure 2-15 illustrates a clinical sinus node resetting study that involves the introduction of progressively more premature atrial stimulated impulses (A2) after every eighth to tenth sinus impulse (A1) during a stable sinus rhythm (A1-A1) with measurement of the first (A2-A3) spontaneous return cycle after the stimulus.

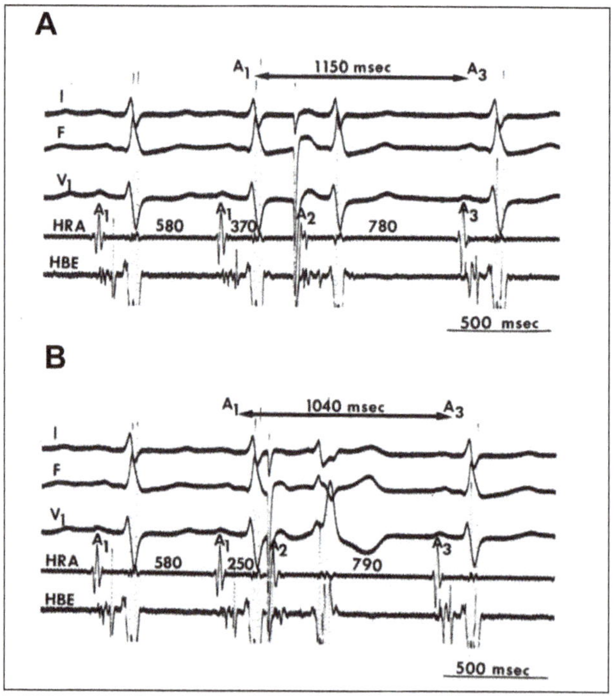

Figure 2-15 Atrial premature stimulation to assess sinus node resetting properties. ECG leads I, aVF (F), and V_1, high right atrial (HRA) electrogram, and His bundle electrogram (HBE). (Reproduced from Josephson ME. *Josephson's Clinical Cardiac Electrophysiology: Techniques and Interpretations* (5th ed.). Philadelphia, PA: Wolters Kluwer; 2016.)

In Panel A, the sinus cycle length (A1-A1) is 580 ms and A2 is applied at a premature coupling interval of 370 ms (indicated by interval from A1-A2 above the HRA recording). The A2-A3 return cycle is 780 ms, indicating reset ([A1-A2 + A2-A3] (1150 ms) < [2 × A1-A1] (1160 ms). In Figure 2-15, Panel B, the A1-A2 is reduced to 250 ms and the A2-A3 is 790 ms, also showing reset (A1-A2+A2-A3 (1040 ms) < 2 x A1-A1 (1160 ms).

As described in Figure 2-14, A2-A3 CL is determined by both conduction and automaticity properties. Measuring the following CL, A3-A4 (not shown in Figure 2-14) allows assessment of automaticity without antegrade conduction delay from the premature impulse assuming that the effects of the premature activation lasts more than one CL.

Figure 2-16 shows a typical sinus node response pattern and its interpretation from a clinical study. Panel A plots data consistent with a fully compensatory pause at long, premature CLs and a resetting response at shorter premature CLs. The relationship between the premature CLs (A1-A2) on the abscissa and return cycle lengths (A2-A3) on the left ordinate is similar to the format in Figure 1-11.

The spontaneous sinus cycle length of 800 ms is indicated by the dashed horizontal line. The upper diagonal line indicates the range of responses that are equivalent to a compensatory pause (see Figure 1-11 for explanation). The measured response to different premature stimulation CLs is divided into several zones.

Zone I: Fully compensatory response. Zone I (green circles in Panel A) consists of the range of A1-A2 premature coupling CLs at which the return cycle (A2-A3) is fully compensatory and the points fall along the diagonal line (A1-A2 + A2-A3 = 2 × A1-A1), Zone I occurs in response to premature atrial impulses occurring in the last 20% to 30% of the spontaneous CL and most likely represents collision of the prematurely stimulated impulse with the sinus impulse (shown in Figure 2-14, Panel A).

Zone II: Resetting response. The points falling below the diagonal line in Figure 2-16, Panel A (red circles) indicate occurrence of resetting (A1-A2 + A2-A3 < 2 × A1-A1). The response in Zone II is the range of premature coupling intervals where the stimulated premature impulse, A2, reaches the pacemaker and depolarizes it, causing it to initiate its next impulse earlier than expected (shown in Figure 2-14, Panels B and C), which results in A3, the return cycle at the atrial recording site (A3 in Figure 2-14). A2-A3 can remain constant throughout Zone II, producing a plateau, or A2-A3 may increase sometimes after a plateau, as in Figure 2-16, Panel A.

The relationship in Figure 2-16, Panel A differs in two aspects from the one described in Figure 1-10 and plotted in Figure 1-11, where the stimulus was applied and measurements made directly at the pacemaker site. In Figure 2-16, Panel A, the zone of compensatory pause (Zone I) is longer for the sinus node resetting response because collision of

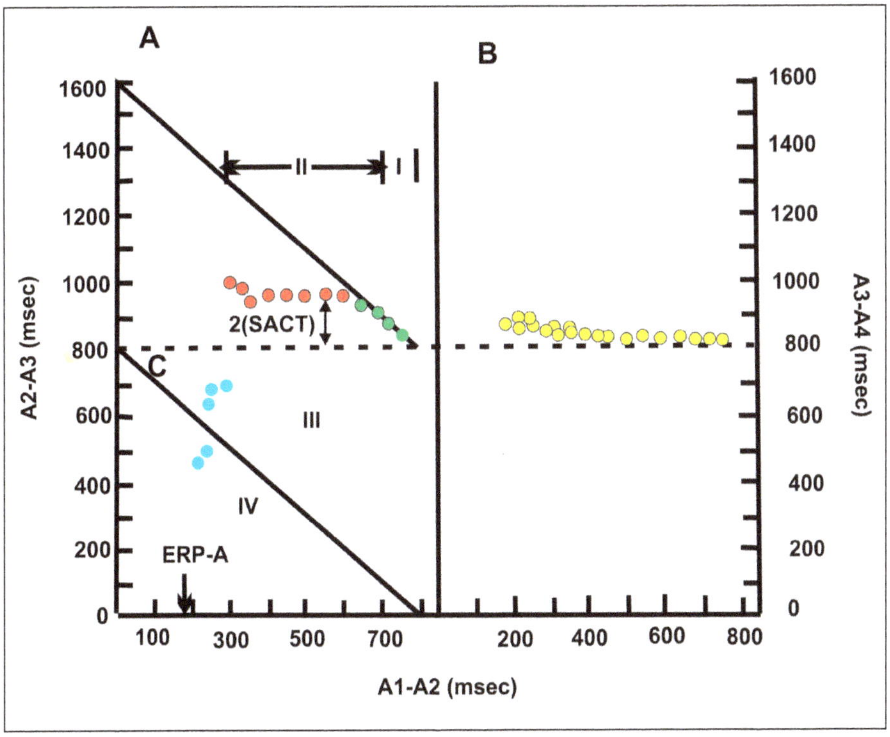

Figure 2-16 Graphic display of sinus node response to atrial premature stimulation.

stimulated and pacemaker impulses are more likely to occur within the perinodal region interposed between stimulus and pacemaker site (shown in Figure 2-14, Panel A). Also, the return cycle (A2-A3) is longer than the spontaneous CL (red circles are above the dashed horizontal, (vertical arrow) even when the spontaneous CL of the pacemaker is not predicted to be lengthened.

Sinoatrial conduction time (SACT). The difference between A2-A3 and the spontaneous CL (A1-A1, double headed arrow in Figure 2-16, Panel A) is usually interpreted to reflect total conduction time of the premature impulse into the node and conduction time of the reset sinus impulse out of the node (2 × SACT) (see also Figure 2-14, Panels B–D). However, an increase in the return pacemaker cycle length still remains a possible cause, particularly when there is sinus node disease (see below). If the A2-A3 interval increases as shown in Figure 2-16, Panel A, at A1-A2 less than 400 ms, additional conduction delay of earlier premature impulses in the perinodal region is likely to be responsible.

In clinical studies evaluating sinus node resetting, it has been conventionally assumed for simplicity that conduction into the sinus node (from stimulation site to pacemaker) is equal to conduction time out of the node (from pacemaker to stimulation site) and that the return cycle length of the pacemaker is not affected, resulting in the calculation of sinoatrial conduction time (SACT) as

$$\frac{(\text{A2-A3}) - (\text{A1-A1})}{2}$$

This measurement is taken during the plateau phase of Zone II when stimulation is performed as close to the node as feasible (Figure 2-16, vertical arrow). However, as explained above, these assumptions may not always be correct, and the accuracy of this measurement is limited by possible differences in conduction time of the premature impulse into and out of the node, changes in sinus node automaticity, and pacemaker shift.

The second return cycle. Figure 2-16, Panel B plots the second return cycle (A3-A4) against the premature coupling interval A1-A2. This relationship provides insight into changes in automaticity or pacemaker shift. Measured values (yellow circles) remain nearly constant for A1-A2 coupling intervals from 800–400 ms in this example, but increase slightly for coupling intervals less than 400 ms. An A3-A4 that is the same as A1-A1 indicates that automaticity of the sinus node is not suppressed, although it is possible that any suppression during A2-A3 quickly dissipates before the second return cycle.

Using the second return cycle to improve the SACT calculation. SACT can be overestimated when A3-A4 is greater than the A1-A1 because this suggests depression of automaticity. When this occurs, the SACT calculated from A2-A3 yields an overestimation, since depression of sinus node automaticity is not taken into account in this measurement. Comparing A2-A3 to A3-A4 as the basic sinus cycle length (and not A1-A1) might help remove the influence of pacemaker depression on SACT calculation. If A3-A4 is shorter than A1-A1 (and it is not caused by reentry), there is likely a shift in the pacemaker toward the atrial margin of the node causing a decrease in conduction time from node to atrium. Such a shift also might be detected by a change in the atrial electrogram or P wave, indicating a change in exit of the impulse from the node. Although there is also the possibility of acceleration of the pacemaker depolarization, based on laboratory data this seems to be unlikely.

Panel C (Zones III and IV): Interpolation and effective refractory period. In Figure 2-16, Panel C, the diagonal line represents complete interpolation of the premature impulse; at any point on this line, the sum of the intervals A1-A2 + A2 – A3 = A1-A1, which is 800 ms. Complete interpolation means that the premature impulse did not reach the pacemaker to depolarize it early (no reset), nor did it collide with the pacemaker impulse to prevent that impulse from depolarizing the atrium resulting in a compensatory pause as in Zone I (see explanation in Figure 1-10, Panel E). The A1-A2 interval at which complete interpolation is observed may define the effective refractory period of the most peripheral perinodal region. Block of the premature impulse in this region does not necessarily cause the sinus impulse to encounter refractory tissue on its exit from the sinus node if it arrives here after the perinodal region recovers (Figure 2-14, Panel E).

Zone III. In Figure 2-16, Panel C, the points that are above the diagonal line represent incomplete interpolation. A1-A2 + A2-A3 is slightly longer than the spontaneous CL (800 ms) indicating some influence of the premature stimulus on the sinus node pacemaker. A2-A3 is still significantly shorter than the spontaneous CL, so it is unlikely to result from an effect of the stimulated impulse (A2) directly on the sinus node pacemaker. Incomplete interpolation may be caused by partial penetration of the premature impulse through the perinodal region before it blocks without reaching the pacemaker site. Because of this penetration, there is delay of the reset sinus impulse, A3, exiting the sinus node in the partially refractory perinodal region. This is a form of concealed conduction of the prematurely stimulated impulse.

Zone IV sinus node reentry. Sinus node reentry (Figure 2-16, Panel C) is represented by points below the line of complete interpolation where A1-A2 + A2-A3 is less than A1-A1.The stimulated premature impulse propagates in a circuitous pathway within the node and returns to activate the atrium with a shorter CL than the spontaneous CL. The atrial activation sequence and P-wave morphology are often identical to sinus rhythm. Sinus node reentry is further described in Chapter 10.

Examples of Arrhythmias Caused by Alterations in Sinus Node Automaticity

Arrhythmias originating in the sinus node result from an increase (sinus tachycardia) or decrease (sinus bradycardia) in normal automatic impulse initiation. These changes in impulse initiation are based on the principles discussed in Figure 1-2 involving alterations in spontaneous diastolic depolarization (SDD), maximum diastolic potential (MDP), threshold potential (TP), and action potential duration (APD).

Unlike ectopic arrhythmias, where the responses to electrical stimulation and pharmacological agents are often helpful in determining electrophysiological mechanisms (described in Chapter 3), stimulation protocols and drugs are not necessary to identify automaticity as being a mechanism of most sinus arrhythmias. Diagnosing an abnormal rhythm from the ECG as originating in the sinus node implies an alteration in automaticity as being an underlying mechanism. An exception is supraventricular tachycardia caused by reentry in the sinus node. This arrhythmia is briefly described in Chapter 10. The response to stimulation and drugs can, however, identify abnormalities in sinus node pacemaker function.

SINUS TACHYCARDIA

Figure 2-17 shows a sinus tachycardia with a heart rate of 120 bpm. The P waves are positive in leads I, II, III, and aVF, and negative in aVR and aVL, consistent with an origin in the sinus node. Other ECG changes in Figure 2-17 include a right bundle branch block pattern, a rightward shift in the QRS axis (+90 degrees), S waves in leads I and aVL, and Q waves in lead III.

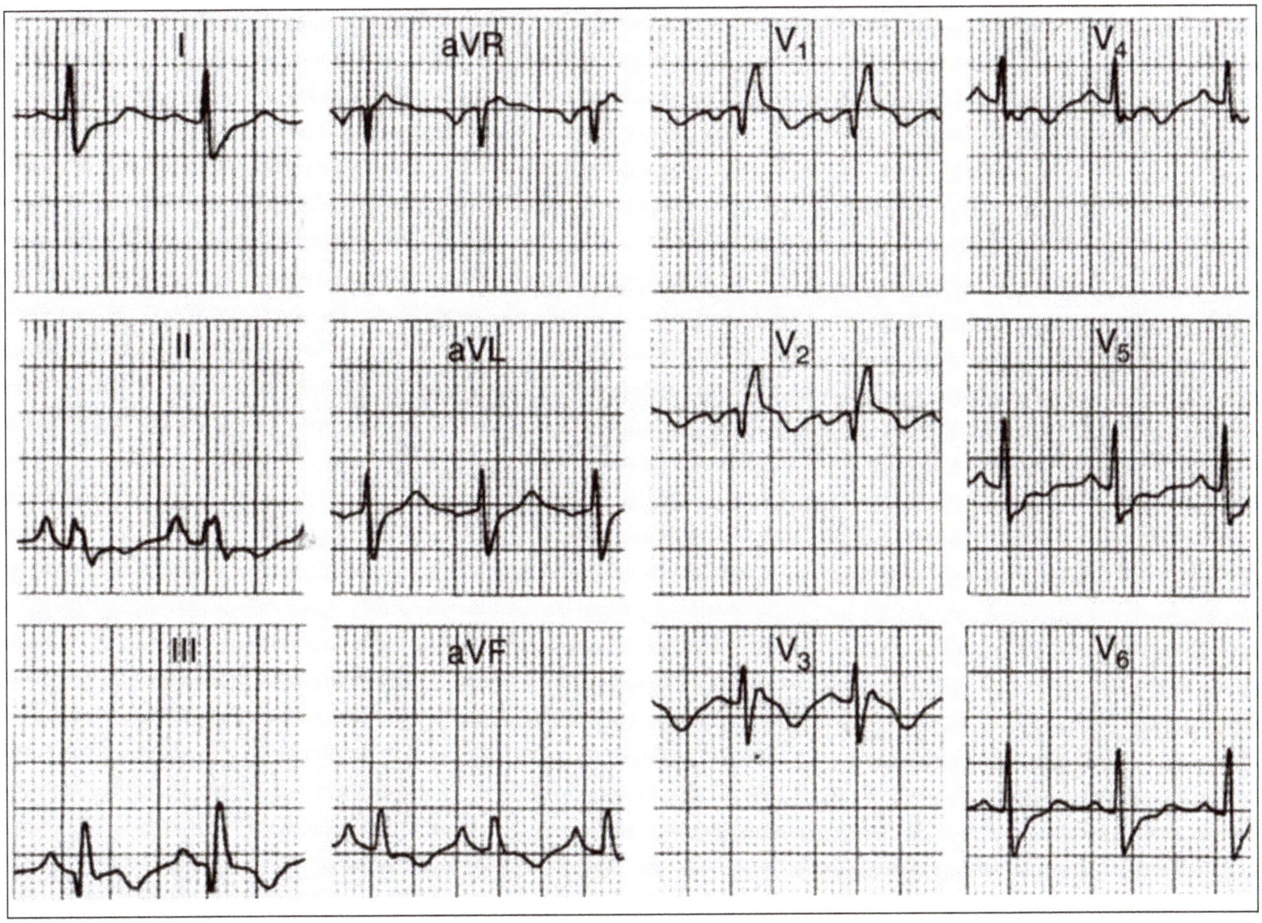

Figure 2-17 A 12-lead ECG from a 50-year-old male with sinus tachycardia. (Reproduced from Wellens HJJ, Conover M. *The ECG in Emergency Decision Making*. St. Louis, MO: Saunders Elsevier; 2006.)

Although sinus tachycardia is a normal response to exercise, the sinus tachycardia in this patient is in response to an acute pulmonary embolism, indicated by symptoms of dyspnea, pleuritic chest pain, and syncope. It is caused by enhanced sympathetic activity and reduced parasympathetic activity, which enhances SDD and reduces MDP (Figure 1-2) described in Chapter 1. This imbalance of the autonomic nervous system is mostly a reflex response to the acute hemodynamic changes. Systemic arterial hypoxia may also activate sympathetic reflexes. In addition, the release from platelets of humoral factors such as serotonin and other substances such as thrombin and vasoactive peptides affect the sinus rate by increasing SDD.

Sinus tachycardia occurs in a number of other clinical situations, either as a reaction to normal physiological stimuli such as fever, hypotension, anxiety, exertion, or pregnancy, or in response to pathological stimuli such as thyrotoxicosis, anemia, pulmonary emboli, myocardial ischemia, heart failure, and shock. It should be a reason for the physician to look for a cause. The general features of tachycardia are a rate of 100–180 bpm with regular P-P intervals, and normal-contour P waves that can sometimes become peaked. The common cause is enhanced sympathetic effects and/or reduced parasympathetic effects on the sinus node pacemakers. However, the inciting stimulus for the autonomic imbalance differs for the different situations. The common electrophysiological effect is enhanced sinus node pacemaker activity from an increased slope of the pacemaker potential (SDD) caused by enhanced sympathetic activity and decreased parasympathetic activity and possibly a decrease in the MDP resulting from vagal withdrawal, as explained in Figure 1-2.

A separate clinical syndrome, inappropriate sinus tachycardia (also called nonparoxysmal or permanent sinus tachycardia) has no obvious cause. This arrhythmia may manifest as a nonparoxysmal tachycardia arising in the sinus node, with a resting rate of 100 bpm or more in a supine or sitting position or an average rate of 90 bpm or more in a 24-hour ambulatory ECG. In some of these patients tachycardia may be due to abnormal autonomic function. In clinical studies sinus node response to catecholamines (beta stimulation with isoproterenol or low-grade exercise) may be enhanced while response to vagal stimulation may be depressed. There also may be enhanced intrinsic pacemaking in the sinus node in cases where a persistent elevation in the sinus rate is observed after (pharmacological) autonomic denervation with a β-blocker and atropine. Tachycardia independent of the ANS may result from changes in characteristics of membrane channels involved in automaticity (called remodeling) to increase the net inward pacemaker current (Figure 2-6). For example, in a familial form of inappropriate sinus tachycardia, a gain in function mutation in the pacemaker gene *HCN4* has been found.

SINUS BRADYCARDIA

The ECG in Figure 2-18 was taken from a 45-year-old male admitted to the coronary care unit with an acute inferior myocardial infarction. It shows sinus bradycardia (heart rate ~ 48 bpm), a prolonged PR interval (300 ms), ST elevation in leads II, III, and aVF, and ST depression in leads I, aVR, and aVL. The ST elevation and positive T wave in lead V_4R indicate a proximal occlusion of the right coronary artery.

Sinus bradycardia may occur in the patient with chest pain with an occlusion of the right coronary artery or a proximal branch of the circumflex, both which may supply the region of the sinus node. It is associated with enhanced vagal activity that decreases inward I_f and I_{NCX} and increases outward I_{KACh} (Figure 2-6), decreasing the slope of SDD and increasing MDP (Figure 1-2). Enhanced parasympathetic activity may be a neural reflex response to ischemia (Bezold-Jarisch reflex, coronary chemoreflex). Ischemia may also stimulate the large number of vagal ganglia that populate the sinus node. Ischemia of the sinus node cells may also slow impulse initiation by increasing an outward K^+ current that is activated by a decrease in intracellular ATP (I_{KATP}).

Sick Sinus Syndrome

The ECG in **Figure 2-19** is from a patient with sick sinus syndrome, a condition associated with abnormalities in both sinus node automaticity and conduction. The rhythm is of sinus origin with normal appearing P waves and a PR interval of 180 ms. Sinus bradycardia is evident with a heart rate of 38–42 bpm. Slow sinus rate can be explained by the basic mechanisms that cause decreased automaticity described in Figure 1-2.

In addition to sinus bradycardia, long, intermittent sinus pauses can occur, as shown in the ECG in **Figure 2-20** taken from another patient with sick sinus syndrome. Lead II at the bottom shows a period of sinus rhythm at a rate of 75 bpm After the fifth sinus beat, there is a sudden pause of 2200 ms indicated by the horizontal bar, terminated by an escape impulse caused by normal automaticity in the AV junction (normal QRS not preceded by a P wave; see Chapter 3).

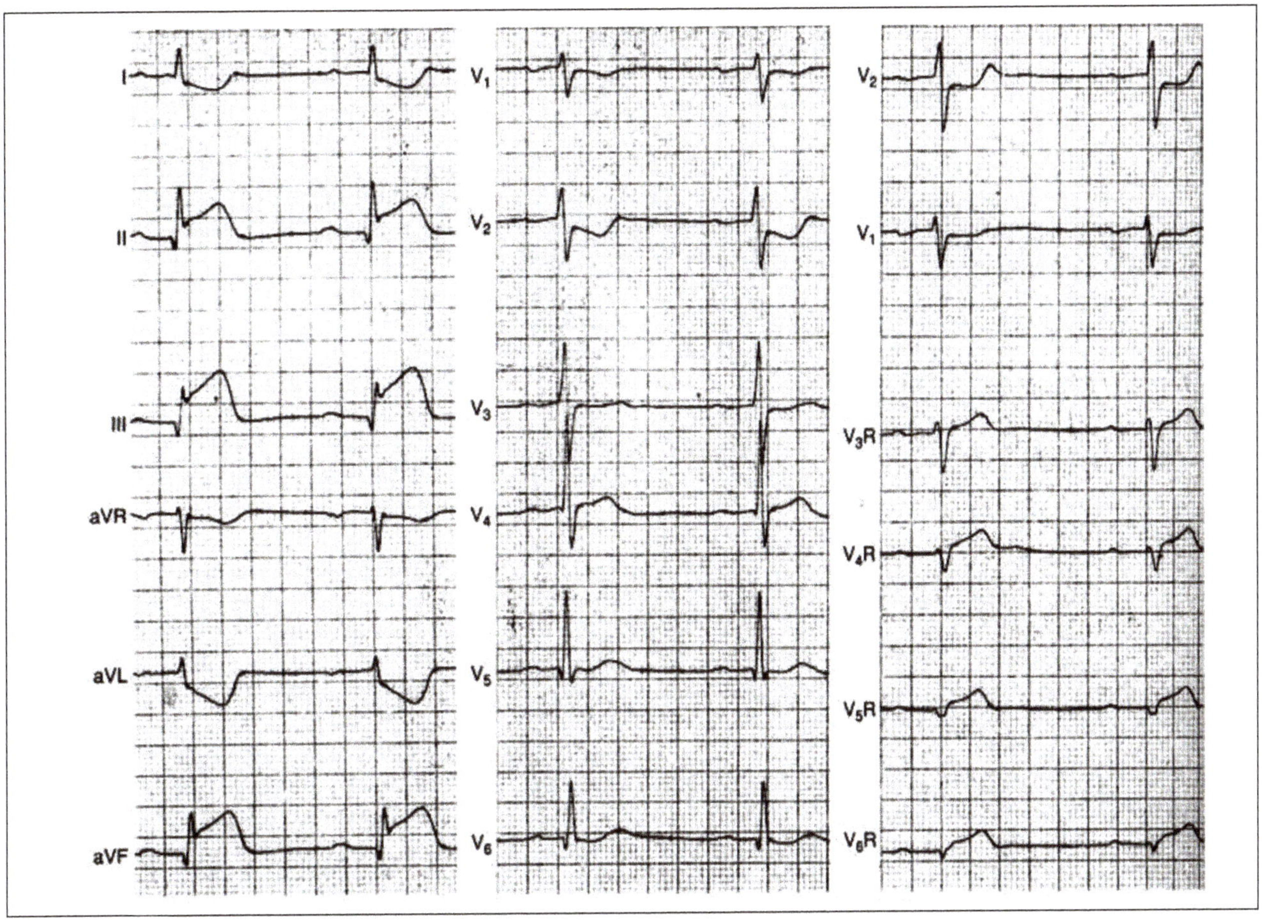

Figure 2-18 A 12-lead ECG from a 45-year-old male with an acute inferior myocardial infarction. (Reproduced from Wellens HJJ, Conover M. *The ECG in Emergency Decision Making.* St. Louis, MO: Saunders Elsevier; 2006.)

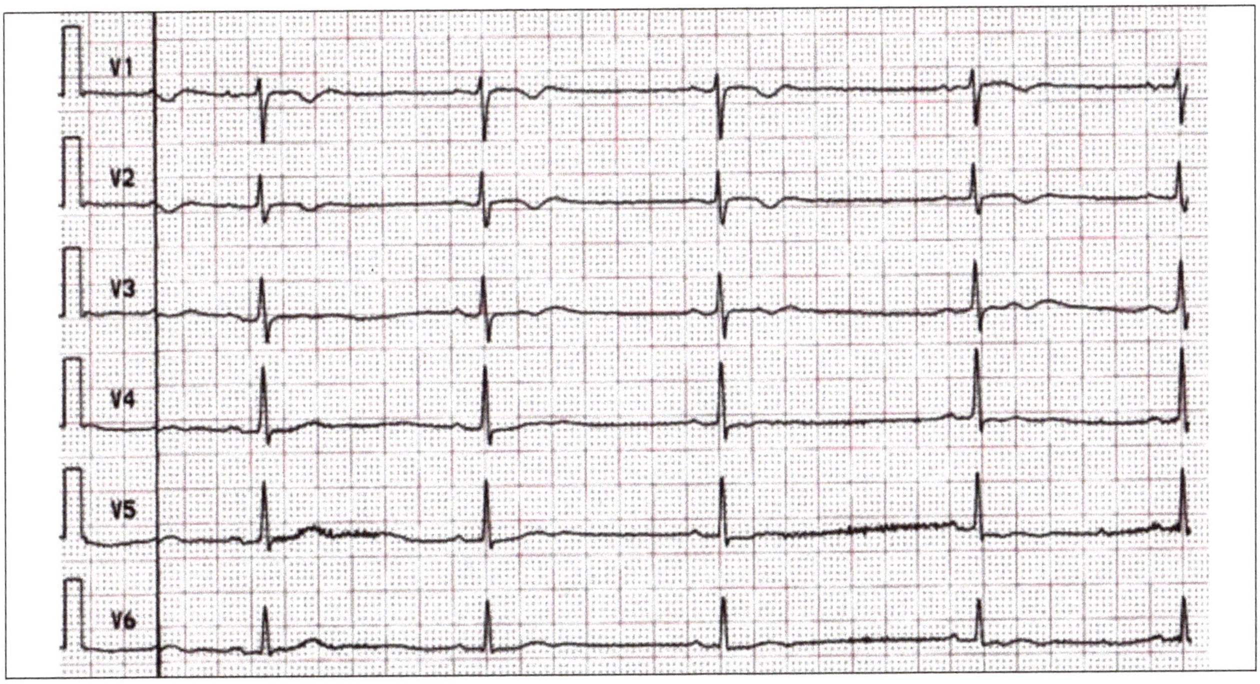

Figure 2-19 ECG leads V_1–V_6 showing sinus bradycardia associated with sick sinus syndrome.

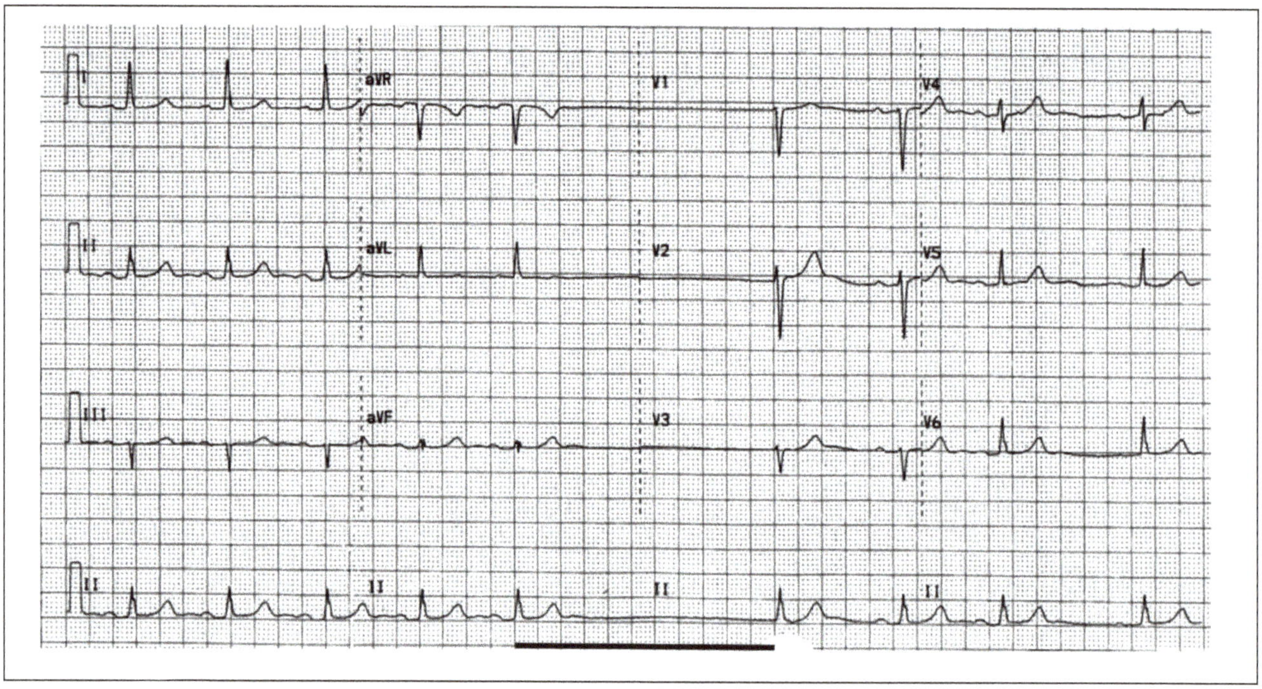

Figure 2-20 A 12-lead ECG from a patient with sick sinus syndrome.

The escape interval is longer than would normally be expected from overdrive suppression of a junctional pacemaker during sinus rhythm, indicating that sick sinus syndrome may be associated with enhanced overdrive suppression of latent pacemakers.

In some patients with sick sinus syndrome, periods of bradycardia may also alternate with periods of tachyarrhythmias (sinus bradycardia–tachycardia syndrome), the tachycardia usually being paroxysmal atrial fibrillation.

Changes Due to Aging

Sick sinus syndrome is usually associated with pathological changes in the sinus node characterized by fibrosis, sinus node degeneration leading to a loss of pacemaker cells, and changes in ion channel function. Some (but not all) of these changes may be associated with the normal aging changes in nodal structure and function. The pathological changes cause a decrease in sinus node automaticity and slowing of conduction in the node and perinodal region with conduction block of sinus impulses to the atrium (sinoatrial conduction block). It is difficult to distinguish between decreased automaticity and sinoatrial conduction block on the 12-lead ECG without simultaneous direct recordings from the sinus node. Persistent and regular sinus bradycardia shown in Figure 2-19 is likely a result of decreased automaticity. Sudden pauses shown in Figure 2-20 are thought to result from sinoatrial conduction block, since sudden failure of pacemaker activity is considered unlikely.

Changes in Ion Channel Function

Sick sinus syndrome arrhythmias may be a consequence of abnormal autonomic nervous system control, alterations in ion channel function of nodal or perinodal cells, or a combination of the two. A slower-than-normal intrinsic sinus rate in some patients after combined sympathetic and parasympathetic pharmacological blockade indicates alterations in properties of pacemaker membrane channels. Reduction of intrinsic pacemaker activity may result from decreased inward currents I_f or I_{NCX} or increases of outward K^+ currents, contributing to the pacemaker potential caused by changes in the properties of the ion channels referred to as "ion channel remodeling" (Figure 2-6). For example, a genetic basis of some familial sinus bradycardias is due to loss of function of I_f due to mutations in *HCN4* channels and/or its critical subunit protein, MiRP1. Interestingly these patients can also have AV block and atrial fibrillation. Reduction in the density of pacemaker cells coupled to peripheral transitional cells caused by disease in concert with the reduction caused by aging may slow the rate of remaining pacemaker cells. When there is a reduced number of pacemaker cells, the density of current flow to each surviving pacemaker cell from surrounding nonpacemaker cells might be increased, inhibiting pacemaker activity, if the source of the current flow (the density of nonpacemaker cells) is relatively unchanged (Figure 1-3). A decreased density of pacemaker cells may also result in insufficient current generated during their automatic firing to depolarize surrounding cells that is necessary for propagation of the impulse away from the pacemaker site, resulting in failure of conduction (block). Conduction disturbances between the sinus node pacemaker and atrial myocardium might also be caused by a reduction of gap junction coupling reducing current flow between myocytes, owing to the infiltration of fibrous tissue or other degenerative changes or by a reduction in Cx43 gap junctions as a consequence of both disease and aging. (The role of gap junctions in conduction and failure of conduction is described in detail in Chapter 9). I_{Na} in perinodal cells might also be decreased because of changes in ion channel function (remodeling), decreasing action potential amplitude and prolonging refractoriness. Alterations in Na^+ channel function in perinodal cells possibly related to gene mutations may contribute to genetically linked sick sinus syndrome. When sinus bradycardia is interspersed among periods of tachyarrhythmias, the tachycardia may also lead to pacemaker ion channel remodeling. Rapid heart rates have been shown experimentally to cause changes in proteins that form ion channels, changing the properties of these channels.

ANS Abnormalities in Sick Sinus Syndrome

Abnormalities in ANS function may sometimes contribute to the arrhythmias of sick sinus syndrome. In some patients, there may be a blunted response to exercise or isoproterenol, indicating a diminished sympathetic influence on the sinus node pacemaker. This might be caused by a decrease in the density of nerve endings, reduction in quantity of β_1 receptors, or by signal transduction abnormalities between the receptors and ion channels.

The response to parasympathetic blockade is more complex. In some patients with sick sinus syndrome, atropine administration fails to accelerate the heart rate or the acceleration is diminished. This is suggestive of decreased parasympathetic as well as sympathetic control. On the other hand, speeding of sinus rate to within the normal range after parasympathetic block, which also can occur in some patients with sick sinus syndrome, indicates that much of the sinus node dysfunction is caused by hyperactive parasympathetics. In addition to causing decreased automaticity, enhanced parasympathetic effects can cause conduction block by decreasing sinus or perinodal action potential phase 0 (decreasing I_{CaL}) and also prolonging time-dependent refractoriness (Figure 2-7) despite shortening action potential duration. Decreased sympathetic influence might have a similar effect.

Effect Electrical Stimulation on Sinus Node Automaticity and Conduction in Sick Sinus Syndrome

Prolonged sinus node recovery time (SRT). Enhanced overdrive suppression of the spontaneous rhythm is characteristic of sinus node dysfunction in sick sinus syndrome and results in abnormal SRTs. Abnormal SRTs are indicated by the shaded area to the left of the line in Figure 2-13, indicating the extent of prolonged SRT at the different spontaneous sinus cycle lengths. Corrected sinus node recovery times (CSRTs) are similarly prolonged. These abnormalities, as well as prolonged SACTs determined by premature stimulation, usually occur in symptomatic patients with sinus bradycardia, sinoatrial exit block, or tachycardia–bradycardia syndrome.

Figure 2-21 shows an example of the exaggerated overdrive sinus node suppression (prolonged SRT) in a patient with sick sinus syndrome.

The first segment of the ECG at the left in each panel is the end of a 1-min period of overdrive at the cycle lengths (CLs) indicated (overdrive stops at the arrows). The sinus CLs following overdrive are indicated by numbers below the recordings. The overdrive CL is progressively decreased from top to bottom records (700 to 320 ms). Overdrive suppression increases from 1400 to 4995 sec at the shortest overdrive CL (bottom record), which is several times longer than the normal SRT (compare to Figure 2-11 and Figure 2-12, where SRT is about 1100 ms). Overdrive suppression of the sick sinus node is also more sensitive to the duration of overdrive than the normal sinus node. With sinus node dysfunction, conduction block of overdrive impulses into the sinus node is likely to occur at longer CLs than in normal subjects, and when it occurs, it leads to a short recovery time (not shown in Figure 2-21).

Enhanced over drive suppression has important clinical implications. When sinus rhythm is interrupted by an atrial tachyarrhythmia in a patient with tachycardia-bradycardia syndrome, cessation of the tachyarrhythmia can be followed by an abnormally long pause of several seconds or more leading to syncope.

Enhanced overdrive suppression of sinus node automaticity and depressed conduction may be caused by abnormal autonomic influences on the node (see above) or by changes in ion channel or Na^+–K^+ pump function caused by ion channel remodeling. Enhanced pump activity and the outward current that it generates in the face of weaker net inward pacemaker current is one possible mechanism.

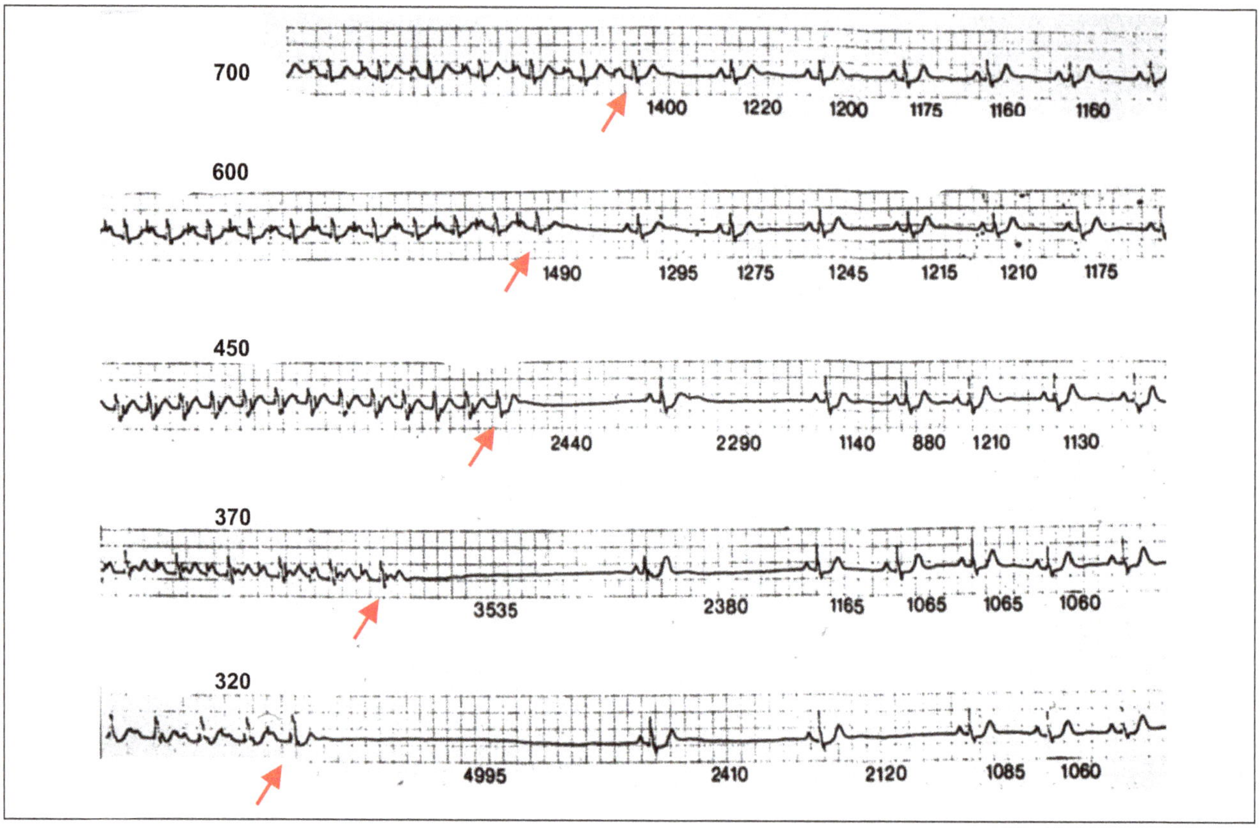

Figure 2-21 ECGs from a patient with sick sinus syndrome recorded during overdrive stimulation. The overdrive stimulation lasted for 1 minute (CL at far left, above). Overdrive stopped at the **arrows**. Numbers below each record indicate post-overdrive CLs in ms (Wellens' ECG collection).

Sinoatrial Conduction Time (SACT) in Sinus Node Disease

As explained in Figure 2-10, increased conduction delay of stimulated impulses into and out of the node with increasing overdrive rate increases the measured SRT. Abnormally prolonged SACT is implied by a Zone I response over a larger range of coupling intervals (compensatory pause, Figure 2-16) during premature stimulation or even failure to reset the sinus node (no Zone II), which occurs in the most severe cases.

An example of such failure to reset the sinus node is shown in **Figure 2-22**, where all the RCLs over a wide range of premature (test) coupling intervals fall along the diagonal line of compensatory pause.

This is most likely the result of prolonged perinodal refractoriness, which prevents premature impulses from penetrating and resetting the sinus node pacemaker.

Additional Sinus Node Bradycardias

A sinus rate <60 bpm is somewhat arbitrarily classified as sinus bradycardia and occurs in a number of other situations where the P waves have a normal contour, sometimes accompanied by irregular sinus cycle length (sinus arrhythmia). Sinus bradycardia can be a normal physiological response to (1) athletic training, (2) underwater diving, (3) vomiting, or (4) sleep, or can result from pathological stimuli such as (5) inferior myocardial infarction, (6) increased intracranial pressure, or (7) hypoxia. This list is not all-inclusive. It can also be a response to drugs such as digitalis or L-type calcium channel blockers such as verapamil, adenosine, and ivabradine. In some instances, it results from enhanced parasympathetic nerve activity and decreased sympathetic nerve activity (1–6 above) caused by different stimuli: for example, baroreceptors (hypertensive carotid sinus syndrome) or the central nervous system (increased intracranial pressure), etc. The electrophysiological effects on sinus node pacemakers that result in slowing of the intrinsic rate are a decreased slope of spontaneous diastolic (phase 4) depolarization and an increased maximum diastolic potential (described in Figure 1-2). Drugs that cause bradycardia do so through a number of different mechanisms, including changes in autonomic nervous system function (digitalis increases vagal activity) and direct effects on ion channels (verapamil decreases I_{CaL}, ivabradine decreases I_f). In any of these situations, factors that slow pacemaker activity may also cause sinoatrial conduction block, contributing to the sinus bradycardia.

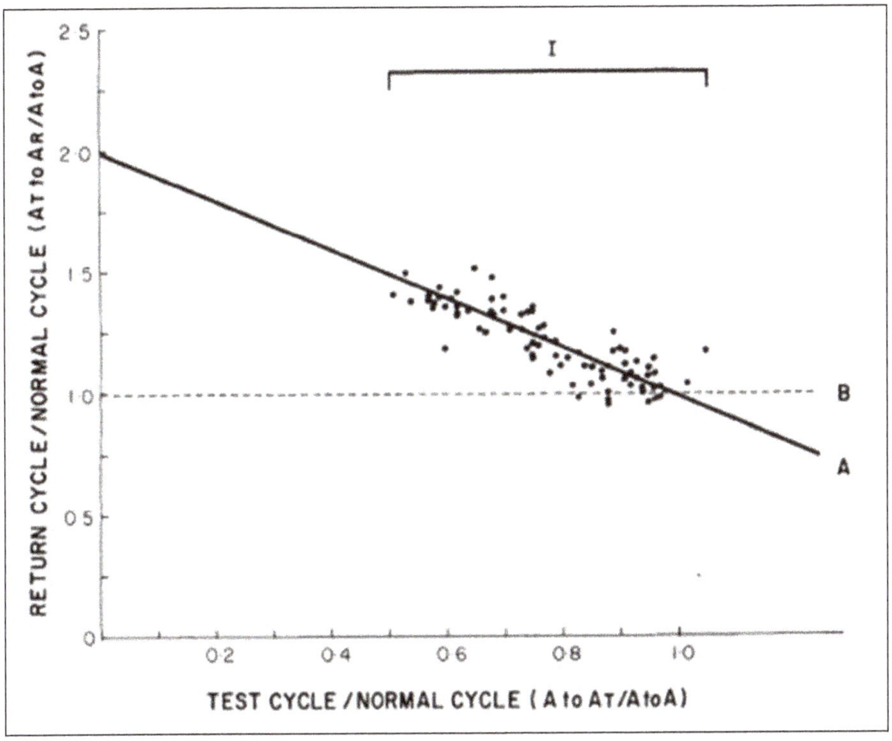

Figure 2-22 The return cycle plotted as a function of the test cycle for a patient with sick sinus syndrome. The ordinate is the normalized return cycle (**A to A** is the spontaneous CL) and the abscissa is the normalized premature (test) cycle. The **diagonal line** is the line delineating a compensatory pause. The **dashed line** (**B**) is the spontaneous CL. (Reproduced from Strauss HC, Saroff AL, et al. Premature atrial stimulation as a key to the understanding of sinoatrial conduction in man: Presentation of data and critical review of the literature. *Circulation.* 1973;47:86–93.)

SUMMARY

The sinus node is a heterogeneous structure with pacemaker cells at its center and latent pacemaker cells around its periphery. The pacemaker cells have special action potentials designed for automatic impulse initiation with spontaneous diastolic depolarization (SDD). SDD is the result of inward (I_f, I_{CaL}, I_{CaT}, I_{NCX}) and outward (I_K, I_{K1}, I_P) membrane currents, but the net current is inward. Phase 0 of the pacemaker cells is the result of I_{CaL}, unlike working myocardial cells with phase 0 caused by I_{Na}. Myocardium at the periphery of the node has transitional properties between nodal pacemaker and atrial cells and forms a perinodal zone.

Several factors control the rate of automaticity of sinus node pacemakers. Activity of the sympathetic nervous system increases automaticity by increasing the inward currents that increase the slope of SDD. Activity of the parasympathetic nervous system decrease inward currents and increase outward currents to decrease SDD and increase the negativity of the maximum diastolic potential (MDP).

A second important factor controlling rate of automaticity is gap junctions. Although electrotonic current flow between cells at the periphery of the node with more negative membrane potentials tend to suppress SDD of central pacemaker cells, a paucity of gap junctions and low-conductance gap junctions keeps this suppression at a minimum so as not to hinder normal sinus node pacemaker activity.

Arrhythmias caused by sinus node normal automaticity can be identified on the 12-lead ECG; impulse origin in the sinus node at abnormal rates, either too fast (>100 bpm, sinus tachycardia) or too slow (<60 bpm, sinus bradycardia). The response of sinus node pacemakers to programmed stimulation provides the foundation for identifying automaticity at ectopic sites. Overdrive stimulation (pacing) causes overdrive suppression of sinus node pacemakers. Programmed premature stimulation results in resetting of sinus node pacemakers, typical of normal automaticity. In the description of the response to stimulation, the influence of conduction delays of stimulated impulses into the node to reach the pacemaker and pacemaker impulses back out of the node influences the measurements that are usually made in the atrium and may not give a true picture of the effects of stimulation on the sinus node pacemaker cells. The responses to premature stimulation can be used to measure conduction time into and out of the node (sinoatrial conduction time, SACT).

SOURCES

Basic Electrophysiology

Biel M, Wahl-Schott C, Michalakis S, Zong X. Hyperpolarization-activated cation channels: From genes to function. *Physiol Rev.* 2009;89:847–885.

Boineau JP, Canavan TE, Schuessler RB, et al. Demonstration of a widely distributed atrial pacemaker complex in the human heart. *Circulation.* 1988;77:1221–1237.

Boineau JP, Schuessler RB, Hackel DB, et al. Widespread distribution and rate differentiation of the atrial pacemaker complex. *Am J Physiol Heart Circ Physiol.* 1980; 239(8):H406–H415.

Boineau JP, Schuessler RB, Roeske WR, et al. Quantitative relation between sites of atrial impulse origin and cycle length. *Am J Physiol Heart Circ Physiol.*1983;245(14): H781–H789.

Boyett MR, Honjob H, Kodama I. The sinoatrial node, a heterogeneous pacemaker structure. *Cardiovas Res.* 2000;47:658–687.

Boyett MR, Honjob H, Kodama I. The sinoatrial node, a heterogeneous pacemaker structure. *Cardiovas Res.* 2000;47:658–687.

Chandler NJ, Greener ID, Tellez JO, et al. Molecular architecture of the human sinus node: Insights into the function of the cardiac pacemaker. *Circulation.* 2009;119:1562–1575.

Courtney KR, Sokolove PG. Importance of electrogenic sodium pump in normal and overdriven sinoatrial pacemaker. *J Molec Cell Cardiol.* 1979;11:787–794.

DiFrancesco D. The role of the funny current in pacemaker activity. *Circ Res.* 2010;106:434–446.

Dobrzynski H, Boyett MR, Anderson RH. New insights into pacemaker activity. Promoting understanding of sick sinus syndrome. *Circulation.* 2007;115:1921–1932.

Efimov, IR, Fedorov VV, Joung B, Lin S-F. Mapping cardiac pacemaker circuits. Methodological puzzles of the sinoatrial node optical mapping. *Circ Res.* 2010;106:255–271.

Fedorov VV, Schuessler RB, Hemphill, et al. Structural and functional evidence for discrete exit pathways that connect the canine sinoatrial node. *Circ Res.* 2009;104:915–923.

Hilgemann DW. New insights into the molecular and cellular workings of the cardiac Na^+/Ca^{2+} exchanger. *Am J Physiol Cell Physiol.* 2004;287:C1167–C1172.

James TN. Structure and function of the sinus node, AV node and His bundle of the human heart: Part I—Structure. *Prog Cardiovasc Dis.* 2002;45:235–267.

Jones SA, Boyett MR, Lancaster. Declining into failure. The age-dependent Loss of the L-type Calcium channel within the sinoatrial node. *Circulation.* 2007;115:1183–1190.

Kerr CR, Strauss HC. The nature of atriosinus conduction during rapid atrial pacing in the rabbit heart. *Circulation.* 1981;63:1149–1157.

Lakatta E. A paradigm shift for the heart's pacemaker. *Heart Rhythm.* 2010;7:559–564.

Lakatta EG, DiFrancesco D. What keeps us ticking: a funny current, a calcium clock, or both? *J Molec Cell Cardiol.* 2009;47:57–170.

Lakatta EG, Maltsev VA, Vinogradova TM. A coupled system of Intracellular Ca^{2+} clocks and surface membrane voltage clocks controls the timekeeping mechanism of the heart's pacemaker. *Circ Res.* 2010;106:659–673.

Lange G. Action of driving stimuli from Intrinsic and extrinsic Sources on in situ cardiac pacemaker tissues. *Circ Res.* 1965;17:449–459.

Lei M, Zhang H, Grace AA, et al. SCN5A and sinoatrial node pacemaker function. *Cardiovasc Res.* 2007;74:356–365.

Mangoni ME, Nargeot JL. Genesis and regulation of the heart automaticity. *Physiol Rev.* 2008;88:919–982.

Robinson RB. The long and short of calcium-dependent automaticity in the sinoatrial node. *Am J Physiol Heart Circ Physiol.* 2011;300:H31–H32.

Saki R, Hagiwara N, Matsuda N, et al. Sodium–potassium pump current in rabbit sino-atrial node. *J Physiol.* 1996;490:51–62.

Schuessler RB, Boineau JP, Bromberg BI. Origin of the sinus impulse. *J Cardiovasc Electrophysiol.* 1996;263–274.

Steinbeck G, Haberl R, Luderitz B. Effects of atrial pacing on atrio-sinus conduction and overdrive suppression in the isolated rabbit sinus node. *Circ Res.* 1980;46:859–869.

Strauss HC, Bigger JT Jr. Electrophysiological properties of the rabbit sinoatrial perinodal fibers. *Circ Res.* 1972;31:490–506.

Tellez JO, Dobrzynski H, Greener ID, et al. Differential expression of ion channel transcripts in atrial muscle and sinoatrial node in rabbit. *Circ Res.* 2006;99:1384–1393.

Truex RC, Smythe MQ, Taylor MJ. Reconstruction of the human sinoatrial node. *Anat Rec.* 1967;759:371–378.

Watanabe EI, Honjo H, Boyett MR, et al. Inactivation of the calcium current is involved in overdrive suppression of rabbit sinoatrial node cells. *Am J Physiol Heart Circ Physiol.* 1996;271(40): H2097–H2107.

Yeh Y-H, Burstein B, Qi Y, et al. Funny current downregulation and sinus node dysfunction associated with atrial tachyarrhythmia. A molecular basis for tachycardia-bradycardia syndrome. *Circulation.* 2009;119:1576–1585.

Clinical Electrophysiology

Asseman P, Berzin B, Desry D, et al. Persistent sinus nodal electrograms during abnormally prolonged postpacing atrial pauses in sick sinus syndrome in humans: sinoatrial block vs overdrive suppression. *Circulation.* 1983;68:33–41.

Brady PA, Low PA, Shen WK. Inappropriate sinus tachycardia, postural orthostatic tachycardia syndrome, and overlapping syndromes. *PACE.* 2005;28:1112–1121.

Gang ES, Reiffel JA, Livelli FD, Bigger JT Jr. Sinus node recovery times following the spontaneous termination of supraventricular tachycardia and following atrial overdrive pacing: A comparison. *Am Heart J.* 1983:105;210–215.

Goldstein RE, Beiser GD, Stampfer M, Epstein SE. Impairment of autonomically mediated heart rate control in patients with cardiac dysfunction. *Circ Res.* 1975;36:571–578.

Jordan J, Yamaguchi I, Mandel WJ. Comparative effects of overdrive on sinus and subsidiary pacemaker function. *Am Heart J.* 1977;93:367–374.

Josephson ME. *Josephson's Clinical Cardiac Electrophysiology: Techniques and Interpretations* (5th ed.). Philadelphia, PA: Wolters Kluwer; 2016.

Morillo CA, Klein GJ, Thakur RK, et al. Mechanism of 'inappropriate' sinus tachycardia:Role of sympathovagal balance. *Circulation.* 1994;90:873–877.

Scheinman MM, Kunkel FW, Peters RW, et al. Atrial pacing in patients with sinus node dysfunction. *Am J Med.* 1976;61:641–649.

Singer W, Shen W-K, Tonette L, et al. Evidence of an intrinsic sinus node abnormality in patients with postural tachycardia syndrome. *Mayo Clin Proc.* 2002;77:246–252.

Stilla A-M, Raatikainena P, Ylitalob A, et al. Prevalence, characteristics and natural course of inappropriate sinus tachycardia. *Europace.* 2005;7:104–112.

Yusuf S, Camm AJ. Deciphering the sinus tachycardias. *Clin Cardiol.* 2005;28:267–276.

Wellens HJJ, Conover M. *The ECG in Emergency Decision Making.* St. Louis, MO: Saunders Elsevier. 2006.

Atrial, A-V Junctional, and Ventricular Normal Automaticity and Automatic Arrhythmias

CHAPTER 3

The previous chapter describes the basic electrophysiology of normal automaticity in the sinus node and how the basic mechanisms can be translated into the clinical electrophysiology of normal and abnormal sinus node function. The sinus node is a prototype for normal automaticity of ectopic pacemaker sites (outside the node) that cause arrhythmias with a normal automatic mechanism as described in this chapter.

SECTION 3A Atrial Normal Automaticity and Automatic Arrhythmias

Normal automaticity occurs at ectopic atrial sites to cause atrial arrhythmias. In this section, the mechanism of atrial automaticity and examples of automatic atrial arrhythmias are described.

Basic Electrophysiological Mechanisms

LOCATION OF ATRIAL PACEMAKERS WITH NORMAL AUTOMATICITY

Atrial cells with the properties of normal automaticity (atrial pacemakers) are distributed throughout the right and left atria, at locations indicated by the red numbers in **Figure 3-1**. Pacemaker cells in most of these regions have the *HCN4* gene for the I_f pacemaker current, which is a marker for normal automaticity.

The specific anatomic locations of the atrial pacemaker sites indicated in red numbers in Figure 3-1 are as follows: adjacent to the anatomical sinus node, some of which may be in the perinodal region (1), along the length of the crista terminalis (CT) (2), in the interatrial septum (3), at the junction of the inferior right atrium and inferior vena cava (IVC) (10), near or on the Eustachian ridge (a remnant of the Eustachian valve of the IVC) (4), at the orifice (os) of the coronary sinus (CS) (5), in the muscle around the mitral and tricuspid valve annulus and muscle that extends into both A-V valves (6 and 7), in atrial muscle in and around the pulmonary veins (PV) (8), in atrial muscle that extends into the vena cavae (9 and 10), and in atrial muscle in the ligament of Marshall, which runs adjacent to the great cardiac vein that empties into the CS (11). Figure 3-1 also shows sites of origin of focal atrial tachycardias (black circles) in a series of 196 cases. Focal origin means arising in a small, circumscribed region. Although the mechanism was not specifically identified for all tachycardias, many may have been caused by automaticity. This same figure will be referred to in the section entitled, Sites of Origin of Focal Atrial Tachycardias.

ELECTROPHYSIOLOGY OF NORMAL AUTOMATICITY IN THE ATRIA

Specific properties of atrial pacemaker action potentials and ionic currents are different from working atrial myocardial cells. Properties of the pacemaker potential or spontaneous diastolic depolarization (SDD) control the rate of impulse initiation, which can cause atrial tachycardias (Figure 1-2).

Transmembrane Action Potentials of Atrial Pacemaker Cells

Transmembrane potentials of typical working atrial muscle cells that comprise the majority of the atria (shown in Figure 2-4, red tracing) have a highly negative resting membrane potential of −80 to −90 mV attributed to the outward membrane current, I_{K1} without any SDD, a rapid phase (0) of depolarization caused by the inward membrane current I_{Na}, a transient outward current (I_{to}) causing initial repolarization, a short plateau caused mainly by the inward membrane current I_{CaL} (although the plateau phase may be absent in some cells), and rapid repolarization caused by outward K^+ membrane currents, I_K, and I_{Kur}.

Electrophysiological Foundations of Cardiac Arrhythmias: A Bridge Between Basic Mechanisms and Clinical Electrophysiology, Second Edition.
 Cardiotext Publishing, ISBN: 978-1-942909-42-2.

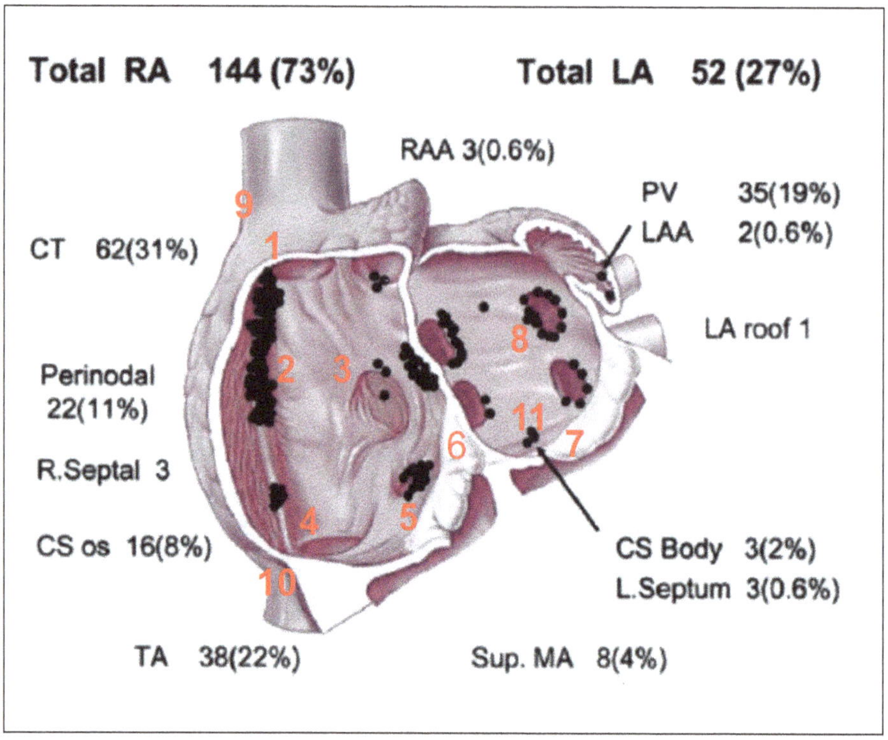

Figure 3-1 Sites of origin of focal tachycardias in 196 cases (number and percentage of total at each site) indicated by **black circles**. **Red numbers** are locations of sites with normal automaticity that we have added to the original figure. RA, right atrium; LA left atrium; CS, coronary sinus; CT, crista terminalis; LAA, left atrial appendage; MA, mitral annulus; PV, pulmonary veins; RAA, right atrial appendage; TA, tricuspid annulus. (Modified from Kistler PM, Roberts-Thomson KC, et al. P-wave morphology in focal atrial tachycardia. Development of an algorithm to predict the anatomic site of origin. *J Am Coll Cardiol.* 2006;48:1010–1017.)

The pacemaker cells with normal automaticity in the atria all have in common the property of spontaneous diastolic depolarization (SDD), although there are some different characteristics in the transmembrane action potentials of cells in different regions of the atria. **Figure 3-2** shows action potentials of a pacemaker cell in the crista terminalis (CT).

These cells have highly negative membrane potentials (~ −80 mV caused by I_{K1}), a rapid phase (0) of depolarization (caused by I_{Na}), an initial sharp phase 1 of repolarization (likely caused by I_{to}) and a plateau phase (caused by I_{CaL}) (Figure 3-2, Panel A). When CT cells develop automaticity such as after exposure to catecholamines (Figure 3-2, Panel B), the transmembrane potential exhibits SDD similar to sinus node pacemakers.

Figure 3-3, Panel A shows the action potentials characteristic of pacemakers at another location, the inferior right atrial-vena caval site. These cells, and those at the orifice of the CS, have somewhat less negative membrane potentials than CT cells (−75 to −70 mV) but still have an I_{Na}-dependent phase 0 and a prominent SDD (D1D2). The membrane currents causing SDD shown in Panel B are described later in this chapter.

Pacemaker action potentials from cells around the A-V valves and in the atrial muscle that extends into the tricuspid and mitral valves have even less negative resting potentials (between −70 and −60 mV caused by I_{K1}) and slower phase 0 depolarization, which is probably caused by both I_{Na} and I_{CaL}.

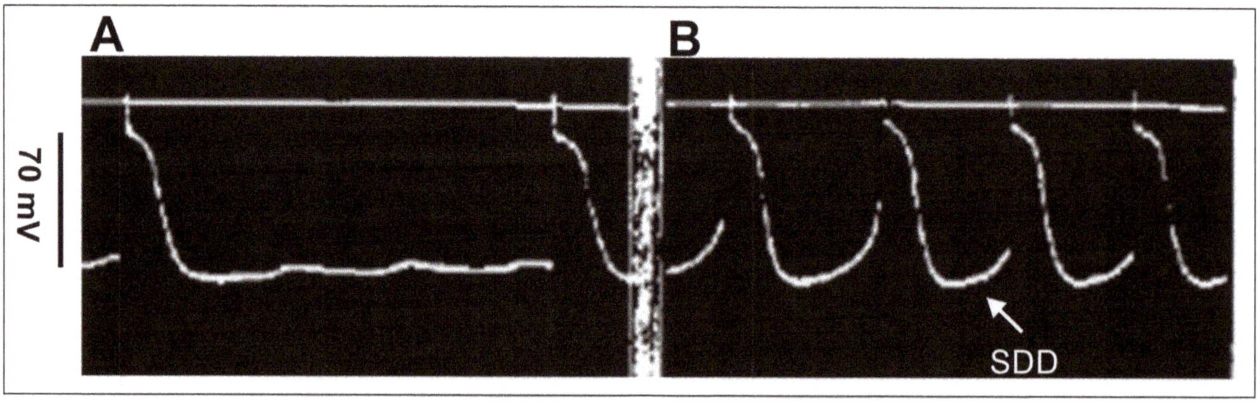

Figure 3-2 Action potentials recorded from a cell in the canine crista terminalis (CT) before (**Panel A**) and after exposure (**Panel B**) to catecholamines. (Reproduced from Hogan PM, Davis LD. Evidence for specialized fibers in the canine right atrium. *Circ Res.* 1968:23;387–396.)

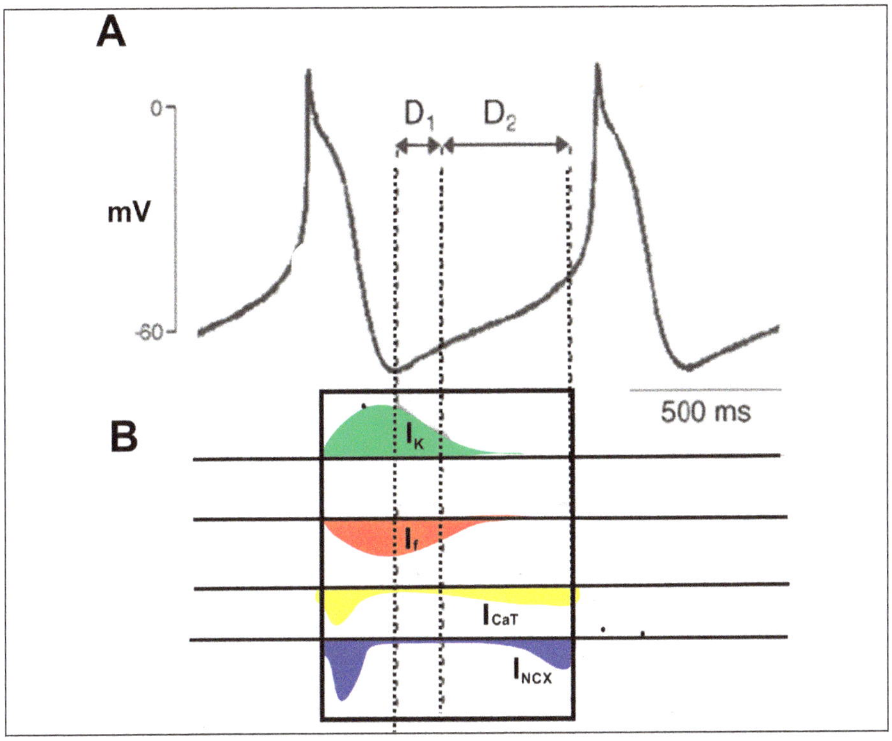

Figure 3-3 **Panel A:** Action potentials of pacemaker cell in feline inferior right atrium. **Panel B:** Membrane currents responsible for the pacemaker potential during the time period enclosed within the rectangle. **Upward shaded area** is outward current, **downward shaded area** is inward current. Magnitude of currents is not drawn to scale. (Modified from Lipsius SL, Huser J, et al. Intracellular Ca2+ release sparks atrial pacemaker activity. *News Physiol Sci.* 2001;16:101–106. Current traces in B have been redrawn. We assume responsibility for any inaccuracies in our drawing.)

The transmembrane potentials of pulmonary vein myocardium in the distal part of the veins, have SDD at a reduced membrane potential, which can be either a normal property of these cells (normal automaticity) or an abnormal property (abnormal automaticity, Chapter 4). Impulse initiation at these sites might also be caused by triggered activity (Chapter 5).

Membrane Currents Causing Automaticity in Atrial Pacemaker Cells

The membrane channels and currents causing normal automaticity in atrial cells have some similarities to those in the sinus node (Figure 2-6). Figure 3-3, Panel B shows a diagram of the currents contributing to the atrial pacemaker potential in pacemaker cells in the inferior right atrium. Diastolic depolarization consists of two phases: an early, rapid, and short-lasting depolarization and a later, slower, and longer-lasting depolarization (D_1 and D_2, respectively, in Figure 3-3, Panel A). The early, rapid depolarization (D_1) is the result of the inward I_f pacemaker current (downward red) and decay of the outward I_K current (the membrane current that causes repolarization; upward green). The I_f pacemaker current has characteristics similar to I_f in the sinus node, is activated upon repolarization, and decreases as membrane potential becomes less negative during the D_1 period of SDD. The longer-lasting, slower depolarization (D_2) is a result of the inward Na^+–Ca^{2+} exchanger current, I_{NCX} (downward blue). I_{NCX} is initially generated during phases 2 and 3 of repolarization, triggered by the release of Ca^{2+} from the sarcoplasmic reticulum (SR) by L-type calcium current (described as Ca^{2+}-induced SR Ca^{2+} release). Inward Ca^{2+} current through I_{CaT} channels (downward yellow) contributes to the terminal segment (D_2) of the pacemaker potential and triggers a secondary release of Ca^{2+} from the SR that generates I_{NCX} during SDD. More detailed descriptions of SR function, Ca^{2+}-induced Ca^{2+} release, and generation of I_{NCX} can be found in Chapter 5.

Some atrial pacemakers may even lack I_f and depend primarily on the Na^+–Ca^{2+} exchanger current for generation of SDD. The role of I_{CaL} (described for the sinus node in Figure 2-6) in pacemaking is uncertain and not shown in Figure 3-3. Whether this model applies to pacemaker cells in other regions of the atria that do not have the two well-defined components of diastolic depolarization, such as in the CT, is not known. Other currents not shown in Figure 3-3 that influence SDD are the Na^+-K^+ pump current (I_p) (Figure 2-6) and the K^+ current that sets the resting potential (I_{K1}), both of which can provide outward current during phase 4 depolarization.

Autonomic Nervous System (ANS) and Rate of Impulse Initiation

The ANS is the most important factor controlling the rate of automatic impulse initiation by ectopic atrial pacemakers that cause arrhythmias. The changes in the spontaneous rate of automatic impulse initiation depend on electrophysiological parameters described in Figure 1-2: the maximum diastolic potential (MDP), the threshold potential (TP), and the slope of the pacemaker potential (SDD).

The atria are innervated by both parasympathetic and sympathetic divisions. The density of nerve endings in different regions varies accounting for regional differences in magnitude of effects of the ANS. Activation of the sympathetics accelerates the firing rate mainly by increasing the slope of SDD (Figure 3-2). Sympathetic nerve activation increases inward I_f and I_{NCX}, which enhances SDD. An increase in I_{CaL} caused by sympathetic activation may sometimes be involved in the acceleration of rate, either by contributing to inward current during SDD or by increasing Ca^{2+} in the SR, which leads to an increase in I_{NCX}. These changes in membrane currents are due to the interactions of norepinephrine released from sympathetic nerve terminals with β_1-adrenergic receptors.

Conversely, parasympathetic activation slows the spontaneous rate of atrial pacemaker cells by decreasing SDD through a decrease in I_f and I_{NCX} (Figure 1-2, Panel A). Acetylcholine (ACh) decreases I_{CaL} and as a result, SR Ca^{2+} release, thereby decreasing I_{NCX}. ACh also increases outward K^+ currents I_{KAch}, and I_{K1}. This effect results in an increase in MDP, and decrease in SDD that also contributes to the slowing of pacemaker rate (Figure 1-2, Panel B). The effects of ACh are a result of its actions on muscarinic (M_2) receptors. When the effects of parasympathetic stimulation are sufficiently intense, pacemaker activity may stop but resumes when stimulation ceases.

ELECTRICAL STIMULATION OF ATRIAL PACEMAKERS

The response of atrial pacemakers to electrical stimulation conforms to the general effects described in Figure 1-6 and Figure 1-7.

Overdrive Stimulation

The effects of overdrive stimulation on normal automatic impulse initiation in the sinus node are described in Figure 2-9, Figure 2-11, and Figure 2-12. Similarly, in the atria there is a transient period of suppression after a period of overdrive stimulation. The duration of suppression is directly related to rate and duration of overdrive, and is typically followed by a gradual decrease (warm up) in automatic cycle length (CL) until the pre-overdrive rate is attained. Overdrive stimulation does not stop pacemaker activity. Overdrive suppression is attributed to increased intracellular Na^+ entering the cell during the action potential phase 0 (I_{Na}) and increased outward I_p generated by the Na^+-K^+ pump (Figure 1-6). Some of the overdrive suppression may also result from increased intracellular Ca^{2+} and release of ACh from vagal nerve endings that are activated by the electrical stimuli as described for the sinus node. Overdrive suppression may be greater in pacemaker cells with a strong I_{Na}-dependent phase 0 such as the CT pacemakers (Figure 3-2) than in cells with a weaker I_{Na} such as pacemakers in the A-V valves and around the valvular annuli. Less Na^+ enters the cells with a weaker I_{Na} during overdrive and there is less stimulation of the Na^+–K^+ pump.

Conduction delay into and out of ectopic atrial pacemaker sites should be taken into account when interpreting the overdrive suppression response, as described for the sinus node in Figure 2-10. The effects of overdrive on automatic atrial tachycardia are illustrated later in this chapter.

Programmed Premature Stimulation

The response of automatic pacemakers to premature stimulation is described in Figure 1-10 and Figure 1-11. Premature stimulation of atrial pacemakers is followed by compensatory pauses or resetting depending on their coupling intervals. Since atrial pacemakers may be surrounded by a region of slow conduction similar to the perinodal region of the sinus node, there may be similar influences of conduction into and out of the pacemaker site as described for the sinus node (Figure 2-14).

It is important to emphasize that premature stimulation does not start nor terminate pacemaker activity. This is an important property that distinguishes normal automaticity from delayed afterdepolarization (DAD)-triggered activity (Chapter 5) and reentry (Chapter 9).

RESPONSE OF AUTOMATICITY TO PHARMACOLOGICAL AGENTS

Certain pharmacological agents can sometimes be used to ascertain if normal automaticity is the cause of an atrial arrhythmia. Their effects on normal automaticity have been well documented in experimental studies and differ from their effects on other arrhythmogenic mechanisms.

Impulse initiation by atrial pacemakers is transiently accelerated by β_1 agonists and transiently slowed by parasympathomimetic agonists (see section above on ANS). The response to β_1 agonists does not distinguish automaticity from DAD-triggered activity (Section II, Chapter 5) that is also transiently accelerated. However, a key point is that ACh or parasympathomimetic drugs slow or stop pacemaker activity, which then resumes when the effect declines. Other arrhythmogenic mechanisms described in subsequent sections (Chapters 5 and 6 and Chapter 11: Atrioventricular (A-V) Junctional Reentrant Arrhythmias) can be slowed and then stopped by parasympathomimetic effects. They do not recur until something happens that reinitiates the arrhythmogenic mechanism (e.g., a burst of sympathetic activity or a premature impulse arising from another location).

The response to adenosine can distinguish normal atrial automaticity from other mechanisms by transiently slowing impulse initiation. If automatic impulse initiation stops, it then resumes when adenosine levels decline. Adenosine can terminate triggered activity and some kinds of reentry that do not resume when adenosine levels decline. Adenosine acts on adenosine A_1 receptors in atrial pacemakers (as it does in sinus node pacemakers), which are coupled to ion channels by guanine nucleotide-binding inhibitory protein, G_i. This results in activation of the K^+ channel that is also activated by ACh, the cyclic AMP (cAMP)-independent ACh/adenosine-regulated potassium current, which is designated $I_{KAch,Ado}$. Adenosine increases this outward K^+ current which opposes the inward depolarizing current during the pacemaker potential and slows the rate of SDD (see Figure 3-3).

Some of the antiarrhythmic drugs that block the Na^+ current (I_{Na})—e.g., Vaughan Williams Class IA (quinidine and procainamide) and B (lidocaine)—can decrease atrial automaticity by decreasing I_f and shifting the threshold potential for activation of I_{Na} (which causes phase 0), to less negative levels. Other arrhythmogenic mechanisms are also depressed. Class IV L-type Ca^{2+} channel-blocking drugs (e.g., verapamil) have little effect on SDD in normally automatic atrial cells, because I_{CaL} plays only a small role in SDD. The lack of response may be helpful in differentiating normal automaticity from abnormal automaticity that is slowed or stopped by L-type Ca^{2+} channel-blocking drugs (Chapter 4).

In the future, a specific I_f channel-blocking drug might help in identifying normal automaticity. Ivabradine does block I_f to slow sinus node automaticity and has been tested clinically for this purpose. Its effects on other normally automatic pacemakers has not been completely documented. This drug may also act on other ion channels.

Examples of Arrhythmias Caused by Atrial Automaticity

Normal automaticity at ectopic sites in the atria can cause arrhythmias by two basic mechanisms; slow escape rhythms after suppression of the dominant sinus node pacemaker, and rapid tachycardias caused by acceleration of atrial impulse initiation.

AUTOMATIC ATRIAL ESCAPE RHYTHMS

Figure 3-4 shows an example of an atrial escape rhythm. At the top left, a sinus rhythm is present with an upright P wave. After slowing of the sinus rhythm, the cycle length prolongs and the P waves change. Toward the middle of the top recording, the P waves are now inverted at a longer cycle length representing the expression of an atrial pacemaker that appeared after sinus slowing. The PR interval shortened to 0.14 sec from the PR interval of 0.16 sec during sinus rhythm. Thereafter, P waves show changes during subsequent atrial impulses indicating further changes in the atrial pacemaker site. Occasionally, there is a sinus P wave with a shorter cycle length.

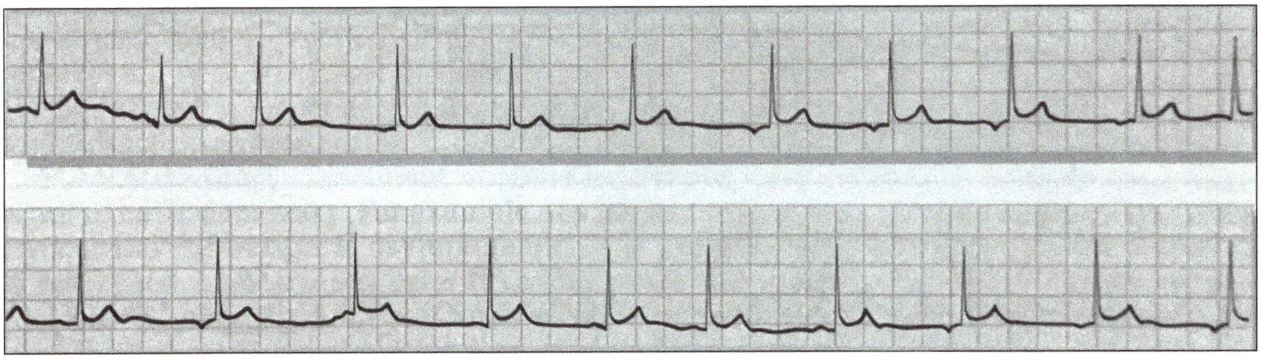

Figure 3-4 Atrial escape rhythm. (Reproduced from Libby P, Bonow RO, Mann DL, et al. *Braunwald's Heart Disease*. Philadelphia PA: Saunders Elsevier; 2008.)

Atrial escape rhythms such as the one shown in Figure 3-4, occur after slowing of the sinus rate or absence of sinus node activity. The change in P-wave morphology along with the decrease in PR interval is indicative of a shift of the pacemaker site to the inferior region of the right atrium (see Figure 3-7). Transient sinus slowing or arrest may have no clinical significance if latent pacemakers promptly escape to prevent ventricular asystole. Wandering atrial pacemakers can occur in the very young and also in athletes with slow sinus rates.

Atrial escape impulses are a relatively rare occurrence in humans despite the experimental studies that show atrial ectopic pacemakers to be second in the hierarchy of pacemakers, after the sinus node. In humans, A-V junctional pacemakers usually control the rhythm when there is failure of sinus node impulse initiation (described later in this chapter). Parenthetically, although we have designated this to be an example of normal atrial automaticity, there is no confirming proof that it is. Atrial escape rhythms might also be caused by abnormal automaticity (Chapter 4). That distinction can be made in case of overt atrial disease which is a cause of abnormal automaticity. The other arrhythmogenic mechanisms, afterdepolarizations and reentry, usually cause tachycardias and not slow escape rhythms.

AUTOMATIC ATRIAL TACHYCARDIA

Figure 3-5 shows an automatic atrial tachycardia which begins at the downward-pointed arrows with the change in P-wave morphology from the sinus P wave (upward-pointed arrow). The atrial tachycardia rate is 130 bpm. P waves are inverted in leads II and III (also in aVF, which is not shown), indicating that the atrial impulses are not arising in the sinus node but rather inferiorly in the right atrium (Figure 3-6, Figure 3-7, and Figure 3-8 describe the P-wave morphology based on site of impulse origin). Each P wave is followed by a normal QRS. The P-R interval is about 80 ms, which is slightly shorter than during sinus rhythm.

This ECG alone does not indicate the mechanism for the tachycardia. It is estimated that about half of all atrial tachycardias are caused by automaticity, the remainder by triggered activity (Chapter 6) or reentry (Chapter 10). Automatic atrial tachycardia may be paroxysmal (intermittent) or incessant (tachycardia occurring more than 50% of the time). Both intermittent and incessant tachycardia can occur in young patients without atrial disease, although each can also occur in patients with diseased atria. Incessant tachycardia can eventually cause cardiomyopathy resulting from structural remodeling caused by the persistent rapid rate.

Electrophysiological Characteristics of Automatic Atrial Tachycardia

Table 3-1 summarizes the characteristics of automatic atrial tachycardia. In this table, features that specifically identify the arrhythmia mechanism as normal automaticity are indicated by asterisks (*) and bold font. Features indicated by plus signs (+) may also be characteristic of tachycardias caused by other mechanisms. Each of the characteristics of automatic atrial tachycardia in Table 3-1 is described in detail after the table.

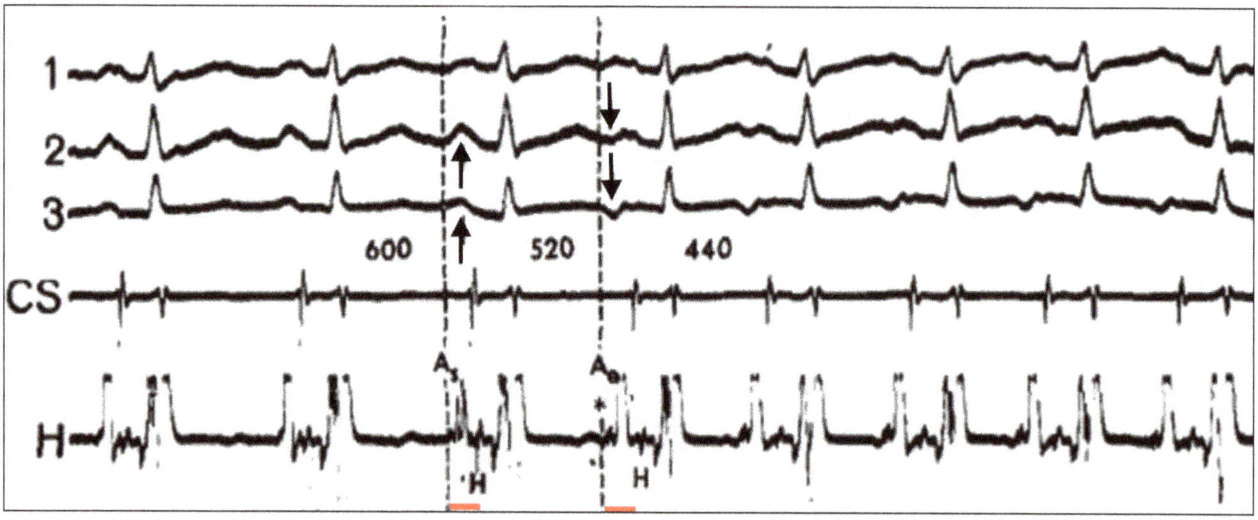

Figure 3-5 Automatic atrial tachycardia. Leads I, II, and III, and electrograms from the coronary sinus (CS) and His bundle region (H). **Upward arrow** indicates sinus impulse, onset of atrial tachycardia indicated by **downward arrow**. Numbers above CS recording are CLs, horizontal red bars below H electrogram indicate A-H interval (A-V nodal conduction time). (Reproduced from Goldreyer BN, Gallagher JJ, et al. The electrophysiologic demonstration of atrial ectopic tachycardia in man. *Am Heart J.* 1973;85:205–215.)

Table 3-1 Characteristics of Automatic Atrial Tachycardia

1. The first complex of tachycardia occurs late in the cardiac cycle. Unlike an escape rhythm, it is not necessarily related to a sinus pause or absence of sinus node activity (+).
2. Tachycardia onset is not associated with atrial or A-V nodal conduction delay. Onset is not related to a prolonged P-R interval (+).
3. Onset of tachycardia is often characterized by "warm up" (+). Spontaneous termination may be preceded by slowing of rate (+).
4. The P-R interval increases as atrial rate increases (cycle length decreases) (+).
5. Tachycardia has a focal origin with a P wave that differs from the sinus P wave and is characteristic of the site of origin (+).
6. Tachycardia may be initiated by sympathetic stimulation especially during exercise (+). The rate of tachycardia is accelerated by sympathetic stimulation (+).
7. **Parasympathetic nerve stimulation by vagal maneuvers may transiently slow tachycardia but does not terminate it. Ventricular rate may slow because of atrial slowing and transient A-V block (*).**
8. **Adenosine transiently slows atrial rate but does not terminate tachycardia. Ventricular rate may slow, both because of atrial slowing and transient A-V block (*).**
9. Tachycardia is not affected by an L-type Ca^{2+} channel-blocking drug (+).
10. **Tachycardia cannot be initiated by overdrive or premature stimulation (*).**
11. **Tachycardia usually exhibits overdrive suppression following overdrive stimulation but is not terminated (*).**
12. **Tachycardia can be reset by premature stimulation but not terminated (*).**
13. **Tachycardia is not terminated by cardioversion (*).**

(*) Features set in bold with an asterisk (*) specifically identify the arrhythmia mechanism as normal automaticity.

(+) Features indicated by plus signs (+) may also be characteristic of tachycardias caused by other mechanisms.

Onset Occurs Late in the Cardiac Cycle

The first complex of tachycardia occurs late in the cardiac cycle (Table 3-1, #1). This is a general characteristic of an automatic mechanism. The onset of automatic tachycardia shown in Figure 3-5 illustrates this point. The initial three complexes are sinus impulses with normal P waves (upward arrow), QRS complexes, and P-R intervals occurring at a CL of 600 ms. The fourth complex (downward arrow) is the beginning of atrial tachycardia. It has an altered P-wave morphology (inverted P wave in lead III, indicating an origin in the inferior right atrium) and occurs late; the CL between the last sinus P wave and the first P wave of tachycardia is 520 ms.

The long CL at onset reflects the period required for enhanced SDD of the ectopic pacemaker to reach threshold and initiate an impulse (Figure 1-2, Panel A). However, a long sinus cycle or sinus pause is not absolutely necessary, as it would be for an escape impulse, because SDD of the atrial pacemaker is accelerated, often by sympathetic stimulation, for example during exercise. Tachycardia is not initiated by a premature impulse early in the cycle, which is often a feature of tachycardia caused by triggered activity dependent on DADs (Chapter 5) or atrial or A-V nodal reentry (Chapter 10 and Chapter 11).

Absence of Prolonged P-R Interval or A-V Conduction Delay during Tachycardia Onset

Onset of tachycardia is not associated with atrial or A-V nodal conduction delay (Table 3-1, #2). These features, if present, would usually be indicative of reentry (Chapter 10), since the occurrence of reentry is dependent on altered conduction. In Figure 3-5 the onset of the atrial tachycardia is not associated with any change in the A-H interval on the His bundle electrogram (H), indicating that no change has occurred in the measured A-V nodal conduction time (length of horizontal red bar is the same for last sinus impulse and first tachycardia impulse). In contrast, the A-H interval is prolonged when supraventricular tachycardia is caused by A-V nodal reentry (Chapter 11).

Warm Up

In Figure 3-5, after the first long coupled atrial impulse at the CL of 520 ms, tachycardia continues because of enhanced automaticity in the atrial pacemaker that has a faster rate (CL 440 ms) than the sinus node pacemaker. Sinus node automaticity is then overdrive suppressed by the ectopic pacemaker.

The CL of the automatic tachycardia may sometimes progressively shorten for several cycles until its ultimate rate is achieved (warm up; Table 3-1, #3—not shown in Figure 3-5). Warm up is not specific for automatic tachycardia but can also occur with DAD-dependent triggered activity (Chapter 5) or reentrant tachycardias having tissue in the tachycardia circuit sensitive to sympathetic stimulation, such as A-V nodal tissue (Chapter 11). Warm up of an automatic tachycardia results from the combination of sympathetic enhancement of SDD (perhaps caused by a fall in blood pressure) and gradual removal of the effects of overdrive suppression also caused by sympathetic stimulation. Warm up may not be noticeable with faster tachycardias.

The rate of atrial pacemaker automaticity causing tachycardia at rest rarely exceeds 175 impulses/min and may be as slow as 100 impulses/min. The range of rates is faster than the intrinsic rate of atrial pacemakers and likely reflects the stimulating effects of changes in autonomic tone with an increased net sympathetic effect. Alterations in pacemaker channel properties that enhance net inward pacemaker current (remodeling) might also cause a more rapid rate.

Often, prior to termination of automatic tachycardia, the rate gradually slows. Gradual slowing can also occur with triggered activity and reentry.

P-R Interval Prolongs as Tachycardia Rate Increases

As the CL of tachycardia decreases, A-V nodal delay of atrial impulses conducting to the ventricles increases causing prolongation of the P-R interval (Table 3-1, #4). This characteristic is a result of normal, rate-dependent slowing of conduction in the A-V node. However, it is not specific for automaticity as the mechanism of atrial tachycardia, since triggered atrial tachycardias and focal atrial reentrant tachycardias may show the same relationship. With each of these mechanisms, atrial impulses conduct through the A-V node to the ventricles and the normal, rate-dependent slowing of conduction in the A-V node occurs.

Focal Origin with Abnormal P-Wave Morphology

An automatic atrial tachycardia has a focal origin with a P wave that is different than the sinus P wave and is characteristic of the site of origin (Table 3-1 #5). Impulse initiation occurs in a small circumscribed region of the atria known as a focus. These arrhythmias are called focal tachycardias. The focus is estimated to be about 2–4 mm^2 (exact measurements have not been made). Focal origin is not specific for automaticity but can occur with the other arrhythmogenic mechanisms, such as triggered activity and atrial reentry in a small circuit.

Sites of origin of focal atrial tachycardias. The sites of origin of focal atrial tachycardias in a clinical electrophysiological study including 196 cases are shown on a schema of the heart (Figure 3-1, dark black circles and black numbers) at the beginning of this section. 73% of tachycardias originated at right atrial sites, and 27% at left atrial sites. Since the complete electrophysiological characterization described in Table 3-1 needed to demonstrate automaticity was not done in this series, these data are not specific for automatic tachycardias. Nevertheless, since a large number of focal tachycardias are automatic, these sites likely reflect the origin of automatic tachycardias. Sites of origin also correlate for the most part with the locations of atrial cells with the property of normal automaticity (Figure 3-1, red numbers). The most frequent origin in this series is along the crista terminalis (CT, 31% of tachycardias, site 2). The next most frequent site is adjacent to the tricuspid annulus (TA, 22%, site 6), followed by tachycardias originating in perinodal pacemakers (11%, site 1).

Other sites of origin with decreasing frequency are orifices of the PVs in 19% of cases in this series (site 8); os of the coronary sinus (CS) near the apex of Koch's triangle (8%, site 5) or from the muscle extending deeper into the CS into the left atrium (2%, site 11); right and left atrial septa (3% and 0.6%, site 3), adjacent to the mitral annulus (MA) (4%, site 7); and the right and left atrial appendages (RAA and LAA, respectively; 0.6% each). Although not shown in this figure, tachycardias also may originate in the superior vena cava (site 9) and in atrial myocardium adjacent to the His bundle (parahisian).

P-wave morphology is characteristic of atrial site of origin. The P wave associated with automatic atrial tachycardia differs from the sinus P wave and is characteristic of the site of origin (Table 3-1, #5). The P waves of the initial and subsequent automatic tachycardia impulses are most frequently the same, indicating a single site (focus) of origin different from sinus rhythm (Table 3-1, #5). This characteristic may also occur with triggered activity caused by DADs (Chapters 5 and 6). It contrasts to most forms of reentrant supraventricular tachycardia in which initial and subsequent P waves are different since reentry is often initiated from a location that differs from the location where the reentrant circuit occurs (Chapter 10). Occasionally, automaticity may arise at multiple sites that compete with each other and show different P-wave characteristics.

High lateral right atrium. In general, as shown in **Figure 3-6**, atrial tachycardias arising in the high lateral right atrium (perinodal region, atrial appendage, or high CT) depolarize the right atrium before the left, in a superior to inferior direction (red star and arrow). There are positive P waves in leads I, II, III, V_1, and V_6 with a duration of ~100 ms, with the P wave being most positive in lead II. Because the site of origin is near the sinus node, the P wave is similar to the sinus P wave. Tachycardias originating in this region may sometimes be diagnosed as inappropriate sinus tachycardia owing to similarities in P-wave morphology to sinus P waves.

Inferior right and left atrium. Tachycardias arising in the inferior part of the atria (**Figure 3-7**) such as the inferior CT, CS, or near the TA or valve have negative P waves in leads II and III. This results from inferior-to-superior atrial activation (red star and arrow).

An additional clue to the site of origin is the P-wave duration. Tachycardias having their origin near the interatrial septum have narrow P waves (<100 ms) because of nearly simultaneous activation of right and left atria (Figure 3-7, left panel).

Superior aspect of the left atrium. Tachycardias arising in the superior aspect of the left atrium (**Figure 3-8,**

asterisk, left panel) are associated with P waves that are negative in lead I and positive in leads II and III. In case of left lateral wall location, the P wave is higher in lead III than lead II and has a width of 100 ms or more because of sequential activation of first the left and then the right atrium. A positive P wave in V_1 indicates a posterior site near the PVs.

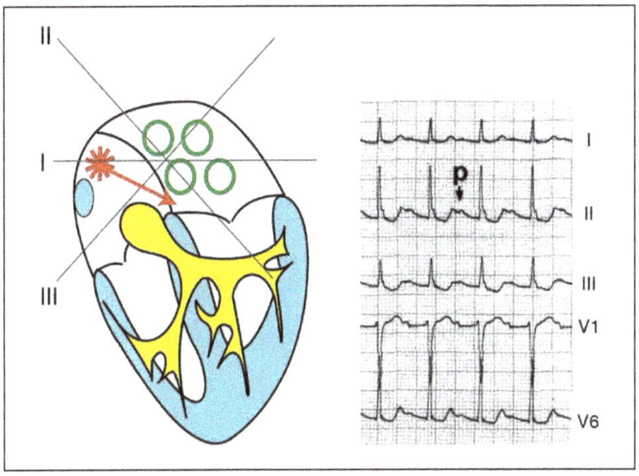

Figure 3-6 High lateral right atrial focus (**red asterisk at left**). **Arrow** shows direction of activation. Concomitant ECG at the **right** (Wellens' ECG collection).

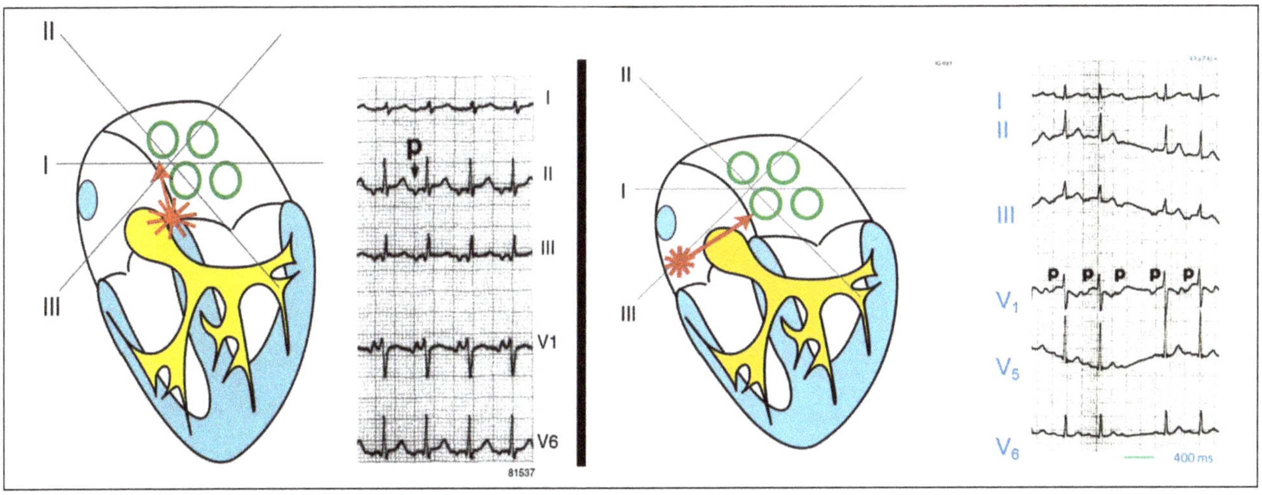

Figure 3-7 **Left:** Inferior atrial focus in or close to the interatrial septum (**asterisk**). **Right:** Inferior lateral focus (**asterisk**). The direction of activation is indicated by **arrows**. ECGs are at the **right** of each diagram (Wellens' ECG collection).

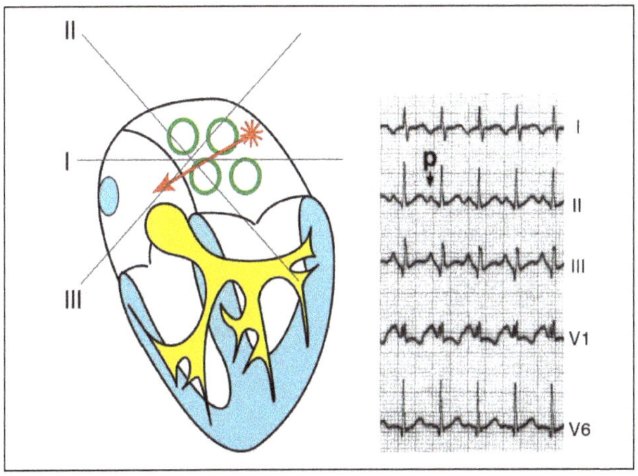

Figure 3-8 Left; superior lateral left atrial focus (**asterisk**) and direction of activation (**arrow**). ECG at the **right** (Wellens' ECG collection).

Effects of Sympathetic Stimulation

Automatic atrial tachycardia is often initiated by sympathetic stimulation (Table 3-1, #6). Initiation depends on sympathetic nerve activity to enhance SDD of the ectopic pacemaker (Figure 1-2, Panel A), and occurs during exercise or other causes of increased sympathetic activity. This explains why tachycardias can be initiated in the clinical laboratory by treadmill exercise or administration of isoproterenol.

The rate of automatic tachycardia is accelerated by sympathetic activity. **Figure 3-9** shows an automatic tachycardia accelerating from 150 bpm at rest (Panel A) to greater than 250 bpm with exercise (Panel B). In these patients, frequent occurrence of the arrhythmia may lead to a dilated cardiomyopathy.

The increase in rate is a result of increased slope of SDD of the pacemaker caused by a net increase in inward current. Initiation or acceleration of tachycardia by sympathetic stimulation, however, is not specific for normal automaticity. It can occur with other arrhythmogenic mechanisms, particularly triggered activity caused by DADs (Chapter 5).

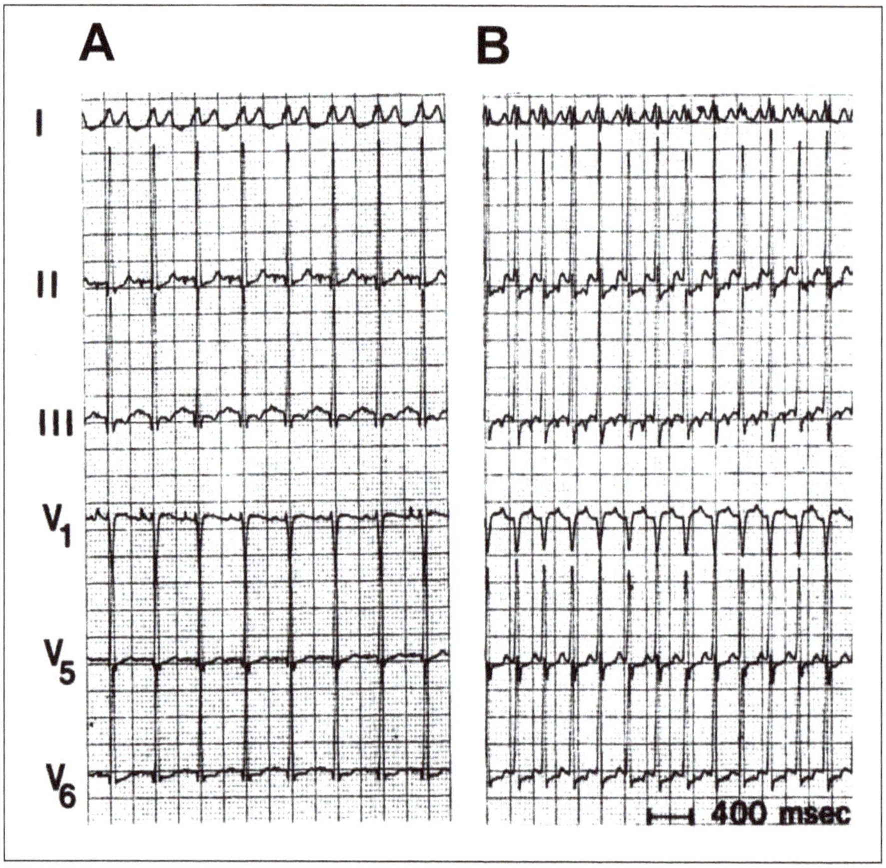

Figure 3-9 ECG showing incessant atrial tachycardia at rest (**Panel A**) and during exercise (**Panel B**).

Effects of Parasympathetic Stimulation

Transient slowing without termination by parasympathetic activation is a specific identifier of automatic atrial tachycardia (Table 3-1, #7) as shown in **Figure 3-10**. Vagal activation by carotid sinus massage (CSM) causes prolongation of the P-P interval and transient inhibition of the atrial pacemaker by decreasing SDD and increasing MDP (Figure 1-2, Panels A and B). It also causes A-V block due to vagal effects on A-V nodal conduction. However, the atrial tachycardia is not terminated. It continues after massage is stopped at the right of the figure. The slowing of atrial rate is independent of the effects of vagal activation to slow or block conduction in the A-V node. Slowing of conduction in the A-V node is the cause of slowing and stopping supraventricular tachycardias caused by A-V nodal reentry (Chapter 11). Triggered atrial tachycardias caused by DADs are also slowed and terminated by vagal stimulation (Chapter 5).

Adenosine

Administration of adenosine (Table 3-1, #8) transiently slows the rate of automatic atrial tachycardia but does not terminate it, as shown in **Figure 3-11**. Adenosine (12 mg) was administered just prior to the beginning of the recording. In addition to slowing the atrial rate, as seen in the electrogram recorded from the high right atrium (HRA, arrows), A-V block also occurred, as is evident in lead V_1 and the His bundle electrogram (HBE).

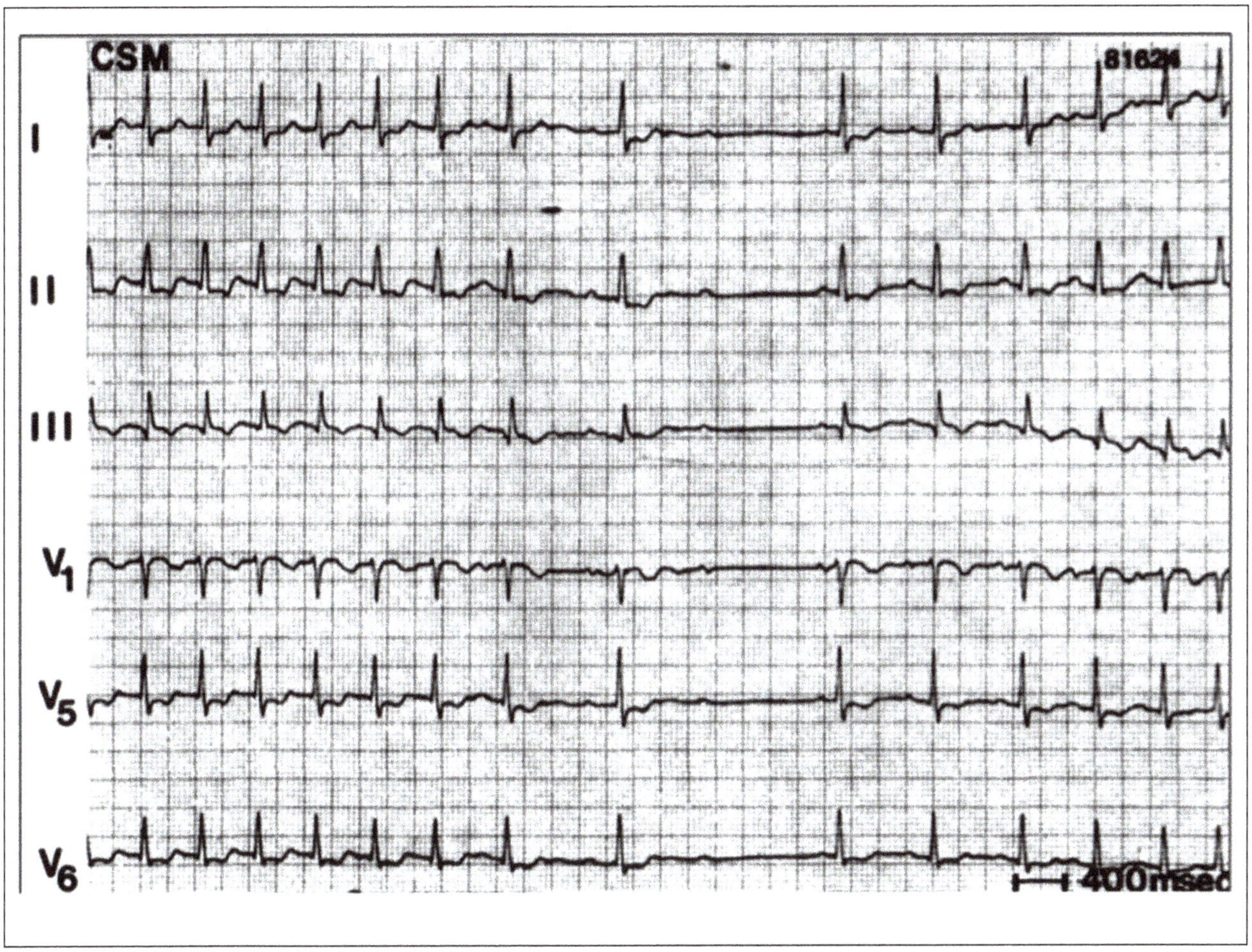

Figure 3-10 Effects of carotid sinus massage (CSM) on automatic atrial tachycardia (Wellens' ECG collection).

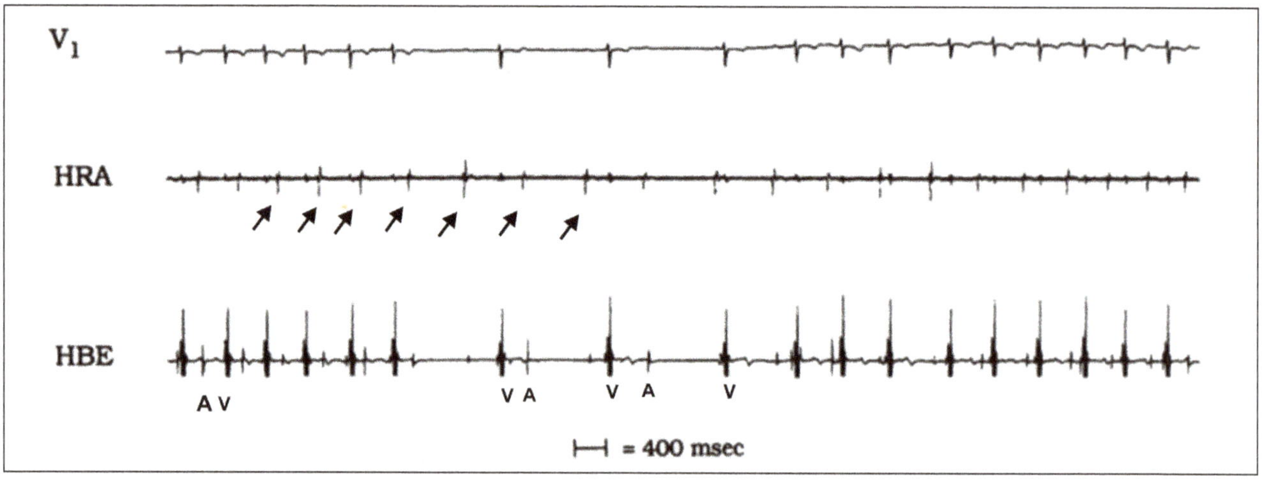

Figure 3-11 ECG surface lead V_1, electrogram from high right atrium (HRA), and His bundle electrogram (HBE) after administration of adenosine. **Arrows** point to atrial deflections. A, atrial electrogram; V, ventricular electrogram. (Reproduced from Engelstein ED, Lippman N, et al. Mechanism-specific effects of adenosine on atrial tachycardia. *Circulation.* 1994;89:2645–2654.)

A-V block occurs because of the pharmacologic effects of adenosine to depress A-V nodal conduction, but its slowing of the atrial rate is not caused by adenosine's actions on the A-V node. Rather, slowing is caused by the decrease of SDD that adenosine causes in pacemaker cells. The effects of adenosine last for only seconds because it is rapidly metabolized; once the adenosine is dissipated, automaticity returns to the pre-drug level. Adenosine can also antagonize the effects of sympathetic nerve activity on pacemaker activity.

Adenosine is therefore useful in distinguishing among arrhythmogenic mechanisms causing supraventricular tachycardia. It terminates tachycardia that is dependent on A-V nodal reentry by causing transient A-V nodal conduction block (Chapter 11), and it terminates tachycardia caused by DAD-dependent triggered activity by suppressing DADs (Chapter 6). It probably has little effect on focal atrial tachycardia caused by small atrial reentrant circuits (Chapter 10).

The effects of adenosine on abnormal automaticity (Chapter 4) in the atria are unknown. Therefore, it cannot be used to distinguish between normal and abnormal automaticity.

Effects of L-type Ca^{2+} Channel-Blocking and Other Antiarrhythmic Drugs

Class IV (Vaughan Williams classification) L-type Ca^{2+} channel-blocking drugs (e.g., verapamil) may slightly slow atrial tachycardia caused by normal automaticity commensurate with the small role of I_{CaL} in the atrial pacemaker SDD (Figure 3-3), but they do not terminate it (Table 3-1 #9). Class IV drugs also may not have significant effects on atrial tachycardia caused by focal atrial reentry (Chapter 10). They should, however, terminate atrial tachycardia caused by abnormal automaticity (Chapter 4), DAD-dependent triggered activity (Chapter 5), and A-V junctional reentry that involves the A-V node as part of the reentrant circuit (Chapter 11).

Class IA and B (Na^+-channel blockers), Class II (β-receptor blockers), and Class III (I_K blockers) antiarrhythmic drugs can slow automatic atrial tachycardia. Class IA and B decrease I_f pacemaker current and shift the threshold potential for phase 0 to less negative values. Class II reduces sympathetic effects on the atrial pacemakers, and Class III lengthens the action potential duration (see Figure 1-2). The slowing effect is not specific for automatic tachycardias and might also occur for triggered and reentrant tachycardia.

Overdrive Stimulation

Automatic atrial tachycardia cannot be started by overdrive stimulation (Table 3-1, #10 and #11). Overdrive stimulation during tachycardia causes transient suppression related to the rate and duration of overdrive similar to the sinus node with warm up over several CLs following termination of overdrive (see Figure 1-6 for description of the mechanisms). Tachycardia cannot be terminated by overdrive. Although by no means the same as overdrive, cardioversion is another form of intense stimulation that does not stop automatic tachycardia because it does not inhibit the pacemaker SDD.

Premature Stimulation

Automatic atrial tachycardias cannot be started by premature stimuli (Table 3-1, #10 and #12). They can be reset but not terminated by premature stimuli. The responses of compensatory pause and resetting of automatic pacemakers to premature stimulation is explained in Figures 1-10 and in the graphical display in Figure 1-11.

SUMMARY

Normal automaticity is a property of atrial cells at special locations throughout the right and left atria. Membrane currents that cause SDD in those cells are similar to those in sinus node pacemakers and include inward currents I_f and I_{NCX} and outward current I_K.

β_1-adrenergic agonists accelerate automatic impulse initiation, which is not a specific response of normal automaticity, since they also accelerate triggered activity and A-V nodal reentry. Parasympathetic stimulation or parasympathomimetic agents transiently slow or stop automaticity that returns after stimulation is ended, unlike DAD-triggered activity and A-V nodal reentry, which are terminated. Adenosine transiently slows and stops automaticity which returns when adenosine levels decline while it terminates DAD-triggered activity and A-V nodal reentry. L-type Ca^{2+} channel-blocking drugs have little effect on normal automaticity because of the small role of I_{CaL} in the pacemaker potential. The lack of effect may help differentiate normal from abnormal automaticity that is suppressed by these drugs. Na^+-channel blockers such as procainamide slow normal automaticity but also suppress other arrhythmogenic mechanisms.

The response of atrial pacemakers to electrical stimulation is characteristic of normal automaticity: transient overdrive suppression following overdrive stimulation and resetting after premature stimulation. Automaticity is neither started nor terminated by electrical stimulation.

Automatic atrial arrhythmias are caused by two primary mechanisms: ectopic pacemaker escape and acceleration of ectopic pacemaker impulse initiation causing tachycardia. An escape mechanism occurs after suppression of the dominant sinus node pacemaker. Tachycardia results from enhancement of atrial pacemaker SDD. The characteristics of automatic atrial tachycardia that distinguish it from other mechanisms causing supraventricular tachycardias are outlined in Table 3-1.

SOURCES

Basic Electrophysiology

Bassett AL, Fenoglio JJ Jr, Wit AL, et al. Electrophysiologic and ultrastructural characteristics of the canine tricuspid valve. *Am J Physiol.* 1976;230:1366–1385.

Euler DE, Jones SB, Gunnar WP et al. Cardiac arrhythmias in the conscious dog after excision of the sinoatrial node and crista terminalis. *Circulation.* 1979;59:468–475.

Jones SB, Euler DE, Hardie E et al. Comparison of SA nodal and subsidiary atrial pacemaker function and location in the dog. *Am J Physiol Heart Circ Physiol.* 1978;3(4):H471–H476.

Jones SB, Euler DE, Randall WC, et al. Atrial ectopic foci in the canine heart: Hierarchy of pacemaker automaticity. *Am J Physiol Heart Circ Physiol.* 1980;7:H788–H797.

Jones SA, Yamamoto Y, Tellez T et al. Distinguishing properties of cells from the myocardial sleeves of the pulmonary veins. A comparison of normal and abnormal pacemakers *Circ Arrhythmia Electrophysiol.* 2008;1:39–48.

Lerman BB, Belardinelli L. Cardiac electrophysiology of adenosine: Basic and clinical concepts. *Circulation.* 1991;83:1499–1509.

Randall WC, Rinkema LE, Jones SB, et al. Functional characterization of atrial pacemaker activity. *Am J Physiol Heart Circ Physiol.* 1982;242(11):H98–H106.

Rozanski GJ, Lipsius SL, Randall WC. Functional characteristics of sinoatrial and subsidiary pacemaker activity in the canine right atrium. *Circulation.* 1983;67:1378–1387.

Rozanski GJ, Lipsius SL, Randall WC, Jones SB. Alterations in subsidiary pacemaker function after prolonged subsidiary pacemaker dominance in the canine right atrium. *J Am Coll Cardiol.* 1984;4:535–542.

Rubenstein DS, Lipsius SL. Mechanisms of automaticity in subsidiary pacemakers from cat right atrium. *Circ Res.* 1989;64:648–657.

Wit AL, Fenoglio JJ Jr, Wagner BM, Bassett AL. Electrophysiological properties of cardiac muscle in the anterior mitral valve leaflet and the adjacent atrium in the dog: Possible implications for the genesis of atrial dysrhythmias. *Circ Res.* 1973;32:731–745.

Wit AL, Cranefield PF. Triggered and automatic activity in the canine coronary sinus. *Circ Res.* 1977;41:434–445.

Yamamoto M, Dobrzynski H, Tellez J, et al. Extended atrial conduction system characterised by the expression of the HCN4 channel and connexin45. *Cardiovas Res.* 2006;72:271–281.

Clinical Electrophysiology

Badhwar N, Kalman JM, Sparks PB, et al. Atrial tachycardia arising from the coronary sinus musculature; Electrophysiological characteristics and long-term outcomes of radiofrequency ablation. *J Am Coll Cardiol.* 2005;46:1921–1930.

Gillette PC, Garson A. Electrophysiologic and pharmacologic characteristics of automatic ectopic atrial tachycardia. *Circulation.* 1977;56:571–575.

Gonzalez MD, Contreras LJ, Jongbloed MRM, et al. Left atrial tachycardia originating from the mitral annulus-aorta junction. *Circulation.* 2004;110:3187–3192.

Higa S, Tai C-T, Lin Y-J, et al. Focal atrial tachycardia. New insights from noncontact mapping and catheter ablation. *Circulation.* 2004;109:84–91.

Kalman JM, Olgin JE, Karch M, et al. "Cristal tachycardias": Origin of right atrial tachycardias from the crista terminalis Identified by intracardiac echocardiography. *J Am Coll Cardiol.* 1998;31: 451–459.

Kistler PM, Sanders P, Hussin A, et al. Focal atrial tachycardia arising from the mitral annulus. Electrocardiographic and electrophysiologic characterization. *J Am Coll Cardiol.* 2003;41:2212–2219.

Kistler PM, Sanders P, Fynn SP, et al. Electrophysiological and electrocardiographic characteristics of focal atrial tachycardia originating from the pulmonary veins. Acute and long-term outcomes of radiofrequency ablation. *Circulation.* 2003;108:1968–1975.

Lindsay BD. Focal and macroreentrant atrial tachycardia: From bench to bedside and back to the bench again. *Heart Rhythm.* 2007;4:1361–1363.

Marchlinski F, Callans D, Gottlieb C, et al. Magnetic electroanatomical mapping for ablation of focal atrial tachycardias. *Pacing Clin Electrophysiol.*. 1998;21:1621–1635.

Matsuyama T, Innoue S, Tanno KK, et al. Ectopic nodal structures in a patient with atrial tachycardia originating from the mitral valve annulus. *Europace.* 2006:8;977–979.

Ouyang F, Ma J, Ho SY, et al. Focal atrial tachycardia originating from the non-coronary aortic sinus; Electrophysiological characteristics and catheter ablation. *J Am Coll Cardiol.* 2006;48:122–131.

Saoudi N, Cosio F, Waldo A, et al. Classification of atrial flutter and regular atrial tachycardia according to electrophysiologic mechanism and anatomic bases: A statement from a joint expert group from the working group of arrhythmias of the European Society of Cardiology and the North American Society of Pacing and Electrophysiology. *J Cardiovasc Electrophysiol.* 2001;12:852–866.

Scheinman MM, Basu D, Hollenberg M. Electrophysiologic studies in patients with persistent atrial tachycardia. *Circulation.* 1974;50:266–273.

SECTION
3B

Atrioventricular (A-V) Junctional Normal Automaticity and Automatic Arrhythmias

Normal automaticity in the atrioventricular (A-V) conduction pathway, causes A-V junctional arrhythmias. This section describes the electrophysiological properties of automaticity in the junction and gives several examples of automatic arrhythmias arising in this region.

Basic Electrophysiological Mechanisms

LOCATION OF A-V JUNCTIONAL PACEMAKERS WITH NORMAL AUTOMATICITY

The A-V junction is the normal anatomical and electrical connection between atria and ventricles. This broader functional term includes the anatomical A-V node, the myocardial connections between the atria and the node, the connection between the node and the bundle of His, and the bundle of His itself. All these regions have normal pacemaker activity that can cause A-V junctional arrhythmias.

A-V Junctional Conduction System

The A-V junctional conduction system (yellow) is located at the base of the right atrium within the triangle of Koch, shown by connecting the green circles in **Figure 3-12**. This is a triangular region bounded by the coronary sinus ostium (CSO), tendon of Todaro (TT) (a continuation of the valve of the inferior vena cava), and the tricuspid annulus and valve (TA), proximal to the central fibrous body (CFB).

The A-V node component of the A-V junction, often referred to as the compact A-V node (CN) has two extensions (left and right) that course towards the attachments of the mitral and tricuspid valves. The rightward extension (RE in the figure) is the most prominent. It extends toward the narrow region of myocardium (the isthmus) between the coronary sinus and the tricuspid valve and is called the inferior (posterior) nodal extension. The leftward extension (LE) forms a conducting pathway between the left atrial side of the interatrial septum and the nodal tissue (CN) or nodal-His region (NH). The role of these extensions in the formation of reentrant circuits that cause A-V nodal reentrant tachycardia is described in Chapter 11.

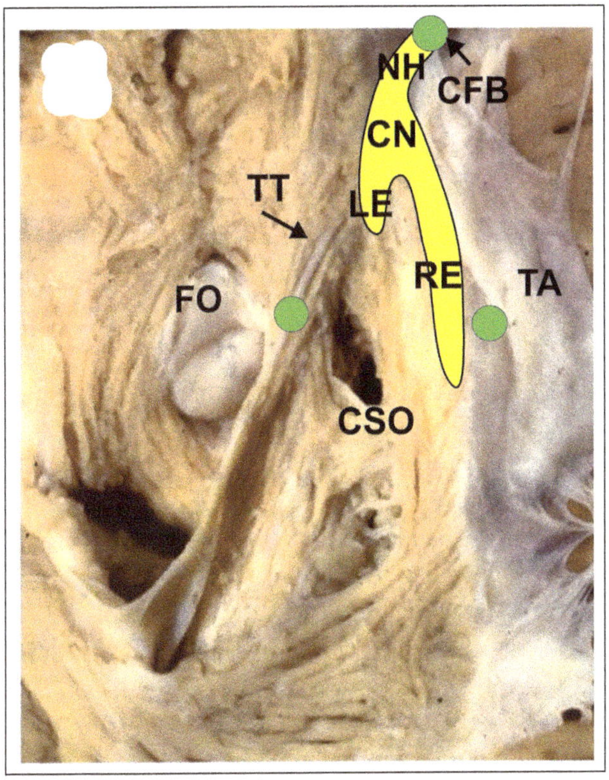

Figure 3-12 Anatomy of the inferior right atrium and A-V junction. (Figure kindly provided by Dr. Jose Angel Cabrera and Dr. Damian Sanchez-Quintana.)

The Compact Node and Extensions

The compact A-V node (CN), also referred to as the A-V node (Figure 3-12) is formed by a "knot" of interwoven, spindle shaped myocardial cells (diameter of about 5–10 um [micrometers]), smaller than working atrial and ventricular cells, that are generally "pale" in microscopic appearance because of the paucity of myofibrils. These nodal cells are connected to each other by gap junctions comprised of several different kinds of connexin proteins (Cx). In humans there is only a small amount of the high-conductance Cx43 gap- junction protein, through which relatively large currents flow that support rapid conduction in the ventricles. The node contains an abundance of the low-conductance Cx45 and Cx32 gap junctions, which contribute to the slow conduction in this region because of the poor electrical coupling it provides among A-V nodal myocytes. The rightward extension (RE) contains cells similar to those in the CN, small and closely packed with an interweaving architecture. It has more Cx43 gap junctions than the CN as well as Cx40 and Cx45 gap junctions. The leftward extension (LE) also has a microscopic structure similar to the CN, contains little Cx43 and more Cx45 gap junctions.

Transitional Cells

The CN and its extensions are surrounded by transitional cells that connect it to the atria. The morphology of these cells is intermediate in microscopic structure (size and myofibrils) between atrial and nodal cells (sometimes referred to as "AN" cells, see Figure 3-13). At the apex of the triangle of Koch, where the CN merges with the His bundle (NH), the transitional cells are longer than nodal cells, have a larger diameter (but not as large as His bundle cells) and are arranged parallel to each other. In this region, the lower NH region is surrounded by fibrous tissue of the CFB, which insulates it from surrounding atrial myocardium. This penetrating part of the transitional node leaves the fibrous tissue as the bundle of His on the crest of the ventricular septum (not shown in Figure 3-12). The myocytes of the His bundle resemble Purkinje cells of the ventricular conducting system with a larger diameter and more myofibrils than the CN cells, and they contain the higher-conductance connexin Cx40 gap-junction proteins in addition to Cx45. From the bundle of His, the left and right bundle branches of the ventricular conducting system are formed (see Section 3C, Ventricular Normal Automaticity and Automatic Arrhythmias).

ELECTROPHYSIOLOGY OF NORMAL AUTOMATICITY IN THE A-V JUNCTION

A-V Junctional Action Potentials

Figure 3-13 shows representative action potentials of cells from different regions of the A-V junction.

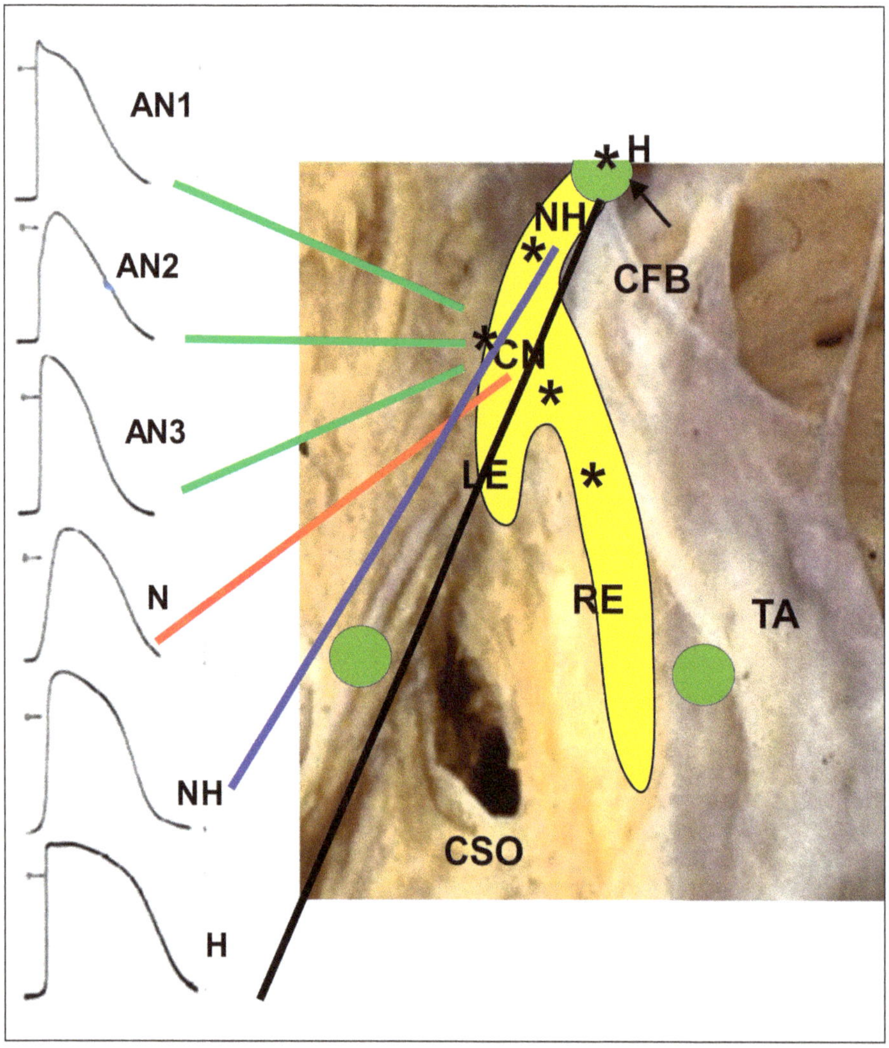

Figure 3-13 Action potentials (**at the left**) from A-V junction of rabbit heart. Lines connect action potentials to schematic of A-V junctional anatomy described in Figure 3-12. **Asterisks** indicate sites of normal automaticity. (**Left side** of figure showing action potentials are reproduced from Billette J. Atrioventricular nodal activation during periodic premature stimulation of the atrium. *Am J Physiol Heart Circ Physiol.*1987; 21:H163–H177. We have related these action potentials to diagram at the right.)

Compact A-V Node (CN); Nodal (N) Action Potential

Action potentials from the CN are designated as the A-V nodal (N) action potentials. The N action potential has distinctive features due to membrane currents specific to these cells. Action potentials in the nodal extensions may have similar characteristics (not shown in the figure).

The N action potential in Figure 3-13 arises from a less negative resting potential (approximately -60 mV) than atrial and ventricular cells. There is a reduced amount of I_{K1}, which is the primary membrane current causing the more negative resting potentials (~ -80 to -90 mV) of working atrial and ventricular myocytes. The depolarization phase (0) of the N action potential is much slower (5–15 V/s), and it has a lower overshoot (~ +10 mV) than working myocardial cells (+15–20 mV) because the main inward current during the N action potential upstroke (phase 0) is the "slow" L-type calcium current (I_{CaL}) instead of the "fast" sodium current (I_{Na}) of working myocardial cells. The combined effects of a weak inward depolarizing current during phase 0 (I_{CaL}) and low- conductance gap junctions (Cx45) cause the slow propagation through the CN (about 10 cm/s).

The delayed rectifier current, I_K, is responsible for repolarization of the N action potential along with inactivation of I_{CaL}. Recovery of I_{CaL} is both voltage and time-dependent. It outlasts repolarization, accounting for the refractory period of the node extending beyond complete repolarization, similar to the perinodal cells of the sinus node (Figure 2-7).

Atrio-Nodal (AN) Transition Cells Between Compact Node and Atrium

The atrio-nodal transitional cells between CN and atrium (labeled AN1-3 in Figure 3-13) have several different action potential characteristics that are transitional between atrial and CN. Transitional cells have more negative resting potentials than N cells due to increased I_{K1} and a strong electrotonic interaction with atrial cells (but still less negative than atrial cells). They also have faster upstrokes (phase 0) than N cells due to increased I_{Na} (but still slower than atrial cells).

Transitional Cells Between the Compact Node and His Bundle (NH cells)

As the CN transitions to the His bundle (NH cells in Figure 3-13), action potentials with characteristics intermediate between nodal and His bundle occur. The resting potential becomes more negative (~-75 mV) because of increased I_{K1}, and phase 0 is more rapid due to an increased contribution of I_{Na} compared with nodal cells. His bundle action potentials (H in Figure 3-13) have many features of Purkinje cells, with even more negative resting potentials (–75 to –85 mV), faster I_{Na}-dependent phase 0, an I_{CaL}-dependent plateau phase, I_K-dependent repolarization, and voltage-dependent recovery of excitability—i.e., refractory periods last until cells are repolarized.

Automaticity and Pacemaker Potential (SDD)

Automaticity occurs at different sites along the A-V junctional pathway (black asterisks in Figure 3-13), including AN, CN, LE and RE, NH, and H. **Figure 3-14** (top recording, AVN) shows the pacemaker potential or spontaneous diastolic depolarization (SDD, arrow) and automaticity recorded from an N cell in the CN (AVN) in an isolated superfused canine A-V junction. The lower recording (HB) shows action potentials from a cell in the His bundle, which has less SDD (arrow). (The AVN was disconnected from the HB in this experiment). This illustrates the hierarchy of pacemakers with nodal cells having a faster automatic rate than His bundle cells.

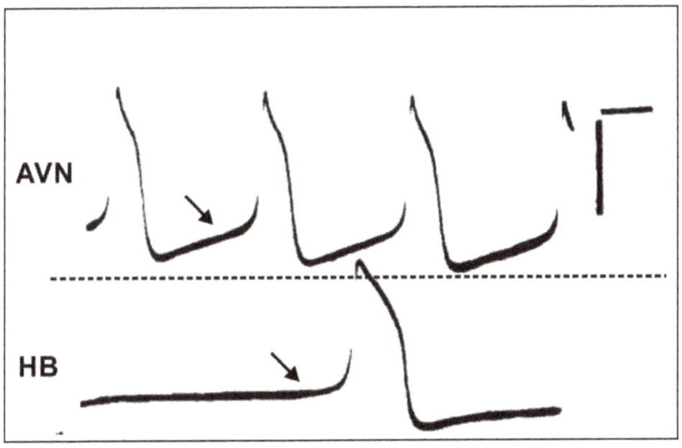

Figure 3-14 Action potentials of canine A-V node (CN) (upper recording, AVN) and from His bundle cell (HB) in lower recording. (Reproduced from Tse WW. Effect of epinephrine on automaticity of the canine atrioventricular node. *Am J Physiol.* 1975;229;34–37.)

Pacemaker Currents in the Compact Node

The membrane currents responsible for automaticity of N cells in the CN and cells in the RE extension are similar to the currents in the sinus node (see Figure 2-6). There is an inward I_f pacemaker current (HCN_4 mRNA, and I_f channel protein expression have been documented). I_{NCX} also contributes inward current along with I_{CaL}. The outward currents shown in Figure 2-6 are likely to also participate. The reduced I_{K1} mentioned above with regard to the N resting potential facilitates pacemaker depolarization as it does in sinus node, since outward current through this channel is reduced. Weak coupling to adjacent atrium diminishes the inhibitory electrotonic influence of the atrium on pacemaking in the atrio-nodal (AN) regions and right extension (RE), just as poor coupling of the sinus node pacemakers to surrounding atrial myocardium facilitates sinus node impulse initiation. Within the node, weak electrical coupling between the N and AN cells may facilitate N automaticity for the same reason.

Clinical ablation procedures intended to block conduction in A-V junctional pathways, uncouple the A-V node from atrium and can result in the appearance of automatic junctional rhythms, which may be atrio-nodal or A-V nodal in origin. This unintended "experiment" has demonstrated that coupling of the node to atrial myocardium suppresses normal nodal automaticity.

Pacemaker Currents at Other Sites

The AN and NH transitional region and the His bundle are additional sites that have normal automaticity. The mechanism for the pacemaker potential (SDD) has not been specifically elucidated for these regions. The pacemaker potential in NH cells is likely to involve currents prominent in both nodal and Purkinje cells such as I_f, I_{NCX}, and I_K (Figure 2-6). Membrane currents causing automaticity in Purkinje cells of the ventricular conducting system are described in Section 3C, Ventricular Normal Automaticity and Automatic Arrhythmias. The mechanism for the Purkinje cells, which involves a greater contribution of I_f and smaller contributions of intracellular Ca^{2+} and I_{NCX}, may also apply to the His bundle (see Figure 3-31).

Control of Rate of A-V Junctional Automaticity

In keeping with the concept of the hierarchy of pacemakers (Figure 1-4), the intrinsic rate of automaticity of A-V junctional cells in experimental studies is slower than that of atrial pacemakers and faster than the automatic rate in the ventricular conducting system. Within the A-V junction, the compact node has a faster intrinsic rate (~30–55 impulses/min) than the His bundle (~30–40 impulses/min). The autonomic nervous system (ANS) is a modulating influence on automaticity (see below). A-V junctional pacemakers are normally overdriven by the sinus node, which has a faster intrinsic rate. The general principles governing shifts of pacemaker site from the sinus node to the A-V junction are the same as described in Figure 1-8. A-V junctional escape occurs when sinus node overdrive is decreased. A-V junctional pacemaker acceleration (to a faster rate of impulse initiation than the sinus node and atrial pacemakers) causes a shift of the pacemaking site to the A-V junction.

ANS and A-V Automaticity

Sympathetic stimulation. Automaticity is accelerated by sympathetic stimulation through β_1 receptor activation at all A-V junctional pacemaker sites. **Figure 3-15** illustrates the effects of β_1-adrenergic stimulation to accelerate SDD and automatic activity of an atrial-nodal (AN) transitional cell from the canine heart.

Different regions of the A-V junction may have different sensitivities to adrenergic stimulation. There is some evidence that during junctional rhythm originating in the NH region, the site of impulse initiation shifts to the CN during adrenergic stimulation due to a greater acceleration of impulse initiation in the CN.

Effects of adrenergic stimulation can result in rapid automatic clinical arrhythmias originating in the A-V junction. This occurs if the acceleration in the A-V junctional rate is greater than that of the sinus node or other ectopic sites that are also accelerated by the increased sympathetic activity. The molecular mechanisms for enhancement of the pacemaker current in the A-V node are similar to the sinus node: β_1-receptor enhancement of I_f, larger deactivation of I_K, increased I_{NCX} caused by an increase in calcium release from the sarcoplasmic reticulum, and increased I_{CaL} and I_{CaT}. The role of I_{NCX} and calcium currents in pacemaker activity in the His bundle is uncertain, but this region likely has an I_f pacemaker current that is increased by sympathetic activity.

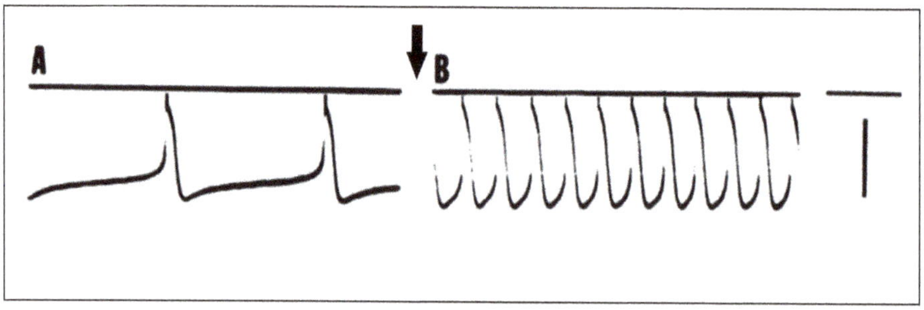

Figure 3-15 Effects of adrenergic stimulation on AN cell from canine heart. **Panel A** shows the control spontaneous firing rate. **Panel B** shows the faster rate after epinephrine (administered at **arrow**). Calibration shown at right border horizontal bar, 1.0 sec; vertical bar, 50 mV. (Reproduced from Tse WW. Adrenergic potentiation on spontaneous activity of canine paranodal fibers. *Am J Physiol Heart Circ Physiol.* 1984;16:H415–421.)

Parasympathetics (vagus). The A-V node is highly innervated by the parasympathetic nervous system via the vagus nerve. The His bundle is innervated less, partly explaining why vagal activation has a greater effect to suppress automaticity in the node than in the His bundle.

In addition, there is a stronger effect of acetylcholine (ACh) released from vagal nerve endings on pacemaker currents in A-V node than His bundle, resulting in a greater suppression of automaticity in the A-V node than in the His bundle.

In **Figure 3-16**, automaticity in the A-V nodal (N) cell in the top trace is completely suppressed by ACh (administered at the arrow) while the pacemaker automaticity in the His bundle cell in the bottom trace is little affected. ACh increases I_{KACh} outward current and decreases I_f pacemaker current—both actions causing a decrease in pacemaking in the A-V node, but not a prominent effect in the His bundle.

When His bundle automaticity is accelerated by sympathetic activity, ACh can slow it—a process called accentuated antagonism. This occurs even though automaticity in the His bundle has much less sensitivity to ACh under more normal circumstances. On the basis of the different effects of the parasympathetics on pacemakers in different regions of the A-V junction, the site of a junctional automatic pacemaker is predicted to shift to the His bundle during vagal activation, which suppresses A-V nodal automaticity more than His bundle automaticity.

Pharmacological Agents

Adenosine. A-V nodal (N) cells have adenosine receptors and the $I_{KACh/Adeno}$ ion channel, which responds to adenosine by increasing outward I_K. Adenosine can also decrease inward currents, I_{CaL}, and I_f. The net effect of adenosine is a decrease in inward current that is instrumental in slowing A-V nodal conduction and causing conduction block that terminates reentrant A-V nodal tachycardia (see Chapter 11). The same effects should also slow or transiently stop automaticity by a decrease in net inward pacemaker current. Thus, the response of A-V junctional automaticity to adenosine would be similar to the response of sinus node or atrial pacemakers. The automatic rhythm resumes once adenosine has been metabolized.

In contrast to its effects on A-V nodal pacemakers, the effects of adenosine on His-Purkinje pacemakers are not so clearly defined. Adenosine might slow automatic impulse initiation mainly when automaticity is enhanced by sympathetic stimulation, by an anti-adrenergic action. In the absence of sympathetic activity, adenosine has little effect.

Calcium channel blocking drugs. Drugs like the L-type Ca^{2+}-channel blocker, verapamil are also predicted to have a differential effect on A-V nodal compared with His bundle automaticity. In A-V nodal (N) cells the upstroke (phase 0) is a result primarily of inward I_{CaL}. Thus, verapamil may decrease A-V nodal automatic rate by shifting the threshold potential (TP) for activating I_{CaL} to more positive levels (Figure 2-2, Panel C), and by decreasing the I_{CaL} contribution to the pacemaker potential.

In contrast, the action potentials of His bundle cells have a phase 0 that is predominantly dependent on I_{Na}, which is not significantly affected by therapeutic concentrations of verapamil. His bundle pacemaker currents, if similar to more peripheral Purkinje fibers in the ventricle (see Figure 3-31), would not be expected to be significantly reduced by L-type calcium-channel blocking drugs, since I_{CaL} plays only a minor role, if any, in automaticity.

Radio Frequency (RF) Current—Heat

Heat is another stimulus that induces or accelerates SDD in A-V nodal cells. The heat generated by radiofrequency (RF) current during ablation procedures can cause accelerated A-V junctional rhythms that arise in or near to the compact A-V node.

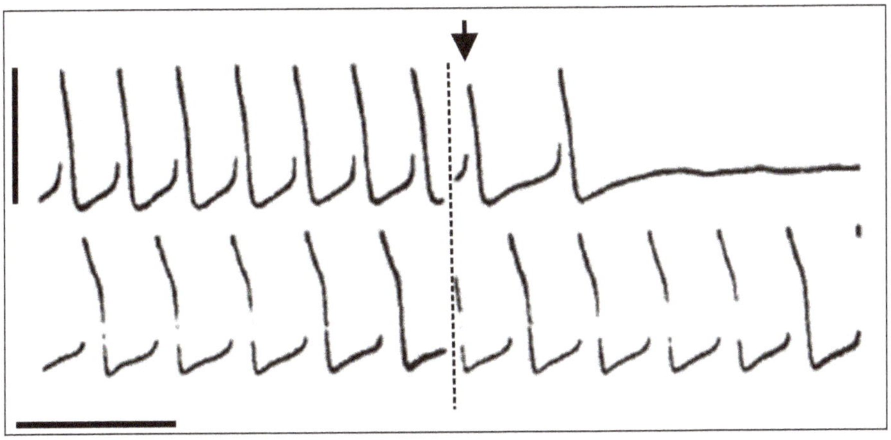

Figure 3-16 Action potentials recorded simultaneously from A-V node (N cells) (**top trace**) and His bundle (**bottom trace**) in canine A-V junction before and after (**arrow**) exposure to ACh. Vertical dashed line indicates a break in the recording (Reproduced from Tse WW. Suppressive effect of acetylcholine on automaticity of canine atrioventricular node. *J Electrocardiol.* 1982;15:233–240.)

RELATIONSHIP OF AUTOMATICITY TO CONDUCTION BLOCK IN THE A-V JUNCTION

Failure of impulse conduction from the atria to the ventricles, leading to complete A-V conduction block, can occur due to spontaneous diastolic depolarization (SDD) in the His bundle, which decreases the membrane potential and affects conduction by reducing available Na^+ channels for activation. Some background electrophysiology of conduction is necessary to understand this mechanism. A detailed description of the mechanism of impulse conduction is in Chapter 9 (Figure 9-4). A brief summary is given here.

In myocardial cells that have an I_{Na}-dependent phase 0 depolarization such as in the His bundle, the level of negativity of the membrane potential at which phase 0 arises (level of the resting potential, phase 4) has an important effect on I_{Na}. As explained in more detail in Chapter 4, Figure 4-5, the intensity of I_{Na} (quantity and rapidity) decreases as the membrane potential from which phase 0 arises, decreases (becomes less negative) because the Na^+ channels in the cell membrane are inactivated and lose the ability to allow the inward flow of I_{Na}. The intensity of I_{Na} is directly related to the speed of impulse conduction because it provides the axial current that excites cells in the direction of propagation (Figure 9-4). As I_{Na} decreases and phase 0 rapidity and amplitude decrease, conduction slows and at a critical low level of I_{Na} conduction stops.

Phase 4 Block Is the Mechanism for Bradycardia-Dependent A-V Block

SDD in the His-Purkinje system affects conduction because membrane potential is decreasing during phase 4. Conduction block in the His bundle caused by SDD, leads to a particular kind of A-V conduction block, called phase 4 block. The term "phase 4 block" indicates that conduction of an impulse arriving in the His-Purkinje system during phase 4, blocks because of SDD. It can also be thought of as bradycardia-dependent block, since it is usually initiated by a long cycle length (CL) or period of bradycardia, which accentuates SDD by allowing it to progress to less negative levels of membrane potential. (Block in the A-V node during phase 4 of N cells can occur without SDD because of the time-dependent recovery of excitability. It is not referred to as phase 4 block).

Phase 4 block has a different mechanism than phase 3 block. Phase 3 block is physiological or functional block that occurs when a supraventricular impulse arrives in Purkinje cells while action potentials are in early phase 3 of repolarization, during which the effective refractory period occurs. The phase 3 block occurs because I_{Na} that is inactivated during phase 0 is not sufficiently recovered to allow impulse conduction. This phenomenon occurs at short CLs (tachycardia-dependent block). The effects of repolarization on I_{Na} and conduction block are described in detail in Figure 9-6.

Figure 3-17 shows paroxysmal (sudden onset) bradycardia-dependent (phase 4) A-V block in a patient with a normal baseline ECG. The first three impulses from the left are of sinus origin at a CL of 760 ms. A-V block occurs after a conducted atrial premature impulse (unfilled arrow beneath the aVF recording, coupling interval 560 ms). The small vertical arrows point out the blocked P waves. The asterisks indicate an escape rhythm. The prolonged P-P interval of 840 ms after the atrial premature impulse occurred because the premature impulse reset the sinus node (see Figure 2-14). This long CL enabled SDD in the His bundle to progress to less negative levels, leading to the conduction block in that region. The site can be localized by recording a His bundle electrogram (HBE) in which His bundle depolarization follows atrial depolarization but is not followed by ventricular depolarization (an example of a HBE recording is shown in Figure 3-24). The origin of the escape rhythm is below the site of block. A-V conduction resumes near the end of the recording (last three impulses).

Phase 4 Block in Normal and Diseased Myocardium

In the normal His-Purkinje system, rapid conduction occurs because of the high negative level of resting membrane potential during phase 4 where there is a strong I_{Na} responsible for phase 0 of the action potential. For conduction to block, I_{Na} must be reduced. Action potentials generated by SDD conduct more slowly than those arising from a steady negative level of resting potential, this is because some Na^+ channels are partly inactivated at the reduced level of membrane potential, and thus I_{Na} is weaker. If the focus of SDD and automaticity is small, it is unlikely that the slowly conducting action potentials generated in the focus will have any noticeable influence on activation of the rest of the His-Purkinje system. Once the impulse leaves the focus, it excites Purkinje cells with normal conduction due to steady, highly negative resting membrane potentials and normal action potentials. However, if there is disease in a significant region characterized by reduced membrane potentials and reduced I_{Na}, conduction block of impulses arising at the end of phase 4 depolarization can occur to cause paroxysmal A-V block. **Figure 3-18** shows how this phenomenon occurs in a model of phase 4 block caused by SDD. The figure shows action potential recordings from four contiguous regions in the His-Purkinje system (A–D).

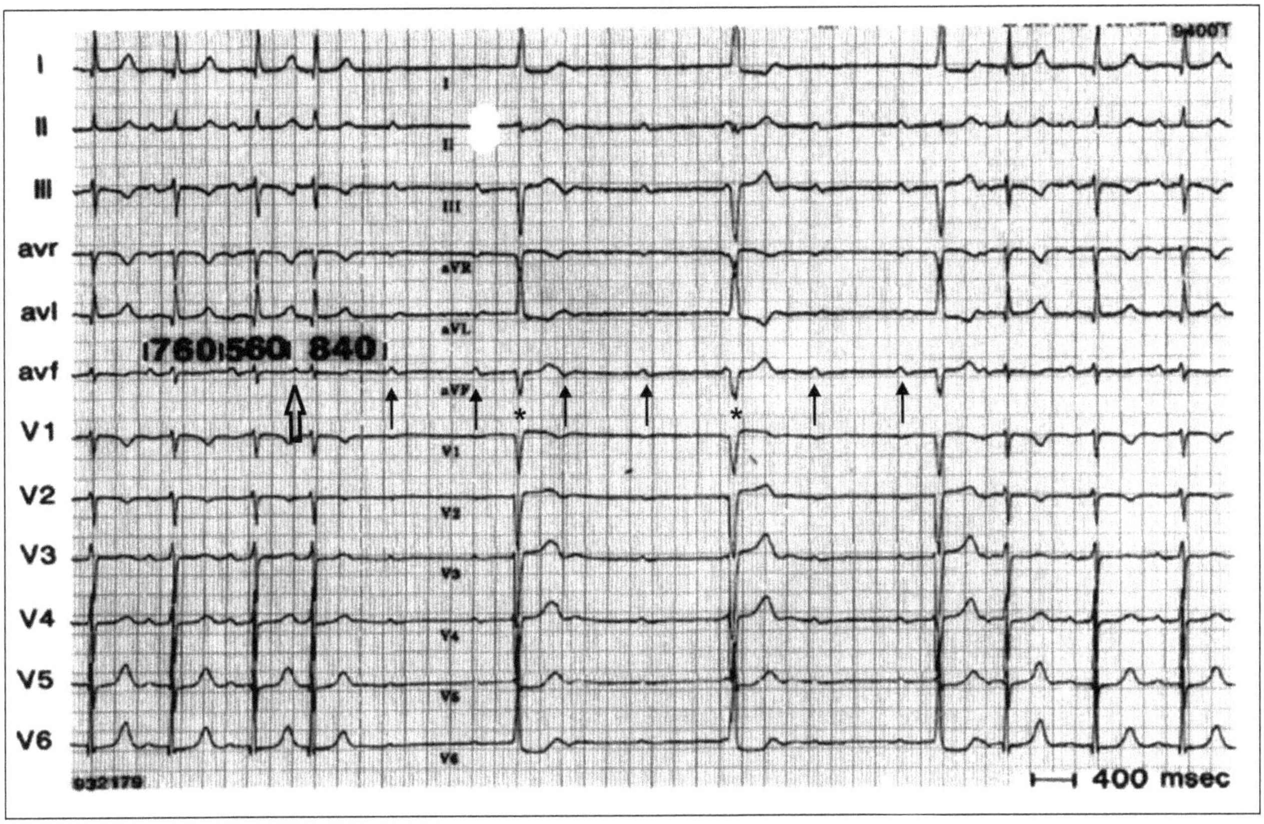

Figure 3-17 ECG recorded during paroxysmal (phase 4) A-V block (Wellen's ECG collection).

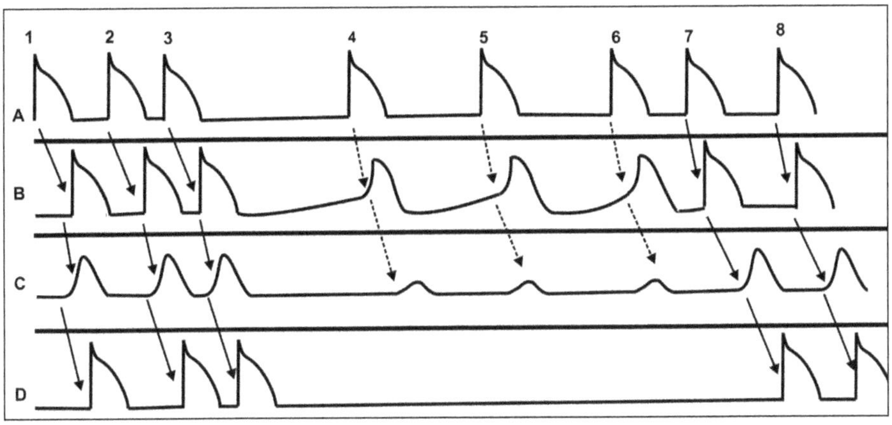

Figure 3-18 Mechanism for phase 4 block.

Regions A and B in the proximal His bundle are relatively normal. Region C that is more distal is abnormal and has a reduced (less negative) membrane potential, decreased action potential amplitude, and slowed phase 0 due to partial I_{Na} inactivation. Region D is distal to the abnormal region and has normal resting and action potentials.

Action potentials 1 and 2 are generated during conduction of sinus impulses into the His bundle in the sequence pointed out by the arrows; excitation of the proximal regions A and B followed by conduction through the diseased Region C and on to Region D indicated by the black arrows.

Action potential 3 in Region A represents a supraventricular premature impulse that successfully propagates through the conducting system, in the direction from A to D (arrows). It is followed by a long cycle caused by resetting of the dominant (sinus) pacemaker. This is the long CL that allows SDD to occur after action potential 3 in Region B.

Action potential 4 is an impulse of sinus origin that conducts into Region A after the long cycle. It arrives in region B during phase 4 depolarization (SDD) (impulse 4). Action potential 4 that occurs when region B is excited during phase 4 depolarization has a reduced phase 0 (I_{Na}). The decreased I_{Na} is unable to excite the cells in Region C (dashed arrow). An additional factor contributing to block is that Purkinje cells with less negative membrane potentials are more difficult to excite (Figure 9-7). This leads to block of conduction (dashed arrow) with failure of propagation to Region D. Failure to propagate the impulse in the His bundle to Region D results in A-V block. It can also result in bundle branch block if more distal in the conducting system.

Action potentials 5 and 6 occurring during a period of bradycardia, also block before reaching Region D. Once SDD occurs in Region B (after action potential 3), the rate of impulses from spontaneous phase 4 depolarization increases (subsequent action potentials 4, 5, and 6) because of the decreased influence of the Na^+–K^+ pump due to long cycles. Action potentials 5 and 6 from Region A, also arrive in region B after SDD depolarization (dashed arrows), which have a reduced phase 0, and therefore cannot excite Region C, leading to persistence of block at the slow heart rate.

Persistent block is favored if the input to Region B occurs at long cycles, allowing more enhanced spontaneous phase 4 depolarization. However, this is not always the case; sometimes shorter cycles can also be associated with persistent block. For example, supraventricular CL may shorten because of enhanced sympathetic activity from the baroreceptors or decreased coronary perfusion if blood pressure decreases, both of which also enhance SDD and decrease overdrive suppression, so phase 4 block might continue.

Action potential 7 conducts to Region D. Restoration of conduction requires suppression of spontaneous phase 4 depolarization. This can be caused by a premature supraventricular or ventricular impulse that activates the region at a short CL. Action potential 7 in Region A occurs prematurely, and as a result activates Region B before SDD reduces the membrane potential. Therefore, action potential 7 in Region B has a larger I_{Na} and a faster and larger phase 0 and is able to excite Region C (solid arrow), leading to resumption of conduction to the distal Region D.

Action potential 8 in Region A is likewise able to conduct because spontaneous phase 4 depolarization is now suppressed in Region B. Other factors that suppress spontaneous phase 4 depolarization can also improve conduction. For example, in experimental studies, low doses of procainamide, which suppress SDD, were able to increase phase 0 even though this drug in higher doses can decrease I_{Na}.

ELECTRICAL STIMULATION OF A-V JUNCTIONAL PACEMAKERS

Overdrive Suppression

Typical of normal automaticity, overdrive stimulation transiently suppresses A-V junctional pacemakers with a subsequent return to the original automatic rate, the amount of suppression being related to the rate and duration of overdrive. It does not initiate or terminate automatic A-V junctional rhythms (see Figure 1-6).

Overdrive suppression is less in A-V nodal cells compared with His bundle pacemakers because of cell differences in membrane currents. A-V nodal cells have action potentials and pacemaker currents similar to the sinus node with less negative resting potential and Ca^{2+} (I_{CaL})-dependent action potential phase 0. His bundle pacemakers have more negative resting potentials and Na^+ (I_{Na})-dependent phase 0 (Figure 3-13). Overdrive of the mostly I_{CaL}-dependent action potentials of A-V nodal cells is not expected to activate as much Na^+–K^+ pump current (I_p) as in His bundle cells because less Na^+ enters the nodal cells during overdrive. The different responsiveness of A-V nodal cells and His bundle pacemakers can be used to help determine the site of origin of A-V junctional rhythms in the clinical setting as described in the sections on clinical arrhythmias.

Programmed Premature Electrical Stimulation

There are no experimental laboratory data describing the resetting response of junctional pacemakers to premature stimulation. Resetting of A-V nodal pacemakers likely has similar characteristics to sinus node resetting, including conduction delay into and out of the pacemaker site (Figure 2-14). Resetting of His bundle pacemakers is likely to be similar to Purkinje fiber pacemakers described in the section on ventricular automaticity later in this chapter. Like automatic pacemakers at other ectopic sites, junctional automaticity is neither initiated nor terminated by programmed premature stimulation.

The properties of automaticity in different regions of the A-V junction are summarized in Table 3-2 at the end of this section on A-V junction.

Examples of Arrhythmias Caused by Alterations in A-V Junctional Automaticity

Normal automaticity in the A-V junction can cause slow escape rhythms when the rate of impulses entering the A-V junction from the dominant sinus node pacemaker is decreased. Normal automaticity in the A-V junction causes rapid tachycardias when the slope of SDD is enhanced.

AUTOMATIC A-V JUNCTIONAL ESCAPE RHYTHMS

Figure 3-19 shows an ECG from a patient with sick sinus syndrome and is an example of A-V junctional escape. The first two impulses at the beginning of the record are of sinus origin, at a CL of 800 ms. They are characterized by normal P-QRS complexes in all leads. The second sinus impulse is followed by a pause of 1200 ms, which is terminated by an impulse with a QRS that is almost identical to the sinus QRS but which is not preceded by a P wave, an A-V junctional escape impulse. Possible retrograde atrial depolarization is likely concealed in the T wave, which has a slightly altered shape compared to the sinus T wave. The normal QRS morphology indicates that depolarization arises in the A-V junction, either the A-V node or His bundle. The P wave follows the QRS. This characteristic indicates that conduction time to the atria from the pacemaker site is longer than conduction time to the ventricles, resulting in ventricular depolarization before atrial depolarization. The first junctional escape impulse is followed by another junctional impulse (CL is 1400 ms). Sinus rhythm then reoccurs until there is another long pause, again followed by a junctional impulse (last impulse at the right). The progressive shortening of sinus CLs prior to the pause indicates that sinoatrial Wenckebach with exit block causes the pause.

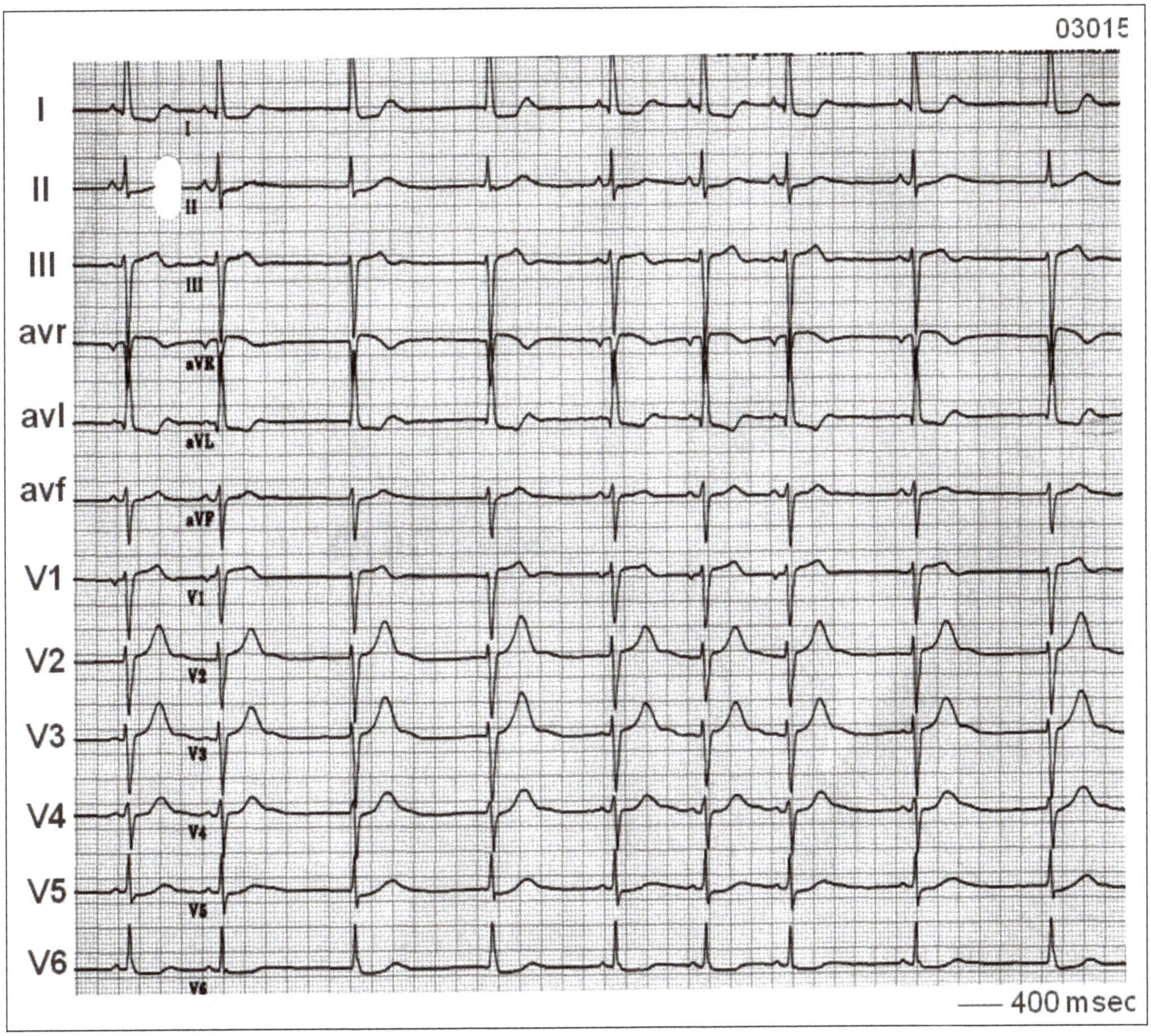

Figure 3-19 A 12-lead ECG showing A-V junctional escape (Wellens' ECG collection).

A-V junctional escape impulses and rhythms occur when the usually dominant sinus node impulse fails to reach and depolarize the junction, either transiently or for a prolonged period of time. This may result from failure of sinus impulse initiation, sinus automatic rate slowing below the automatic A-V junctional rate, or conduction block in the pathway between the sinus node pacemaker and atrium. The resultant decrease in overdrive suppression allows the A-V junctional pacemaker to escape after a pause. Although experimentally, atrial pacemakers rank second below sinus node pacemakers in the pacemaker hierarchy, the A-V junction usually is the location of the pacemaker in humans after sinus node dysfunction.

The QRS and P Waves of Junctional Escape Rhythms

The QRS of junctional escape rhythms is usually of normal configuration, reflecting conduction in a normal pattern over the ventricular conducting system from the junctional focus, unless there is disease in the ventricular conducting system. The junctional focus may control the atrial depolarization characterized by narrow, inverted P waves in leads II, III, and aVF because of retrograde atrial activation. The P-wave amplitude in lead I is usually small and of variable contour. The frontal axis of the P wave is generally between −60° and −80°. P-wave configuration in the precordial leads is variable, with inverted P waves in none, some, or all precordial leads. P waves occasionally precede but are usually superimposed on, or follow the QRS. Should the atria remain under the control of an independent focus such as the sinus node in heart block, P waves reflect the site of that focus.

A-V Junctional Escape Rhythm Rates

A-V junctional escape rhythms occur at the inherent physiologic rate of junctional pacemakers and are also modified by resting autonomic tone (**Figure 3-20**). In humans, the intrinsic rate of an escape rhythm arising in the A-V node is about 30–55 bpm, while the rate of an escape rhythm arising in the His bundle (intrahisian) is about 30–40 bpm. However, as seen in Figure 3-20, there is considerable variability and overlap, since autonomic influences that affect rate vary in different patients. Rates of A-V junctional pacemakers are in general faster than pacemakers below the His bundle, in the ventricular bundle branches or peripheral Purkinje system, indicated by the infra-His bundle rates of 15–40 bpm in Figure 3-20.

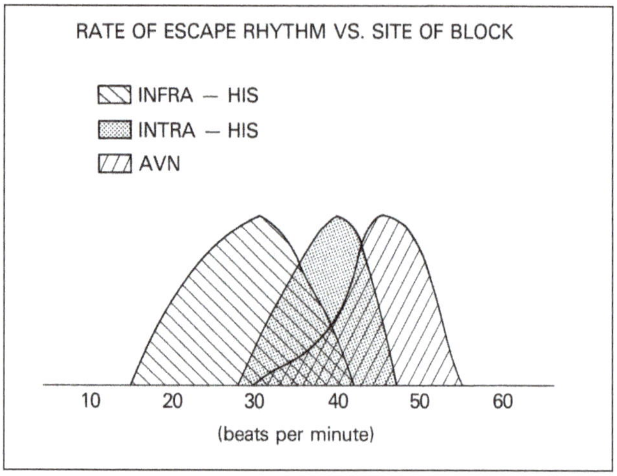

Figure 3-20 Range of rates of escape rhythms in a series of patients with A-V block located to different regions in the A-V conducting system by His bundle recording: A-V node (AVN), His bundle (intrahisian), and below the His bundle (infrahisian). The pattern of shading according to the scale above indicates the likely pacemaker location. (Reproduced from Josephson ME. *Josephson's Clinical Cardiac Electrophysiology: Techniques and Interpretations* (5th ed.). Philadelphia, PA: Wolters Kluwer; 2016.)

ACCELERATED AUTOMATIC A-V JUNCTIONAL RHYTHMS AND TACHYCARDIA

Junctional impulse initiation at rates above 70 bpm is classified as accelerated junctional rhythm or junctional tachycardia, since the rates are faster than the intrinsic rates of a junctional pacemaker. These rhythms occur when the junctional automatic rate exceeds the sinus rate.

Accelerated A-V Junctional Rhythm

Figure 3-21 shows an accelerated junctional rhythm in a patient with no cardiac abnormalities except for the arrhythmia and the absence of cardiac drugs. The first impulse is of sinus origin with a normal P-R interval. The second impulse has a junctional origin (normal QRS), preceded by a nonconducted sinus P wave (PR interval is too short for the QRS to be caused by a conducted atrial impulse). This first junctional impulse is not premature but occurs after a long CL that is characteristic of automaticity, the long CL allowing SDD to proceed to the threshold potential. The junctional rhythm then accelerates for the next four impulses (warm up) at a rate of about 104 bpm. Retrograde conduction from the junctional focus leading to negative P waves in leads II and III is present with increasing ventricular to atrial (V-A) conduction time. Then, a pause occurs for no apparent reason. After the pause, an accelerating junctional rhythm reoccurs.

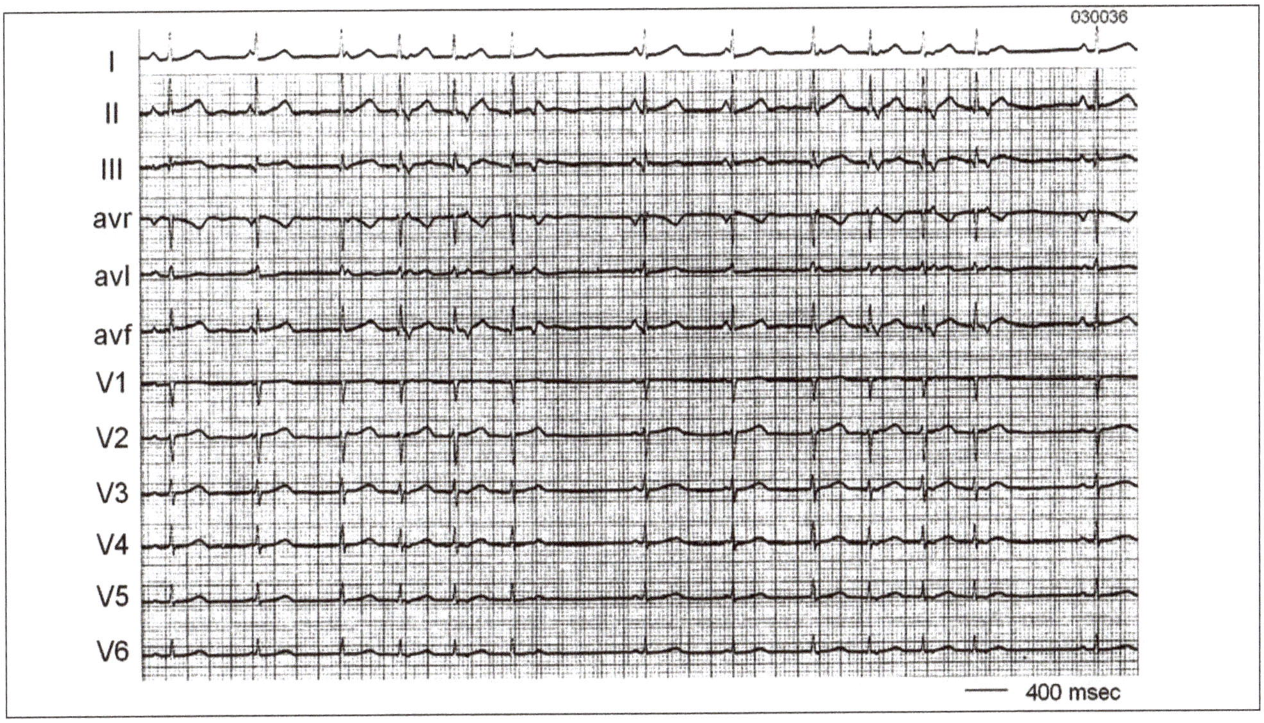

Figure 3-21 A 12-lead ECG showing an accelerated junctional rhythm (Wellens' ECG collection).

The increase above the intrinsic rate of the junctional pacemaker in Figure 3-21 may result from enhanced sympathetic and/or reduced parasympathetic activity. Acceleration of a junctional pacemaker may also occur in patients receiving digitalis, after open-heart surgery, or in the presence of electrolyte disturbances.

A-V Junctional Tachycardia

Figure 3-22 shows the ECG of an A-V junctional tachycardia accompanying an acute inferior myocardial infarction caused by occlusion of the right coronary artery, a branch of which often perfuses the A-V node. Periodically during tachycardia, sinus impulses are conducted to the ventricles (best seen in lead II where an upright P wave precedes the QRS for impulses 2, 5, and 8). The QRS morphology of the junctional impulses is almost the same as the QRS of the sinus impulses. Lead V_1 shows some ventricular aberration because of the shorter R-R interval following the conducted sinus impulses. The rate of impulse initiation in the A-V junction is about 120 per min, faster than the accelerated junctional rhythm in Figure 3-21. Impulse initiation may be accelerated by ischemia with concomitant release of norepinephrine from local sympathetic nerve endings. Sinus bradycardia or sinoatrial exit block may exist concomitantly because of ischemia of the sinus node.

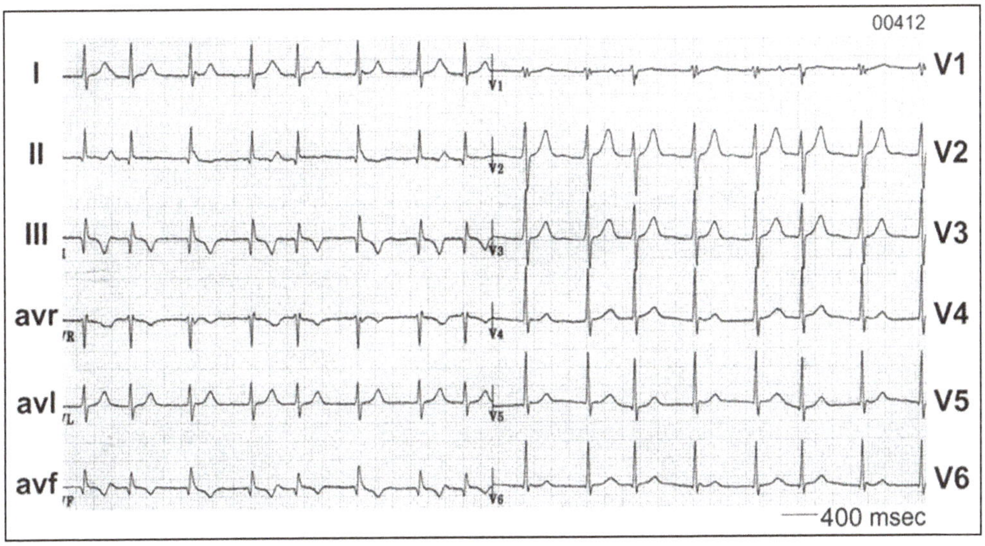

Figure 3-22 A 12-lead ECG showing a junctional tachycardia (Wellens' ECG collection).

Junctional Ectopic Tachycardia (JET)

The junctional tachycardia shown in **Figure 3-23** has some different characteristics than the rhythms shown in Figures 3-21 and 3-22. It is classified as a junctional ectopic tachycardia (JET) even though the accelerated junctional rhythm in Figure 3-21, and the junctional tachycardia in Figure 3-22, are also ectopic.

Junctional ectopic tachycardia is distinguished from the junctional tachycardia shown in Figure 3-22 by the clinical setting in which it occurs. It is most frequently seen in infancy in association with congenital cardiac defects, postoperatively after surgery near the A-V junction when it is often incessant, and in adults with congenital heart defects. It also occurs in adults in the absence of heart disease. In adults, it is usually not incessant but can last from several seconds to hours. Another distinguishing feature is the rapid, irregular rate (about 100–250 bpm in adults; 150–275 bpm in infants). Automatic junctional tachycardia initiation is not related to a premature atrial impulse and prolonged A-V nodal conduction as often occurs in reentrant A-V nodal tachycardia (Chapter 11).

In the junctional ectopic tachycardia shown in Figure 3-23, the first three junctional complexes at the left are aberrantly conducted and atrioventricular dissociation is present. Tachycardia continues with an irregular ventricular CL of 320–360 ms (rate of 165–180 bpm). Each QRS which has a normal morphology, is preceded by a His bundle electrogram (H in the HBE recording), indicating an origin either in the A-V node or proximal His bundle (see section on His bundle recordings). At the atrial level (HRA) the frequency is half of that at the His level indicating 2-to-1 conduction between the A-V junction and the atrium. The mechanism for the irregularity of the ventricular rate is unknown; it is not related to atrial capture.

A-V DISSOCIATION AND JUNCTIONAL RHYTHMS

When A-V dissociation occurs during accelerated junctional rhythms or tachycardia, it is supportive of an automatic junctional mechanism. A-V dissociation occurs when the atria remain under the control of a sinus node or atrial pacemaker while the ventricles are driven by an independent junctional pacemaker (Figure 3-22, leads I and II show the positive P waves of the sinus node pacemaker). Such independence of atrial and ventricular activation can exist in the presence of normal A-V conduction if the atrial impulse arrives at the A-V node when it is refractory from a prior junctional impulse. Atrial capture of the ventricles for one or more cycles can occur when atrial impulses arrive at the A-V junction after recovery of excitability resulting in incomplete A-V dissociation (see Figure 3-22, in which sinus impulses are conducted to the ventricles in lead II, impulses 2, 5, and 8). Retrograde conduction can also occur from the junctional focus to the atria (Figure 3-21, see lead II, impulses 4, 5, and 6 from the left). The presence of A-V dissociation is evidence for an automatic junctional mechanism since it excludes atrial tachycardia (automatic or reentrant) as well as A-V reentrant tachycardia, all of which have related atrial and ventricular activity.

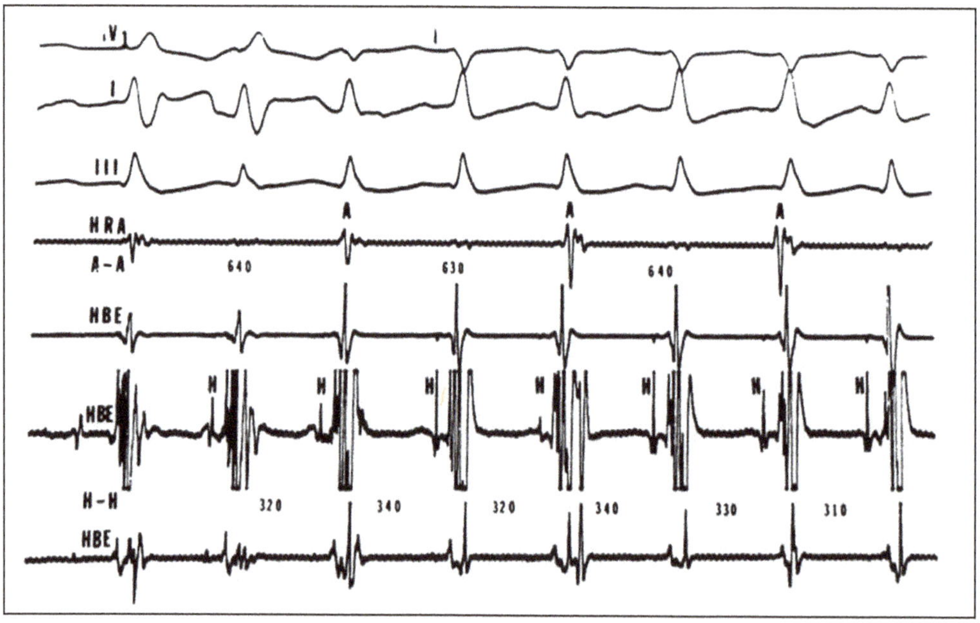

Figure 3-23 ECG leads V_1, I, and III, bipolar electrograms from the high right atrium (HRA) and His bundle (HBE) during JET. The atrial (A-A intervals) and ventricular CL (R-R intervals) are shown below the HRA and HBE recordings. (Reproduced from Ruder MA, Davis JC, et al. Clinical and electrophysiologic characterization of automatic junctional tachycardia in adults. *Circulation*. 1986;73:930–937.)

DETERMINING THE SITE OF ORIGIN OF JUNCTIONAL ARRHYTHMIAS

Limitations of the Relationship of the P Waves to the QRS

In the past, A-V junctional rhythms had been classified into upper, middle, and lower A-V nodal rhythms based on the relationship of the P waves to the QRS. It was assumed that if the origin was in an automatic focus in the upper or atrio-nodal (AN) region (upper nodal rhythms), P waves would precede QRS complexes because of rapid access of junctional impulses to the atria and delayed conduction through the A-V node to the ventricles. For rhythms arising in a focus in the mid-nodal (N) region (mid-nodal rhythms), P and QRS complexes coincide because retrograde conduction time to the atria and antegrade conduction time to the ventricles would be approximately equal. For rhythms arising in an automatic focus in the lower node (NH) or His bundle (H) (lower nodal rhythms), the QRS would precede the P wave since conduction retrograde through the A-V node would delay access to the atria until after the junctional impulse had entered the ventricles.

This classification, however, is not accurate, since variations in antegrade and retrograde conduction times can alter the predicted relationship between P and QRS. For example, a rhythm arising in the mid-nodal region might have P waves preceding the QRS if there is excessive delay in antegrade activation to the ventricles, or P waves following the QRS if there is delay in retrograde activation to the atria. Therefore, additional criteria are helpful in locating the junctional focus to either the A-V node (although upper cannot usually be distinguished from middle) or lower node-His bundle. These criteria include the characteristics of the His bundle electrogram and the response to autonomics, adenosine, and electrical stimulation. Many of these criteria are summarized in Table 3-2 at the end of this section on A-V automaticity.

His Bundle Recordings and Location of an Automatic Junctional Focus

Ideally, locating an A-V junctional pacemaker would best be accomplished by recording electrical activity directly from the different components of the junction and constructing activation maps during an arrhythmia. Unfortunately, this approach is not feasible because of the difficulty in recording an extracellular signal from the A-V node in clinical studies. The reason is that the small magnitude of extracellular current flow because of the small size of the node and low amplitude slow action potentials are difficult to detect with standard electrogram recording techniques.

Recordings from an electrode catheter positioned at the A-V junction, called a His bundle electrogram (HBE), show atrial activity in the low right atrial septum at the atrial margin of the A-V node (A), and His bundle activity (H), but not "true" A-V nodal activity, which occurs between the two (**Figure 3-24**). Ventricular activation in the region of the catheter (V) is also evident. The time interval between the A and H electrograms (A-H interval) indicates conduction from the low atrial recording site, through the A-V node to the His bundle-recording site. The time interval from the H electrogram to the V electrogram (H-V interval) indicates conduction time from the His bundle recording site to ventricular myocardium in the region of the catheter.

In Figure 3-24, in the left panel (labeled "proximal"), the catheter is placed in a position so as to record an electrogram from the proximal His bundle (near its junction with the lower node). In the right panel ("distal"), the catheter is in a position to record from the His bundle towards the bifurcation of the bundle branches. As a result, the His bundle deflection in this distal recording occurs with more of a delay after the atrial deflection (A-H interval of 130 ms) than the electrogram from the proximal bundle (A-H interval of 70 ms). The A-H interval for the distal recording site includes both A-V nodal and some His bundle conduction time while the A-H interval for the proximal recording site is determined mainly by A-V nodal conduction time.

In contrast, the H-V interval at the proximal recording site includes conduction through most of the His bundle and is longer (100 ms) than the distal recording site which includes only that part of the conducting system distal to that site (40 ms).

The HBE does not identify A-V nodal electrical activity, which is not recorded. The HBE usually can only verify that a pacemaker is in the A-V junction and usually cannot distinguish between A-V nodal and His bundle origin. In a limited number of situations it can localize the pacemaker to the His bundle. The following examples illustrate the utility of the HBE in localizing an A-V junctional pacemaker.

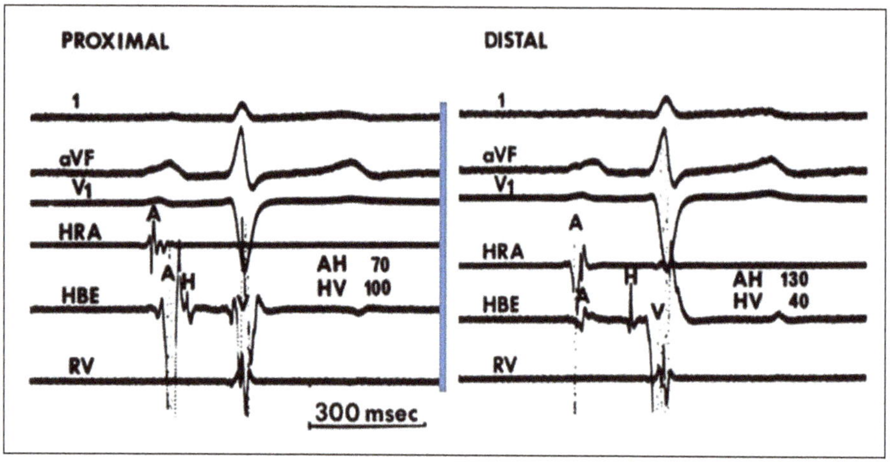

Figure 3-24 His bundle electrograms (HBE) with catheter position at the proximal His bundle (**left**), catheter position at the distal His bundle (**right**). ECG leads 1, aVF, and V_1 and intracardiac recordings from an electrode catheter in the high right atrium (HRA), at the A-V junction (HBE), and right ventricular apex (RV). The HBE recording includes an atrial electrogram (A), an electrogram from the bundle of His (H) and ventricle (V). A-H and H-V intervals are labeled. (Reproduced from Josephson ME. *Josephson's Clinical Cardiac Electrophysiology: Techniques and Interpretations* (5th ed.). Philadelphia, PA: Wolters Kluwer; 2016.)

Origin Proximal to the HBE Recording Site

A junctional escape rhythm after failure of sinus node impulse initiation is shown in **Figure 3-25**. The QRS complex is normal. The origin is not in the atrium since the atrial electrogram (HRA) occurs after the onset of the QRS in the surface leads. The origin of this rhythm in the A-V junctional region is indicated by a His bundle electrogram (H in the HBE recording) that precedes each ventricular depolarization (RVA, bottom recording), showing an origin proximal to the HBE recording site. The interval between His electrogram and ventricular electrogram is 45 ms, which is within the normal range for conduction of a sinus impulse when the His bundle catheter is positioned in a mid to distal His bundle location (Figure 3-24). These features (H deflection preceding the ventricular depolarization with a normal conduction interval) occur when junctional impulse initiation is proximal to the HBE recording site with normal propagation from the site of initiation past the recording site to the ventricles. Further distinction between proximal His bundle and A-V nodal origin in this case is not possible.

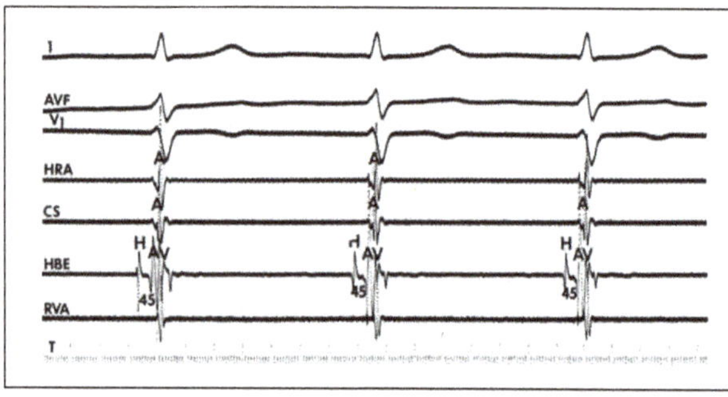

Figure 3-25 Junctional escape rhythm. ECG leads I, aVF, and V_1, and electrograms from high right atrium (HRA), coronary sinus (CS), His bundle region (HBE), and right ventricular apex (RVA). The HBE includes an H deflection indicating His bundle activity, A indicating atrial activity, and V indicating ventricular activity. (Reproduced from Josephson ME. *Josephson's Clinical Cardiac Electrophysiology: Techniques and Interpretations* (5th ed.). Philadelphia, PA: Wolters Kluwer; 2016.)

Origin Distal to the HBE Recording Site

An H-V interval during junctional rhythm that is shorter than the H-V interval during a conducted sinus impulse or an H electrogram superimposed on the ventricular electrogram usually indicates impulse origin distal to the His bundle recording site with retrograde His bundle activation. The retrograde conduction time from the site of impulse origin is less than antegrade conduction time through the His bundle. If the QRS complexes are normal in this situation, it can be assumed that impulse origin is in the distal His bundle, before the origin of the bundle branches. If impulse initiation is not in the A-V junction but rather in the ventricles, the QRS would be aberrant, ventricular depolarization would occur before His bundle depolarization and the His bundle electrogram might not be discernible because it would be buried in the larger ventricular electrogram.

Origin in the Mid or Upper A-V Node

The rapid retrograde conduction to the atria in Figure 3-25, with atrial activation in the high right atrium (HRA) and coronary sinus region (CS) coinciding with the ventricular electrogram, favors an origin in the mid or upper A-V node. However, as previously explained, the relationship of atrial to ventricular activation is not an accurate predictor since retrograde and antegrade conduction may vary in different cases. In this example, the retrograde conduction from a His bundle pacemaker might be more rapid than anterograde conduction if a "fast" A-V nodal pathway is traversed in the retrograde direction (see Chapter 11 for a description of slow and fast A-V nodal conduction pathways).

Complete Block Within the His Bundle

With complete block in the A-V node, when the pacemaker is in the lower A-V node distal to the site of block or proximal His bundle, a His bundle electrogram (recorded distal to the site of block) occurs prior to a normal QRS similar to the recordings during sinus node failure as previously described in Figure 3-25. On the other hand, if complete block is in the His bundle, distal to the recording site, a His bundle electrogram can be recorded after each blocked atrial impulse. If the QRS of the escape rhythm is normal, the pacemaker is in the His bundle distal to the site of block.

In the case of complete heart block shown in **Figure 3-26** (atrial rate (AR) of 110 beats/min and a ventricular rate (VR) of 46 beats/min), the His bundle recording catheter is positioned at the site of conduction block within the His bundle, and therefore, records His bundle activity both proximal and distal to the site of block. The His bundle recording shows an H_1 deflection after each atrial depolarization (P wave) (black arrows) with an AH (PH) interval of 130 ms, representing atrial conduction through the AV node to the recording site just proximal to where block occurs. The His bundle deflection H_2 that precedes each normal QRS (R) (unfilled arrows) results from automaticity in the His bundle just distal to the site of block. The H_2-V interval that represents conduction time from the His bundle pacemaker to the ventricular muscle is approximately normal for a distal catheter location, indicating that the pacemaker is located in the distal His bundle.Origin of Junctional Tachycardias

The same principles previously discussed apply to more rapid junctional rhythms. For the junctional ectopic tachycardia shown in Figure 3-23, a His bundle electrogram (H) in the second from the bottom HBE recording, occurs before each normal QRS with a normal H-V interval, indicating that the automatic focus is in the A-V node or proximal His bundle. A more distal location would be suggested by a shortened H-V interval or simultaneous H and V deflections as described above.

Locating the Automatic Focus by ANS Response: Parasympathetic Activation and Block

The response of a junctional arrhythmia to changes in ANS activity, particularly the parasympathetic nervous system, can localize an automatic focus to either the A-V node or His bundle. Junctional rhythms originating in the A-V node are slowed by parasympathetic activation (e.g., carotid sinus massage [CSM]) and accelerated by parasympathetic block (atropine). Parasympathetic stimulation or block has little or no effect on junctional rhythms originating in the His bundle. These properties are based on the more extensive parasympathetic innervation of the A-V node than His bundle and the greater effect of ACh on pacemaker activity in A-V node than His bundle described in Figure 3-16 and Table 3-2.

A-V Nodal Pacemaker Response

Figure 3-27 shows an A-V nodal pacemaker response to atropine in a patient with complete A-V block and a junctional rhythm (normal QRS). The top recording shows the control rhythm with a sinus rate of 65 bpm and a junctional rate (HR) of 40 bpm. After atropine administration (bottom record), both sinus and junctional impulse initiation accelerated, sinus to 165 bpm and junctional (HR) to 75 bpm, while A-V block was maintained. The junctional acceleration is the response expected of an A-V nodal pacemaker.

Lower Nodal or His Bundle Pacemaker Response

In **Figure 3-28**, the junctional pacemaker in another patient with complete heart block is little affected by vagal activation and block, consistent with a lower nodal or His bundle pacemaker.

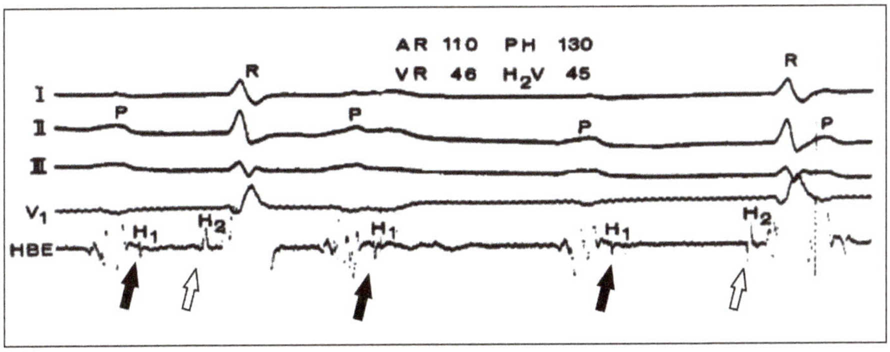

Figure 3-26 ECG leads I, II, III, and V_1 and an His bundle electrogram (HBE) recorded during complete heart block. (Reproduced from Rosen KM, Dhingra RC, et al. Chronic heart block in adults. Clinical and electrophysiological observations. *Arch Intern Med.* 1973;131:663–672.)

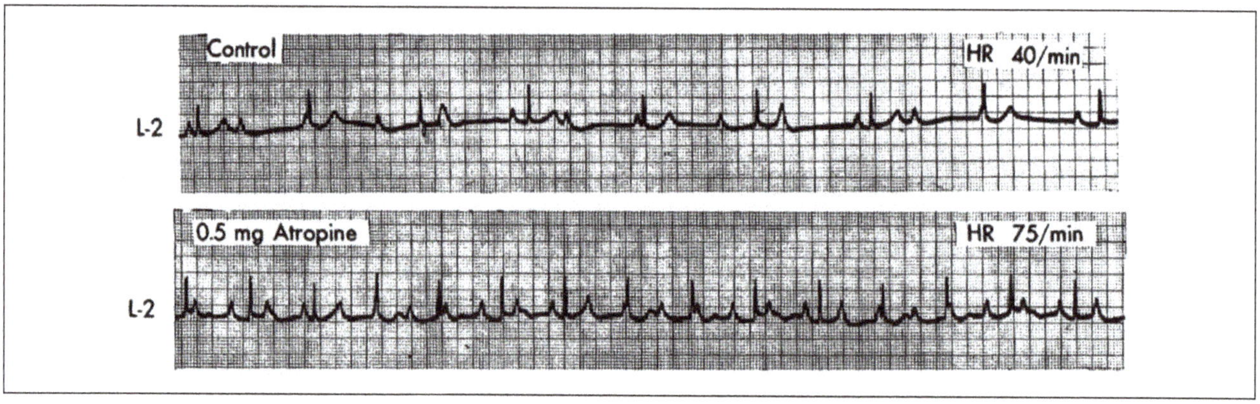

Figure 3-27 ECG lead 2 in a patient with complete A-V bock before (Control) and 3 min after administration of 0.5 mg of atropine. HR, ventricular heart rate. (Reproduced from Narula OS, Scherlag BJ, et al. Analysis of the A-V conduction defect in complete heart block utilizing His bundle electrograms. *Circulation*. 1970;41;437–448.)

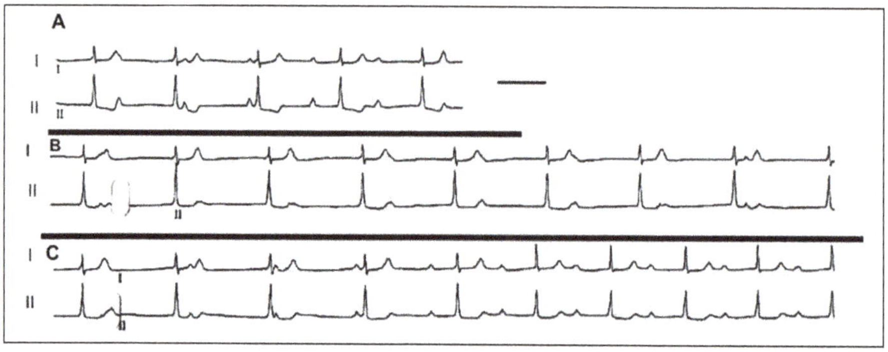

Figure 3-28 ECG leads I and II showing complete A-V block. **Panel A:** Control. **Panel B:** Carotid sinus massage. **Panel C:** Atropine.

Figure 3-28, Panel A shows the control rhythm with complete heart block, a normal QRS, and a ventricular rate of around 40 bpm. In Panel B, during application of carotid sinus massage (CSM) to enhance vagal activity, the ventricular rate slows only slightly while sinus rate is markedly slowed. In Panel C, after the administration of atropine just prior to the recording, the junctional rate is little changed from control, although there is a significant increase in the sinus rate by the end of the record.

Junctional Tachycardia and Parasympathetic Effects

The same differential effect of vagal activation and block on the A-V node and His bundle pacemakers is expected to occur with accelerated junctional rhythms and tachycardia as just described for slow A-V junctional escape rhythms. Carotid sinus massage has variable effects on junctional ectopic tachycardia (JET), having no effect in some patients consistent with His bundle automaticity, and transiently slowing tachycardia in others consistent with A-V nodal automaticity (Table 3-2). In other patients, tachycardia can be terminated, consistent with delayed afterdepolarization (DAD)-dependent triggered activity (see Chapter 6).

Sympathetic Stimulation

Since β-adrenergic stimulation increases automaticity in both A-V node and His bundle, acceleration of the rate of junctional rhythms occurs with sympathetic stimulation (exercise, for example) or β_1-adrenergic agonists and slows with β_1-adrenergic blockers, no matter the site of origin within the A-V junctional region. Adrenergic stimulation with exercise or isoproterenol can initiate junctional ectopic tachycardia and increase their rate consistent with effects on pacemakers either in the A-V node or His bundle.

Response to Adenosine and Other Drugs to Locate Automatic Focus

Adenosine

A different response of A-V nodal and His bundle pacemakers to adenosine can distinguish between an A-V nodal and His bundle pacemaker location. A-V nodal cells have adenosine receptors. If the junctional pacemaker is located in the A-V node during complete A-V block, adenosine transiently slows or suppresses SDD and the ventricular rate.

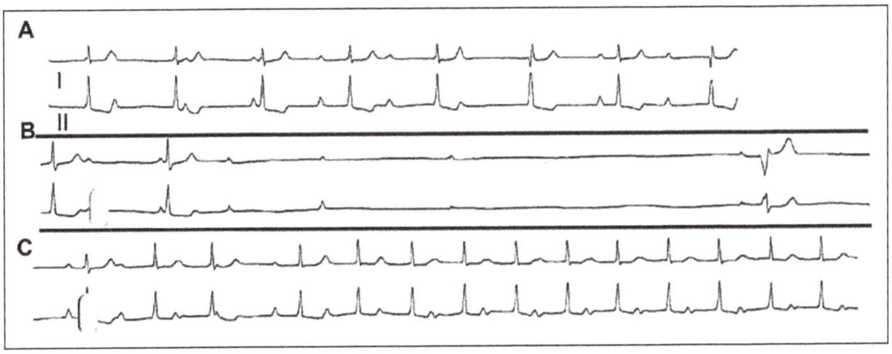

Figure 3-29 ECG leads I and II showing complete A-V block. **Panel A** shows control rhythm, **Panel B** shows the effects of adenosine, and **Panel C** recovery after adenosine.

The response to adenosine of a junctional pacemaker in the A-V node is illustrated In **Figure 3-29**. Panel A shows control ECG recordings from a patient with complete heart block (sinus rate is 75 bpm, junctional rate is 50 bpm). In Panel B, adenosine administration suppresses the junctional as well as the sinus node pacemaker; as is expected of a pacemaker in the A-V node. Panel C shows the return of rapid junctional and sinus rates after the adenosine effect dissipated due to a reflex response to the decreased blood pressure that occurred with adenosine.

Lack of an adenosine effect on the junctional rhythm suggests location of an A-V junctional pacemaker in the His bundle. Adenosine has minimal effect on pacemakers in the ventricular conducting system in the absence of sympathetic stimulation, and the same response would be expected for a His bundle pacemaker.

Adenosine sometimes terminates A-V junctional tachycardia demonstrating that this arrhythmia has multiple mechanisms. Transient slowing occurs when the pacemaker is in the A-V node. Lack of an effect occurs when the pacemaker is in the His bundle. When a junctional arrhythmia is terminated by adenosine it is likely to be caused by DAD- triggered activity that is described in Chapter 5.

Verapamil

Drugs that blocks L-type Ca^{2+} channels and decrease I_{CaL}, such as verapamil, also have differential effects on A-V nodal and His bundle automaticity. I_{CaL} plays a major role in A-V nodal action potential phase 0 depolarization and contributes to the pacemaker potential, similar to the sinus node. On the other hand, it has a much lesser role in automaticity originating from the His bundle. I_{CaL} is not involved in His bundle phase 0 depolarization and conduction and plays less of a role in the pacemaker potential causing normal automaticity.

Therefore, although clinical data is not available, when automaticity is the mechanism, verapamil is expected to slow both escape junctional rhythms and junctional tachycardias originating in the A-V node but not suppress junctional automatic rhythms or tachycardias originating in the His bundle. Verapamil can also stop junctional tachycardia when it is caused by DAD-triggered activity since DADs are suppressed by verapamil (Chapter 5).

Lidocaine

Lidocaine, which is a Na^+ channel-blocking drug, also has a differential effect on junctional arrhythmias. It slows Purkinje cell pacemaker activity (assumed to have a similar mechanism as His bundle automaticity), thereby slowing the automatic rate of a His bundle junctional pacemaker, while having minimal effects on an A-V nodal junctional pacemaker. The different effects can be explained by the lack of participation of I_{Na} in the generation of A-V nodal action potentials and a lesser role of I_f in nodal automaticity; whereas I_{Na} plays a major role in Purkinje cell action potentials and I_f is an important current for Purkinje cell automaticity (Figure 3-31). Lidocaine slows automaticity to a large extent by decreasing I_f. In assessing the responses of junctional rhythms to lidocaine, it is important to consider the role of ischemia. Tissue in the junction can be depressed by pathophysiology such as ischemia, which may enhance lidocaine's A-V nodal depressant effects on both conduction and automaticity.

Overdrive Stimulation to Locate an A-V Junctional Automatic Focus

A-V junctional pacemakers show transient suppression after overdrive, typical of the effects of overdrive on automaticity. Two factors may distinguish between an A-V nodal pacemaker and a His bundle pacemaker. One is the dependence of overdrive suppression on the location of the site of stimulation, and the second is the different sensitivity of the A-V node and His bundle to stimulation (Table 3-2).

Site of stimulation. The site of stimulation influences access of the stimulated impulses to the pacemaker site. For this reason, the site of stimulation might sometimes be useful in differentiating A-V nodal location from His bundle location of a junctional pacemaker. Overdrive pacing from the atria is expected to more easily access an A-V nodal pacemaker than a His bundle pacemaker especially at rapid overdrive rates. If rapid pacing from an atrial site has more of a suppressive effect on the junctional pacemaker than rapid pacing at the same rate, from a ventricular site, the pacemaker is likely to be in the A-V node or A-V node-atrial region. Rapid ventricular pacing might result in conduction block of retrograde impulses in the A-V junction before they reached the pacemaker site while rapid pacing from the atria is more likely to reach the pacemaker site with block occurring distal to that site.

On the other hand, if the pacemaker is located in the lower node (NH) or His bundle, rapid pacing from the ventricles is likely to have more of an suppressive effect than pacing from the atria at the same rate since it is more likely than some atrial paced impulses will block in the A-V junction before reaching the pacemaker site than ventricular-paced impulses.

Sensitivity to overdrive suppression. Another feature that distinguishes A-V nodal from His bundle pacemakers is a different sensitivity to overdrive. The effects on A-V nodal pacemakers are likely to be less than on His bundle pacemakers owing to the nature of their action potentials. I_{CaL}-dependent depolarization phase 0 in A-V nodal cells results in less Na^+ loading during overdrive similar to the sinus node than in His bundle cells with a Na^+-dependent depolarization phase 0. His bundle pacemakers are expected to respond with greater suppression, similar to the effects of overdrive on pacemakers in the more distal conducting system (Figure 1-7 and Section 3C on Ventricular Normal Automaticity and Automatic Arrhythmias).

However, the exact location of the pacemaker cannot always be certain since modification of the overdrive effect by disease of the junction cannot be discounted. In most cases, since the data are from patients with heart block, pathophysiology such as ischemia might make an A-V nodal pacemaker more sensitive to overdrive so it cannot be distinguished from a His bundle pacemaker.

Accelerated Junctional Rhythms and Tachycardias

The effects of overdrive stimulation on accelerated junctional rhythms and tachycardias are complicated since multiple mechanisms cause these arrhythmias. While some of these arrhythmias respond to overdrive with the typical features of overdrive suppression indicative of an automatic mechanism, some show overdrive acceleration, which is characteristic of abnormal automaticity (see Chapter 4) or DAD-dependent triggered activity (Chapter 5). Failure to initiate or terminate some junctional tachycardias by overdrive stimulation is also suggestive of an automatic mechanism. However, some junctional tachycardias are initiated and terminated by stimulation because they are caused by either DAD-induced triggered activity (Chapter 5) or reentry (Chapter 11).

Programmed Premature Stimulation

There are little data available describing the response of A-V junctional pacemakers to premature stimulation protocols. Some ectopic junctional tachycardias are initiated and terminated by premature stimuli, which would indicate DAD-triggered activity as their mechanism rather than automaticity. Occasionally, a resetting response to premature impulses has been observed which might be expected of normal automaticity. The characteristics of resetting are predicted to be dependent on the site of stimulation relative to the pacemaker site as described for overdrive suppression. When the stimulation site is separated from the pacemaker site by some A-V nodal tissue (e.g., ventricular stimulation with an upper nodal pacemaker), there is more conduction delay of both the premature impulse to the pacemaker site and the reset spontaneous impulse to the measurement site. In this situation, the resetting curves likely resemble the one for sinus node in Figure 2-14, with the return cycle greater than the spontaneous cycle because of the conduction delays. On the other hand, ventricular stimulation of a His bundle pacemaker might entail minimal conduction delay and the return cycle would more closely mimic the automatic cycle.

COMPARISON OF A-V NODE AND HIS BUNDLE PACEMAKER CHARACTERISTICS

Table 3-2 summarizes and compares the characteristics of A-V junctional pacemakers in the A-V node and His bundle that were previously described. These characteristics can be used to determine the site and mechanism of impulse initiation of an automatic arrhythmia arising in the A-V junction.

Table 3-2 Comparison of A-V Node and His Bundle Pacemaker Characteristics

	A-V Node Automaticity	His Bundle Automaticity
Intrinsic Rate (impulses/min)	30–55	30–45
Sympathetic acceleration	++++	+++
Parasympathetic inhibition	++++ (does not terminate)	Little effect
Adenosine inhibition	++++ (does not terminate)	+?
I_{CaL} block inhibition	++++ (can terminate)	Little effect
I_{Na} block inhibition	Little effect	++++ (can terminate)
Overdrive suppression	+++ (does not terminate)	++++ (does not terminate)
Premature stimulation	+++ (does not terminate)	+++ (does not terminate)

++++ is an indication of the qualitative magnitude in each area

BYPASS TRACT AUTOMATICITY

In addition to the normal A-V conducting system, there are other connections between atria and ventricles in some patients, called "accessory pathways" or "bypass tracts." They provide an alternative conducting pathway of atrial impulses to the ventricles, which sometimes enables them to bypass the A-V node and His bundle (see Chapter 11). Automatic impulse initiation can occur in cells of some of these bypass tracts to cause escape rhythms or tachycardias. We classify these arrhythmias as normally automatic since automaticity appears to be a normal property of bypass tract cells although transmembrane potentials showing SDD have not been recorded.

The heat generated by RF current used to ablate bypass tracts causes automatic arrhythmias. It is likely to be a stimulus accelerating SDD as it does in A-V nodal cells.

SUMMARY

Action potentials and automaticity in different regions of the A-V conducting system, have different characteristics. The distinguishing features of the nodal (N) cells in the compact node (CN) are the less negative resting potential, and a slow phase 0 depolarization that is dependent on $I_{CaL.}$ SDD likely resembles the sinus node with a small role for I_f and a larger role for I_{CaL} and I_{NCX}. The lower node (NH region) and His bundle have more negative resting membrane potentials, a faster phase 0 depolarization that has a significant I_{Na} component, and a greater role for I_f than I_{NCX} in generating SDD.

The intrinsic rate of impulse initiation is faster in the atrio-nodal (AN) and CN regions than in the His bundle. Automaticity is accelerated in all regions by sympathetic stimulation. Parasympathetic stimulation suppresses automaticity (but does not stop it entirely) in the AN and CN regions while His bundle automaticity is little affected. Likewise, adenosine transiently suppresses automaticity in the AN and CN region while having little effect on automaticity in the His bundle. Automaticity in the A-V node (CN) is stopped by Ca^{2+}-channel blockers (verapamil) but not by Na^+-channel blockers (lidocaine), while automaticity in the His bundle shows the opposite effects. Overdrive stimulation has less of a suppressant effect on A-V node SDD because of the minimal contribution of Na^+ current to the action potential, than His bundle automaticity that has Na^+ current-dependent phase 0.

Automatic arrhythmias arising in the A-V junction are caused by two primary mechanisms: pacemaker escape and acceleration of pacemaker impulse initiation.

Escape rhythms occur after suppression of sinus node impulse initiation and/or conduction such as in sick sinus syndrome. ECG characteristics can identify an automatic focus in the A-V junction, but cannot usually pinpoint the exact origin. The intrinsic heart rate of (escape) rhythms arising in the A-V node is about 30–55 bpm, while the heart rate when the pacemaker is in the His bundle is about 30–40 bpm, although there is considerable overlap. A His bundle electrogram (HBE) can locate the focus to the A-V junction, but only distinguishes an A-V nodal from a His bundle origin when there is A-V block in the His bundle with a His electrogram following the blocked atrial depolarization. Programmed stimulation or response to autonomic agonists or drugs that block different ion channels can be used to distinguish between an A-V node and His bundle site of impulse initiation.

Accelerated A-V junctional rhythms (~100 bpm) and A-V junctional tachycardias (~120–150 bpm) are both a result of enhanced SDD either in the A-V node or His bundle. Junctional ectopic tachycardia (JET) can reach a rate of ~250 bpm. They are not initiated by a premature impulse as are DAD-triggered and A-V reentrant tachycardias. A junctional origin is indicated by a normal QRS that is not preceded by a sinus P wave. P-wave and HBE characteristics are the same as for slower junctional rhythms previously described. A-V dissociation is indicative of an automatic mechanism.

Tachycardias arising in the A-V node are suppressed by parasympathetic stimulation, adenosine, and Ca^{2+}-channel blocking drugs, all of which do not have significant effects on arrhythmias arising in the His bundle (Table 3-2). The response to overdrive stimulation can also confirm an automatic mechanism and locate the site of origin. The effects on A-V nodal pacemakers are likely to be less than on His bundle pacemakers.

SOURCES

Basic Electrophysiology

Anderson RH, Ho SY. The morphology of the specialized atrioventricular junctional area: The evolution of understanding. *Pacing Clin Electrophysiol.* 2002;25:957–966.

Dobrzynski H, Nikolski VP, Sambelashvili AT, et al. Site of origin and molecular substrate of atrioventricular junctional rhythm in the rabbit heart. *Circ Res.* 2003;93:1102–1110.

Hariman RJ, Chen C-M. Recording of diastolic slope from the junctional area in dogs with junctional rhythm. *Circulation.* 1983;68:636–643.

Hucker WJ, McCain ML, Laughner JI, et al. Connexin43 expression delineates two discrete pathways in the human atrioventricular junction. *Anat Rec.* 2008;291:204–215.

Hucker WJ, Nikolski VP, Efimov IR. Autonomic control and innervation of the atrioventricular junctional pacemaker. *Heart Rhythm.* 2007;4:1326–1335.

Li J, Greener ID, Inada S, et al. Computer three-dimensional reconstruction of the atrioventricular node. *Circ Res.* 2008;102: 975–985.

Meijler FL, Janse MJ. Morphology and electrophysiology of the mammalian atrioventricular node. *Physiol Rev.* 1988;68:608–639.

Rosen MR, Danilo P Jr, Weiss RM. Actions of adenosine on normal and abnormal impulse initiation in canine ventricle. *Am J Physiol Heart Circ Physiol.*1983;13:H715–H721.

Scherlag BJ, Lazzara R, Helfant RH. Differentiation of "A-V junctional rhythms." *Circulation.* 1973;48:304–312.

Clinical Electrophysiology

Aravindakshan V, Kuo C-S, Gettes LS. Effect of lidocaine on escape rate in patients with complete atrioventricular block: A. Distal His bundle block. *Am J Cardiol.* 1977;40:177–183.

Boyle NG, Anselme F, Monahan K, et al. Origin of junctional rhythm during radiofrequency ablation of atrioventricular nodal reentrant tachycardia in patients without structural heart disease. *Am J Cardiol.* 1997;80:575–580.

Castellanos A, Sung RJ, Castillo CA, et al. His bundle recordings in diagnosis of impulse formation in Kent and Mahaim tracts. *Br Heart J.* 1976;38:1173–1178.

Collins KK, Van Hare GF, Kertesz NJ, et al. Pediatric nonpost-operative junctional ectopic tachycardia. Medical management and interventional therapies. *J Am Coll Cardiol.* 2009;53:690–697.

Cosio FG, Anderson RH, Kuck K-H, et al. Living anatomy of the atrioventricular junctions. A guide to electrophysiologic mapping. A consensus statement from the Cardiac Nomenclature Study Group, Working Group of Arrhythmias, European Society of Cardiology, and the Task Force on Cardiac Nomenclature from NASPE. *Circulation.* 1999;100:e31–e37.

Fisch C, Knoebel SB. Junctional rhythms progress in cardiovascular diseases. *J Am Coll Cardiol.* 1970;13:141–158.

Garson A, Gillette PC. Junctional ectopic tachycardia in children: Electrocardiography, electrophysiology and pharmacologic response. *Am J Cardiol.* 1979;44:298–302.

Hamdan M, MD, Van Hare GF, Fisher W, et al. Selective catheter ablation of the tachycardia focus in patients with nonreentrant junctional tachycardia. *Am J Cardiol.* 1996;78:1292–1297.

Hariman RJ, Gomes JAC, El-Sherif N. Recording of diastolic slope with catheters during junctional rhythm in humans. *Circulation.* 1984;69:485–491.

Inoue S, Becker AE. Posterior extensions of the human compact atrioventricular node. A neglected anatomic feature of potential clinical significance. *Circulation.* 1998;97:188–193.

Knoebel SB, Fisch C. Accelerated junctional escape: A clinical and electrocardiographic study. *Circulation.* 1974;50:151–158.

Konecke LL, Knoebel SB. Nonparoxysmal junctional tachycardia complicating acute myocardial infarction. *Circulation.* 1972;45:367–374.

Kuo C-S, Reddy CP. Effect of lidocaine on escape rate in patients with complete atrioventricular block: B. Proximal His bundle block. *Am J Cardiol.* 1981;47:1315–1320.

Lee KL, Chun HM, Liem LB, Sung RJ. Effect of adenosine and verapamil in catecholamine-induced accelerated atrioventricular junctional rhythm: Insights into the underlying mechanism. *Pacing Clin Electrophysiol.* 1999; 22[Pt.I]:866–870.

Lerman BB, Belardinelli L. Cardiac electrophysiology of adenosine: Basic and clinical concepts. *Circulation.* 1991;83;1499-1509

Lerman BB, Josephson ME. Automaticity of the Kent bundle: Confirmation by phase 3 and phase 4 block. *J Am Coll CardioI.* 1985;5:996–998.

Lerman BB, Wesley RC, DiMarco JP, et al. Antiadrenergic effects of adenosine on His-Purkinje automaticity. Evidence for accentuated antagonism. *J Clin Invest.* 1988;82:2127–2135.

Matsushita T, Chun S, Sung RJ. Influence of isoproterenol on the accelerated junctional rhythm observed during radiofrequency catheter ablation of atrioventricular nodal slow pathway conduction. *Am Heart J.* 2001;142:664–668.

Narula OS, Narula JT. Junctional pacemakers in man. Response to overdrive suppression with and without parasympathetic blockade. *Circulation.* 1978;57:880–889.

Padanilam BJ, Manfredi JA, Steinberg LA, et al. Differentiating junctional tachycardia and atrioventricular node re-entry tachycardia based on response to atrial extrastimulus pacing. *J Am Coll Cardiol.* 2008;52:1711–1717.

Pick A, Dominguez P. Nonparoxysmal A-V nodal tachycardia. *Circulation.* 1957;16:1022–1032.

Rosen KM. Junctional tachycardia: Mechanisms, diagnosis, differential diagnosis, and management. *Circulation.* 1973;47:654–664.

Scheinman MM, Gonzalez RP, Cooper W, et al. Clinical and electrophysiologic features and role of catheter ablation techniques in adult patients with automatic atrioventricular junctional tachycardia. *Am J Cardiol.* 1994;74:535–572.

Shepard RK, Natale A, Stambler BS, et al. Physiology of the escape rhythm after radiofrequency atrioventricular junctional ablation. *Pacing Clin Electrophysiol.* 1998;21:1085–1092.

SECTION

3C Ventricular Normal Automaticity and Automatic Arrhythmias

Normal automaticity that occurs in specific regions of the ventricles causes ventricular arrhythmias. In this section, ventricular normal automaticity and automatic ventricular arrhythmias are described.

Basic Electrophysiological Mechanisms

LOCATION OF VENTRICULAR PACEMAKERS WITH NORMAL AUTOMATICITY

Normal automaticity in the ventricles occurs in Purkinje cells that form the specialized ventricular conducting system. Normal automaticity is not a property of ventricular muscle.

Purkinje Cell Pacemaker Distribution and Structure

The ventricular specialized conducting system branches from the His bundle to form the left and right bundle branches. The left bundle branch fans out down the left side of the ventricular septum to form the anterior and posterior fascicles and sometimes a third radiation in the mid septal region, the septal fascicle. The right bundle branch courses on the right side of the septum and extends for some distance before dividing into a subdivision that usually passes through the moderator band and other parts extending over the endocardial surface. Both the right and left bundle branches and fascicles that emanate from them are enclosed in fibrous sheaths. As the fascicles course more distally, the fibrous sheath that surrounds them is lost and the Purkinje cells form an extensive subendocardial network.

Purkinje cells in the His bundle and bundle branches have a larger diameter, fewer contractile elements, and more abundant glycogen particles in their cytoplasm compared to ventricular muscle cells. In the most distal conducting system that forms the subendocardial network, Purkinje cells more closely resemble ventricular muscle with increased myofibrils and less cytoplasmic glycogen. The exact anatomical distribution is uncertain because of the structural similarity to contractile muscle, but they are presumed to cover much of the endocardial surface. Transitional cells of the subendocardial Purkinje network make contact with ventricular muscle forming Purkinje–muscle junctions that lead to ventricular muscle activation. The isoforms of connexin (Cx) in the ventricular conducting system are Cx45 and Cx40 in the proximal bundle branches, the same as in the His bundle. In the more distal conducting system, Cx43 occurs in addition to Cx45 and Cx40 (ventricular muscle has primarily Cx43). The connexins in the conducting system have a large conductance that favors rapid impulse propagation.

ELECTROPHYSIOLOGY OF NORMAL AUTOMATICITY IN THE VENTRICLES

Characteristics of the Purkinje Cell Action Potential

A Purkinje cell action potential (PF) is diagrammed in **Figure 3-30** in comparison with action potentials of the sinus node (SAN) (Chapter 2), atrium (ATR) and A-V node (AVN) (Chapter 3, Sections 3A and 3B).

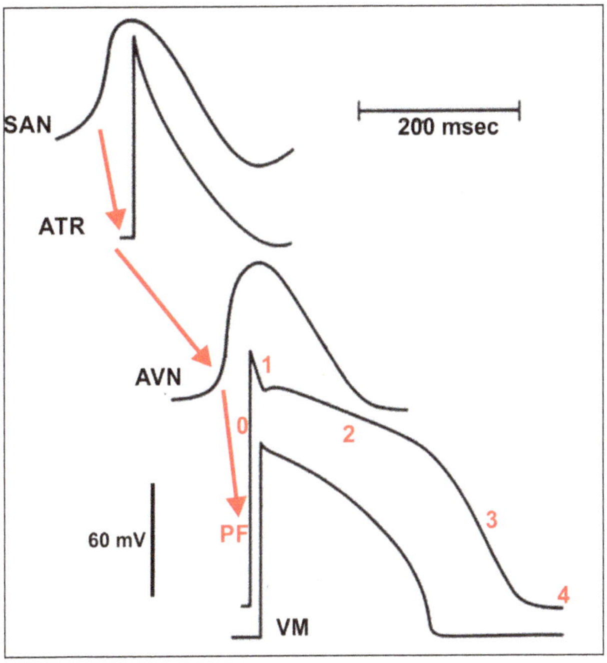

Figure 3-30 Action potentials from Purkinje cell (PF), sinus node cell (SAN), atrial muscle cell (ATR), A-V nodal cell (AVN), and ventricular muscle cell (VM). The phases of the Purkinje action potential labeled with **red numbers**. **Red arrows** point out the sequence of activation. Time and voltage scales indicated.

As Figure 3-30 illustrates, Purkinje cells have a more negative resting potential, (~−85 to −90 mV) than sinus node, A-V node, and His bundle cells due to a larger potassium current (I_{K1}), a more rapid rate of phase 0 depolarization resulting from a large sodium current (I_{Na}) (a cause of rapid impulse conduction), an initial fast repolarization (phase 1) resulting from the transient outward current (I_{to}), a longer, well-defined plateau (phase 2) caused by the long-lasting calcium current (I_{CaL}), and a rapid repolarization (phase 3) resulting from inactivation of I_{CaL} and activation of the delayed rectifier current (I_K comprised of I_{Kr} and I_{Ks}).

The duration of the plateau phase (phase 2) is the main determinant of the Purkinje fiber action potential duration and effective refractory period that is voltage- dependent. The action potential duration and refractory periods increase from His bundle to the distal bundle branches, from which point they decrease until contact is made with ventricular muscle. Action potential duration and refractory periods in general are longer on the right side of the conduction system than on the left. They are also longer than in ventricular muscle cells. The region of maximum action potential duration is sometimes referred to as the "gate," which can be the site of block of premature impulses. During moderately rapid atrial rates (~150 bpm) right bundle branch block (RBBB) occurs before left bundle branch block (LBBB) because of the longer refractory period (phase 3 block; see Figure 9-6). However, at more rapid rates (~180 bpm) LBBB is more prominent. The cause for the reversal is unknown.

Purkinje Cell Pacemaker Potential

Purkinje cells have a pacemaker potential caused by a net inward current (comprised of several inward and outward currents) that causes spontaneous diastolic (phase 4) depolarization (SDD) under appropriate conditions. The top tracing of **Figure 3-31** shows a diagram of action potentials of an automatic Purkinje cell in which SDD is evident (arrow). Below are diagrams of the membrane currents contributing to diastolic depolarization with downward deflections indicating inward currents and upward deflections indicating outward currents similar to Figure 2-6 that displays pacemaker currents in the sinus node. The currents comprising the pacemaker potential in Purkinje cells have some similarities to the sinus node but are not identical.

Inward currents. The primary inward current is the "funny" (I_f) pacemaker current (red). I_f channels are deactivated (closed) during the action-potential upstroke (phase 0) and initial plateau phase of repolarization (phase 2) but are activated as repolarization brings the membrane potential to levels more negative than about −60 mV. Diastolic depolarization begins at a more negative membrane potential than in the sinus node (around −80 mV). Since the activation kinetics are slow, the channels continue to activate throughout diastole, leading to an increasing inward current that contributes to the SDD (Figure 3-31). The I_f current is carried primarily by Na^+ but also has a K^+ component. The I_f channel then deactivates as the upstroke (phase 0) of the spontaneous action potential occurs. The I_f pacemaker current is more prominent in Purkinje cells than in sinus node cells.

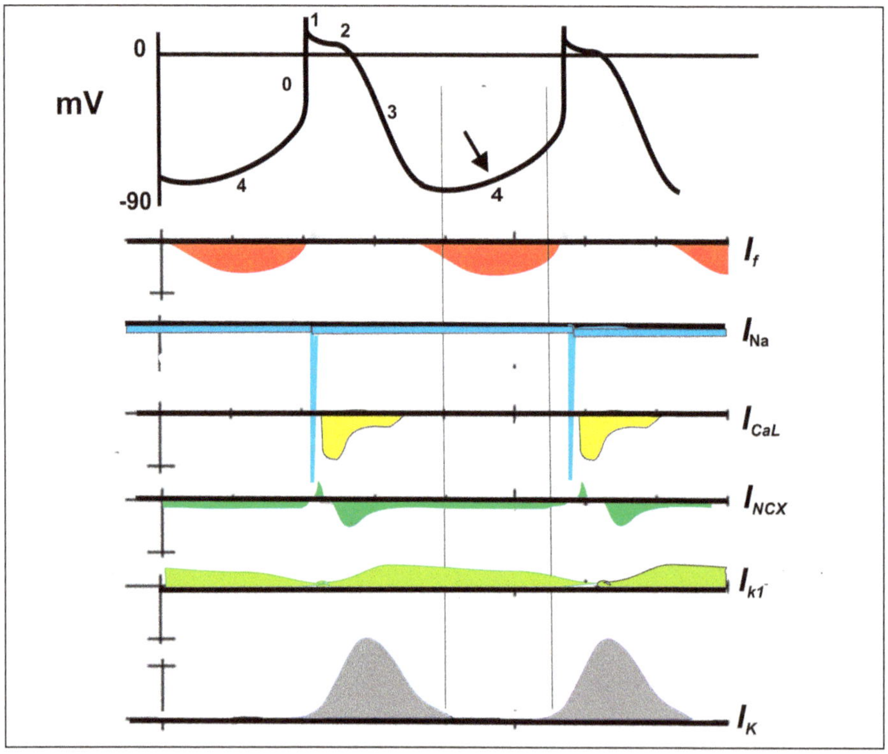

Figure 3-31 Diagram of membrane currents contributing to spontaneous diastolic depolarization (SDD, **arrow**) in Purkinje cells.

Another inwardly directed membrane current that contributes to the pacemaker potential is a Na^+ current called the window or late Na^+ current. The rapid inward current I_{Na} that causes phase 0 of the action potential is indicated by the large, blue, downward spike in the I_{Na} record. The late Na^+ current is a small persistent inward Na^+ current that follows inactivation of the rapid Na^+ current (indicated by the steady blue following the blue spike in the I_{Na} trace).

The Na^+–Ca^{2+} exchange current (I_{NCX}, dark green) that is described in the sections on sinus, atrial, and A-V node pacemakers may also be involved in generation of SDD. Possible contributions of I_{CaL} (yellow) and I_{CaT} (not shown) to the Purkinje cell pacemaker potential still need clarification.

Outward currents. Outward currents also contribute to the pacemaker potential in Purkinje cells. The delayed rectifier potassium current (I_K, Figure 3-31, gray) is activated during the action potential and is a major factor in causing repolarization because it flows outward from the cell, making the inside more negative. I_K channels that participate in repolarization begin to inactivate toward the end of repolarization as membrane potential becomes more negative, leading to a decrease in the repolarizing I_K current. Decay of the I_K current continues after repolarization because the channels slowly inactivate at the negative level of membrane potential. This ongoing inactivation leads to a decrease in outward current that contributes to the overall increase in net inward current of the pacemaker potential.

I_{K1} (light green) is another potassium channel/current that contributes to the pacemaker potential. This current is not prominent in sinus or A-V nodes but is prominent in Purkinje cells. I_{K1} is the major potassium conductance during diastole and is responsible for the high (negative) resting potential. The I_{K1} channels have the property of inward rectification, such that the conductance and outward current flow is large at negative membrane potentials near the potassium equilibrium potential (E_K) and decreases at less negative membrane potentials. Therefore, as the membrane potential depolarizes during the pacemaker potential, the outward current flow through the I_{K1} channels decreases, and this contributes to the increase in net inward current of the pacemaker potential. The presence of a large I_{K1} can partly explain the relatively slow intrinsic automatic rate of Purkinje cells. At the beginning of the period of SDD, net inward current is decreased by the I_{K1} outward flow which decreases later on during pacemaker depolarization.

The outward current generated by the Na^+–K^+ exchange pump (I_P) is present throughout diastole. It is another current that opposes SDD.

Control of Automatic Rate

The intrinsic pacemaker rate of Purkinje cells (the term "Purkinje fibers" is sometimes used which indicate a group of Purkinje cells) is less than the rate of atrial and A-V junctional pacemakers. The rate decreases from about 40–50 impulses/min at the junction with the His bundle, to 25–30 impulses/min in the peripheral Purkinje cells. The rate is more rapid in the distal left ventricular conducting system than the right. Automaticity in the peripheral Purkinje cells that have gap-junction connections with ventricular muscle is suppressed by electrotonic current flow from the muscle in a manner similar to suppression of sinus node automaticity by adjacent non-automatic atrial cells diagrammed in Figure 1-3.

Autonomic Nervous System (ANS) Effects

The ANS is an important controller of automaticity in the ventricular specialized conducting system. The entire conducting system is richly innervated by sympathetic nerves and sparsely innervated by parasympathetic nerves. Purkinje cells have mainly β_1-adrenergic receptors and very few muscarinic (M_2) receptors. Activation of the sympathetic nerves accelerates automaticity by increasing the net inward pacemaker current to increase the slope of spontaneous diastolic depolarization (see Figure 1-2A). The molecular mechanism is similar to the effects of β_1 activation by norepinephrine at the supraventricular pacemaker sites as previously described. It is mainly a result of earlier and faster activation of I_f and increased I_{NCX} through augmenting intracellular Ca^{2+} cycling. Ventricular tachycardia originating in the Purkinje system occurs when the automatic rate is accelerated more than the rate of supraventricular pacemakers.

The parasympathetics may have a small effect to decrease Purkinje cell automaticity since acetylcholine (ACh) decreases inward I_f pacemaker current, but this doesn't seem to have much physiological importance. An exception is when pacemaker activity is accelerated by sympathetic activation; then, parasympathetic activation can slow the automatic rate by decreasing the acceleration effect of the sympathetics by accentuated antagonism.

Mechanical Effects from Stretching

Stretch of the Purkinje system enhances automatic activity and might occur in akinetic areas after acute ischemia, in ventricular aneurysms, or in bulging, failed ventricles. Stretch-induced automaticity may result from the activation of stretch-activated membrane channels and/or production of enhanced Ca^{2+} release and Ca^{2+} waves. Both can cause an inward current during diastolic bulging. Ischemia can also enhance automaticity by increasing net inward diastolic current.

ELECTRICAL STIMULATION OF VENTRICULAR (PURKINJE) PACEMAKERS; OVERDRIVE AND PREMATURE STIMULATION

Purkinje cells have a prominent response to overdrive. Following a period of overdrive, automaticity is suppressed and gradually returns with time. Longer periods of overdrive or more rapid rates of overdrive, result in a longer period of overdrive suppression. The basic mechanism of overdrive suppression is described in Chapter 1. Purkinje cells have a large inward I_{Na} that controls inward Na^+ movement, and a Na^+–K^+ pump that generates a strong pump current (I_p), accounting for the strong overdrive suppression (see Figure 1-6 and Figure 1-7). It is one way by which Purkinje automaticity is suppressed by supraventricular pacemakers.

The effects of programmed premature stimulation on automatic pacemakers is described in Chapter 1 (see Figure 1-10). Like automatic rhythms in atria and A-V junction, premature stimulation neither initiates nor terminates ventricular automaticity in ventricular pacemakers. Purkinje cell pacemakers are reset by premature stimulation with a return CL that is about the same as the spontaneous CL, indicating no major effect of premature activation on SDD. The resetting response resembles the curve shown in Figure 1-11. Conduction delays sometimes influence the resetting response in the ventricles in a similar way to that already described in the resetting response of the sinus node (see Figure 2-14). Such conduction delays can occur across the muscle Purkinje junction when the stimulus site is in the ventricles. Significant delays are less likely when the conduction system is stimulated directly.

PHARMACOLOGICAL AGENTS AND VENTRICULAR PACEMAKERS

Although adenosine may slow automaticity in isolated Purkinje cells in the experimental laboratory, it does not reduce the idioventricular rate in patients with heart block, and therefore probably has little effect on the ventricular (Purkinje) pacemaker mechanism. The lack of response to adenosine distinguishes ventricular arrhythmias caused by normal automaticity from some of the arrhythmias caused by DAD-triggered activity which are suppressed by adenosine (see Chapter 5).

Drugs that block Na^+ channels, like lidocaine or procainamide (e.g., Class I antiarrhythmic drugs in the Vaughan Williams classification), decrease automaticity in Purkinje cells. These drugs have little effect on A-V nodal automaticity and therefore may help distinguish between an A-V nodal and His–Purkinje origin of ventricular arrhythmias. Automaticity in Purkinje cells is decreased as a result of shifting the threshold potential for activation of the Na^+ current to less negative levels and reducing net inward current of the pacemaker potential by decreasing I_f (see Figure 1-2).

L-type Ca^{2+}-channel blockers (e.g., verapamil) have little effect on normal automaticity of Purkinje cells because of the small role of I_{CaL} in genesis of the pacemaker current. However, it has a strong depressant effect on abnormal automaticity described in Chapter 4.

Examples of Arrhythmias Caused by Alterations in Ventricular Automaticity

Normal automaticity in the ventricle can cause slow escape rhythms, accelerated ventricular rhythms, or specific types of ventricular tachycardia.

VENTRICULAR ESCAPE RHYTHMS

The ECG in **Figure 3-32** is from a patient with complete heart (A-V) block; the sinus node impulse is unable to pass through the A-V junction to excite the ventricles. The ECG shows A-V dissociation, with no relationship between automatic firing of the sinus node pacemaker (P-wave rate of about 85 bpm) and the pacemaker in the ventricles (QRS rate of 35 bpm). The ventricular rate is typical for a normally automatic distal Purkinje pacemaker. However, in some cases the escape rate may be significantly slower. The QRS is 120 ms wide and has a configuration indicating a pacemaker in the left posterior (inferior) fascicle.

In the presence of complete block, activation and overdrive suppression of latent pacemakers with normal automaticity distal to the site of block is removed, enabling a site in the A-V junction or ventricular conducting system to become the pacemaker of the ventricles. A-V junctional pacemakers (in the A-V node and His bundle) are described in the previous section of this chapter. When A-V block is in the distal His bundle or both bundle branches (bilateral bundle branch block), pacemaker escape occurs in the bundle branches distal to the site of block or in the distal Purkinje system.

In the absence of complete A-V block, ventricular escape rhythms are rare. Clinically, sinus bradycardia or arrest associated with enhanced vagal activity or sick sinus syndrome usually leads to escape of an A-V junctional pacemaker because of their faster intrinsic rate (Figure 3-20).

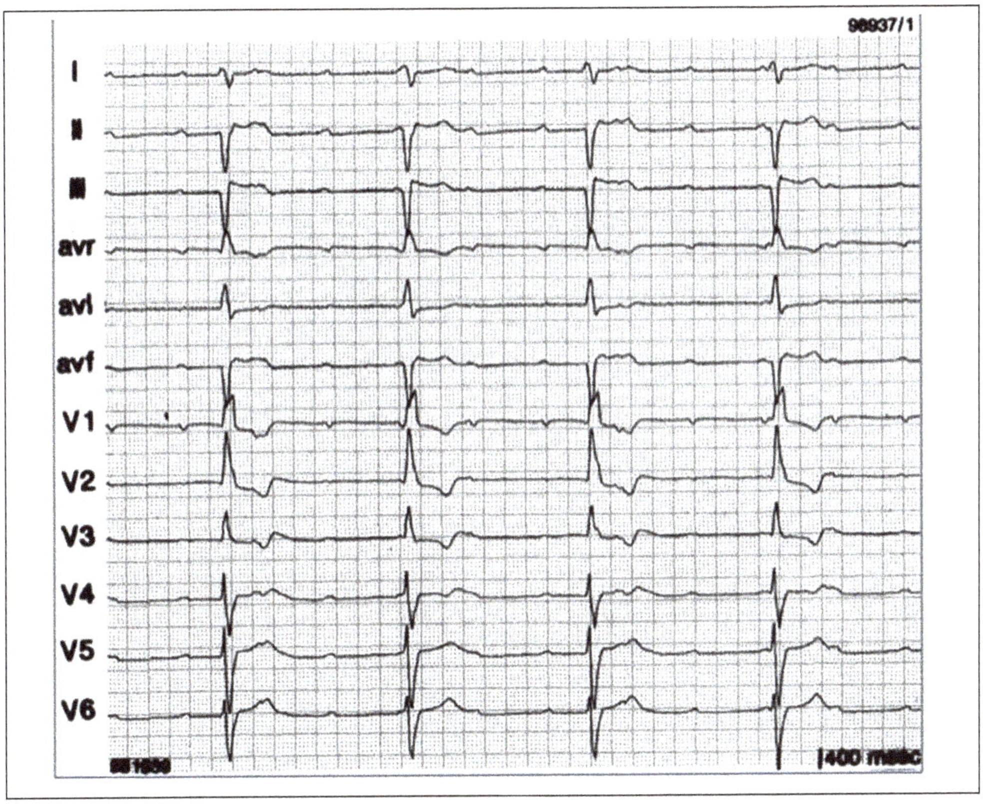

Figure 3-32 A 12-lead ECG recorded from a patient with complete heart block (Wellens' ECG collection).

It is possible that abnormal automaticity (see Chapter 4) in ventricular muscle or Purkinje cells with reduced resting potentials might sometimes cause the ventricular escape rhythm in complete A-V block. This might occur if there is significant disease in the conducting system or ventricles that causes reduction of the resting membrane potential. The response to overdrive stimulation described below can distinguish between normal and abnormal automaticity.

Site of Origin of Escape Rhythms

QRS Morphology

The morphology of the QRS in the 12-lead ECG indicates the site of origin of ventricular pacemakers, not only for escape rhythms but also for premature ventricular depolarizations, accelerated ventricular rhythms, and tachycardias described below.

The QRS morphology reflects the regions activated earliest because of the pacemaker location. A right-sided origin produces a LBBB morphology because the right ventricle is activated prior to the left, whereas a left-sided origin produces a RBBB pattern because the left ventricle is activated first. On the left side, the pacemaker can be located in any of the fascicles. Origin in the anterior (superior) fascicle results in a RBBB with right-axis deviation, and origin in the posterior (inferior) fascicle results in a RBBB with left-axis deviation. A septal origin, either in a septal fascicle or the network formed by ramifications from the anterior and posterior fascicles supplying the septum is characterized by a narrower QRS (100–120 ms). The closer the pacemaker is to the origin of the left bundle, the narrower the QRS and the less marked is the RBBB, since there is quick access of the impulse into the right bundle branch. Likewise, the closer the pacemaker is to the origin of the right bundle, the narrower the QRS and the less prominent is LBBB because of rapid access to the left-sided conducting system. A distal origin of a pacemaker in the conducting system is characterized by a broad QRS (QRS ≥ 120 ms) since ventricular muscle is depolarized earlier than the conducting system.

In Figure 3-32, the QRS is aberrant and broad (duration 120 ms) with a RBBB pattern, indicating an origin in the posterior (inferior) fascicle of the distal left ventricular conducting system. The ECG in **Figure 3-33** also shows complete A-V block and A-V dissociation with a fascicular escape rhythm. Ventricular impulse origin is proximal in the left bundle branch indicated by the narrower QRS complexes with a RBBB pattern (duration 110 ms). The rate is faster than in Figure 3-32, about 50 bpm. This is related to the more proximal location of the pacemaker (the rate decreases from proximal to distal conducting system), although other factors such as autonomic tone may also be involved.

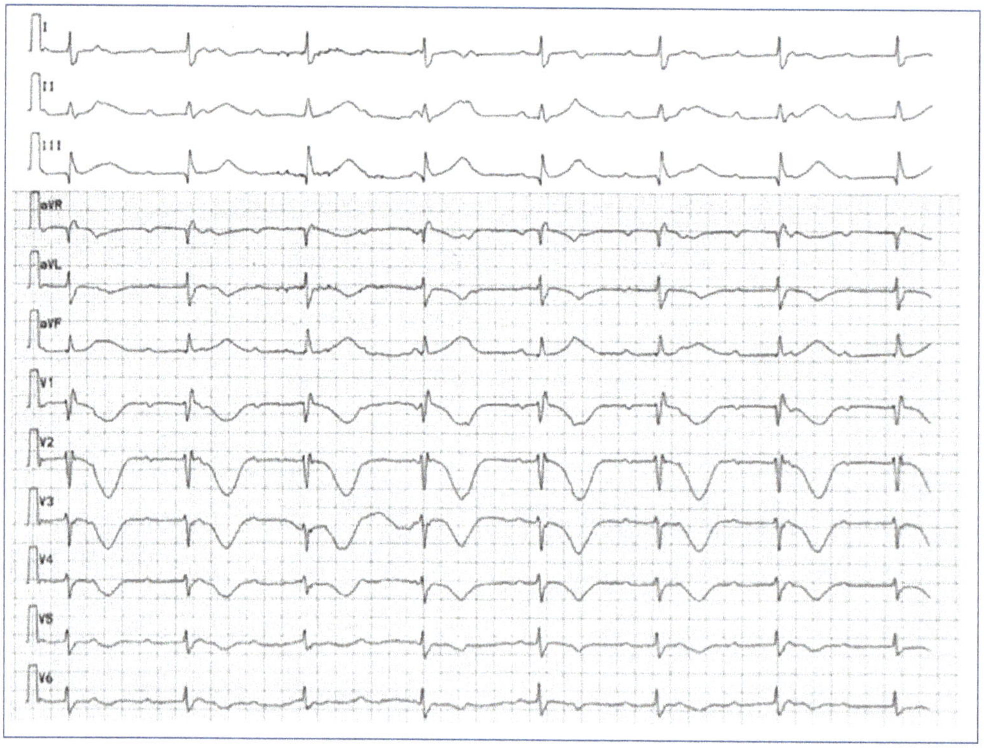

Figure 3-33 A 12-lead ECG recorded from a patient with complete heart block and a fascicular ventricular rhythm. There are T-wave abnormalities in the precordial leads (Wellens' ECG collection).

His Bundle Recordings

As described for A-V junctional rhythms, His bundle recordings in conjunction with the ECG may sometimes assist in localizing the pacemaker site in the ventricular conducting system. When the pacemaker is distal in the His bundle or conducting system, for example after bilateral bundle branch block, the H deflection in the His bundle electrogram (HBE) is associated with atrial depolarization and not with the ventricular complex. In this case, the QRS morphology, not the HBE, provides the necessary information for locating the pacemaker site.

HBEs can be useful for localizing the pacemaker site when block is in the proximal segment of the bundle of His, or proximal to the His bundle in the A-V node. As previously described (Figure 3-25), when the pacemaker is just distal to the block, in the lower node or His bundle, the H deflection occurs prior to each QRS with a normal QRS morphology and an H-V interval (conduction time from His bundle to ventricular activation) appropriate for the catheter location (proximal or distal, Figure 3-24). On the other hand, when impulse origin is at a distal His bundle or fascicular site, the His bundle is activated retrogradely from that site. The position of the H deflection with relation to ventricular depolarization then depends on the relative antegrade conduction time from the pacemaker site to the ventricles and retrograde conduction time from the pacemaker site to the His bundle.

In **Figure 3-34**, Panel A, a ventricular complex in the HBE recording, from a pacemaker in the left-anterior superior-fascicle, is associated with a His bundle electrogram (Hr) preceding ventricular activation and an H-V interval that is significantly shorter (20 ms) than the typical H-V interval associated with a sinus impulse (45 ms). The reason is diagrammed in Panel Aa′. The site of the pacemaker is indicated by the red asterisk. The His bundle (recording site is indicated by yellow circle) is depolarized by the retrograde impulse from the fascicular site of impulse formation (dashed white arrow) with conduction time through the fascicles to the His bundle being shorter than antegrade conduction time to ventricular myocardium (red arrows) across the Purkinje-ventricular muscle junctions.

Electrograms can also be recorded from the fascicle itself by moving the electrode catheter to a more distal position. In this case, the interval to the ventricular electrogram resulting from antegrade propagation from an impulse of fascicular origin is significantly shorter (< 25 ms) than the supraventricular His to ventricular deflection, which is 45–60 ms.

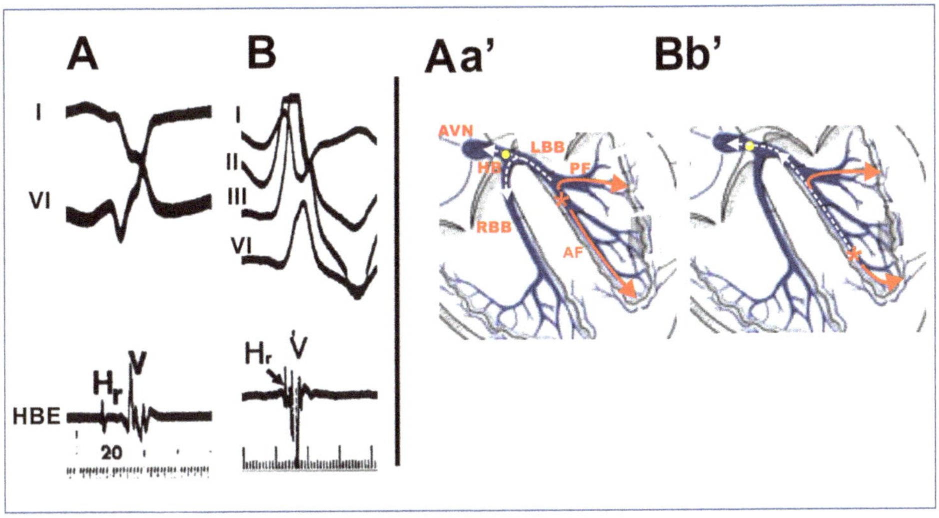

Figure 3-34 **Panels A and B:** ECGs and intracardiac electrogram from His bundle region (HBE). V, ventricular electrogram; Hr, His bundle with retrograde conduction. **Panels Aa' and Bb':** Diagrams of activation patterns of the left bundle branch (LBB) that correspond to the electrograms in the **left panel**. Pacemaker location indicated by asterisks in the proximal (**Panel Aa'**) and distal (**Panel Bb'**) bundle branch. AF, anterior fascicle: HB, His bundle branch; PF, posterior fascicle; RBB, right bundle branch. **Yellow circle** = HB recording site. **White dashed arrows** indicate retrograde activation, **red arrows** indicate antegrade activation.

In Figure 3-34, Panel B, there is a wide aberrant QRS with a RBBB pattern indicating an impulse origin in the distal left conducting system. When the pacemaker site is more distal in the conducting system, the His bundle or fascicular deflection occurs after the onset of the surface QRS since the proximal conducting system is activated retrogradely, either simultaneously or after antegrade ventricular activation. The His deflection (Hr, arrow in Panel B) occurs after the onset of the QRS. As diagrammed in Panel Bb′, where the distal pacemaker site is indicated by the red asterisk, the His bundle (yellow circle indicates HBE recording site) is activated retrogradely from the distal pacemaker site (dashed white arrow). Antegrade conduction of the impulse (red arrow) starts to depolarize the ventricles prior to retrograde activation of the His bundle because of a shorter conduction time to the ventricles than retrograde to the His bundle. In some cases, the His bundle deflection can be completely masked by the simultaneous depolarization of the ventricles.

Effects of Electrical Stimulation

Overdrive Suppression

Pacemakers with normal automaticity in the ventricular conducting system in patients with complete A-V block respond to overdrive stimulation of the ventricles with characteristic overdrive suppression. After a period of overdrive, the first spontaneous cycle is longer than the pre-overdrive cycle length (overdrive suppression) and then there is a gradual return to the original cycle length of the ventricular rhythm over the next 5–10 cycles. The amount of suppression is directly related to the rate and duration of overdrive.

Overdrive suppression of ventricular (Purkinje) pacemakers is greater than that of the sinus node because of the greater amount of Na^+ entering ventricular pacemaker cells during overdrive than sinus node cells.

Figure 3-35 compares the magnitude of maximum pacemaker overdrive suppression in the sinus node (left axis) and ventricular (labeled "subsidiary") pacemaker site (right axis) in patients with complete heart block. The mean maximum ventricular (subsidiary) pacemaker recovery time (vertical bar with asterisks at the right) is significantly greater than the mean maximum sinus node recovery time (vertical bar at the lower left).

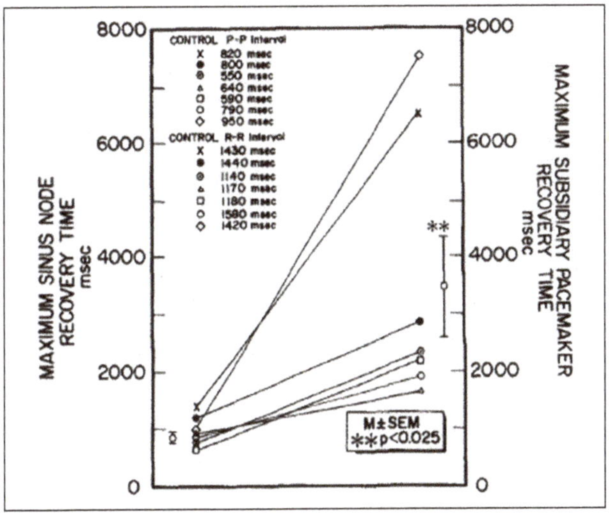

Figure 3-35 Maximum sinus node and ventricular pacemaker recovery times in patients with complete heart block in whom both the atrial and ventricular pacemaker were overdriven at a range of stimulation rates. Maximum sinus node recovery time (first cycle following overdrive stimulation) is on the **left axis** and maximum ventricular pacemaker recovery time for the same patients (first cycle following ventricular stimulation) is on the **right axis**. **Diagonal lines** connect maximum sinus overdrive suppression to maximum subsidiary overdrive suppression for each patient. The control P-P and R-R intervals for each patient prior to overdrive suppression are in the **upper left corner**. (Reproduced from Jordan J, Yamaguchi I, et al. Comparative effects of overdrive on sinus and subsidiary pacemaker function. *Am Heart J.* 1977;93:367–374.)

As described in Chapter 4, abnormal automaticity is not overdrive suppressed. Therefore, the response of the pacemaker in Figure 3-35 does verify a normal automatic mechanism.

Premature Stimulation

The response to premature stimulation of ventricular (Purkinje) pacemakers with normal automaticity expressed during complete heart block conforms with the description above. There is a narrow range of premature coupling intervals that are followed by compensatory pauses because of failure of the prematurely stimulated impulse to reach the pacemaker, and also a range of coupling intervals that reset the pacemaker. The reset cycle length is equal to the spontaneous cycle length when the stimulus is applied directly to the conducting system (His bundle) and often longer than the spontaneous cycle length when applied to the ventricles because of conduction delays across the Purkinje ventricular muscle junction. The shortened return cycle may sometimes occur when there is very early premature stimulation of the ventricle. The shortened return cycle is caused by shortening of the premature action potential duration (the duration of the action potential is cycle length-dependent, Figure 7-7), especially at slow rhythms when the action potential duration of the basic rhythm is long. Early premature impulses do not terminate the automatic rhythm.

Effects of Autonomic Mediators and Adenosine

Sympathetic stimulation or administration of β_1-adrenergic agonists such as isoproterenol increases the slope of SDD of Purkinje cell pacemakers (inward I_f and I_{NCX} pacemaker currents are increased), accelerating pacemaker rate of firing, and the ventricular rate when there is complete heart block. Parasympathetic stimulation has little effect. Adenosine may have no effect or slightly slow the rate transiently depending on the level of adrenergic stimulation of the pacemaker. Adenosine has little if any direct effect on ventricular pacemaker channels but can antagonize the effects of β_1 stimulation. In general, these characteristic responses of normal automaticity to pharmacological agents are not necessary to identify it as the mechanism for ventricular escape rhythms. However, they can help identify normal automaticity as a cause of some ventricular tachycardias described in the next section.

VENTRICULAR PREMATURE DEPOLARIZATIONS AND ACCELERATED VENTRICULAR RHYTHMS

Ventricular Premature Depolarizations

Ventricular premature depolarizations (VPDs) (also referred to as premature ventricular contractions or PVCs) appear as impulses of ventricular origin during a supraventricular rhythm (arrows in **Figure 3-36**). They may occur as single impulses or as several consecutive ventricular depolarizations forming couplets (2 impulses), triplets (3 impulses), or salvos (4–6 impulses). Three or more in a row constitute ventricular tachycardia. They can be caused by any of the mechanisms for arrhythmias, normal or abnormal automaticity, triggered activity, or reentry. VPDs caused by normal automaticity may be associated with a number of different cardiac diseases, can be a toxic manifestation of drugs, or can be idiopathic, possibly having a genetic basis.

VPDs caused by normal automaticity are focal. In any given patient, they can all arise from the same site of origin (unifocal) or from different sites of origin (multifocal). If conduction of the impulse originating in a single focus follows variable pathways, the arrhythmia can mimic a multifocal source.

Automatic VPDs intervene during sinus rhythm because of the acceleration of SDD of a ventricular (Purkinje) pacemaker and do not require a sinus pause (Figure 3-36). SDD reaches threshold potential for one or more impulses, prior to arrival of a sinus or supraventricular impulse. SDD is then suppressed by following supraventricular impulses. The sympathetic nervous system or drugs that have sympathomimetic effects are common causes of VPDs because they enhance the inward pacemaker currents. For example, VPDs commonly occur during exercise. The acceleration of SDD may be sporadic since the level of sympathetic activity fluctuates.

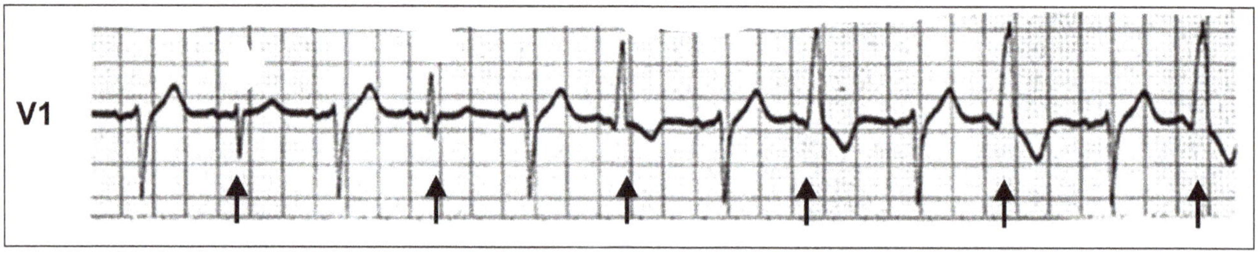

Figure 3-36 Ventricular premature depolarizations (**arrows**).

The ECG characteristics of VPDs caused by normal automaticity do not distinguish them from VPDs caused by abnormal automaticity in partially depolarized ventricular muscle or Purkinje cells (see Chapter 4) but can distinguish them from VPDs caused by triggered activity (Chapter 5) or reentry (Chapter 9). VPDs caused by automaticity usually have a variable coupling interval to the previous sinus impulse. Early-occurring VPDs can occur on the T wave of the previous supraventricular impulse resulting in the "R on T" phenomenon, which in the ischemic heart can precipitate ventricular fibrillation. The sinus impulse does not in any way cause an automatic VPD as would be the case with triggered or reentrant VPDs where the coupling interval between the VPD and prior initiating sinus impulse is often fixed. These mechanisms for fixed coupling are described in Chapters 5 and 9.

Fusion QRS complexes, another feature of automatic impulse initiation in the ventricles, can occur, resulting from activation of part of the ventricles by the supraventricular wavefront and part by the wavefront initiated by the ventricular pacemaker. The morphology of the fusion complexes can vary depending on the coupling interval to the previous sinus impulse. In Figure 3-36, the VPDs (arrows) with long coupling intervals show a fusion QRS (QRS 2, 4,and 6 from the left) while the QRS of the last 2 VPDs results entirely from ventricular activation from the ventricular pacemaker (no fusion) since its early firing activates the ventricles before arrival of the supraventricular impulse.

In some situations, conduction of the supraventricular impulse into the ventricular focus is blocked, while conduction out of the focus is not (unidirectional conduction block mechanisms described in Chapter 9), leading to a parasystolic focus. Such a parasystolic focus can be identified by variable coupled VPDs where the inter-ectopic intervals are some multiple of the basic rate of the automatic parasystolic focus.

Accelerated Idioventricular Rhythms

Normal automaticity also causes transient ventricular arrhythmias with rates of approximately 60–100 bpm that are faster than the intrinsic escape rate of 35–45 bpm but not as fast as ventricular tachycardia, which is greater than about 100–120 bpm. These rhythms are referred to as accelerated idioventricular rhythms (AIVR) when there are three or more consecutive ventricular impulses. An example is shown in **Figure 3-37.**

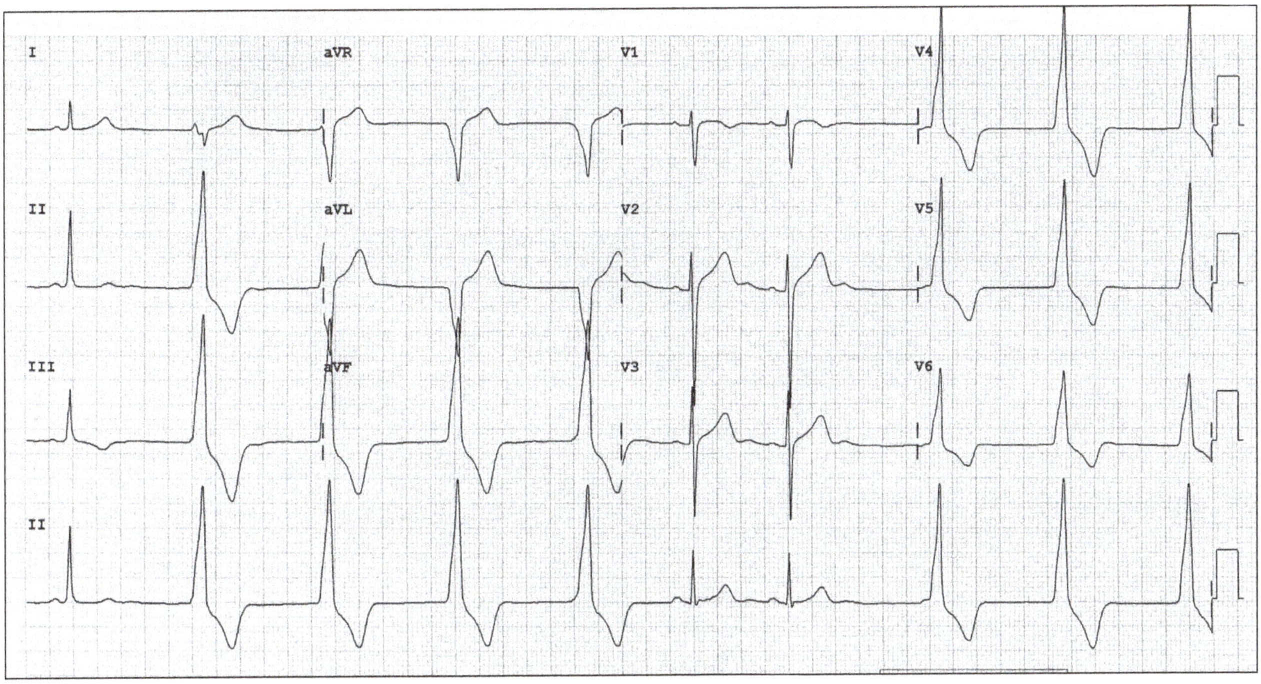

Figure 3-37 A 12-lead ECG showing accelerated idioventricular rhythm (60 bpm) (AIVR). (Reproduced from Burns E. ECG clinical case emergency medicine; Life in the fast lane, https://litfl.com/ecg-library)

In the ECG in Figure 3-37, the first impulse at the left in the bottom rhythm strip (lead II) is a fusion complex between a sinus and ventricular impulse (see below). Impulses 2–5 show a ventricular pacemaker firing at a CL of around 1000 ms, which is faster than the normal escape rate. Sinus impulses reach and overdrive the ventricular pacemaker before SDD reaches threshold, during impulses 6 and 7, at a sinus CL of 800 ms. Sinus CL then increases to greater than 1200 ms because of sinus arrhythmia (spontaneous increasing and decreasing sinus CL), allowing again for escape of the ventricular pacemaker (impulse 8) at a long coupling interval reflecting the time for SDD to reach threshold. The sinus arrhythmia causing appearance and disappearance of the AIVR may be caused by periodic increases in vagal activity that is prominent in trained athletes.

In AIVR, the atria are activated by impulses originating in the sinus node and the ventricles by the impulses originating in the accelerated ventricular (Purkinje) pacemaker, the varying rate depending on the presence of intact A-V conduction after a sinus P wave. This feature accounts for the intermittent appearance of the arrhythmia.

The AIVR in Figure 3-37 is likely to be caused by normal automaticity since it occurred in a heart with no overt cardiac abnormalities, rather than by abnormal automaticity associated with cardiac disease (see below). The cause of the accelerated pacemaker firing is not always obvious in AIVR. A possible candidate is enhanced sympathetic activity to the ventricles. AIVR can also accompany disturbances in serum electrolytes such as hypokalemia, which enhances Purkinje cell SDD.

AIVR is also associated with isoarrhythmic A-V dissociation and fusion complexes. Fusion complexes are a hallmark of an automatic pacemaker. In Figure 3-37, the first QRS at the left in the lead II recording results from fusion between the sinus and ventricular wavefronts. Fusion is indicated by the altered QRS; compare the QRS morphology with the QRS morphology of a sinus impulse that is the sixth impulse from the left. The short PR interval preceding it is too short to have been caused by an impulse conducted from the atrium. If the ventricular rate is faster than the atrial rate and retrograde AV conduction is present, there can be retrograde activation of the atria for long periods of time without fusion. In the absence of retrograde conduction, the ventricular pacemaker does not disturb the atrial rate.

AIVR can also be caused by abnormal automaticity in the setting of ischemia, infarction or reperfusion of an occluded coronary artery where partial depolarization of the resting membrane potential occurs to less negative levels (Chapter 4).

Site of Origin of VPDs and Accelerated Ventricular Rhythms

The same features of the QRS morphology of escape rhythms, provide information on the origin of VPDs and accelerated ventricular rhythms. Similarly, the explanation of the relationship of His bundle electrograms to ventricular depolarization also applies. Both VPDs and accelerated rhythms can arise anywhere in the ventricular conducting system. Electrical mapping has also been able to locate the site of origin of VPDs, confirmed by their disappearance after ablation of the site.

Effects of Electrical Stimulation

VPDs caused by automaticity cannot be initiated by overdrive stimulation but can be transiently suppressed. This response distinguishes an automatic mechanism from a delayed afterdepolarization (DAD) -triggered mechanism, which can cause VPDs initiated by overdrive (Chapter 5). The response of VPDs caused by reentry to overdrive is difficult to predict (Chapter 9). Likewise, AIVR caused by normal automaticity is not initiated by overdrive but is expected to be transiently suppressed. No data are available on the effects of premature stimulation, but one would expect the resetting response that is characteristic of normal automaticity. Automatic AIVR is not generally initiated or terminated by premature stimulation.

Effects of Autonomic Mediators and Adenosine

The responses of VPDs and AIVR to autonomic mediators, adenosine or other pharmacological agents are not required to identify normal automaticity as the causative mechanism. It is likely that normal automaticity causing these arrhythmias would exhibit similar responses as escape rhythms described above, and tachycardias described in the next section.

IDIOPATHIC FOCAL VENTRICULAR TACHYCARDIA

Idiopathic focal ventricular tachycardia can occur in the absence of structural heart disease (although the term "idiopathic" is used for a variety of tachycardias, some in fact, may in fact be associated with undetected disease). It is often exercise-induced, but can also occur without exercise. It sometimes might be related to genetic changes in pacemaker channels.

Exercise-Induced Ventricular Tachycardia

The ECG in **Figure 3-38** shows exercise-induced ventricular tachycardia. Clinical presentation can include bouts of unsustained repetitive monomorphic tachycardia and frequent premature beats in addition to tachycardia. The arrhythmia is not usually associated with exercise-induced ischemia; there is an absence of ST segment changes. The CL of tachycardia is generally between 300–400 ms, somewhat longer than reentrant ventricular tachycardia (see Chapter 12). The ECG in Figure 3-38 is characterized by a LBBB pattern with right inferior axis consistent with an origin of tachycardia in the outflow tract of the right ventricle (RVOT). The QRS configuration is smooth with a large voltage. There is a QS complex in aVL that suggests an origin towards the septum.

Ventricular Tachycardia and Sympathetic Activation; Exercise-Enhanced Pacemaker Activity

The normal electrophysiological response of the heart to exercise is acceleration of the sinus rate from the effect of norepinephrine to increase SDD of the sinus node pacemaker. Although latent pacemakers are also exposed to sympathetically released norepinephrine at the same time which increases net inward pacemaker current, the enhanced sinus rate normally remains sufficiently rapid to suppress them. The resulting rhythm is sinus tachycardia. In order for ventricular pacemakers to assume control of the heart during sympathetic activation to cause ventricular tachycardia, the increase in ventricular pacemaker automaticity must be greater than the increase in sinus node or supraventricular pacemaker automaticity (Figure 1-8, Panel C). Enhanced sympathetic activity also causes DADs and triggered activity that have a faster rate than the sinus node, another mechanism for exercise-induced ventricular tachycardia (Chapter 5). The mechanism causing tachycardia, whether automaticity or triggered activity cannot be ascertained from the ECG alone. Electrophysiology properties described below can be used to distinguish between the two mechanisms.

Not only is ventricular impulse initiation faster than the sinus node when automatic exercise-induced tachycardia occurs, but the rates (180–200 bpm) are faster than the rates that ventricular pacemakers can attain with maximum sympathetic stimulation in normal hearts that do not have exercise-induced ventricular tachycardia. For example, in patients with heart block in the A-V node (and presumably normal ventricular conducting system), the maximum ventricular rate during and after exercise only increases to around 70–100 bpm. It is not known whether the faster rate response in patients with ventricular tachycardia results from a higher density of sympathetic nerve endings at the ectopic site or a greater effect of β_1-receptor stimulation on pacemaker currents at this site. Genetic factors may also be responsible in some cases.

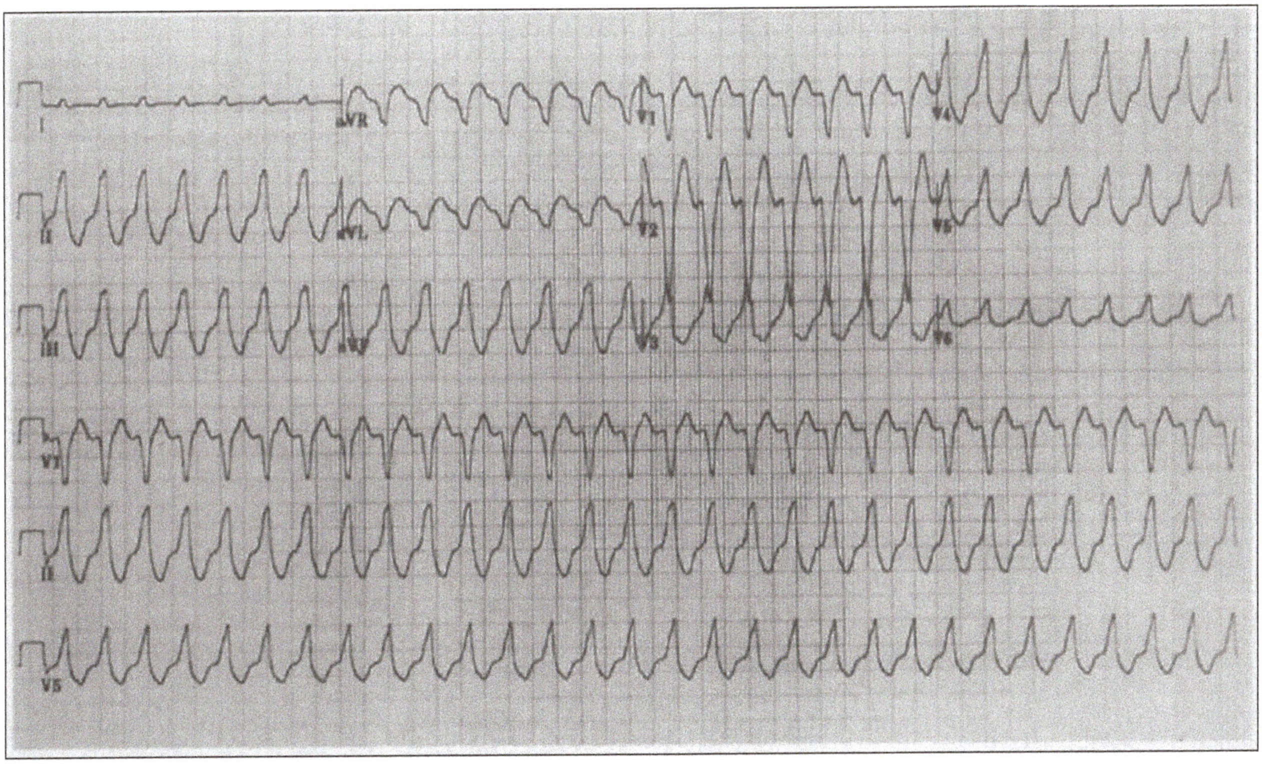

Figure 3-38 A 12-lead ECG showing an exercise-induced ventricular tachycardia. (Reproduced from Varma NJ, Josephson ME. Therapy of "Idiopathic" ventricular tachycardia. *J Cardiovasc Electrophysiol.*1997;8:104–116.)

Electrophysiological Properties of Exercise-Induced Ventricular Tachycardia Caused by Normal Automaticity

As indicated earlier, there are two mechanisms that can cause exercise-induced ventricular tachycardia: normal automaticity, and DAD-induced triggered activity. Each mechanism has characteristics that enables it to be distinguished from the other. The characteristics of automatic exercise tachycardia are described here. In Chapter 6,Table 6-1, the characteristics of triggered exercise tachycardia are detailed and compared to automatic tachycardia.

Initiation by exercise or a β_1-adrenergic agonist. Automatic tachycardias are initiated by exercise-enhanced sympathetic activation which results in adrenergic β_1-receptor stimulation. In **Figure 3-39**, the induction of ventricular tachycardia by infusion of the β_1-agonist isoproterenol in a patient who has exercise-induced automatic ventricular is shown in Panel C, replicating the spontaneous onset of tachycardia during a period of exercise outside the laboratory.

Onset of tachycardia is preceded by shortening of the sinus CL to 400 ms but the increase in sinus rate does not cause the enhanced automaticity responsible for the tachycardia. (Remember that SDD is suppressed by overdrive; Figure 1-6). The first impulse of tachycardia may occur at varying coupling intervals to the last sinus impulse when caused by automaticity since it is not related to the increase in rate.

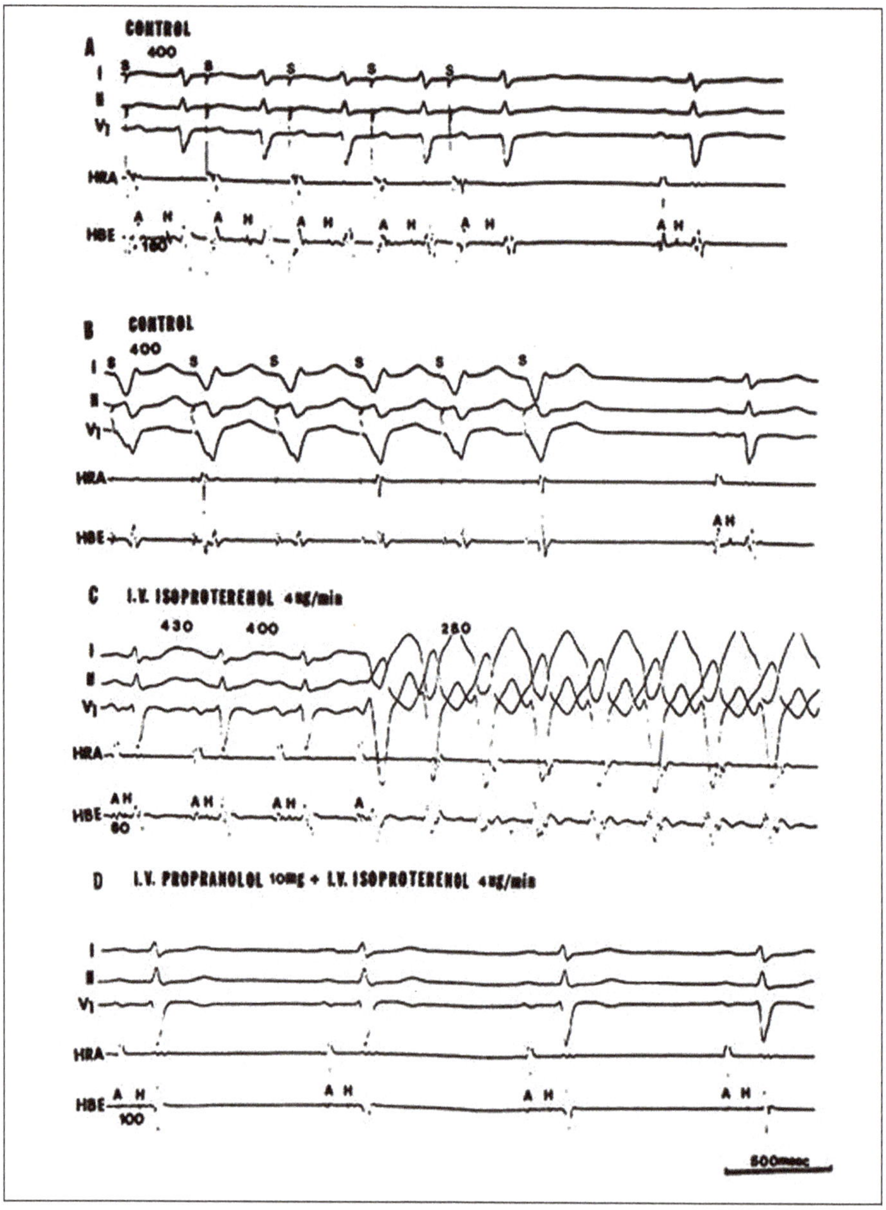

Figure 3-39 Initiation of automatic exercise tachycardia. Leads I, II, and V_1, and high right atrial (HRA), and His bundle (HBE) electrograms are displayed. **Panels A** and **B:** Pacing in the high right atrium (HRA) and right ventricle. **Panel C:** Intravenous infusion of isoproterenol 4 mg/kg. **Panel D:** β-adrenergic blockade with intravenous propranolol (0.2 mg/kg). (Reproduced from Sung RJ, Keung EC, et al. Effects of β-adrenergic blockade on verapamil-responsive and verapamil-irresponsive sustained ventricular tachycardias. *J Clin Invest.* 1988;81:688–699.)

Simply increasing the heart rate with atrial (Panel A) or ventricular (Panel B) pacing at a CL of 400 ms (the same as the sinus CL at which tachycardia appears during exercise and during isoproterenol infusion) does not initiate the arrhythmia eliminating the increase in rate as initiating tachycardia. Isoproterenol no longer initiates tachycardia after administration of propranolol, which blocks the β_1-adrenergic receptors (Panel D).

In contrast, exercise-induced ventricular tachycardia caused by DAD-triggered activity is initiated by the exercise-induced increase in sinus rate, which increases DAD amplitude (Chapter 5). The pacing in Panels A and B of Figure 3-39 would have initiated tachycardia if it was caused by DAD-triggered activity (see Figure 6-25).

Overdrive and Programmed Premature Stimulation

Overdrive and programmed premature stimulation do not start or stop automatic exercise-induced tachycardia, consistent with the properties of automatic arrhythmias. **Figure 3-39**, Panels A and B, demonstrates the failure of overdrive stimulation to initiate tachycardia. Premature stimulation also does not induce this arrhythmia (not shown). Both overdrive and premature stimulation can initiate DAD-triggered tachycardia (Table 6-1).

Figure 3-40 shows the failure of electrical stimulation to terminate exercise-induced automatic tachycardia. At the beginning of the record, a period of overdrive is shown at a CL of 280 ms followed by a premature stimulus at a coupling interval of 240 ms. Transient suppression of tachycardia that follows allows the appearance of a supraventricular impulse (narrow QRS complex) after overdrive before tachycardia resumes. A second period of overdrive (S) has the same effect.

Exercise-induced ventricular tachycardia caused by DAD-triggered activity can be terminated by overdrive or premature stimulation (Chapter 6, Table 6-1).

Adenosine and parasympathetics. Exercise-induced automatic ventricular tachycardia is not terminated by adenosine, a response that can identify this mechanism. Automatic tachycardia may be transiently suppressed by adenosine consistent with the slowing effect of adenosine on ventricular automaticity during adrenergic stimulation. The slowing may allow the sinus node to become the dominant pacemaker even though sinus rate is also slowed by adenosine (**Figure 3-41**, Panel A), but the automatic tachycardia quickly resumes as the effects of adenosine dissipate (Panel B).

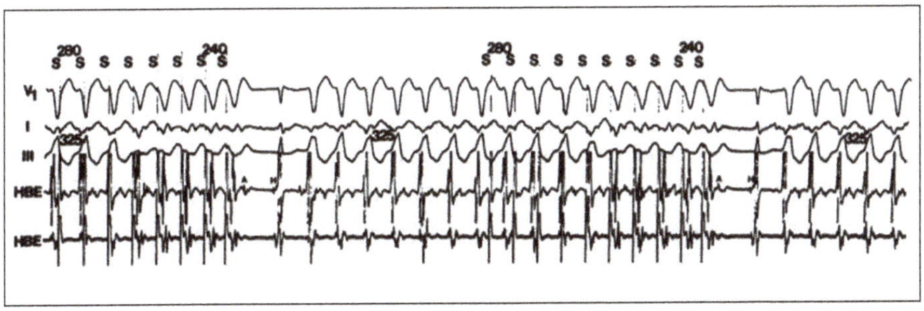

Figure 3-40 ECG leads V_1, I, III, and HBEs (HBE) recorded during isoproterenol-induced automatic ventricular tachycardia (CL 325 ms), overdrive stimulation (S) at CL 280 ms, followed by a premature stimulus (CL 240 ms). (Reproduced from Sung RJ, Keung EC, et al. Effects of β-adrenergic blockade on verapamil-responsive and verapamil-irresponsive sustained ventricular tachycardias. *J Clin Invest.* 1988;81:688–699.)

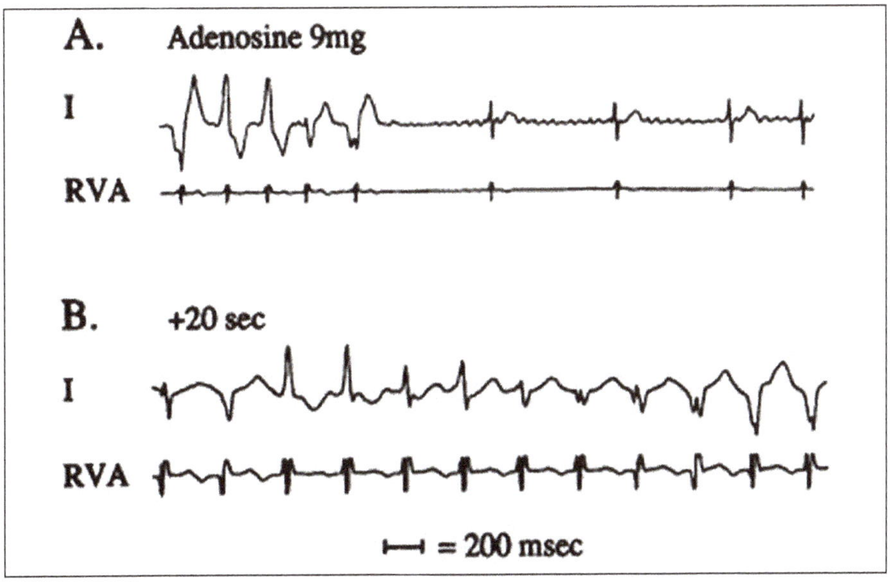

Figure 3-41 Surface lead I and intracardiac recordings from the right ventricular apex (RVA) in a patient with ongoing exercise-induced VT. Adenosine administered before recordings in **Panel A**. **Panel B** shows recordings made 20 sec after adenosine administration. (Reproduced from Lerman BB. Response of nonreentrant catecholamine-mediated ventricular tachycardia to endogenous adenosine and acetycholine. Evidence for myocardial receptor-mediated effects. *Circulation.* 1993;87:382–390.)

Adenosine does terminate DAD-dependent-triggered exercise-induced tachycardia, distinguishing this mechanism from automaticity (Chapter 6, Figure 6-24 and Table 6-1).

Automatic exercise-induced ventricular tachycardia is also not terminated by vagal activation although it might be slowed. ACh has little direct effect on the pacemaker currents in Purkinje cells, although it can reduce the stimulating effects of the sympathetics by accentuated antagonism. Triggered tachycardia caused by DADs may sometimes be terminated consistent with a suppressant effect of ACh on sympathetic-induced DADs, another distinguishing feature between the two mechanisms (Chapter 6, Table 6-1).

Verapamil. Exercise-induced automatic ventricular tachycardia is not terminated by L-type Ca^{2+} channel-blocking drugs such as verapamil, since the L-type Ca^{2+} channel plays only a minor role in the genesis of the pacemaker potential in ventricular (Purkinje) pacemakers. Exercise-induced tachycardias caused by DADs are terminated because of the prominent role L-type Ca^{2+} currents play in the genesis of DADs (Figure 5-2). The lack of response of tachycardia to an L-type Ca^{2+} channel-blocking drug also eliminates the possibility of abnormal automaticity that might occur in ventricular muscle as a mechanism for this tachycardia (Chapter 4).

Idiopathic focal ventricular tachycardia not related to exercise. Some idiopathic focal ventricular tachycardias caused by enhanced normal automaticity are not exercise-induced. They are not initiated or terminated by programmed stimulation. β-receptor blocking drugs only slightly slow their rate. Adenosine also does not affect the rate as expected for noncatecholamine-enhanced automaticity.

Site(s) of origin of exercise-induced tachycardia. The most prevalent site of origin of exercise-induced ventricular tachycardia, either automatic or triggered, is the right ventricular outflow tract (RVOT) endocardially above the infundibulum, at the entrance to the outflow tract on the interventricular septal surface. **Figure 3-42** shows the anatomy of this region (area outlined by dashed white lines). The ECGs at the left are from a tachycardia originating in the posterior of the region and the ECGs at the right during tachycardia originating at the anterior of the region. In general, RVOT tachycardias have a LBBB morphology with a right inferior axis and a QS in aVL. The more rightward the axis, the more anterior the origin of tachycardia (ECG on right). Conversely, the less rightward the axis, the closer the origin to the posterior right ventricle (ECG on left).

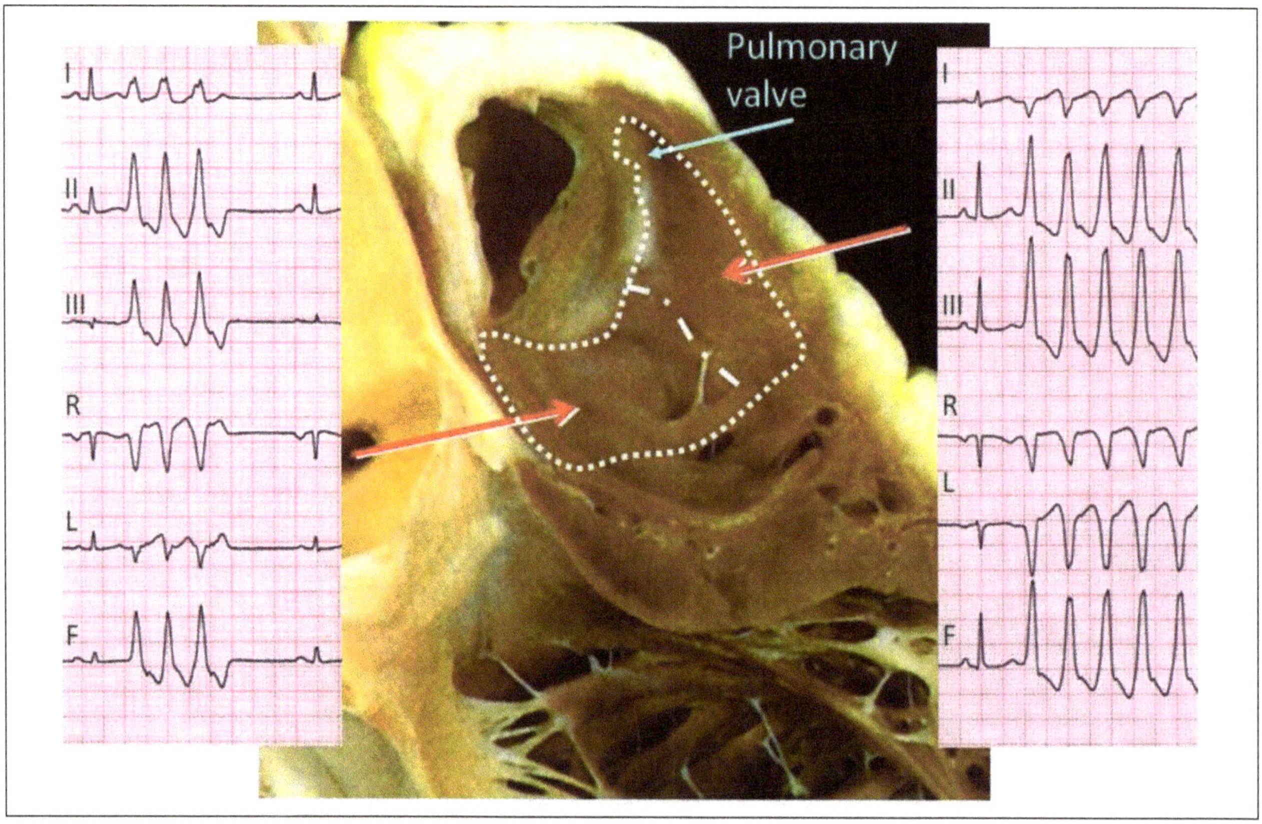

Figure 3-42 Right ventricular outflow tract outlined by the **dashed lines**. ECGs from two different sites (indicated by the **red arrows**) recorded during exercise-induced monomorphic ventricular tachycardia. (Figure kindly provided by Jose Angel Cabrera and Damian Sanchez-Quintana.)

Apart from the right ventricular outflow tract, other sites of origin of focal idiopathic tachycardias, both exercise- and nonexercised-induced, include (1) sleeves of myocardium connected to the RVOT, extending along the pulmonary artery above the pulmonary valve; (2) the right ventricular inflow tract; (3) the left ventricular outflow tract (LVOT) in the superior basal region of the left interventricular septum or left ventricular free wall; (4) ventricular myocardium extending above the aortic annulus at the aortic sinuses of Valsalva; (5) the vicinity of the mitral annulus; (6) the papillary muscles in both left and right ventricles; and (7) the epicardial surface of the left ventricle at the cardiac crux.

Role of Purkinje Cells

In general, similar to the origin of escape and accelerated ventricular rhythms caused by automaticity, focal idiopathic tachycardias are expected to originate in the Purkinje cells of the ventricular conducting system since they have the property of normal automaticity. However, Purkinje cells have not been located at all of the sites of focal idiopathic tachycardia. Since the structure of the subendocardial Purkinje cells cannot be differentiated from ventricular muscle by standard anatomical methods, regions in which Purkinje cells have not been described may in fact have subendocardial Purkinje cells. Normal automaticity may also arise in embryological remnants of pacemaker tissue that remain in some regions such as the RVOT.

Automatic Fascicular Tachycardias

Automatic focal ventricular tachycardia may also arise in Purkinje cells with enhanced automaticity in the fascicles of the conduction system (fascicular tachycardia). Some tachycardias are exercise-induced and some are not. The left bundle branch has a faster automatic rate and is more likely to be the site of origin of automatic fascicular tachycardia than the right. Tachycardias originating in the fascicles have a narrower QRS (<120 ms) than tachycardias originating more distally. They also have a bundle branch block pattern. **Figure 3-43** (top panel) shows an automatic fascicular tachycardia with a CL of 540 ms provoked by exercise. The ECG has a RBBB pattern and shows that tachycardia arises in or close to the left anterior (superior) fascicle.

A His bundle deflection (arrows, bottom panel) appears almost simultaneous with the onset of the QRS. As explained in Figure 3-34, with a distal origin in the fascicle, retrograde conduction time to the His bundle can be about the same as antegrade conduction to the ventricles.

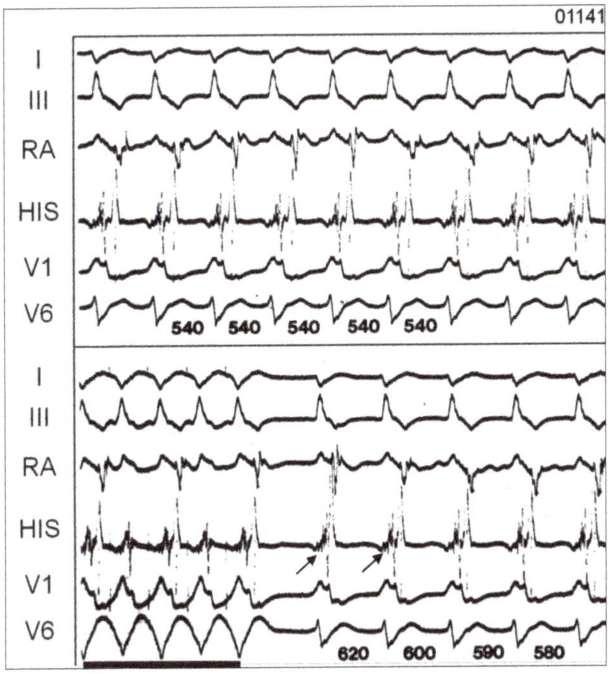

Figure 3-43 ECG leads I, III, V_1, and V_6, and electrograms from the right atrium (RA), and His bundle during exercise-induced fascicular tachycardia (**top panel**) and the end of a period of overdrive stimulation (**horizontal bar** under V_6) (**bottom panel**) (Wellens' ECG collection).

Effects of Electrical Stimulation

Automatic fascicular tachycardias are not initiated or terminated by overdrive or premature stimulation but can be overdrive suppressed, consistent with an automatic mechanism. Figure 3-43 (bottom panel) shows the effects of overdrive on automatic tachycardia. A 1-minute period of overdrive at a rate of 160 bpm (only the last five underlined stimulated impulses are shown at the left) is followed by transient overdrive suppression with a gradual shortening of the post overdrive CL from 620 back to 540 ms.

Effects of Autonomic Agonists, Adenosine, and Verapamil

The typical response expected of normal automaticity to these drugs can confirm an automatic mechanism as a cause of fascicular tachycardia. Catecholamines increase automatic fascicular tachycardia rate by accelerating SDD, similar to the other automatic ventricular rhythms described in this section. Adenosine may slow tachycardia transiently when it is related to increased sympathetic activity or may not have any significant effect when sympathetics are not involved. Tachycardias are not significantly influenced by parasympathetic activation or L-type Ca^{2+} channel-blocking drugs because of their minimal effect on SDD in Purkinje cells.

Ventricular (Purkinje) Automaticity as Triggers of Tachycardias and Fibrillation

Premature impulses arising in the distal conducting system as indicated by a Purkinje fiber potential in electrode catheter recordings can initiate rapid tachycardias or fibrillation. Although such impulse origin in Purkinje cells might be caused by enhanced normal automaticity, it also might arise from other arrhythmogenic mechanisms. The mechanism has not been elucidated.

SUMMARY

Normal automaticity in the ventricles that causes arrhythmias occurs in Purkinje cells (fibers) of the conducting system and not in ventricular muscle. Purkinje cells have SDD caused mainly by inward I_f pacemaker current and a declining I_K outward current during phase 4. The Na^+–Ca^{2+} exchanger current that plays a prominent role in SDD of sinus and A-V nodal pacemakers appears to be less important.

The intrinsic pacemaker rate of Purkinje cells decreases from about 40–50 bpm at the junction with the His bundle, to 25–30 bpm in the periphery. The ANS accelerates SDD and automatic rate primarily by increasing inward I_f. The parasympathetics have only a small effect to decrease Purkinje automaticity. Adenosine has little effect unless automaticity is enhanced by sympathetic stimulation, in which case it may slow impulse initiation transiently. Ca^{2+} channel-blocking drugs have little effect.

Overdrive stimulation increases Na^+–K^+ pump current (outward I_P) causing CL-dependent overdrive suppression. Premature impulses cause resetting of pacemaker activity. Automatic impulse initiation is neither started nor stopped by electrical stimulation.

Automatic arrhythmias are caused by either pacemaker escape or acceleration of pacemaker impulse initiation. Pacemaker escape occurs during complete heart block. Acceleration of SDD can cause VPDs, AIVR, and VT.

Automatic exercise-induced tachycardia is initiated by sympathetic activation or β_1-adrenergic stimulation that enhances SDD. Automatic exercise-induced tachycardia is neither started nor stopped by overdrive and programmed premature stimulation. Automatic exercise-induced tachycardia is not terminated by adenosine, parasympathetic stimulation, and verapamil.

SOURCES

Basic Electrophysiology

Biel M, Wahl-Schott C, Michalakis S, Zong X. Hyperpolarization-activated cation channels: From genes to function. *Physiol Rev.* 2009;89:847–885.

Boyden PA, Hirose M, Dunn W. Cardiac Purkinje cells. *Heart Rhythm.* 2010;7:127–135.

Dangman KH, Hoffman BF. The effects of single premature stimuli on automatic and triggered rhythms in isolated canine Purkinje fibers. *Circulation.* 1985:71:813–822.

Kerzner J, Wolf M, Kosowsky B, Lown B. Ventricular ectopic rhythms following vagal stimulation in dogs with acute myocardial infarction. *Circulation.* 1973;XLVII:44–50.

Klein HO, Lebson R, Cranefield PF, Hoffman BF. Effect of extrasystoles on idioventricular rhythm. Clinical and electrophysiologic correlation. *Circulation.* 1973;47:758–764.

Krellenstein DJ, Pliam MB, Brooks McC, Vassalle M. On the mechanism of idioventricular pacemaker suppression by fast drive. *Circ Res.* 1974;35:923–934.

Lerman BB, Wesley, RC Jr., DiMarco JP, et al. Antiadrenergic effects of adenosine on His-Purkinje automaticity. Evidence for accentuated antagonism. *J Clin Invest.* 1988;82: 2127–2135.

Mangoni M, Nargeot J. Genesis and regulation of the heart automaticity. *Physiol Rev.* 2008;88:919–982.

Pliam MB, Krellenstein DJ, Vassalle M, Brooks McC. Influence of the sympathetic system on the pacemaker suppression which follows overdrive. *Circulation.* 1973;48:313–321.

Rardon DP, Bailey JC. Adenosine attenuation of the electrophysiological effects of isoproterenol on canine cardiac Purkinje fibers. *J Pharmacol Exp Ther.* 1984;228(3):792–798.

Reiser J, Anderson GJ. Differences in automaticity between Purkinje strands from right and left dog ventricle. *Am J Physiol Heart Circ Physiol.* 1980;239(8): H247–H251.

Rosen MR, Danilo P Jr, Weiss RM. Actions of adenosine on normal and abnormal impulse initiation in canine ventricle. *Am J Physiol.* 1983;244:H715–H721.

Weld FM, Bigger JT Jr. The effect of lidocaine on diastolic transmembrane currents determining pacemaker depolarization in cardiac Purkinje fibers. *Circ Res.* 1976;38:203–208.

Clinical Electrophysiology

Buxton AE, Waxman HL, Marchlinski FE, et al. Right ventricular tachycardia: Clinical and electrophysiologic characteristics. *Circulation.* 1983;68:917–927.

Callans DJ, Volker M, Schwartzman D, et al. Repetitive monomorphic tachycardia from the left ventricular outflow tract: Electrocardiographic patterns consistent with a left ventricular site of origin. *J Am Coll Cardiol.* 1997;29:1023–1027.

Crawford T, Mueller G, Good E, Jongnarangsin K, et al. Ventricular arrhythmias originating from papillary muscles in the right ventricle. *Heart Rhythm.* 2010;7:725–730.

Delacretaz E, Stevenson WG, Ellison K, et al. Mapping and radiofrequency catheter ablation of the three types of sustained monomorphic ventricular tachycardia in nonischemic heart disease. *J Cardiovasc Electrophysiol.* 2000;11:11–17.

de Soyza N, Bissett JK, Kane JJ, et al. Association of accelerated idioventricular rhythm and paroxysmal ventricular tachycardia in acute myocardial infarction. *Am J Cardiol.* 1974;34:667–670.

Dixit S, Gerstenfeld EP, Lin D, et al. Identification of distinct electrocardiographic patterns from the basal left ventricle: Distinguishing medial and lateral sites of origin in patients with idiopathic ventricular tachycardia. *Heart Rhythm.* 2005;2:485–491.

Doppalapudi H, Yamada T, McElderry T, et al. Ventricular tachycardia originating from the posterior papillary muscle in the left ventricle. A distinct clinical syndrome. *Circ Arrhythmia Electrophysiol.* 2008;1:23–29.

Gallagher JJ, Damato AN, Lau SH. Electrophysiologic studies during accelerated idioventricular rhythms. *Circulation.* 1971;44: 671–677.

Gonzalez RP, Scheinman MM, Lesh MD, et al. Clinical and electrophysiologic spectrum of fascicular tachycardias. *Am Heart J.* 1994;128:147–156.

Good E, Desjardins B, Jongnarangsin K, et al. Ventricular arrhythmias originating from a papillary muscle in patients without prior infarction: A comparison with fascicular arrhythmias. *Heart Rhythm.* 2008;5:1530–1537.

Grimm W. Accelerated idioventricular rhythm: epidemiology, pathophysiology, immediate evaluation and management, long-term management, experimental, and theoretical developments. *Cardiac Electrophysiol Review.* 1997;1/2:97–101.

Josephson ME. *Josephson's Clinical Cardiac Electrophysiology: Techniques and Interpretations,* (5th ed.). Philadelphia, PA: Wolters Kluwer; 2016.

Kanagaratnam L, Tomassini G, Schweikert R, et al. Ventricular tachycardias arising from the aortic sinus of Valsalva: An under-recognized variant of left outflow tract ventricular tachycardia. *J Am Coll Cardiol.* 2001;37:1408–1414.

Klein L, Shih HT, Hackett K, et al. Radiofrequency catheter ablation of ventricular tachycardia in patients without structural heart disease. *Circulation.* 1992;85:1666–1674.

Lopers G, Stevenson WG, Soejima K, et al. Identification and ablation of three types of ventricular tachycardia involving the His-Purkinje system in patients with heart disease. *J Cardiovasc Electrophysiol.* 2004;15:52–58.

Morady F, Kadish AH, DiCarllo L, et al. Long-term results of catheter ablation of idiopathic right ventricular tachycardia. *Circulation.* 1990;82:2093–2099.

Stevenson WG, Soejima K. Catheter ablation for ventricular tachycardia. *Circulation.* 2007;115:2750–2760.

Sung RJ, Shen EN, Morady F, et al. Electrophysiologic mechanism of exercise-induced sustained ventricular tachycardia. *Am J Cardiol.* 1983;51:525–530.

Tada H, Tadokoro K, Ito S, et al. Idiopathic ventricular arrhythmias originating from the tricuspid annulus: Prevalence, electrocardiographic characteristics, and results of radiofrequency catheter ablation. *Heart Rhythm.* 2007;4:7–16.

Takumi Y, McElderry HT, Okada T, et al. Idiopathic focal ventricular arrhythmias originating from the anterior papillary muscle in the left ventricle. *J Cardiovasc Electrophysiol.* 2009;20:866–872.

Wellens HJJ, Conover M. *The ECG in Emergency Decision Making.* St. Louis, MO: Saunders Elsevier; 2006.

CHAPTER 4

Abnormal Automaticity: Basic Principles and Arrhythmias

As the term implies, abnormal automaticity is not a normal property of myocardial cells and only occurs in myocardium with electrophysiological properties altered by pathology. How cardiac disease causes this mechanism for arrhythmias and examples of the arrhythmias it can cause are described in this chapter.

Basic Electrophysiological Mechanisms of Abnormal Automaticity

ELECTROPHYSIOLOGY OF ABNORMAL AUTOMATICITY

Abnormal automaticity occurs in diseased myocardium. The pathology results in distinct changes in electrophysiology. Although in the clinical literature any form of automaticity at ectopic sites is sometimes referred to as "abnormal automaticity," we reserve the use of this term to identify this abnormal electrophysiological mechanism.

Working atrial and ventricular myocardial cells generate the contractile force of the heart, but do not normally have the property of spontaneous diastolic (phase 4) depolarization (SDD) and automaticity—and therefore do not initiate spontaneous impulses to cause arrhythmias. However, under pathological conditions, working myocardial cells can acquire the property of automaticity. The primary mechanism involves partial depolarization of the resting potential to less negative levels.

Latent pacemaker cells with normal automaticity, particularly Purkinje cells in the ventricular specialized conducting system, can also acquire the property of abnormal automaticity when their resting potential is sufficiently depolarized from normal levels. In these cells, the abnormal automaticity is caused by a different mechanism than normal automaticity.

In addition, experimental laboratory studies on isolated tissues suggest that upregulation of ion channels (e.g., increased expression) that participate in the normal pacemaker mechanism and are normally expressed at very low levels in working myocardial cells, can cause a type of abnormal automaticity. However, the involvement of this mechanism in the genesis of clinical arrhythmias awaits documentation.

The description in this chapter focuses on abnormal automaticity caused by partial depolarization of the resting membrane potential.

Abnormal Automaticity Caused by Depolarization of the Resting Membrane Potential

Overview of the Mechanism

Working myocardial cells have the ion channels that cause SDD in pacemakers with normal automaticity described in Chapters 2 and 3. However, these channels do not cause automaticity in working cells. A large potassium channel (I_{K1}) conductance generates a strong outward K^+ current that is the basis for the highly negative resting potential in both working atrial and ventricular myocytes (approximately −80 to −90 mV). A strong outward I_{K1} current opposes any inward depolarizing current(s) during diastole that might lead to spontaneous diastolic depolarization. Although I_f pacemaker channels do occur in working muscle, they are present at lower levels than in normal pacemaker cells and are not activated during the normal action potential because of the highly negative resting potential.

When the resting potentials of working myocardial cells are reduced sufficiently (become less negative), SDD can occur and cause impulse initiation by the mechanism of abnormal automaticity. The descriptive phrase, depolarization-induced abnormal automaticity, is used throughout this section to refer to this overall mechanism.

Impulse Initiation by Depolarization-Induced Abnormal Automaticity

Initiation of abnormal automaticity by depolarization of the resting membrane potential in a laboratory experiment is demonstrated in the diagrams of transmembrane potentials of a working ventricular muscle cell shown in **Figure 4-1**.

Electrophysiological Foundations of Cardiac Arrhythmias: A Bridge Between Basic Mechanisms and Clinical Electrophysiology, Second Edition.
 Cardiotext Publishing, ISBN: 978-1-942909-42-2.

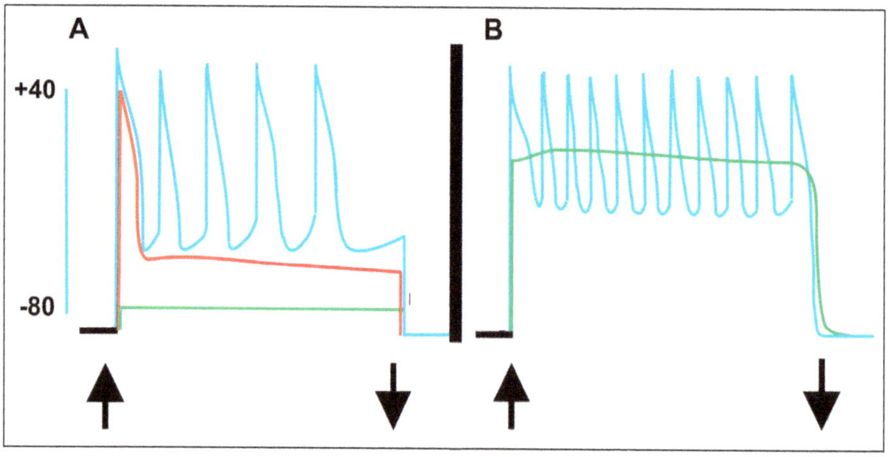

Figure 4-1 Diagram of effect of reducing membrane potential of a working ventricular muscle cell on automatic impulse initiation.

In Figure 4-1, the resting membrane potential at the left (black trace) in Panel A is around -90 mV. The upward arrow shows onset of three different long-lasting membrane potential depolarizations for 5 sec (green, red, and blue traces) that were induced by electrical current pulses. The downward arrow shows when the current pulses were turned off. Membrane potential is first decreased to −85 mV (green trace) without initiating an action potential because it does not reach the threshold potential. Next, the red trace shows the effects of reducing membrane potential to around −65 mV, which stimulates one action potential, but there is no sustained automaticity during the maintained depolarization at this level. Reduction of membrane potential to ~ −60 mV results in abnormal automatic firing (blue trace) until the membrane potential returns to its initial level when the current pulse is turned off (downward pointing arrow). In Panel B, reduction of the membrane potential to a less negative level of -50 mV (at upward arrow) results in a more rapid automatic rate (blue trace) that stops when the current pulse is turned off (downward arrow). However, reduction of the membrane potential to an even less negative level of around −40 mV at the upward arrow (green trace) does not result in automaticity. This sequence demonstrates a general property of depolarization-induced abnormal automaticity; it occurs at a threshold level of reduced membrane potential, the rate increases as membrane potential is depolarized to less negative levels until a level is reached at which abnormal automaticity does not occur. A similar response to membrane depolarization occurs in working atrial cells.

Latent pacemakers that are normally automatic at high (more negative) levels of membrane potential such as Purkinje cells in the ventricular conducting system, also acquire the property of abnormal automaticity when the membrane potential is reduced (see Figure 4-3, Panel C). The abnormal automaticity is caused by a different mechanism (described below) than the normal automaticity. In Purkinje cells, automaticity may also occur over the range of membrane potentials intermediate between the normal high level (around −90 mV) and the low level at which abnormal automaticity occurs (around −60 mV). At these intermediated levels of membrane potential, there is no sharp distinction between normal and abnormal automaticity. Such a distinction is not a problem in atrial or ventricular myocytes, in which normal automaticity does not occur.

Effects of Disease on Resting Membrane Potential

Abnormal automaticity due to depolarization of the membrane potential can occur in a pathological environment. The resting membrane potential is mainly a function of the relationship of extracellular and intracellular K^+ concentrations, $[K^+]$, and the relative permeability of the cell membrane to K^+ (K^+ conductance) according to the Goldman-Hodgkin-Katz Equation. The concentration and membrane conductance of other ions such as Na^+ and Ca^{2+} also contribute, but to a lesser extent. An outward K^+ current flows through membrane channels (I_{K1}) down an electrochemical gradient as the most important cause of the resting membrane potential. A less negative membrane potential can be caused by a decrease in intracellular $[K^+]_i$, an increase in extracellular $[K^+]_o$ or a decrease in membrane permeability to K^+ (decrease in I_{K1} conductance). A decrease in intracellular $[K^+]_i$ might occur during ischemia as K^+ leaks out of the cells into the extracellular space. This might also increase extracellular $[K^+]_o$ if the leaked K^+ is not quickly washed away by the local circulation. The conductance of the I_{K1} channel decreases as membrane potential decreases because of its property of inward rectification, decreasing the I_{K1} current and further decreasing the resting potential. A decrease in I_{K1} caused by changes in function of this ion channel (remodeling) is also the cause of a decreased membrane potential in different kinds of disease.

Figure 4-2 illustrates the importance of I_{K1} alterations in the development of depolarization-induced abnormal automaticity. It shows results of an experimental study in which the amino acids that form the I_{K1} channel in guinea pig ventricular muscle cells were altered to reduce the channel's conductance and resting membrane potential. Panel A (upper left) shows the normal stimulated ventricular muscle action potential occurring at a resting potential of slightly less than −80 mV along with the normal ECG in Panel C.

Panel B, after conductance of I_{K1} was reduced, shows an abnormally automatic ventricular muscle cell at a depolarized membrane potential of −60 mV. The abnormal automaticity was accompanied by ventricular arrhythmias as shown in the ECG in Panel D.

A similar reduction in I_{K1} conductance in diseased working myocardium results in depolarization-induced abnormal automaticity. Examples from the atrium and from Purkinje cells are displayed in **Figure 4-3**. Panel A shows a normal human working atrial muscle cell action potential with a resting membrane potential of −82 mV with no evidence of pacemaker activity. Panel B shows action potentials recorded from diseased human atria with a depolarized membrane potential (~−50 mV). SDD is evident (arrow), causing abnormal automaticity.

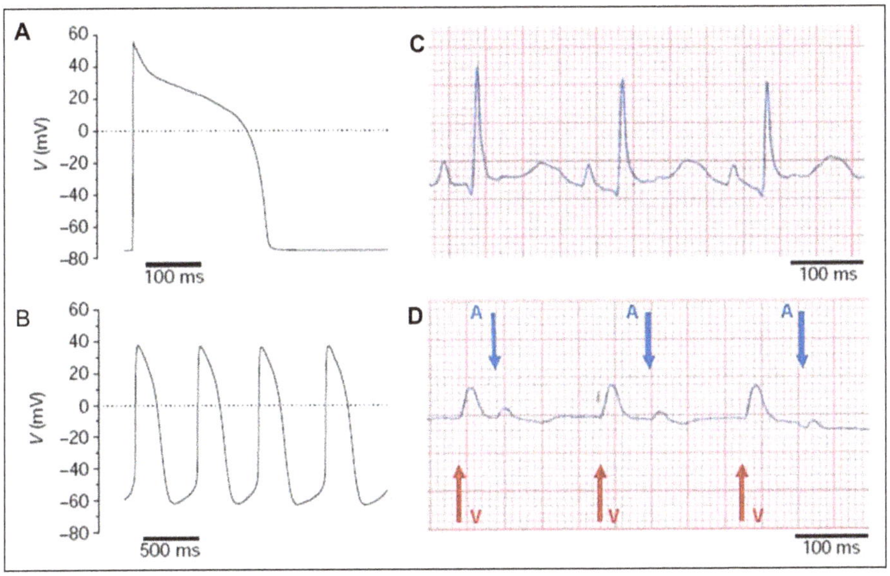

Figure 4-2 Action potentials and ECG recorded from guinea pig ventricular muscle cell. **Panels A** and **C** show recordings from a normal heart. **Panels B** and **D** show effects of reducing I_{K1}. A, atrial depolarization; V, ventricular depolarization. (Reproduced from Miake J, Marbán E, et al. Biological pacemaker created by gene transfer. *Nature*. 2002;419:132–133.)

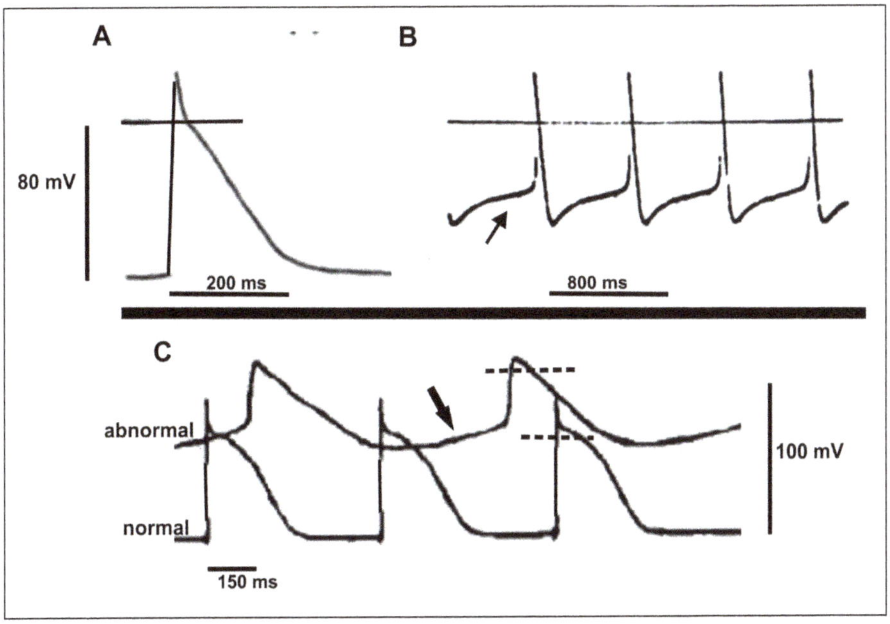

Figure 4-3 **Panel A:** Normal human working atrial muscle action potential. **Panel B:** Diseased human atrium action potentials with abnormal automaticity (**arrow** points to SDD). (Record kindly provided by Dr. M.R. Rosen.) **Panel C:** Normal Purkinje cell action potentials (**bottom recording**) and abnormal automaticity in a subendocardial Purkinje cell in the infarcted region (**top recording**) (**arrow** points to SDD). Horizontal **dashed lines** are 0 potentials for **upper and lower recordings**.

Panel C shows Purkinje cell action potentials recorded from the infarcted canine heart. A normal action potential recorded from normal tissue bordering the infarct is displayed in the lower recording (MDP is ~ −90 mV). In the upper recording are action potentials from a subendocardial Purkinje cell in the infarcted region (abnormal) showing reduction in the membrane potential (~ −60 mV) and abnormal automaticity.

Other mechanisms for pathologic membrane depolarization. An increased membrane permeability to Na^+, which is low at the normal resting potential, also decreases the resting membrane potential because of the entry of increased positive charges into the cell. This might occur in ischemia and other cardiac diseases.

Myocardial cells might also be partially depolarized by the flow of electrotonic current from an adjacent region with a much less negative level of membrane potential. One example is at an infarct border zone. In the infarcted region, depolarized cells with less negative membrane potentials that may be inexcitable because of Na^+-channel inactivation (see Figure 4-5) can sometimes provide the electrotonic current to induce abnormal automaticity in myocardium adjacent to the ischemic and infarcted regions that has more negative membrane potentials and is excitable. The mechanism is similar to the laboratory experiment diagrammed in Figure 4-1. The electrotonic current acts similarly to the applied current pulse to reduce the level of the membrane potential of bordering cells (see Figure 1-3, red arrow in right panel) causing them to initiate abnormally automatic impulses.

A reduced level of membrane potential is not the only criterion for defining this kind of abnormal automaticity. If this was so, the automaticity of the sinus node would have to be considered abnormal. An important distinction between abnormal automaticity at a low level of membrane potential and normal automaticity is that the membrane potential of cells showing the abnormal type of automaticity is reduced from their own normal high level. For this reason, we do not classify automaticity in the A-V node or A-V valves, where membrane potential is normally low, to be abnormal automaticity, although the mechanism for automaticity may be similar.

Membrane Currents Involved in Depolarization-Induced Abnormal Automaticity

A simplified diagram of the membrane currents that cause abnormal automaticity when membrane potential is decreased in working myocardial cells is shown in **Figure 4-4**. The diagram does not show the time courses or the magnitudes of the currents.

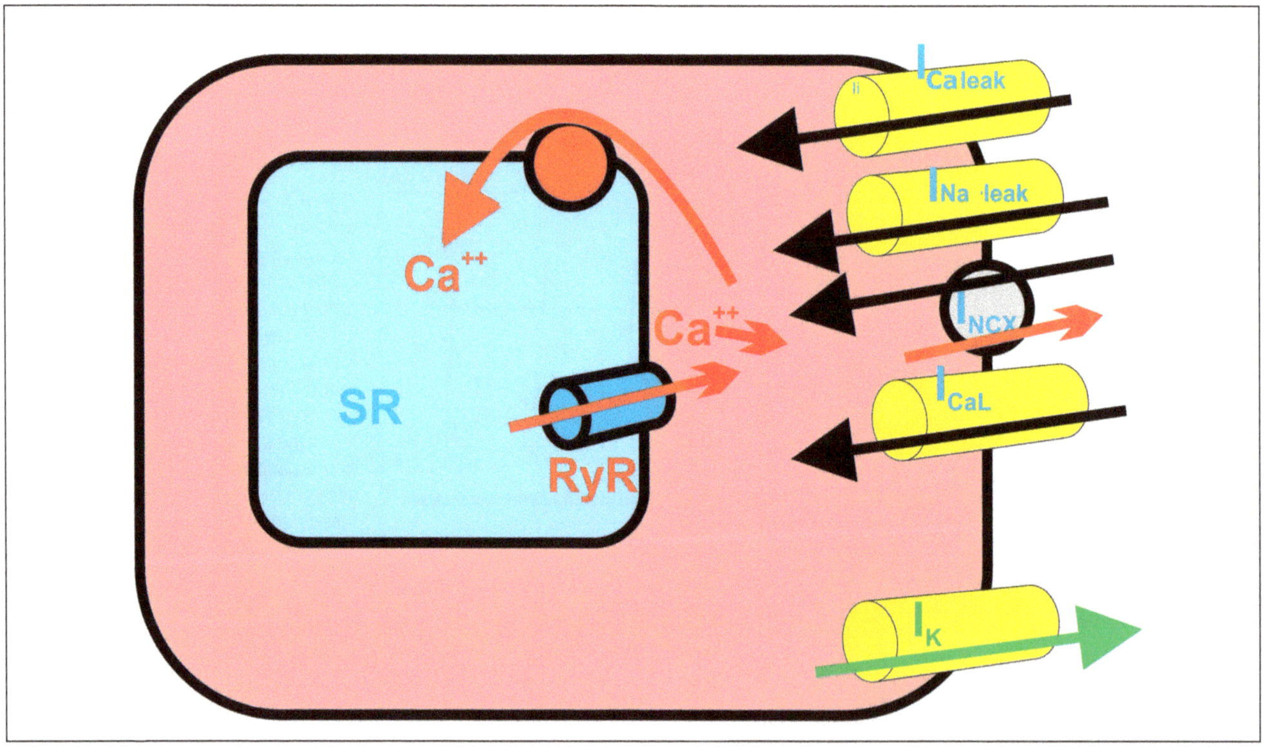

Figure 4-4 Diagram showing membrane currents involved in depolarization-induced abnormal automaticity in a ventricular myocardial cell. **Pinkish area** is myoplasm surrounded by sarcolemma. Within the cell, the **blue region** represents sarcoplasmic reticulum (SR). **Arrows** show direction of current flow.

Inward I_{Na}, I_{CaL}, I_{NCX} currents; decreased outward I_{K1}. At the depolarized level of membrane potential (for example normal membrane potential of –85 mV depolarized to –60 mV by pathology), both the inward leakage of Na^+ and Ca^{2+} (background currents) as well as I_{NCX} provide inward current (Figure 4-4, black arrows). They have a significant depolarizing influence since they are not opposed by a strong outward I_{K1}, which is reduced at the low level of membrane potential and by pathology. Ca^{2+} also enters the cell by I_{CaL} during action potentials (black arrow). Myoplasmic Ca^{2+} is pumped into the SR (red circle and curved red arrow). I_{NCX} is driven by the Ca^{2+} release from the SR through RyR2 channels (dark blue cylinder, straight red arrow) following each contraction and removed from the cell by the Na^+–Ca^{2+} exchanger (grey circle, red arrow) (also see Figure 2-6, Figure 3-3). As the action potential repolarizes due to I_K (green arrow), the driving force on inward $I_{NCX,}$ which is the negative level of the membrane potential, increases leading to SDD. In addition, during repolarization after a spontaneous action potential, I_K deactivates as membrane potential becomes more negative. The resultant decrease in repolarizing outward current (green arrow) contributes to the net increase in the inward current causing SDD.

Inward I_f. The role of inward current supplied by I_f in abnormal automaticity is uncertain. SDD in atrial cells with low (depolarized) membrane potentials occurs in two phases (see Figure 4-3, Panel B), with an initial fast rate of depolarization followed by a slower rate of depolarization similar to normal latent atrial pacemakers at higher levels of membrane potential (see Figure 3-3). The initial fast rate of depolarization may result from a contribution from the I_f pacemaker current, which may be upregulated in diseased atrial myocardium. The second phase of diastolic depolarization is likely caused by Ca^{2+}-induced Ca^{2+} release from the SR and the resultant I_{NCX} inward current, similar to that shown in Figure 3-3. Any role of the I_f pacemaker current in depolarization-induced automaticity in ventricular cells is also likely to be minor because of the low level of these channels expressed in ventricular muscle, although as in the atrial cells, they may be upregulated in some diseases.

In normal latent pacemakers such as Purkinje cells, the I_f channel/current, which is the predominant pacemaker current (Figure 3-31), has a gating mechanism controlling channel's opening and closing that is dependent on the transmembrane voltage. The channels are closed at membrane potentials positive to –60 mV, such as after the upstroke (phase 0) and during the early phases of repolarization of a normal action potential. The channels open in response to the increasingly negative potentials that occur during repolarization, leading to the generation of the inward pacemaker current. When the steady-state membrane potential of Purkinje cells is reduced from its normal level of around –90 mV to around –60 mV or less (Figure 4-3, Panel C), this normal pacemaker current is probably not activated significantly since most of the channels are closed at these levels of membrane potential. The abnormal automaticity that occurs, therefore, is not caused by I_f as is normal automaticity in these cells. The mechanism for abnormal automaticity in Purkinje cells is likely similar to that of depolarized atrial or ventricular myocardium described above.

Characteristics of Phase 0 Depolarization in Abnormal Automaticity

The upstroke (phase 0 depolarization) of the action potential in depolarization-induced abnormally automatic working myocardium has different characteristics than the phase 0 of normal cells. These different characteristics are due to the effects of the steady-state depolarization of the resting potential on the function of the Na^+ and Ca^{2+} channels.

Figure 4-5 shows the effects of reducing the resting membrane potential (depolarization) on phase 0 and Na^+ channel function. At the top is a diagram of the cell membrane with accompanying action potentials below. Na^+ channels are pictured as controlled by "gates": m is the activation gate that opens when the cell is excited, and h is the inactivation gate that closes during and after phase 0. Going from top to bottom in Panel A, the cell membrane diagram shows the resting state, activated state, and inactivated state. In the resting state (top), at the resting membrane potential, the activation gates (m) are closed and the inactivation gates (h) are open, and there is no current flow. In the activated state, the channel is opened by the activation gates (m), permitting Na^+ current to flow (arrows) during depolarization (phase 0) of the action potential. In the inactivated state that occurs after the peak of the action potential, the channel is closed by the h gate (inactivation) and current ceases to flow. The action potential at the left (Panel A) arises from a highly negative resting potential (–90 mV), and all Na^+ channels function to allow depolarizing current (I_{Na}) to generate a normal action potential with a rapid phase 0 (small arrow). The center (Panel B) represents a diseased area, where the action potential arises from a less negative resting potential caused by decreased I_{K1}. This partial depolarization inactivates a fraction of Na^+ channels by closure of the h gates since inactivation by the h gate is dependent on membrane voltage. It closes some channels at a reduced membrane potential, reducing Na^+ current flow even though activated m gates can open, and reducing the rate of phase 0 depolarization (small arrow). A decrease in the electrochemical gradient (inside of the cell being less negative) also contributes to the reduced I_{Na}. At the right (Panel C), at a more depolarized (less negative) membrane potential, increased Na^+ channel inactivation caused by closure of the h gates that occurs at a reduced membrane potential, results in failure of current to flow and action potential generation (arrow).

In **Figure 4-6**, the L-type Ca^{2+} channel is added to the diagram of the cell membrane.

In Figure 4-6, the L-type Ca^{2+} channel is also depicted as being controlled by an activation gate (d) and an inactivation gate (f), both of which must be in the open state for current to flow through the channel during the plateau phase (2, arrow) of the normal action potential, after the fast Na^+ channel is mostly inactivated (Panel A). At the depolarized level of the membrane potential that results in failure of action potential generation because of the failure of Na^+ channels in Figure 4-5, Panel C, the L-type Ca^{2+} channel can still function (Figure 4-6, Panel B) and provide inward Ca^{2+} current during phase 0 (arrow) that enables a "slow response" Ca^{2+}-dependent action potential to be generated. The occurrence of these action potentials is enhanced by the presence of catecholamines that increases the Ca^{2+} current. In situations where membrane depolarization is not sufficient to inactivate all Na^+ channels, the inward depolarizing phase 0 current may be mixed with both a Na^+ and Ca^{2+} component.

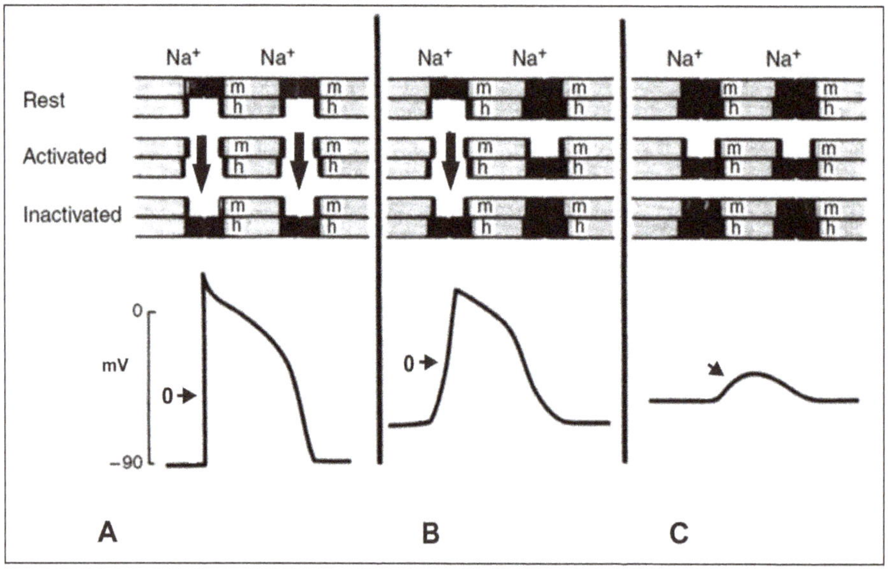

Figure 4-5 Diagram of the effects of decrease in resting membrane potential on the depolarization phase (0) of working myocardial cells. Diagrams of the Na^+ channels are **above** the action potentials. Ca^{2+} channels that also provide inward current have been omitted from the diagram, but are included in the next figure.

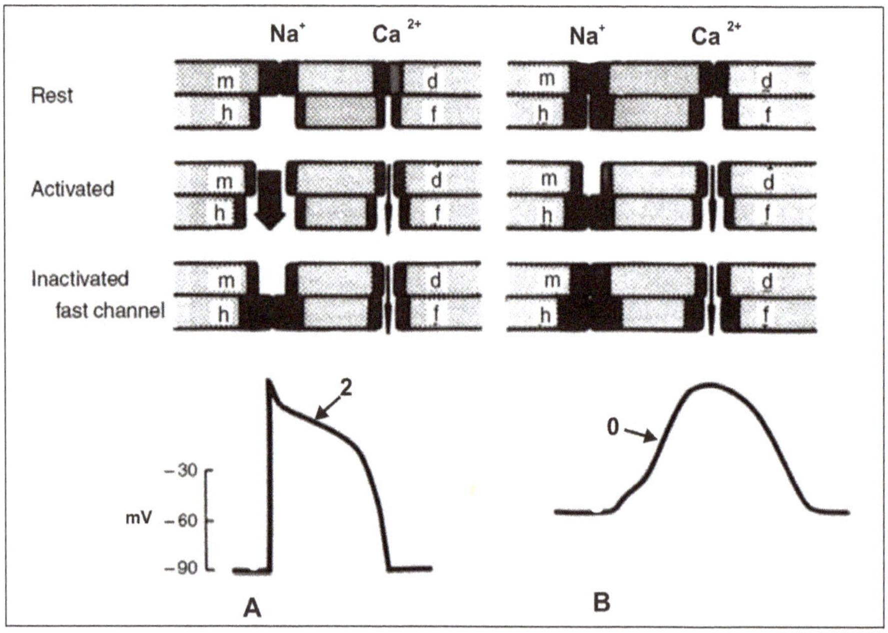

Figure 4-6 Diagram of the effects of decrease in resting membrane potential on the depolarization phase (0) of working myocardial cells. **Panel A:** Na^+ and Ca^{2+} inward currents during normal action potential. **Panel B:** Ca^{2+} inward current at depolarized membrane potential.

A similar conversion of the depolarization phase 0 from fast Na^+ current to a slow L-type Ca^{2+} current also occurs in normally automatic Purkinje cells when they are depolarized to cause abnormal automaticity. The change in properties of phase 0 depolarization in abnormally automatic cells is important in determining the different response of abnormal automaticity to overdrive stimulation and pharmacological agents compared to normal automaticity as described below. It also slows conduction velocity of the impulse that is related to the speed and amplitude of phase 0 depolarization. The importance of this property in causing conduction block and reentry is described in Chapter 9.

Relationship between Depolarized Membrane Potential and Rate of Abnormal Automaticity

As shown in Figure 4-1, an important factor influencing rate of depolarization-induced automaticity is the level of membrane potential to which the cell is depolarized. The less negative the membrane potential, the faster the rate. The increased automatic rate with depolarization is brought about through an acceleration of the pacemaker depolarization (increase in net inward current increases the slope of phase 4) and movement of MDP closer to the threshold potential. (see Figure 1-2 for control of normal automatic rate).

Autonomic Nervous System (ANS)

The rate of depolarization-induced abnormal automaticity is also influenced by the ANS in a similar way as normal automaticity. It is accelerated by sympathetic activation through the effects of norepinephrine on β_1-adrenergic receptors. β_1-adrenergic stimulation enhances a number of different cellular mechanisms, some of which enhance abnormal pacemaker activity and some of which oppose it. Enhanced I_{NCX} (by increased inward I_{CaL} and SR Ca^{2+} loading) accelerates rate, while increased I_K opposes this rate acceleration. Acceleration usually predominates. Parasympathetic activation affects mainly atrial pacemakers, slowing rate by increasing outward acetylcholine sensitive K^+ currents. Therefore, both ventricular and atrial arrhythmias caused by abnormal automaticity are accelerated by exercise, and atrial arrhythmias are slowed by vagal maneuvers, similar to arrhythmias caused by normal automaticity.

When and How Does Abnormal Automaticity Cause Arrhythmias?

Myocardial cells with a propensity for abnormal automaticity do not fire automatically when impulses from the sinus node activate them at a faster rate than their intrinsic abnormal, automatic rate, as is the case for latent pacemakers with normal automaticity.

An abnormal automatic focus manifests itself and causes an arrhythmia when the sinus rate decreases below the intrinsic rate of the abnormally automatic cells. The firing rate of abnormally automatic cells might also be enhanced above that of the sinus node—for example, by depolarization or ANS stimulation leading to arrhythmias in the absence of sinus node suppression.

As described earlier, the rate of impulse initiation by cells with depolarization-induced abnormal automaticity, is dependent on the level of the resting membrane potential. A consequence of this reduction of membrane potential can also be conduction block into or out of the abnormally automatic focus, since conduction is also dependent on the level of the membrane potential (see Figure 9-4). When conduction into the focus is blocked, it is not overdriven by the sinus impulses. This might lead to parasystole if conduction still can occur out of the focus—that is, if block is unidirectional (Figure 9-15). When conduction out of the focus blocks as well, the abnormal automaticity is not expressed as an arrhythmia.

Another factor that influences the ability of abnormally automatic pacemakers to assume the role of dominant pacemaker and cause arrhythmias is the degree to which they are overdrive suppressed by the sinus rhythm, described in the next section.

THE EFFECTS OF ELECTRICAL STIMULATION

Overdrive Suppression of Depolarization-Induced Abnormal Automaticity

Similar to normal automaticity, arrhythmias caused by depolarization-induced abnormal automaticity are neither started nor stopped by overdrive stimulation, an important feature that distinguishes this mechanism from DAD-triggered activity (Chapter 5).

Abnormal automaticity in myocardial cells with depolarized membrane potentials is not overdrive-suppressed to the same extent as normal automaticity that occurs at high negative (normal) levels of membrane potential, such as in some atrial pacemakers (crista terminalis) and in Purkinje cell pacemakers. The amount of suppression of depolarization-induced abnormal automaticity by overdrive is related to the level of membrane potential. **Figure 4-7** compares overdrive suppression in Purkinje cells with different levels of membrane potential.

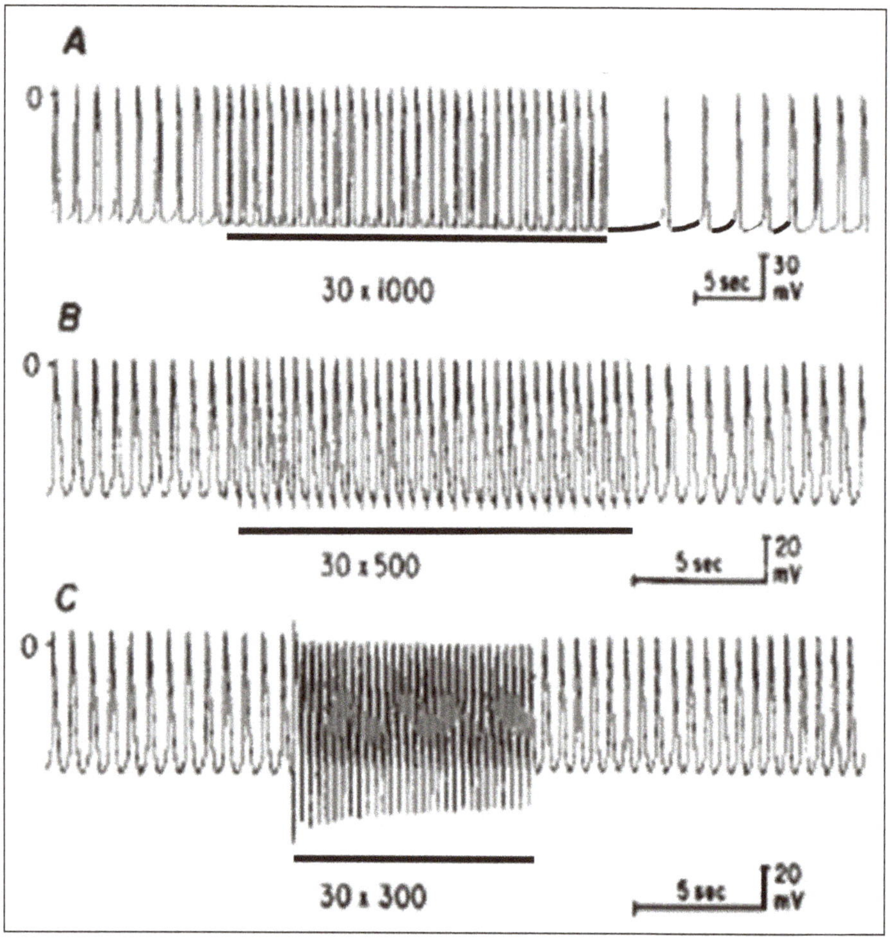

Figure 4-7 Effects of overdrive on normal (**Panel A**) and abnormal automaticity (**Panels B** and **C**). Amplification is increased in **Panels B** and **C** (see mV scale) compared to **Panel A**, and time base is expanded in **Panels B** and **C**. (Reproduced from Dangman KH, Hoffman BF. Studies on overdrive stimulation of canine cardiac Purkinje fibers: Maximal diastolic potential as a determinant of the response. *JACC*. 1983; 2:1183–1190.)

In Figure 4-7, Panel A, the spontaneous firing rate at the left of a Purkinje cell with a high level of membrane potential (~–90 mV) and normal automaticity is followed by a period of overdrive indicated by the horizontal black bar (30 impulses of overdrive at 1000-ms CL). The overdrive suppression following termination of stimulation is indicated by a long CL, about 5 sec, with gradual warm up to the pre-overdrive spontaneous rate, a normal characteristic of overdrive suppression.

Figure 4-7, Panel B shows overdrive of abnormal automaticity at a low level of membrane potential of –60 mV (note amplification in mV has been increased, so action potentials appear the same as in Panel A, even though they have a less negative level of membrane potential and smaller amplitudes). In Panel B, a train of overdrive stimuli (30 impulses at 500-ms CL) indicated by the horizontal black bar is not followed by overdrive suppression.

Figure 4-7, Panel C also shows overdrive of abnormal automaticity in a Purkinje cell at a low level of membrane potential of –60 mV (amplification is also increased as in Panel B). After a train of 30 stimuli at a 300-ms CL (during the period indicated by the horizontal black bar), there is also no overdrive suppression. Rather (although it is difficult to see at the slow recording speed), there is overdrive acceleration; that is, the spontaneous CLs following the overdrive are shorter than the pre-overdrive CL. When the level of depolarized membrane potential is intermediate (for example, –75 to –70 mV), there may be some overdrive suppression that is less than that which occurs at the high level of membrane potential (not shown in the figure).

Mechanism for Lack of Overdrive Suppression

The mechanism for overdrive suppression of normal automaticity is described in Chapter 1. It is dependent on an increase in the electrogenic Na^+/K^+ outward pump current (I_p) to decrease net inward pacemaker current when there is an increase in intracellular Na^+ caused by overdrive (see Figure 1-6). However, as membrane potential is reduced to cause depolarization-induced abnormal automaticity, the Na^+ channel responsible for the action potential upstroke (phase 0) is progressively inactivated and less Na^+ enters the cell during each action potential (see Figure 4-5). Concomitantly less Na^+ also enters the cell during overdrive, resulting in decreased stimulation of the pump and less or no overdrive suppression.

However, long periods of very rapid overdrive can sometimes suppress depolarization-induced abnormal automaticity because sufficient Na^+ eventually enters the cell to stimulate the pump through any remaining functioning Na^+ channels. Although the first CL after overdrive can be slightly prolonged, return to the pre-overdrive CL occurs rapidly instead of gradually, as is the characteristic of normal automaticity. At intermediate levels of membrane potential where there are some functioning Na^+ channels, sufficient Na^+ enters to stimulate the pump during rapid rates of overdrive to cause overdrive suppression.

The same lack of response of depolarization-induced abnormal automaticity to overdrive suppression shortens the time period for an escape impulse to occur from an abnormally automatic pacemaker after sinus node suppression. Because of the lack of overdrive suppression at low membrane potentials, transient slowing of the sinus node might allow an abnormally automatic pacemaker to capture the heart almost immediately for one or more impulses during the period of slowing. In contrast, ectopic pacemakers with normal automaticity would require a longer period of time for escape impulses to occur because they are overdrive suppressed by the sinus node, even during normal sinus rhythm.

Overdrive acceleration (Figure 4-7, Panel C) may be a consequence of increased Ca^{2+} entering during the overdrive, which is extruded by the Na^+–Ca^{2+} exchanger to generate increased I_{NCX} (see Figure 4-4). It is expected that a clinical arrhythmia caused by depolarization-induced abnormal automaticity could be distinguished from one caused by normal automaticity by its lack of suppression by overdrive and even acceleration.

Premature Stimulation and Resetting

Prematurely stimulated impulses reset depolarization-induced abnormal automaticity similarly to normal automaticity. However, one difference may be shortening of the first few CLs following early, prematurely stimulated impulses similar to the overdrive acceleration described above (recall that return CL of normally automatic pacemakers is usually the same as the pre-stimulus CL (Figure 1-10). Abnormal automaticity is neither stopped nor initiated by premature impulses.

PHARMACOLOGY

Depolarization-induced abnormal automaticity has some identical responses to pharmacological agents as normal automaticity but also some different responses. This can help in identifying this mechanism as being the cause of a clinical arrhythmia.

Depolarization-induced abnormal automaticity in the atria and ventricles is accelerated by β_1-adrenergic agonists. It is slowed by cholinergic agonists in the atria. Effects in the ventricle are unknown, but it is likely that there is little effect. These effects are similar to normal automaticity, so response to the ANS or autonomic drugs cannot be used to distinguish between the two.

Depolarization-induced abnormal automaticity is slowed and stopped by L-type Ca^{2+} channel-blocking drugs because of the important role that I_{CaL} plays in phase 0 of the action potential. Block of this channel can decrease SDD (Figure 4-4) and shift the threshold potential for phase 0 to less negative values. It can abolish action potentials in foci of abnormal automaticity, at sufficient concentrations. This response is different from normal automaticity where L-type Ca^{2+} channel-blocking drugs have little effect (except sinus and A-V node pacemakers which have normal automaticity at their normal low levels of membrane potential).

Depolarization-induced abnormal automaticity is little affected by Class I antiarrhythmic drugs (Na^+ channel-blockers such as procainamide and lidocaine) due to the reduced role of I_{Na} in action potentials at the low level of membrane potential. These drugs decrease the I_f pacemaker current, but this current does not have a significant role in abnormal automaticity. These drugs do suppress normal automaticity in latent pacemakers because of the important function of I_f in pacemaker activity.

The effects of adenosine on depolarization-induced abnormal atrial automaticity are likely to be the same as for normal atrial automaticity, where adenosine results in a transient slowing response. Adenosine probably does not affect abnormal automaticity in the ventricles, similar to its lack of effect on normal automaticity.

KEY PROPERTIES OF DEPOLARIZATION-INDUCED ABNORMAL AUTOMATICITY

Table 4-1 summarizes the properties of abnormal automaticity caused by depolarization of the resting membrane potential and compares them with normal automaticity. The differences between the two types of automaticity are indicated in bold. These properties can be useful in identifying the clinical arrhythmias caused by this mechanism for abnormal automaticity.

Table 4-1 Comparison of Properties of Normal and Depolarization-Induced Abnormal Automaticity

	Normal Automaticity of Latent Pacemakers	Abnormal Depolarization-Induced Automaticity
Arrhythmia classification	• Premature impulses • Accelerated idioventricular rhythms • Atrial and ventricular tachycardias • Junctional tachycardias	• Premature impulses • Accelerated idioventricular rhythms • Atrial and ventricular tachycardias • Junctional tachycardias
Onset and termination	Not initiated by acceleration of heart rate or premature impulse	Not initiated by acceleration of heart rate or premature impulse
	Starts with premature impulse late in the CL or during a long CL	• **Starts with premature impulse middle or late in the CL** • **Long preceding CL not necessary**
	No relationship between first tachycardia CL, rate, and duration of tachycardia to previous heart rate	No relationship between first tachycardia CL, rate, and duration of tachycardia to previous heart rate
	Sometimes shows warm up	Sometimes shows warm up
	Sometimes slowing of rate prior to termination	Sometimes slowing of rate prior to termination
	Conduction delay not required	Conduction delay not required
	PR interval directly related to atrial tachycardia rate and site of impulse origin	PR interval directly related to atrial tachycardia rate and site of impulse origin
Origin	**Focal origin, arises in special regions**	**Focal origin, can arise in any region**
	P wave in atrial arrhythmias or QRS in junctional or ventriclular arrhythmias are characteristic of site of origin	P wave in atrial arrhythmias or QRS in junctional or ventricular arrhythmias are characteristic of site of origin
Automatic Nervous System	Initiated and accelerated by sympathetic and β_1 agonists at all sites of origin	Initiated and accelerated by sympathetic and β_1 agonists at all sites of origin
	Slowed but not terminated by parasympathetics (carotid massage) and cholinergic agonists in atria	Slowed but not terminated by parasympathetics (carotid massage) and cholinergic agonists in atria
	Slowing not related to A-V conduction delay or block	Slowing not related to A-V conduction delay or block
	Little effect of parasympathetics in ventricles	Little effect of parasympathetics in ventricles
Pharmacology		
Adenosine	Transient slowing of atrial and junctional arrhythmias not related to A-V nodal delay or block	Transient slowing of atrial and junctional arrhythmias not related to A-V nodal delay or block
	No effect in ventricle	Effect in ventricles not known
Verapamil	**Little effect, minor slowing**	**Slowed or terminated; not related to A-V nodal delay or block**
Na^+ channel-blockers	**Sometimes slows and terminates**	**Little or no effect**
Electrical stimulation	Not initiated by overdrive nor premature stimulation	Not initiated by overdrive nor premature stimulation
	Not terminated by overdrive or premature stimulation	Not terminated by overdrive or premature stimulation
	Overdrive stimulation causes transient suppression	**Overdrive stimulation does not cause suppression and can cause transient acceleration**
	• **Reset by premature stimulation** – **CL following premature impulse is same as spontaneous CL**	• **Reset by premature stimulation** – **CL following premature impulse is same or shorter than spontaneous CL**

*BOLD used to emphasize differences in properties.

Examples of Arrhythmias Caused by Abnormal Automaticity

INCESSANT ATRIAL TACHYCARDIA

Figure 4-8 shows the 12-lead ECG of a patient with incessant atrial tachycardia.

It is characterized by a regular supraventricular rhythm with an atrial rate of 105 bpm and 1:1 A-V conduction. Each P wave is followed by a narrow QRS complex with a normal shape and duration. The P waves are negative in leads I and aVL and positive in all other leads, indicating origin in the high left atrium (see Figure 3-8). This ECG alone does not indicate the tachycardia mechanism.

Responses to Electrical Stimulation and Drugs

The arrhythmia in Figure 4-8 could neither be started nor stopped by overdrive stimulation, premature stimulation, or stopped by cardioversion, indicating that this is an automatic tachycardia but not distinguishing between a normal or abnormal automatic mechanism. Overdrive at very rapid rates (CL <300 ms) transiently suppressed the tachycardia by a small amount. Although depolarization-induced abnormal automaticity should not, in general, be overdrive suppressed (as previously explained in Figure 4-7), very rapid overdrive stimulation can sometimes suppress it. The effects of rapid overdrive are shown in **Figure 4-9**, in another patient with incessant automatic atrial tachycardia (not started or stopped by programmed stimulation or cardioversion), with a rate of 130 bpm (CL of 470 ms). An abnormal automatic mechanism is suggested by the small response to overdrive stimulation.

In Panel A, after a period of overdrive at a CL of 300 ms (stimulated atrial electrograms indicated by the black circles), only the first CL is prolonged to 570 ms (horizontal arrow), but the next CL immediately returns to the tachycardia CL (470 ms). In Panel B, after overdrive at a CL of 100 ms (black circles), the first CL is again prolonged (580 ms), followed by an immediate return to the tachycardia CL (470 ms). As explained above (Figure 4-7), although overdrive suppression of abnormal automaticity may not occur because of the lack of Na^+ entering the cell, at very rapid rates of overdrive for long periods of time, as in Figure 4-9, some Na^+ does enter, resulting in a small amount of suppression. The immediate return to the tachycardia CL without the gradual warm up that is characteristic of pacemakers with normal automaticity (see Figure 1-6 and Figure 1-7) suggests the possibility of abnormal automaticity.

Other tests to distinguish abnormal from normal automaticity include the arrhythmias response to pharmacological agents. Atrial tachycardias caused by abnormal automaticity are not slowed or stopped by Na^+ channel-blocking drugs such as quinidine or procainamide but can be slowed or terminated by verapamil. The atrial tachycardia shown in Figure 4-8 was not affected by the Na^+ channel-blocking drug quinidine. The effects of verapamil were not determined but it should slow or stop abnormal automaticity. Response to other agents are similar to tachycardia caused by normal automaticity, including acceleration by sympathomimetic drugs and transient slowing by cholinergic agonists or adenosine without termination and do not distinguish between these mechanisms.

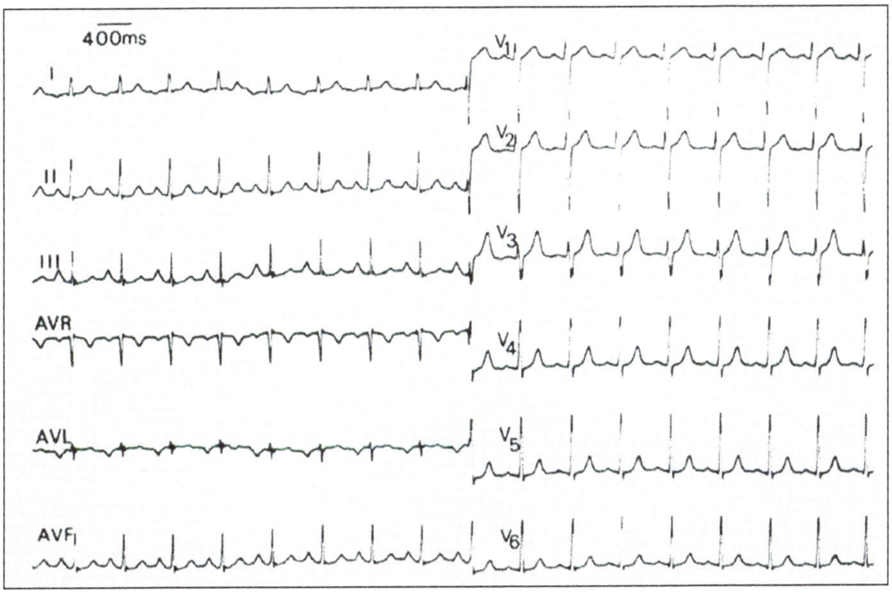

Figure 4-8 A 12-lead electrocardiogram showing incessant atrial tachycardia. (Reproduced from De Baaker JMT, Hauer RNW, et al. Abnormal automaticity as mechanism of atrial tachycardia in the human heart—electrophysiologic and histologic correlation: A case report. *J Cardiovasc Electrophysiol.*1994;5:335–344.)

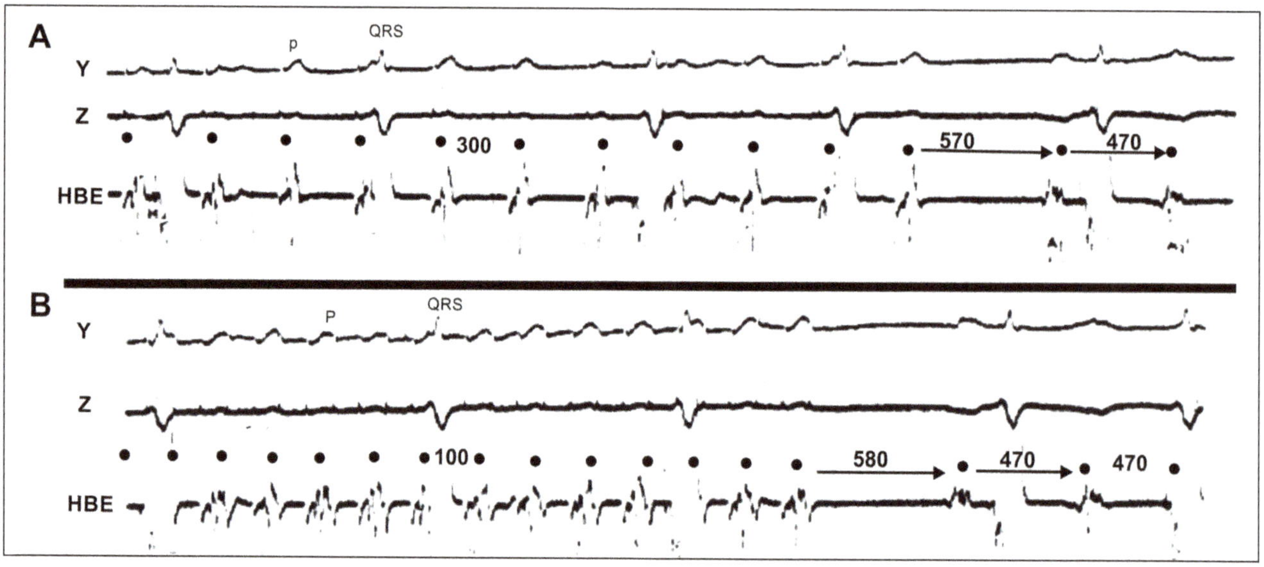

Figure 4-9 Effects of overdrive atrial pacing on chronic incessant atrial tachycardia. Y and inverse Z leads of the Frank orthogonal lead system and an electrogram recorded from the His bundle region (HBE) showing a large atrial deflection. **Panel A** shows overdrive pacing (**black dots**) at a CL of 300 ms. **Panel B** shows overdrive pacing (**black dots**) at a CL of 100 ms. (Record provided by Dr. M. Scheinman.)

Characteristics of Action Potentials at the Site of Arrhythmia Origin

Surgical excision of the tissue after locating the arrhythmia's origin by mapping has been accomplished in a few clinical studies and has identified an abnormal automatic mechanism. The origin of the tachycardia in Figure 4-8 was a focal site in the left atrial appendage. The transmembrane potentials recorded from a surgical specimen excised from the site of origin and superfused in a tissue chamber are shown in **Figure 4-10**.

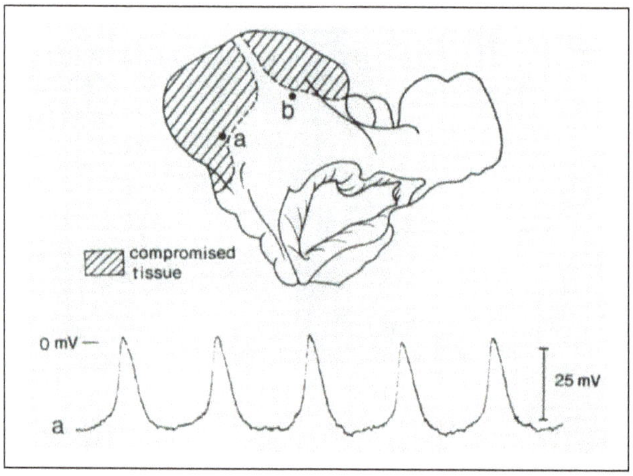

Figure 4-10 Diagram at the top of a specimen of left atrial appendage. The specimen was superfused in a tissue chamber and action potential recorded (shown below) from the site of origin [a] of incessant atrial tachycardia. (Reproduced from De Baaker JMT, Hauer RNW, et al. Abnormal automaticity as mechanism of atrial tachycardia in the human heart—electrophysiological and histologic correlation: A case report. *J Cardiovasc Electrophysiol.* 1994;5:335–344.)

At the top of the figure is a diagram of the excised specimen. The action potentials recorded from site [a] are shown below. The action potentials arise from SDD at a depolarized membrane potential of around −30 mV, and have slow rates of phase 0 consistent with the properties of depolarization-induced abnormal automaticity. The region of origin showed marked pathological changes in structure that likely caused the low membrane potential.

It is uncertain how prevalent this abnormal mechanism is, since the appropriate interventions that might distinguish it from the normal mechanism, e.g., overdrive and verapamil (and surgical excision) usually are not tested. Nevertheless, the origin of focal tachycardias in regions such as the atrial appendages (Figure 3-1) that are not known to have normally automatic cells suggest the likelihood of abnormal automaticity as a mechanism for some tachycardias arising there. Depolarization-induced abnormally automatic tachycardias may occur more frequently in the presence of atrial disease that causes low membrane potentials (Figure 4-5).

ACCELERATED IDIOVENTRICULAR RHYTHM

The arrhythmia in **Figure 4-11** is an accelerated idioventricular rhythm (AIVR) arising in the anteroseptal region in a patient with an acute anterior wall myocardial infarction, occurring after removal of an occluding thrombus. AIVR in myocardial infarction is usually a sign of reperfusion and a marker of reperfusion damage. The timing of the AIVR depends upon the timing of reperfusion and may last for a few minutes. The rate is about 95 bpm, which is greater than the normal rate of a ventricular escape rhythm (30–40 bpm; see Figure 3-32) and less than ventricular tachycardia. The arrhythmia begins with a long coupling interval and is associated with A-V dissociation and fusion QRS complexes. Although in this case the arrhythmia is caused by abnormal automaticity, a similar arrhythmia is described in Chapter 3 (see Figure 3-37) as an example of an accelerated normal automatic pacemaker.

Distinguishing Abnormal and Normal Automaticity in AIVR

Although the ECG features of AIVR in Figure 4-11 are consistent with an arrhythmia caused by automaticity, they do not distinguish between normal and abnormal automaticity. Experimental animal laboratory studies provide additional evidence favoring an abnormal automatic mechanism caused by a low membrane potential in AIVR associated with ischemia, infarction, and reperfusion. In experimental infarction models, this evidence includes:

- AIVR arises from Purkinje cells in the ischemic region with depolarized membrane potentials of −60 to −70 mV.
- AIVR lacks typical overdrive suppression characteristic of normal automaticity.
- AIVR sometimes shows transient acceleration following overdrive.
- AIVR is slowed or suppressed by Ca^{2+} channel-blocking drugs such as verapamil.
- AIVR is not slowed or suppressed by Na^{+} channel-blocking drugs such as lidocaine.

Such data have not been obtained in clinical studies.

ADDITIONAL ARRHYTHMIAS CAUSED BY ABNORMAL AUTOMATICITY

Depolarization-induced abnormal automaticity might cause some junctional tachycardias arising in the His bundle associated with congenital heart surgery or disease of the conducting system.

Some focal ventricular tachycardias associated with cardiac disease such as cardiomyopathies, where membrane potential depolarization is expected to occur, may be caused by depolarization-induced abnormal automaticity. Abnormal automaticity as a cause of these tachycardias has not yet been specifically identified.

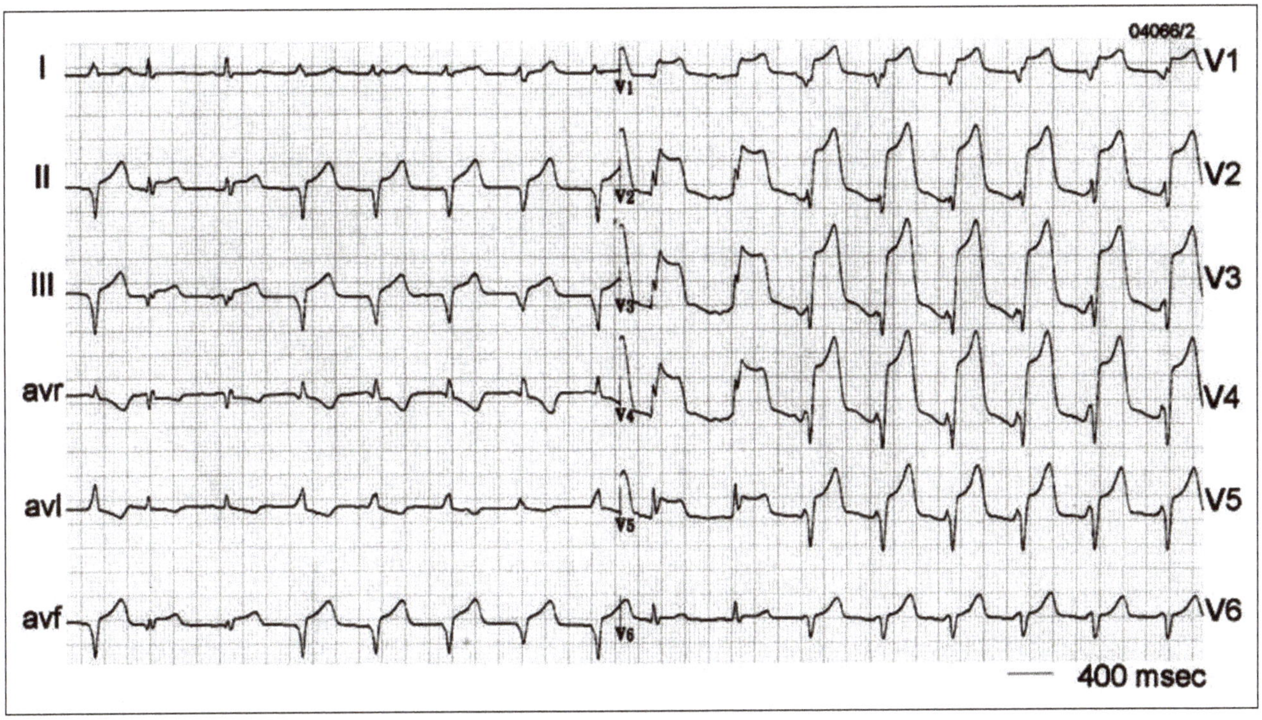

Figure 4-11 A 12-lead ECG showing accelerated idioventricular rhythm (Wellens' ECG collection).

SUMMARY

Abnormal automaticity occurs in diseased myocardial cells, including working ventricular and atrial muscle cells, which do not have the property of normal automaticity. When the resting potentials of working myocardial cells are reduced (become less negative) sufficiently, SDD can occur and cause impulse initiation by the mechanism of depolarization-induced abnormal automaticity. Latent pacemakers that are normally automatic at high (more negative) levels of membrane potential such as Purkinje cells in the ventricular conducting system, also acquire the property of abnormal automaticity when the membrane potential is reduced. The abnormal automaticity is caused by a different mechanism than the normal automaticity.

Abnormal automaticity due to depolarization of the membrane potential occurs in a pathological environment which reduces the negativity of the membrane potential by decreasing intracellular [K^+], increasing extracellular [K^+], or decreasing I_{K1}-channel conductance. An increase in membrane Na^+ permeability can also decrease the membrane potential, as can electrotonic current flow from partially depolarized to more polarized regions. At the depolarized level of membrane potential (for example, normal membrane potential of −85 mV depolarized to −65 mV by pathology), both the inward leakage of Na^+ and Ca^{2+} (background currents) as well as the Na^+–Ca^{2+} exchange current (I_{NCX}) provide inward current contributing to SDD. They have a significant depolarizing influence since they are not opposed by a strong outward I_{K1} that is reduced at the low level of membrane potential and by pathology. I_K deactivation during repolarization is also involved. It is unlikely that the I_f pacemaker current plays a significant role at depolarized levels of membrane potential.

The steady state reduction of the resting potential caused by disease that leads to depolarization-induced abnormal automaticity, inactivates Na^+ channels, decreasing the participation of I_{Na} in generating phase 0 of the action potential. L-type Ca^{2+} channels still function at the depolarized level of the resting potential and therefore, phase 0 depolarization may be mostly dependent on I_{CaL}.

Depolarization-induced abnormal automaticity has unique responses to programmed electrical stimulation and some pharmacological agents that should enable it to be distinguished from normal automaticity in clinical studies. Like normal automaticity, it can be neither started nor stopped by stimulation. It is not overdrive suppressed, as is normal automaticity, because of the reduced amount of Na^+ that enters cells during overdrive and reduced stimulation of I_P. Rapid overdrive stimulation might even cause impulse initiation at shorter CLs after stimulation is stopped (overdrive acceleration) by increasing intracellular Ca^{2+}. Short cycle return responses may also occur after premature stimulation, a response that usually does not occur with normal automaticity.

Depolarization-induced abnormal automaticity is slowed or stopped by Ca^{2+} channel-blocking drugs because of the prominent role that L-type Ca^{2+} current plays in generation of SDD and action potential phase 0. These drugs have little effect on normal automaticity, in which I_{CaL} plays a less prominent role. Na^+ channel-blocking drugs such as procainamide or lidocaine that also decrease I_f have little effect on abnormal automaticity while slowing or stopping normal automaticity.

An example of an arrhythmia caused by abnormal automaticity is incessant atrial tachycardia. Incessant atrial tachycardia caused by abnormal automaticity cannot be started nor stopped by electrical stimulation. It is minimally suppressed by overdrive and might even be accelerated. It is also not affected by Na^+ channel-blocking antiarrhythmic drugs but is slowed by verapamil. Action potentials characteristic of abnormal automaticity have been recorded with a microelectrode in atrial tissue surgically excised at the site of origin of tachycardia.

Accelerated idioventricular rhythm (AIVR) associated with acute myocardial infarction/reperfusion is another arrhythmia that can be caused by abnormal automaticity. The ECG cannot distinguish between normal and abnormal automaticity. Although there is little clinical information pertaining to the mechanism of AIVR in myocardial infarction, experimental laboratory studies attribute it to depolarization-induced abnormal automaticity based on the following: (1) AIVR arises from Purkinje cells in the ischemic region with depolarized membrane potentials (−60 to −70 mV); (2) AIVR lacks typical overdrive suppression characteristic of normal automaticity; (3) AIVR sometimes shows transient acceleration following overdrive; (4) AIVR is slowed or suppressed by Ca^{2+} channel-blocking drugs such as verapamil; and (5) AIVR is not slowed or suppressed by Na^+ channel-blocking drugs such as lidocaine.

SOURCES

Basic Electrophysiology

Cerbai E, Mugelli A. I_f in non-pacemaker cells: Role and pharmacological implications. *Pharmacol Res.* 2006;53:416–423.

Friedman PL, Stewart JR, Wit AL. Spontaneous and induced cardiac arrhythmias in Purkinje fibers surviving experimental myocardial infarction in dogs. *Circ Res.* 1973;33:612–625.

Hoppe UC, Beuckelmann DJ. Characterization of the hyperpolarization-activated inward current in isolated human atrial myocytes. *Cardiovasc Res.* 38;1998;788–801.

Hoppe UC, Jansen E, Sudkamp M, Beuckelmann DJ. Hyperpolarization-activated inward current in ventricular myocytes from normal and failing human hearts. *Circulation.* 1998;97:55–65.

Hordof AJ, Edie R, Malm JR, et al. Electrophysiologic properties and response to pharmacologic agents of fibers from diseased human atria. *Circulation.* 1976;54:774–779.

Ilvento JP, Provet J, Danilo P Jr, Rosen MR. Fast and slow idioventricular rhythms in the canine heart: A study of their mechanism using antiarrhythmic drugs and electrophysiologic testing. *Am J Cardiol.* 1982;49:1909–1916.

Imanishi S, Surawicz B. Automatic activity in depolarized guinea pig ventricular myocardium. Characteristics and mechanisms. *Circ Res.* 1976,39:751–759.

Katzung BG, Morgenstern JA. Effects of extracellular potassium on ventricular automaticity and evidence for a pacemaker current in mammalian ventricular myocardium. *Circ Res.* 1977;40:105–111.

LeMarec HL, Dangman KH, Danilo P Jr, Rosen MR. An evaluation of automaticity and triggered activity in the canine heart one to four days after myocardial infarction. *Circulation.* 1985;71:1224–1236.

Silva J, Rudy Y. Mechanism of pacemaking in *I*K1-downregulated myocytes. *Circ Res.* 2003;92:261–263.

Sridhar A, Dech SJ, Lacombe VA, et al. Abnormal diastolic currents in ventricular myocytes from spontaneous hypertensive heart failure rats. *Am J Physiol Heart Circ Physiol.* 2006;291:H2192–H2198.

Stillitano F, Lonardo G, Zicha, et al. Molecular basis of funny current (If) in normal and failing human heart. *J Mol Cell Cardiol.* 2008;45:289–299.

Wit AL, Bigger JT Jr. Possible electrophysiological mechanisms for lethal cardiac arrhythmias accompanying myocardial ischemia and infarction. *Circulation.* 1975;51 & 52(Suppl. III):96–115.

Zorn-Pauly K, Schaffer P, Pelzmann B, et al. If in left human atrium: A potential contributor to atrial ectopy. *Cardiovasc Res.* 2004;64:250–259.

Clinical Electrophysiology

Gorgels APM, Vos MA, Letsch IS, et al. Usefulness of the accelerated idioventricular rhythm as a marker for myocardial necrosis and reperfusion during thrombolytic therapy in acute myocardial infarction. *Am J Cardiol.* 1988;61:231–235.

Kato M, Dote K, Sasaki S, et al. Intracoronary verapamil rapidly terminates reperfusion tachyarrhythmias in acute myocardial infarction. *Chest.* 2004;126;702-708

Scheinman MM, Basu D, Hollenberg M. Electrophysiologic studies in patients with persistent atrial tachycardia. *Circulation.* 1974;50:266–273.

Sclarovsky S, Strasberg B, Lewin, et al. Multiform accelerated idioventricular rhythm in acute myocardial infarction: Electrocardiographic characteristics and response to verapamil. *Am J Cardiol.* 1993;52:43–47.

Basic Principles of Delayed Afterdepolarizations (DADs) and Triggered Action Potentials

CHAPTER 5

Triggered activity is the second form of impulse initiation listed in the Introduction's Table i-1. "Triggered activity" is the term used to describe impulse initiation that is dependent on afterdepolarizations. It is distinct from automaticity as described in Chapters 1–4, which results from spontaneous diastolic depolarization. Afterdepolarizations are oscillations in membrane potential that follow the primary depolarization phase (0) of an action potential. **Figure 5-1** shows the two types of afterdepolarizations that can cause triggered arrhythmias.

Figure 5-1, Panel A illustrates a delayed afterdepolarization (DAD) (red arrow following action potential 1). It is not initiated until repolarization is complete or nearly complete and therefore is delayed with respect to repolarization. DADs and DAD triggered arrhythmias are the subjects of this chapter and Chapter 6. By way of comparison, in Panel B, the second type of afterdepolarization, referred to as an early afterdepolarization (EAD), is shown by the red arrow following action potential 1. It is manifested as an interruption in repolarization of the action potential and is therefore early with respect to repolarization. (The blue arrow shows normal repolarization.) Early afterdepolarizations and the arrhythmias that they cause are described in Chapters 7 and 8.

An afterdepolarization does not initiate an arrhythmia until its amplitude is large enough to reach the threshold potential for activation of a regenerative inward current that causes an action potential. In Figure 5-1, Panels A and B, this occurs following action potential 2 (second set of red arrows). These action potentials are referred to as triggered action potentials (action potential 3, in green) and the arrhythmias they cause are called triggered arrhythmias. Therefore, for triggered activity to occur, at least one action potential must precede it (in Panels A and B, the trigger is action potential 2) in contrast to automaticity, which can arise de novo in the absence of prior electrical activity. (For example, Figure 1-5 shows an escape rhythm caused by automaticity after sinus node inhibition, the first impulse arises without an immediately preceding "trigger.")

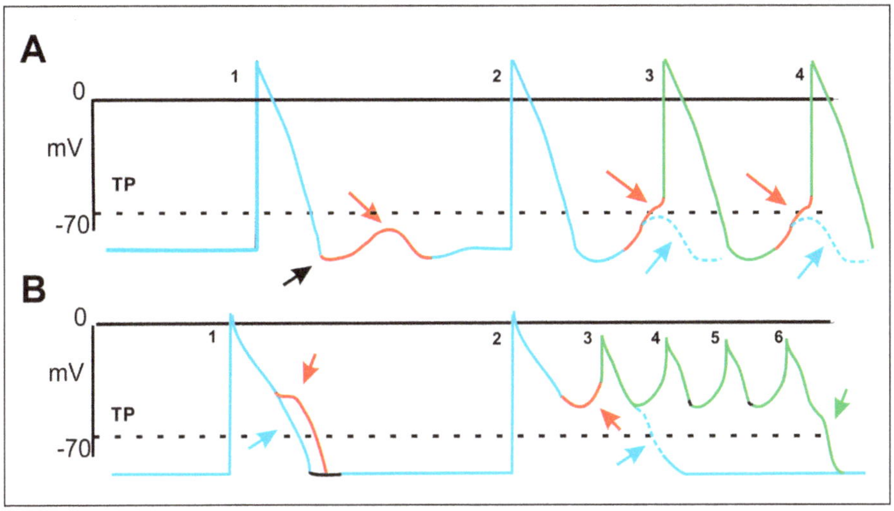

Figure 5-1 There are two types of afterdepolarizations. **Panel A:** Delayed afterdepolarizations (DADs) and DAD-induced triggered action potentials. **Panel B:** Early afterdepolarizations (EADs) and EAD-induced triggered action potentials. Voltage calibration is at the **left** with 0 potential indicated; TP, threshold potential (**dashed line**).

Electrophysiological Foundations of Cardiac Arrhythmias: A Bridge Between Basic Mechanisms and Clinical Electrophysiology, Second Edition.
© 2020 Andrew L. Wit, Penelope A. Boyden, Mark E. Josephson, Hein J. Wellens. Cardiotext Publishing, ISBN: 978-1-942909-42-2.

CHARACTERISTIC APPEARANCE OF DADS AND DAD-TRIGGERED ACTION POTENTIALS

Figure 5-1, Panel A shows the general features of DADs. An action potential of a myocardial cell at the left (in light blue, labeled 1) is followed after complete repolarization by a low-amplitude and short-duration depolarization of the membrane potential (in red with red arrow) that is caused by a transient net inward current during diastole. The afterdepolarization is coupled to and caused by the previous action potential (see below for a description of the mechanism). The DAD may be preceded by an after-hyperpolarization (black arrow following action potential 1), during which the membrane potential becomes transiently more negative than the membrane potential just prior to its initiation. The transient nature of the afterdepolarization clearly distinguishes it from normal spontaneous diastolic (automatic, phase 4) depolarization (SDD), during which the membrane potential declines until an action potential is initiated (Figure 1-1, Panel B).

DAD-Triggered Action Potentials

In Figure 5-1, Panel A, the DAD following action potential 2 is larger, and its depolarization (in red, red arrows) reaches the threshold potential (TP, dashed horizontal line) resulting in a regenerative inward current (Na^+ or Ca^{2+}, depending on the level of the membrane potential) to cause an action potential (action potential 3 in green) called a triggered impulse. The dashed curve in blue and the blue arrow show the time course of the DAD if no triggered action potential had been initiated. This emphasizes that the triggered action potential arises from a DAD. DADs do not always reach threshold (following action potential 1), so that triggerable cells may sometimes be activated regularly (during sinus rhythm) without becoming rhythmically active. The conditions under which they reach threshold are described below. A triggered action potential is also followed by a DAD (red trace and arrow following action potential 3) that may or may not reach threshold. When it does, the first triggered action potential is followed by a second triggered action potential (action potential 4 in green), arising from the DAD caused by the previous action potential. The blue dashed curve associated with action potential 4 shows the membrane potential had the DAD not reached threshold potential. This process can continue, resulting in a series of triggered action potentials that eventually stop when a DAD does not reach threshold potential.

CELLULAR MECHANISMS OF DADS AND DAD-TRIGGERED ACTIVITY: THE ROLE OF CALCIUM

DADs and the triggered activity that they cause result from an oscillatory membrane current originally referred to as the transient inward current (TI or I_{TI}). This current is distinct from the pacemaker current that causes normal automaticity. A distinguishing feature of I_{TI} is that it is associated with abnormalities in intracellular calcium cycling between the sarcoplasmic reticulum (SR) and myoplasm. This intracellular Ca^{2+} cycling normally plays an important role in coupling the action potential to myocardial contraction, a process called excitation-contraction coupling in the forward mode.

Excitation-Contraction (EC) Coupling; Forward Mode

Owing to the importance of Ca^{2+} and SR function in the genesis of DAD-triggered arrhythmias, the normal physiology of EC coupling is first briefly described. Normal EC coupling is sometimes referred to as "forward-mode EC coupling," since excitation (in the form of the action potential) precedes and causes contraction. Ca^{2+} enters the cell during the action potential plateau phase (2) to initiate contraction. Abnormalities that cause DADs and triggered arrhythmias result from "reverse-mode EC coupling," since the Ca^{2+} trigger for contraction from the SR precedes excitation that occurs in the form of a DAD.

Figure 5-2, Panels A and B illustrate the normal movement of Ca^{2+} back and forth between myoplasm (MYO) and sarcoplasmic reticulum (SR) during systole (Panel A) and diastole (Panel B).

The SR is a network of tubular membranes depicted as the red rectangular area in the center of each panel in Figure 5-2. It is the main store of intracellular Ca^{2+} (blue dots). Some of this Ca^{2+} in the SR is free, and some is bound to SR proteins, the most important of which is calsequestrin 2 (Casq2), the cardiac isoform of the protein. Casq2 has a high capacity for binding Ca^{2+} (50%–70% of SR Ca^{2+} is bound to it), but a low affinity for Ca^{2+}; thus, it can readily release free Ca^{2+} when required. Therefore, Casq2 is a major determinant of the ability of the SR to store and release Ca^{2+}, and abnormalities in its function can sometimes cause DAD-triggered arrhythmias.

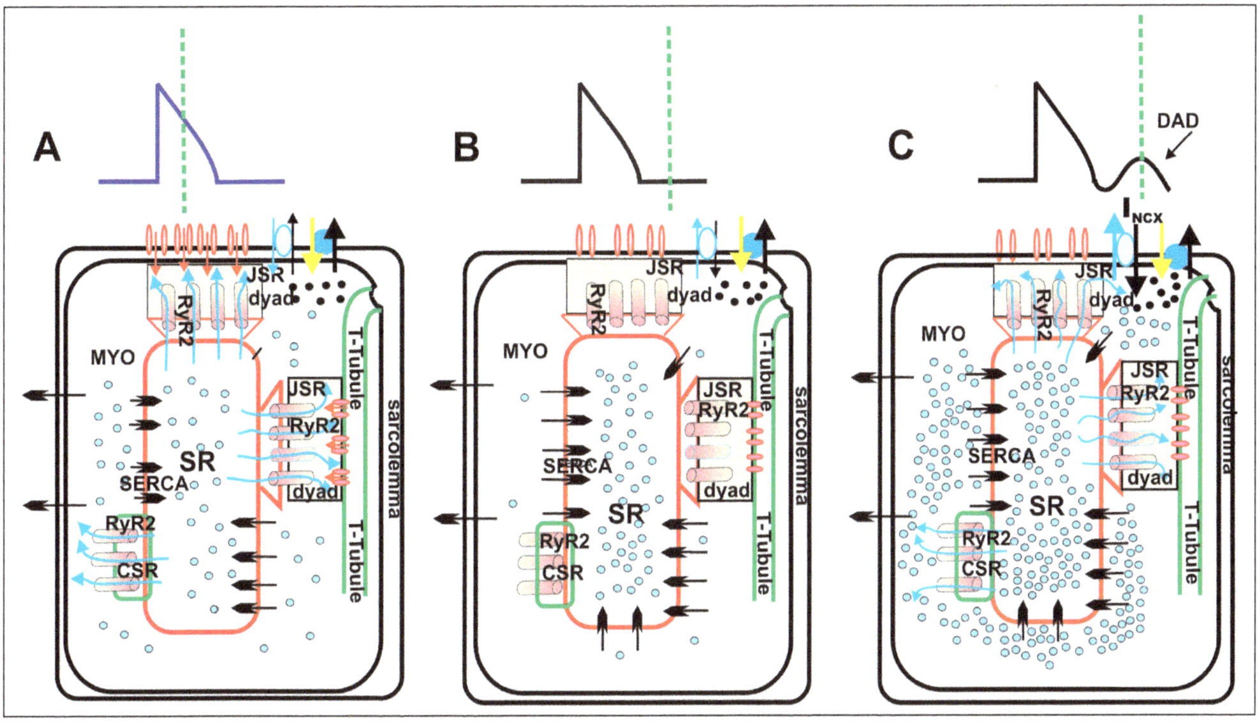

Figure 5-2 Ca^{2+} cycling between myoplasm (MYO) and sarcoplasmic reticulum (SR) in a ventricular muscle. SR outlined in **red**, t-tubules outlined in **green**. CSR; corbular sarcoplasmic reticulum, SR release channels (RyR2) in junctional sarcoplasmic reticulum (JSR). Sarcoplasmic reticulum Ca^{2+} ATPase-dependent pumps (SERCA: **Large black arrowheads**). L-type Ca^{2+} channels: **Small red ovals**. Na^+–Ca^{2+} exchanger: **Light blue oval** in sarcolemma. Na^+–K^+ pump: **Dark blue circle**. Ca^{2+} ions: **Small blue circles**. **Panel A:** Systole (**vertical dashed line** above). **Panel B:** Diastole (**vertical dashed line** above). **Panel C:** DAD formation (in diastole). **Arrows** explained in text.

Free Ca^{2+} is released from the SR into the myoplasm through calcium release channels in the SR membrane (blue arrows, Panel A) called ryanodine receptors (RyR2). The latter are named as such because they were first discovered to respond to the plant alkaloid ryanodine that opens the channels. The number "2" indicates the predominant isoform of the receptor in cardiac myocytes. Ca^{2+} is normally released from the SR during the plateau phase of the transmembrane action potential (Panel A, vertical dashed line on the action potential). The release is triggered mostly by the entrance of Ca^{2+} into the cell via I_{CaL}, through the L-type calcium channel (short red arrows, and small red ovals). This Ca^{2+} binds to the external surface of the RyR2 receptors, opening the Ca^{2+} release channels, a process called Ca^{2+}-induced Ca^{2+} release. The L-type calcium channels are located in invaginations of the sarcolemma forming T tubules that closely abut the junctional sarcoplasmic reticulum (JSR) in terminal cisternae to form dyads. Dyads are also formed where SR abuts non-t-tubular, sarcolemmal membranes (top border). There also may be some net inward Ca^{2+} movement via the Na^+–Ca^{2+} exchanger operating in the forward mode (moves Ca^{2+} into the cell and Na^+ out of the cell) (light blue oval; blue arrow indicates Ca^{2+}, black arrow is Na^+) during the action potential plateau. Notably, the majority of Ca^{2+} that interacts with the contractile proteins in working ventricular and atrial cells, comes from the SR and not directly from Ca^{2+} flux through the L-type channels. The excitation triggers contraction, hence the term "forward" EC coupling.

Ca^{2+} release through the RyR2 operated channels (blue arrows) terminates when SR free Ca^{2+} falls below a threshold level. Ca^{2+}-induced Ca^{2+} release results in about 40%–60% depletion of Ca^{2+} from the SR. RyR2 channel closure may be brought about by an interaction of Casq2 with the channel proteins. Casq2 is the putative SR luminal Ca^{2+} sensor and inhibits RyR2 channel opening when Ca^{2+} is low, causing a temporary state of refractoriness of the channels after each Ca^{2+} release, thus preventing Ca^{2+} release during diastole.

Following the Ca^{2+} release that triggers contraction (Panel A), the myoplasmic Ca^{2+} is reduced by two mechanisms: (1) resequestration into the SR by calcium pumps in the SR membrane (Figure 5-2, Panel B, SERCA, black arrowheads) through active transport with energy supplied by ATPase, and (2) extrusion from the cell mostly by the Na^+–Ca^{2+} exchanger in the sarcolemma operating in the reverse mode at the negative diastolic potential (note reverse direction of the light blue arrow at the blue oval, which represents the Na^+–Ca^{2+} exchanger in Figure 5-2,

Panel B). The function of the exchanger in this reverse mode is described in Chapter 2 in relation to its role in generating an inward current that contributes to the pacemaker potential.

When the Na^+–Ca^{2+} exchanger operates in the reverse mode, it moves more positive charges (3 Na^+, indicated by black arrow in Figure 5-2, Panel B) into the cell than out (1 Ca^{2+}, blue arrow) at diastolic membrane potentials. The movement of Na^+ is down its concentration gradient and generates the energy for moving Ca^{2+} out of the cell against its concentration and electrical gradients (inside 10^{-4} mM free Ca^{2+}, outside 1.8 mM; inside the cell is negative relative to outside the cell, which is positive). The concentration gradient for Na^+ is maintained by the Na^+–K^+ pump that maintains myoplasmic Na^+ at low levels (~ 2–4 mM) (Figure 5-2, Panel B, blue circle, black arrow is Na^+ out of cell in exchange for K^+ into cell, yellow arrow). A small amount of Ca^{2+} is also extruded from the cell by ATPase-dependent sarcolemmal calcium pumps (black arrows at left of the diagram). Under normal circumstances, myoplasmic free Ca^{2+} is reduced to a very low levels during diastole (blue circles) (Figure 5-2, Panel B) resulting in relaxation. Note the steady level of membrane potential during diastole (vertical dashed line) in Panel B.

Spontaneous Diastolic SR Calcium Release and DADs

DADs occur under conditions in which SR Ca^{2+} levels are abnormally elevated called Ca^{2+} overload. They also occur if there are abnormalities in RyR2 function caused by mutations or in acquired pathology (ischemic heart failure) that affects RyR2 receptor function.

Figure 5-2, Panel C shows the mechanism for DADs during Ca^{2+} overload as indicated by the increase in blue circles in Panel C compared to Panels A and B. One cause of Ca^{2+} overload is an increase in Ca^{2+} entering the cell through the L-type Ca^{2+} channels during action potentials, for example, during sympathetic stimulation. Another cause is a decrease in Ca^{2+} extrusion from the cell by the Na^+–Ca^{2+} exchanger as occurs with digitalis toxicity (described in Figure 5-8). Under these conditions, there is increased activity of the SR calcium pumps (Figure 5-2 Panel C, SERCA, black arrows). SERCA senses the increased Ca^{2+} entering the cell (in the myoplasm (MYO) and increases its activity to remove Ca^{2+} from the MYO into the SR in an attempt to maintain the low diastolic level of Ca^{2+} necessary for relaxation. This results in Ca^{2+} "overload" of the SR (blue dots in **Figure 5-2**, Panel C). The SR cannot accommodate this overload and spontaneously releases some of the Ca^{2+} back into the myoplasm through the RYR2 Ca^{2+} release channels after repolarization and during diastole (curved blue arrows); these releases are called calcium sparks since they can be detected by fluorescent microscopy. There is a threshold level of diastolic SR Ca^{2+} that causes RyR2 channels to open, releasing Ca^{2+} into the myoplasm in the absence of membrane depolarization. This process is called store overload-induced Ca^{2+} release. RyR2 receptors may also be sensitive to elevated myoplasmic Ca^{2+}, which causes release channels to open. Furthermore, this diastolic Ca^{2+} release is delayed from the previous major Ca^{2+} release during the action potential plateau that causes contraction because of refractoriness of the release channels that results in the occurrence of DADs to be delayed after complete repolarization. The amount of diastolic Ca^{2+} release from the SR, as well as the rapidity of the release, is related to the amount of Ca^{2+} in the SR. The elevated diastolic Ca^{2+} in the myoplasm is the source of the transient inward (I_{TI}) current that causes DADs (vertical dashed line on action potential above) (described in more detail below). The diastolic release of Ca^{2+} may also be associated with an after-contraction with minimal force following systole, since the contractile mechanism is also activated. Ca^{2+} overload may also be associated with an increase in tonic (diastolic) tension.

The description of Figure 5-2 is an oversimplification of the Ca^{2+} release process. Rather than the SR being one functional unit as shown in Panels A–C, it is many functional units that are formed because the RyR2 channels are clustered and aligned in a specific anatomical pattern to allow for uniform Ca^{2+} release from the SR during the action potential (forward-mode EC coupling). The orderly pattern of RyR2 channels on the SR sets up a series of potential release sites of Ca^{2+} in the cell. When overload of SR occurs to cause DADs, a wave of Ca^{2+} propagates from one ryanodine cluster to another (Ca^{2+} sparks) through the myocyte. The summated Ca^{2+} released causes the DAD that is shown in Figure 5-2, Panel C.

Figure 5-3 shows a ventricular myocyte where a Ca^{2+} wave (indicated by bright fluorescence) has started from spontaneous Ca^{2+} release from the SR (a). This Ca^{2+} wave then propagates the length of the cell (b-p). The increased intracellular Ca^{2+} during the wave is sensed by the Na^+–Ca^{2+} exchanger, which extrudes the Ca^{2+} to produce membrane depolarization as a DAD (see below). This is an example of reverse-mode EC coupling where the increase in myoplasmic Ca^{2+} in the form of a wave, activates Ca^{2+}-dependent membrane ionic current changes.

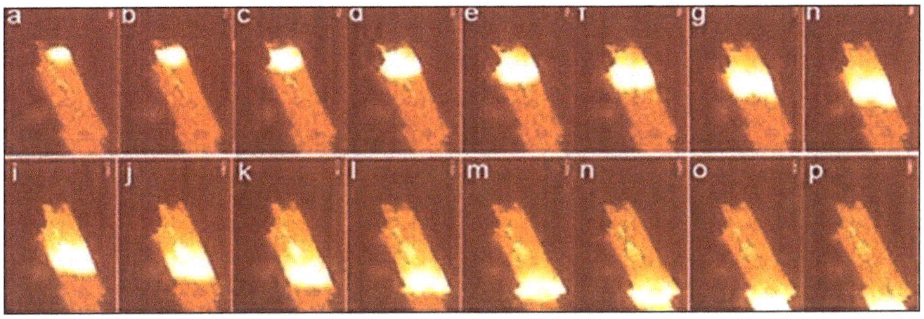

Figure 5-3 Cell-wide Ca^{2+} wave in ventricular myocyte. Images are of a myocyte loaded with a dye that fluoresces with an increase in myoplasmic Ca^{2+}.

In other situations, such as heart failure, ischemic disease, or genetic mutations, SR Ca^{2+} concentration may not be elevated and may even be reduced, but alterations in Ca^{2+} release channel function may still cause transient abnormally high myoplasmic Ca^{2+} levels during diastole that causes DADs. These pathophysiological conditions are described in more detail in the next chapter on DAD arrhythmias.

DADs in Purkinje Cells

Purkinje cells of the ventricular conducting system are more prone to the development of DADs than ventricular muscle, resulting in the Purkinje system being an important source of triggered arrhythmias. Purkinje cells have a microanatomy that is different than ventricular muscle cells depicted in Figure 5-2. In Purkinje cells, t-tubules are absent, and Ca^{2+} entering through the L-type channels propagates as a wave from the influx points to the core of the cell to access the RyR2 receptors that are not in direct contact with the sarcolemma, called the corbular sarcoplasmic reticulum (CSR) (Figure 5-2, Panel A). The special microanatomy of the SR in Purkinje cells with different forms of Ca^{2+} release channels leads to larger Ca^{2+} release from the SR and Ca^{2+} wave propagation. Increased Na^+ entry during the action potential (both during phase 0 and the plateau phase (2) of repolarization) leads to an increase in intracellular Ca^{2+} through the actions of the Na^+–Ca^{2+} exchanger. Increased Ca^{2+} entry during the long plateau phase compared to atrial and ventricular muscle also enhances occurrence of DADs. Purkinje cells also have a weaker I_{K1} than in ventricular muscle. As such, there is less outward current at the resting potential to oppose DADs. DADs are also facilitated by weak gap junctional coupling of Purkinje cells to surrounding myocardium, because Purkinje strands are often separated in bundles from underlying muscle. Normally, muscle cells are tightly coupled in three dimensions to surrounding myocardium. As explained in Figure 1-3, such coupling can prevent membrane depolarization because of the flow of electrotonic current during diastole, in this case inhibiting the formation of DADs in muscle cells.

Relationship Between Diastolic Ca^{2+} and Ionic Currents Causing DADs

In the presence of SR Ca^{2+} overload and excessive Ca^{2+} release from the SR into the myoplasm during diastole, the Na^+–Ca^{2+} exchanger extrudes the elevated Ca^{2+} from the cell in exchange for Na^+ (1 Ca^{2+} for 3 Na^+) generating the net inward current (I_{NCX}) causing the DAD (reverse-mode EC coupling) (Figure 5-2 Panel C, light blue oval, blue arrow is Ca^{2+} moving out of cell, black arrow labeled I_{NCX} is the inward Na^+ current). To reiterate, Ca^{2+} is actively extruded by the Na^+–Ca^{2+} exchanger against a concentration gradient requiring energy expenditure (blue arrow), since free diastolic levels are lower than extracellular concentrations of Ca^{2+} even when intracellular Ca^{2+} is increased in situations where DADs are generated. On the other hand, Na^+ moves down an electrochemical gradient (black arrow) from a higher extracellular to lower intracellular concentration. The energy for Ca^{2+} extrusion comes from the movement of Na^+ ions down this gradient and not the splitting of ATP molecules. The current carried by Na^+ movement causing the DAD is transient and decreases as Ca^{2+} at the internal surface of the sarcolemmal membrane is reduced by the exchanger, hence the nomenclature transient inward current (TI or I_{TI}). I_{NCX} is used synonymously with I_{TI}. The magnitude of I_{NCX} is directly related to the Ca^{2+} that is extruded, and this in turn is directly related to the diastolic Ca^{2+} concentration in the myoplasm.

In addition to I_{NCX}, other inward currents have been proposed to contribute to DADs. One current is a non-specific membrane current, which was originally designated to be the primary TI current. The membrane channel of this current was proposed to be Ca^{2+} sensitive, opening with elevated diastolic Ca^{2+}, with non-specific permeability to cations. Since Na^+ is the predominant cation in extracellular space, it is the primary charge carrier of this current. Another possible contributor to the TI current under certain conditions is a calcium-activated chloride current.

ELECTROPHYSIOLOGIC PROPERTIES OF DADS AND TRIGGERED ACTIVITY

In general, the magnitude of DADs as well as coupling interval to the preceding action potential are related to the diastolic Ca^{2+} levels and the rapidity of Ca^{2+} release from the SR. Therefore, events that change the diastolic Ca^{2+} levels and speed of release affect the occurrence and characteristics of triggered arrhythmias.

Dependence on Action Potential Characteristics

One of the factors that controls the size of DADs and the propensity for occurrence of triggered activity is the characteristics of the action potentials that precede them.

Effects of Action Potential Duration

The duration of the action potential (APD)—time from depolarization to complete repolarization—influences the intracellular and diastolic Ca^{2+} levels that cause DADs. Ca^{2+} enters the cell during the plateau phase of the action potential via I_{CaL}, which inactivates as repolarization proceeds to levels more negative than around −60 mV. Therefore, shortening the action potential duration decreases I_{CaL}, which suppresses DADs while lengthening it increases I_{CaL} and enhances DADs. Changes in action potential duration can be brought about by changes in the repolarizing I_K current (see Figure 7-2 for description of repolarizing membrane currents), a decrease of which prolongs APD, and an increase of which shortens APD. A number of drugs can alter I_K, thereby influencing DADs. For example, Class IA drugs (Vaughan Williams classification) that decrease I_K can increase DAD amplitude by lengthening APD and cause triggered activity in the experimental laboratory and possibly in patients.

Effect of Initial Membrane Potential

The amplitude of DADs is dependent on the level of membrane potential at which they arise. Although they may occur in cells with normal resting potentials of ~ −80 to −90 mV, amplitude can increase as membrane potential becomes less negative. Part of this effect may result from a decrease in outward (I_{K1}) current, which occurs during membrane depolarization, and part may result from an increase in I_{TI} current (I_{NCX}). DADs can occur at low diastolic membrane potentials where normal automaticity does not occur because I_f is inactivated (see Figure 4-3). Therefore, DADs may occur in disease-induced depolarized cells as well as cells with normal levels of membrane potential.

Dependence on Cycle Length (Rate and Prematurity)

The effects of cycle length at which action potentials occur, on DADs and DAD-dependent triggered activity differ from their effects on automaticity. These differences provide a basis for distinguishing triggered arrhythmias from automatic arrhythmias and for using electrical stimulation protocols for identifying triggered activity as a cause of arrhythmias. Some of the key differences are as follows:

- Automaticity of ectopic pacemakers is not initiated by an increase in rate (decrease in cycle length) of the dominant (sinus node) pacemaker or by electrical stimulation and is transiently suppressed by overdrive (overdrive suppression).
- DADs are enhanced by an increase in rate (decrease in cycle length) at which triggerable cells are stimulated. Therefore, triggered arrhythmias can be initiated by decreasing the cycle length and triggered activity can be accelerated by overdrive (overdrive acceleration).

Effect Rate on DAD Amplitude, Coupling Interval, and Triggered Activity

This effect of rate (or triggering cycle length) is illustrated in **Figure 5-4**, which is a diagram of action potentials recorded from a cell with DADs. At the left in each panel, the first three action potentials (in black) occur at a cycle length of 1000 ms. The small black arrows point out the DADs. Such subthreshold DADs might occur during sinus rhythm and not be noticed on the ECG.

In Panel A, the cycle length decreases to 800 ms (blue action potentials) and DAD amplitude increases (blue arrow), but does not reach the threshold for initiating a triggered action potential. In the diagram the cycle length is decreased for 10 sec (double black vertical bars indicate break in time scale; only last 3 sec are shown to the right of the bar) as might occur with an increase in sinus rate or during pacing.

In Panel B, the cycle length is decreased from 1000 ms (black action potentials at left) to 600 ms (blue action potentials). There is an increase in the amplitude of the DADs (blue arrow) that causes one to reach threshold (red arrow), initiating a triggered action potential (red arrow and action potential). The DAD following the triggered action potential does not reach threshold (red arrow at the far right) and triggered activity stops after one impulse. This is analogous to an increase in heart rate or pacing rate triggering a premature impulse.

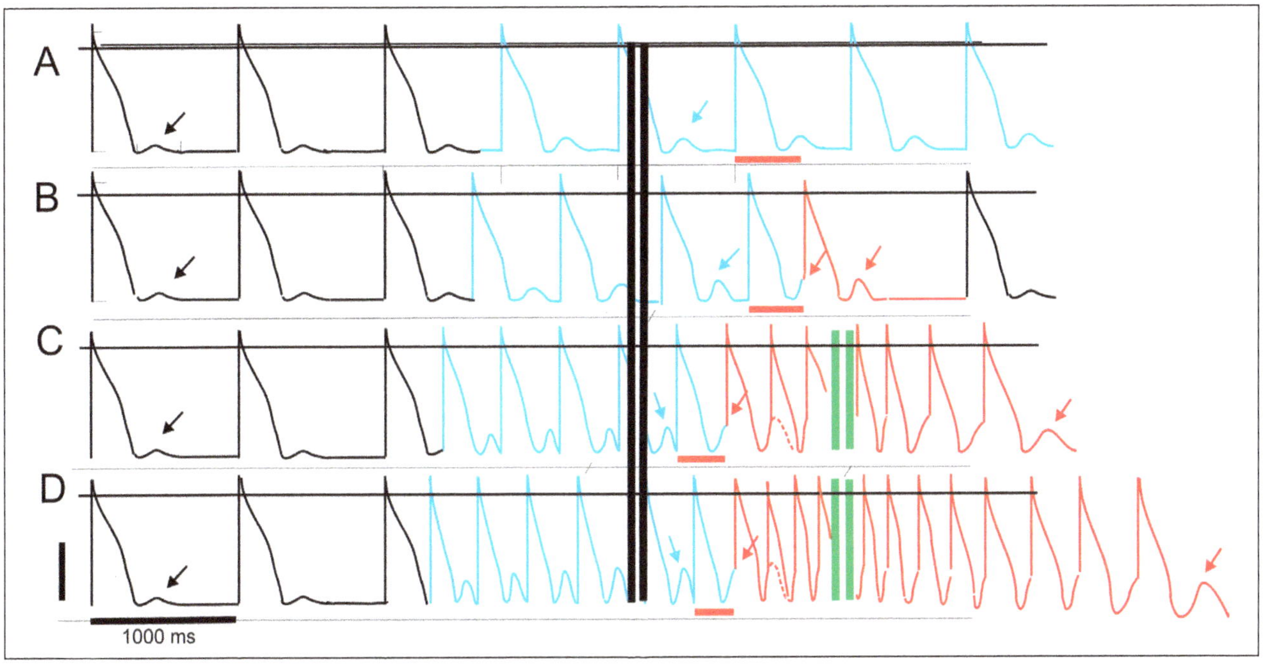

Figure 5-4 Effects of rate expressed as cycle length on DADs and triggered activity.

In Panel C, the cycle length decreases from 1000 ms (black action potentials at left) to 400 ms (blue action potentials). The DAD amplitudes increase even more (blue arrow). A DAD reaches threshold (red arrow) to trigger an action potential (in red) that is followed by a series of triggered action potentials since the DAD after each action potential also reaches threshold potential (dashed red trace indicates DAD of the triggered action potential; green vertical bars indicate a break in the time scale of 10 sec). Triggered activity stops when a DAD fails to reach threshold potential (red arrow at the far right). This is analogous to an increase in spontaneous or stimulated heart rate triggering a tachycardia.

In Panel D, cycle length decreases from 1000 ms (black action potentials at the left) to 300 ms (blue action potentials). The DAD amplitude is even larger (blue arrow). A DAD reaches threshold (red arrow), initiating a triggered action potential (red) that is followed by a DAD (dashed trace) that also initiates a triggered action potential. Each triggered action potential triggers the next one through the same mechanism. After a period of 10 sec—the break in time scale indicated by the green vertical bars—triggered activity terminates, with the last triggered impulse followed by a DAD that does not reach threshold (red arrow at the far right). Panel D also illustrates that the rate of triggered activity is faster and duration is longer when initiated at a shorter cycle length.

The relationship between stimulus cycle length (labeled as activation or triggering cycle length, Act/Trig CL) and DAD amplitude and coupling interval is shown in **Figure 5-5**. The DAD amplitude is shown to increase as cycle length decreases (red circles and line).

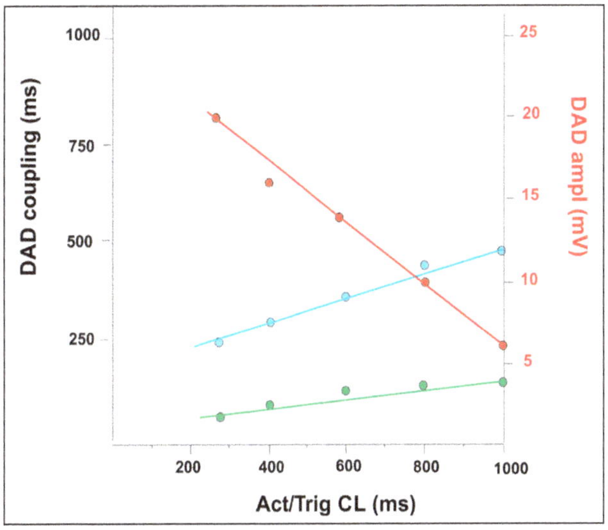

Figure 5-5 Effects of stimulus cycle length expressed as activation or triggering cycle length (Act/Trig CL, abscissa) on DAD amplitude in mV (right ordinate, **red line**) and DAD coupling interval (**green** and **blue lines**).

The direct relationship between stimulus cycle length (Act/Trig CL) and coupling interval of the DAD or first triggered impulse to the action potential upstroke (phase 0) is also shown in Figure 5-5 (blue line). This was also shown in Figure 5-4 where the coupling intervals between the DAD and the preceding action potential decrease as the cycle length decreases. As a result, the coupling interval between the first triggered action potential and the preceding triggering action potential decreases (horizontal red bars in Figure 5-4, Panels B–D) as the stimulus cycle length decreases. The direct relationship is caused by two factors. One is that the peak of the DAD occurs sooner after complete action potential repolarization because of increased speed of Ca^{2+} release from the SR as indicated by the green circles and line. The second is that the APD decreases as the cycle length decreases, which is the usual effect of cycle length on APD owing to an increase in I_p and I_K, outward currents that accelerate repolarization (described in Figure 7-7). (The blue line represents the combination of the two factors).

Single Premature Impulses as Triggers

A decrease of even a single cycle length in the form of a premature impulse also increases the amplitude of DADs and decreases the coupling interval and can trigger impulse initiation as illustrated in **Figure 5-6**.

In Figure 5-6, Panels A–D, action potentials at the left (shown in black) are occurring at a cycle length of 1000 ms and are associated with DADs that are subthreshold (black arrows). In Panel A, a premature action potential at a coupling interval of 800 ms (in blue) is followed by a DAD with a larger amplitude (blue arrow) that is still subthreshold. Likewise, in Panel B, the premature action potential at a coupling interval of 600 ms (in blue) is followed by a DAD with a larger amplitude than in A (blue arrow) but which is also subthreshold. In Panel C, the premature action potential (in blue) at a coupling interval of 500 ms is followed by a DAD that does reach threshold (blue arrow) for triggering an action potential (in red), which is then followed by a short series of triggered action potentials (in red) that terminates with a subthreshold DAD (red arrow at the far right). In Panel D, at a still shorter premature coupling interval of 300 ms, the DAD following the premature action potential (in blue) also reaches threshold (blue arrow) to trigger a longer period of triggered action potentials (in red), (vertical green bars in Panel D indicate a break of 10 sec in the time scale) which terminates with a subthreshold DAD (red arrow at the far right). (Whereas the figure shows a longer period of triggered activity initiated at a shorter coupling interval, this does not always occur.)

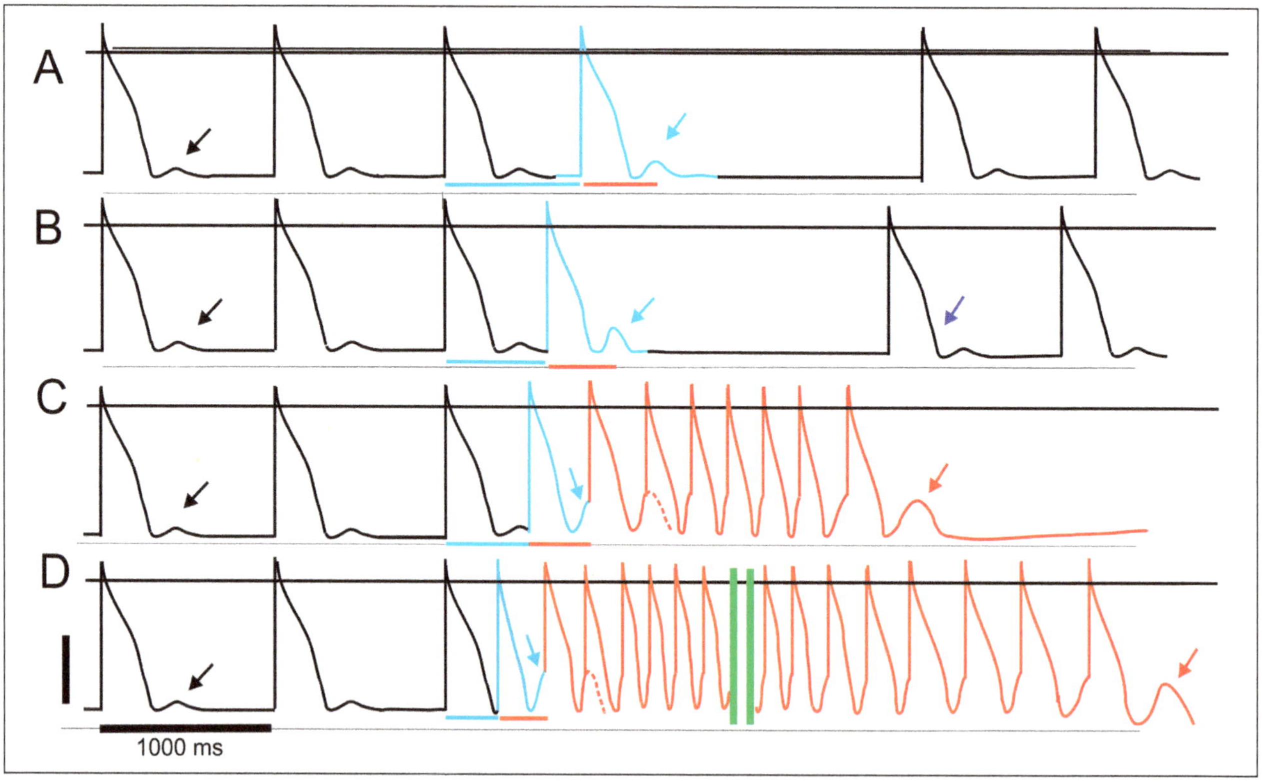

Figure 5-6 Effects of a decrease in a single cycle length (a premature impulse) on DADs and triggered activity.

Similar to the direct relationship between stimulation rate (cycle length) and coupling interval of the DAD described in Figure 5-5, the coupling interval of the DAD and/or the first triggered impulse to the single premature impulse decreases as the premature cycle length decreases. This relationship is shown in Figure 5-6. The blue horizontal bar below the action potentials is the coupling interval of the premature impulse which decreases from Panels A–D. The red horizontal bar is the coupling interval of the peak of the DAD of the premature impulse (A, B) or first triggered impulse (C, D), which also decreases. As with the effects of rate, shortening of the coupling interval of the DAD and first triggered impulse results from shortening of APD and shortening of the interval between peak DAD amplitude and complete repolarization of the preceding action potential.

The effects of rate (cycle length) and premature impulses on the amplitude and coupling interval of DADs is related to their effects on the amount of Ca^{2+} in the myoplasm during diastole. As described above (see Figure 5-2), Ca^{2+} enters the myocardial cell during the plateau phase of the action potential and is taken up into the SR, as well as causing SR Ca^{2+} release. Thus, a greater number of action potentials as occurs with an increase in rate/decreased cycle length results in more Ca^{2+} entering into the cell and the SR, as well as more Ca^{2+} being released from the SR during diastole. The elevated diastolic Ca^{2+} that generates the I_{NCX} or I_{TI} current and the DAD is increased. The rate of release of Ca^{2+} from the SR also increases as SR Ca^{2+} increases, causing DADs to occur earlier relative to repolarization.

Related clinical observations. Although the relationship between the initiation of triggered activity and preceding cycle length described above can often be observed in clinical studies (see Chapter 6), the direct relationship between activation cycle length and coupling interval of the first triggered impulse is not always observed. The increase in rapidity of SR Ca^{2+} release with decreased cycle length that underlies this relationship may reach a maximum beyond which no further increase occurs. The cycle length at which this occurs varies under different conditions and in different tissues. It might sometimes occur at relatively long cycle lengths, and as a result, shortening the cycle length at which tachycardia is initiated in clinical stimulation protocols will not produce the expected decreased coupling interval.

An increase in rate initiating triggered activity causes more Ca^{2+} release than a single premature activation, accounting for the more likely initiation of triggered arrhythmias by overdrive than by premature activation. This contrasts with the characteristics of reentry (the other arrhythmogenic mechanism initiated by stimulation), where premature stimulation is usually more effective in initiating arrhythmias than overdrive (see Chapter 9 for an explanation). The higher level of diastolic Ca^{2+} during more rapid rates of pacing accounts for the observation that it is easier to initiate triggered arrhythmias by premature activation during more rapid pacing rates, since DAD amplitude is closer to threshold. Slow rates often potentiate the initiation of reentry, but in some situations, rapid rates also favor induction of reentry by premature impulses.

Triggered Activity Rate and Duration

The rate of triggered activity is governed by the time it takes for a DAD to depolarize the membrane potential from the maximum diastolic potential (MDP) to the threshold potential for initiating an action potential. Therefore, rate is dependent on the relationship between MDP, rate of DAD depolarization, and threshold potential (similar to rate of automaticity; see Figure 1-2). APD also influences triggered activity rates, with faster rates associated with shorter action potential durations.

Warm Up

The rate of DAD depolarization increases and APD shortens progressively during the initial impulses of triggered activity. Because of the decreased cycle length of the first triggered impulse related to the decreased DAD coupling interval, the second triggered impulse will also have a decreased cycle length because of the decreased coupling interval of the preceding DAD, resulting in more Ca^{2+} entering the cell, increasing the DAD amplitude and decreasing the coupling interval of the next triggered impulse. The increased Ca^{2+} causes a gradual decrease in triggered cycle length (called "warm up") until a steady state is reached (Figures 5-4 and 5-6, Panels C and D).

Another factor that may contribute to the decrease in cycle length during triggered activity is a slow and gradual depolarization of the MDP (membrane potential becomes less negative) moving MDP closer to the threshold potential. This depolarization can result from accumulation of K^+ just outside the cell membrane (coming from the movement of K^+ from intra- to extracellular space carried by the repolarizing I_K), if circulation is not sufficient to rapidly wash it away.

Duration and Termination

As described above, the rate of triggered activity may increase and the duration of the period of triggered activity become longer as the triggering cycle length decreases. These features are also related to the amount of Ca^{2+} entering the cell during the triggering cycle length, with more Ca^{2+} entering at shorter cycle lengths. This relationship can sometimes be seen in clinical studies and provide evidence for DAD-triggered arrhythmias as described in Chapter 6.

Triggered activity can be sustained or paroxysmal. Before terminating spontaneously, it may gradually slow (Panel D in Figure 5-4 and Figure 5-6). The slowing and termination results from an increased activity of the Na^+–K^+ pump and outward I_P. In cells with high (more negative −70 to −90 mV) levels of membrane potential, Na^+ enters during phase 0 of each triggered action potential and is pumped out of the cell by the Na^+–K^+ pump generating I_P as described in Figure 1-6. As the triggered rate speeds up, the amount of Na^+ entering the cell increases. The increase in outward I_P current opposes the inward current causing the DADs, eventually decreasing the rate and amplitude of the DADs, thereby slowing the rate of the triggered action potentials. In addition, I_P moves membrane potential in a negative direction, gradually moving maximum diastolic potential of the DAD further from the threshold for activation of a triggered action potential until triggered activity stops when the peak DAD amplitude does not reach this threshold potential (Figure 5-4, Panel D, and Figure 5-6, Panel D, red arrows at the right). In situations in which the Na^+–K^+ pump is not able to generate sufficient I_P such as in digitalis toxicity where the pump is partially inhibited, other mechanisms related to Ca^{2+} overload effects on ion channels contribute to termination of triggered activity.

After the termination of triggered activity, membrane potential may be more negative (hyperpolarized) than before because of persistent increased I_P. This effect gradually diminishes as I_P returns intracellular Na^+ towards normal. As a result, another episode of triggered activity cannot quickly occur, since the hyperpolarized membrane potential and increased outward I_P prevent DADs from reaching the threshold potential. With time, as I_P diminishes, triggered activity can again be induced. This property is sometimes observed in clinical studies on triggered arrhythmias in which another arrhythmic episode cannot be immediately initiated after initiation and termination of a triggered arrhythmia by electrical stimulation.

Effects of Overdrive Stimulation During Triggered Activity

The factors that govern rate and spontaneous termination of triggered activity are also involved in the response of ongoing triggered activity to overdrive stimulation. These effects are important when considering the effects of overdrive on clinical triggered arrhythmias (**Figure 5-7**).

Figure 5-7 shows a diagram of triggered action potentials after a long period of triggered activity at the left in black. During each action potential, Na^+ (blue arrow) and Ca^{2+} (green arrow) enter the cell, and K^+ (red arrow) leaves the cell. The Na^+–Ca^{2+} exchanger (green oval) generates the TI current by extruding 1 Ca^{2+} for 3 Na^+ ($I_{NCX,}$ downward blue arrow) causing the DADs perpetuating triggered activity. Na^+–K^+ pump activity (blue circle) extrudes 3 Na^+ (upward blue arrow) in exchange for 2 K^+ (downward red arrow).

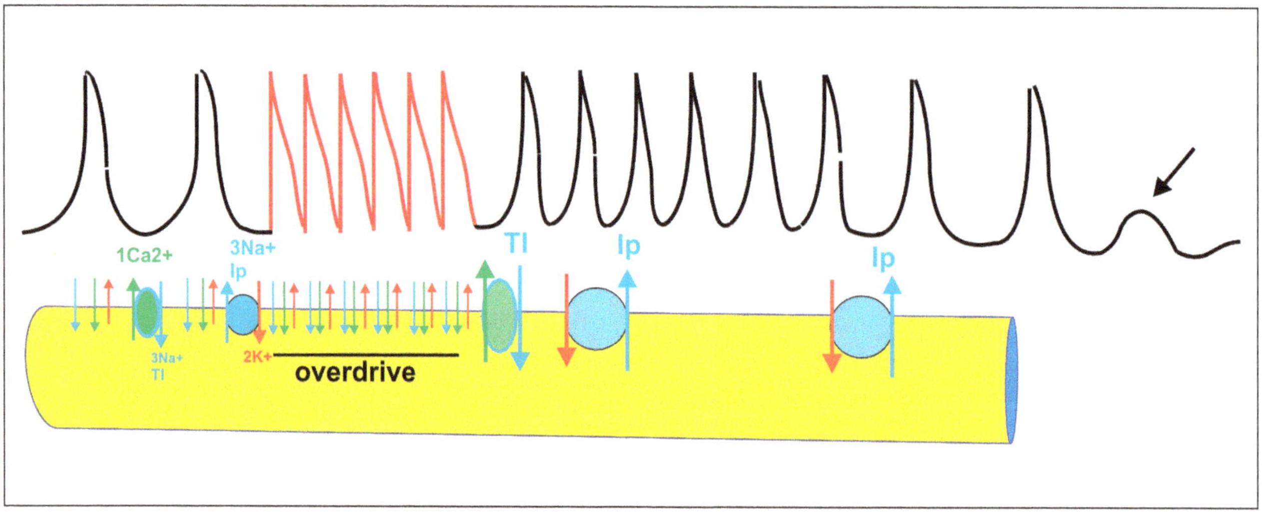

Figure 5-7 Triggered arrhythmia response to overdrive.

The red action potentials show a period of overdrive, during which there is increased Na^+ and Ca^{2+} entering and K^+ leaving the cell during the action potentials. At the end of the period of overdrive (action potentials are black again), there is increased activity of the Na^+–Ca^{2+} exchanger (larger green oval) because of the increased Ca^{2+} that entered during overdrive, enhancing I_{NCX} and TI, causing overdrive acceleration. The Na^+–K^+ pump activity also is increased (larger blue circle), generating more outward I_p that eventually overcomes the increased inward I_{NCX}, causing the DADs to become smaller, and hyperpolarizing the membrane potential until triggered activity stops when a DAD fails to reach threshold potential (arrow at the far right).

Thus, at an appropriate overdrive rate, the overdrive is followed by overdrive acceleration, then slowing, and finally termination. Slower overdrive rates may only cause acceleration followed by a return to the pre overdrive cycle length. Faster overdrive rates may cause immediate termination. As for spontaneous termination, when the Na^+–K^+ pump is partially inhibited by digitalis toxicity (see Figure 5-8), I_p is less important in overdrive termination and increased intracellular Ca^{2+} effects on ion channels may be more important.

Effects of the Autonomic Nervous System

Sympathetic Stimulation

The sympathetic nervous system is an important factor controlling the initiation and rate of DAD-dependent triggered activity. Sympathetic activation or β_1-adrenergic agonist drugs can result in the appearance of DADs in atrial, specialized ventricular (Purkinje) and ventricular muscle cells and likely A-V nodal cells (Figure 6-1). When DADs are already present, sympathetic activation increases the amplitude and rate of depolarization of DADs, decreases their coupling interval and increases the rate and duration of triggered activity.

The sympathetic nervous system exerts its effect on DADs through the effects of norepinephrine to increase Ca^{2+} entry into cells through the L-type Ca^{2+} channels. β_1-receptor activation by catecholamines results in phosphorylation of the L-type Ca^{2+} channels, which increases opening of the channels and L-type Ca^{2+} current, I_{CaL}. RyR2 receptors in SR Ca^{2+} release channels are also phosphorylated, increasing their release activity. Norepinephrine also increases activity of the calcium pump (SERCA) to move more Ca^{2+} into the SR, because phosphorylation of the protein phospholamban removes its inhibitory effects on the pump.

Parasympathetic Suppression

The parasympathetics (vagus nerve) can suppress DADs and triggered activity in atrial, A-V nodal and ventricular tissues (Purkinje fibers and ventricular muscle). In atrial and A-V nodal cells, acetylcholine released from parasympathetic nerve endings acts on the M_2 subtype of muscarinic receptors to slow and terminate triggered activity. This effect is brought about through a G protein-mediated increase in outward K^+ current through K_{ACh} channels. The increase in outward current opposes the inward current during DADs (decreases net inward current) that decreases their amplitudes and makes the membrane potential more negative, preventing DADs from reaching threshold potential. Acetylcholine also decreases inward L-type Ca^{2+} current (I_{CaL}) by suppressing adenylate cyclase to reduce intracellular Ca^{2+} loading. Although ACh does not increase a K_{ACh} channel current in ventricular tissues, it can prevent the increase in cyclic AMP (cAMP) that underlies the formation of DADs under sympathetic stimulation by the process of accentuated antagonism described in Chapter 1.

DADS Caused by Digitalis Toxicity

Digitalis is used as adjunct therapy in heart failure and for rate control in atrial fibrillation. In addition to enhancing automaticity (Chapter 1), the drug can cause arrhythmias due to triggered activity (described in detail in Chapter 6). The mechanism for the arrhythmogenic effect of digitalis to cause DADs and triggered activity is linked to the mechanism for its positive inotropic effects in the atria and ventricles. Digitalis binds to high-affinity isoforms of the Na^+–K^+ pump to block pump activity. In therapeutic amounts, only a small fraction of pumps in the sarcolemma are blocked, with a consequent increase in intracellular Na^+ concentration. The increase in Na^+ concentration throughout the cytoplasm (referred to as the bulk phase) is very small, but the increase in Na^+ concentration in restricted intracellular spaces (an intracellular region that is not in equilibrium with the bulk phase) can be substantial. Such a restricted space important for digitalis effects on contractility and arrhythmogenesis is diagrammed in **Figure 5-8**.

Figure 5-8 illustrates that the restricted space (separated from the bulk phase of the myoplasm) where there can be a substantial increase in Na^+ concentration, is located in the regions where the terminal cisternae of the junctional SR (JSR) abut the sarcolemma membrane. Here, there may be co-localization of L-type Ca^{2+} channels and I_{CaL} (red ovals and arrow), high affinity Na^+–K^+ pumps (large dark blue circle), Na^+–Ca^{2+} exchangers (large light blue oval) and RyR2 receptors, all of which have a role in DAD formation.

In Figure 5-8, Panel A, inhibition of the Na^+–K^+ pump by low doses of digitalis is diagrammed as leading to a small increase in Na^+ in the restricted space (black circles) resulting from a decrease in Na^+ extrusion by the pump (upward black arrow) in exchange for K^+ (downward yellow arrow). Therefore, the Na^+ gradient for the Na^+–Ca^{2+} exchanger (light blue oval, downward black arrow) is reduced and this decreases the thermodynamic energy generated from the movement of Na^+ down its concentration gradient, thereby decreasing energy available for Ca^{2+} extrusion (upward blue arrow). Since Ca^{2+} continues to enter the cell with each action potential via I_{CaL} (downward red arrow), there is a build-up of Ca^{2+} in this restricted space (blue circles) but bulk phase Ca^{2+} does not rise significantly. The increased Ca^{2+} is taken up into the SR by SERCA (large black arrows), increasing SR Ca^{2+} content (blue circles) and subsequently increasing Ca^{2+} release during the action potential, causing the positive inotropic effect. Diastolic membrane potential is not affected since Ca^{2+} release during diastole is minimal (dashed line and action potential above Panel A).

Figure 5-8, Panel B diagrams the digitalis effect in toxic amounts that cause DADs and triggered arrhythmias. The inhibition of a greater fraction of Na^+–K^+ pumps leads to more Na^+ in the restricted space (black circles) and the concomitant greater increase in Ca^{2+} (blue circles) leads to excessive uptake of Ca^{2+} into the SR (large black arrows). The Ca^{2+} overload results in Ca^{2+} release from the SR during diastole (long blue arrows), and the generation of DADs (vertical dashed line in action potential above), and triggered activity because of an increase in I_{NCX} (light blue oval and inward black arrow).

Na^+ accumulation in the restricted space may not be the only mechanism for the positive inotropic and arrhythmogenic effects of digitalis. Digitalis may increase opening of SR Ca^{2+} release channels during diastole through an action on RyR2 receptors, thereby amplifying the effects of the increased Na^+ and Ca^{2+} concentrations. It may also increase entry of Ca^{2+} into the cell through sarcolemmal Na^+ channels. Very high intracellular Na^+ also has a direct effect on the Na^+–Ca^{2+} exchanger, decreasing binding of internal Ca^{2+} to the exchanger that would decrease Ca^{2+} extrusion. It is uncertain if such high levels of Na^+ in cells are reached during clinical digitalis toxicity.

In patients with heart failure, the above effects of digitalis on Ca^{2+} may be amplified. In heart failure there is a decrease in Na^+–K^+ pumps resulting in a greater fraction of the pumps being inhibited by digitalis.

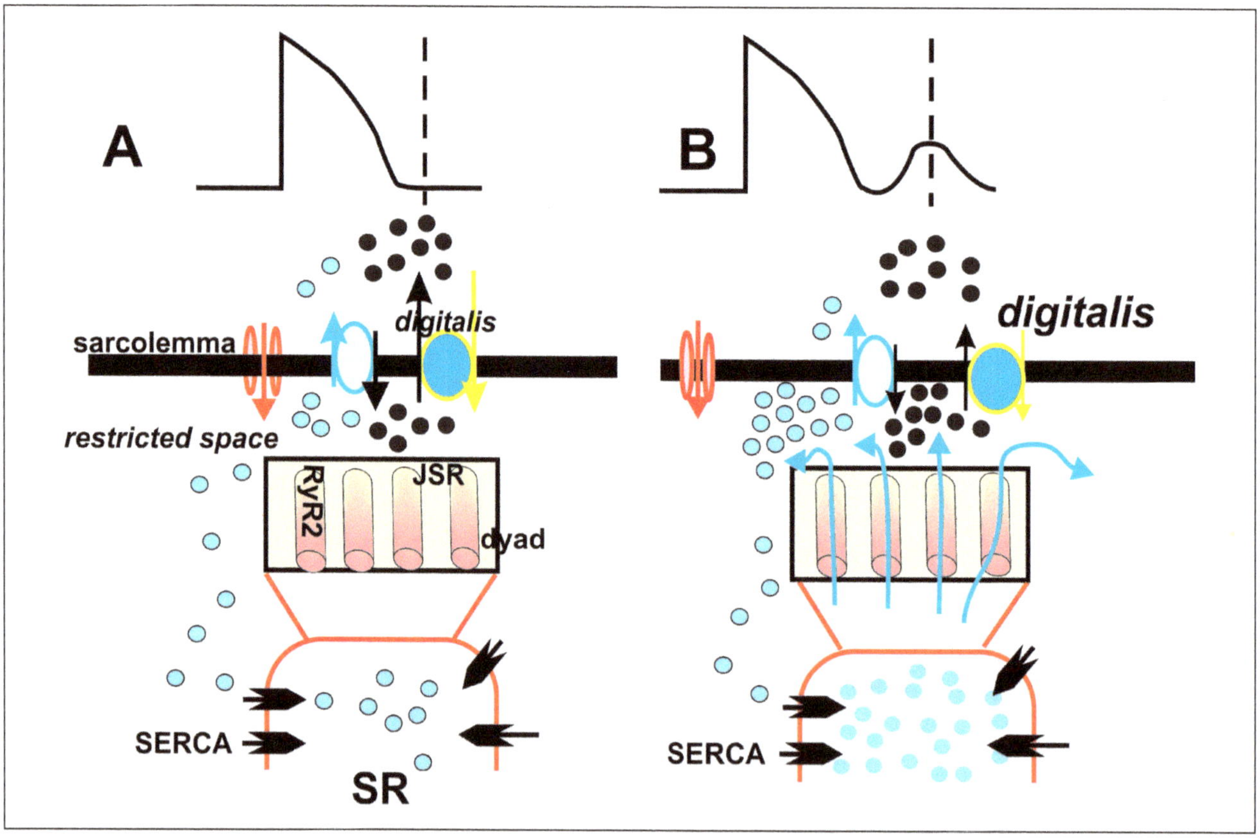

Figure 5-8 Diagram of the restricted space and mechanism for digitalis-induced DADs. **Panel A** diagrams the effects of therapeutic amount of digitalis. **Panel B** diagrams the effects of toxic amount of digitalis.

Pharmacology of DADs and DAD-Induced Triggered Activity

Information on the pharmacology of DADs and triggered activity is extensive and complicated and will not be described in detail. Emphasis here is placed on drug actions that can help identify a triggered mechanism causing a clinical arrhythmia. In general, drugs that decrease Ca^{2+} SR overload are expected to stop triggered activity caused by DADs. Drugs can act at a number of different sites to have this effect.

Of the typical classes of antiarrhythmic drugs (the Vaughan Williams classification), all affect DADs as well as other arrythmogenic mechanisms, and therefore, with the exception of L-type Ca^{2+}-channel blockers, have limited usefulness in identifying triggered activity as a cause of arrhythmias. Some complicated algorithms involving the response of arrhythmias to administration of multiple drugs having Na^+-channel blocking effects may be specific for identifying triggered activity in experimental laboratory animals, but in general are not feasible for identifying mechanisms of clinical arrhythmias.

β_1-Receptor Agonists and Blockers

Because DADs and triggered activity are often caused by sympathetic activation, triggered arrhythmias can be initiated by isoproterenol infusion in the clinical laboratory (which stimulates both β_1 and β_2 receptors) and prevented by drugs that block the β_1 receptor. The effect of isoproterenol is not specific for triggered activity since it can also initiate automatic arrhythmias, which are stopped by β_1-receptor blockade. However, when used along with electrical stimulation protocols, isoproterenol and β-blocking drugs can be helpful in identifying triggered activity.

L-Type Ca^{2+}-Channel Blocking Drugs

L-type Ca^{2+}-channel blocking drugs, such as verapamil, decrease DADs by decreasing Ca^{2+} entry into cells. Although this class of drugs also affects arrhythmogenic mechanisms other than triggered activity, such as abnormal automaticity and certain types of reentry, they can be useful in identifying clinical triggered arrhythmias in conjunction with other arrhythmia characteristics. The next chapter illustrates examples of clinical triggered arrhythmias and the response to L-type Ca^{2+}-channel blocking drugs.

Adenosine

Adenosine is an endogenous nucleoside found in some neurons, platelets, and other sources that has important clinical uses for terminating certain types of tachycardias and can also help identify arrhythmogenic mechanisms as described in Chapter 1. Adenosine acts on a specific subtype of adenosine receptors in the heart (A_1 receptors) to exert its electrophysiologic effects. As described previously, the adenosine receptor is coupled to ion channels and also to adenylyl cyclase through the guanine nucleotide inhibitory protein G_i.

In the atria and sinus node, activation of the A_1 receptor results in an increased outward K^+ current, $I_{ACh/ado}$, independent of cAMP. In the atria, this adenosine-induced increase in K^+ current can decrease DADs and stop-triggered activity that is not catecholamine dependent. Adenosine does not increase K^+ current in the ventricles. Thus, in ventricles, DADs caused by noncatecholamine-related mechanisms, e.g., digitalis or nonspecific pathology, are not inhibited by adenosine.

In both atria and ventricles,(and probably the A-V node) adenosine antagonizes the stimulatory actions of catecholamines on adenylyl cyclase and thereby prevents catecholamine-induced increase in cAMP and I_{Ca}. This inhibits catecholamine-dependent DADs by preventing Ca^{2+} overload and the TI current and terminates triggered activity in both atria and ventricles.

The effects of adenosine in stopping triggered activity—as compared to only transient suppression of automaticity (see Chapter 1)—makes adenosine an important tool for identifying mechanisms of clinical arrhythmias. However, it can also terminate triggered activity caused by catecholamine-induced EADs (see Chapter 8) and reentry involving the A-V node (see Chapter 11).

Drugs used in the experimental laboratory can also influence the function of the SR, either enhancing or suppressing oscillatory movements of Ca^{2+} between the SR and myoplasm. However, they are not available for determining the mechanisms of clinical arrhythmias.

IDENTIFYING DAD-TRIGGERED ACTIVITY AS THE CAUSE OF CLINICAL ARRHYTHMIAS

Identifying the clinical arrhythmias caused by DAD-induced triggered activity relies on the utilization of the basic electrophysiologic and pharmacologic properties described in the previous sections. Although some basic and clinical studies have shown DADs in extracellular monophasic action potential recordings, this is not a feasible method for general clinical use to identify this mechanism since motion artifacts can easily occur that can mimic the appearance of DADs. Each of the following characteristics, if present alone, is usually insufficient to conclude that there is a DAD-triggered mechanism. It often is necessary to demonstrate that an arrhythmia displays several of these characteristics.

ECG Characteristics of Triggered Arrhythmias

The properties of DADs and DAD-triggered activity described in the previous sections, govern the appearance of triggered clinical arrhythmias on the ECG. Such triggered arrhythmias might occur after an increase in the basic (sinus) rate or spontaneously occurring premature impulses because of the effects of short cycle lengths to increase DAD amplitude. The occurrence of triggered impulses or tachycardias are expected to be related to the sinus rate, with a greater likelihood of these arrhythmias at faster sinus rates. The coupling intervals between the first triggered impulse and the cycle length of the triggering impulse are often directly related, a specific characteristic of a triggered arrhythmia. The rate and duration of triggered tachycardia can also be directly related to the triggering cycle length. Once begun, a triggered tachycardia may show a warm-up phase as cycle length progressively shortens, and then, prior to spontaneous termination, there may be a gradual slowing of cycle length. However, these characteristics are not always present and their absence does not negate the possibility of triggered activity. In addition, when they do occur, they are not all specific for triggered activity since arrhythmias caused by other mechanisms (e.g., automaticity or reentry) may also show a warm-up phase and gradual slow down prior to termination. Triggered tachycardias have a focal origin with ECG features related to the site of origin as described for automaticity in Chapter 3.

Electrical Stimulation: Characteristics of DAD-Dependent-Triggered Arrhythmias

As described in Chapters 1–4, electrical stimulation is a valuable tool to identify mechanisms causing arrhythmias. The basic electrophysiologic properties of DADs described in a previous section of this chapter are relevant for the expected clinical effects of electrical stimulation.

Overdrive and Premature Stimulation; Initiation of Triggered Arrhythmias

Overdrive stimulation can be implemented during sinus rhythm in a patient who has spontaneous episodes of an unsustained arrhythmia to determine if the arrhythmia can be induced. The general procedure is described in Chapter 1 and in more detail in *Josephson's Clinical Cardiac Electrophysiology*, Chapters 1 and 2). Both the cycle length and the duration of overdrive can be varied. **Figure 5-9** illustrates an overdrive protocol and its effects on a triggerable focus. In each panel, sinus activation is indicated by the vertical black bars at a cycle length of 500 ms. Overdrive stimulation is indicated by the vertical blue bars and horizontal green line (double slanted bars indicate a break in the time scale during which overdrive stimulation occurs).

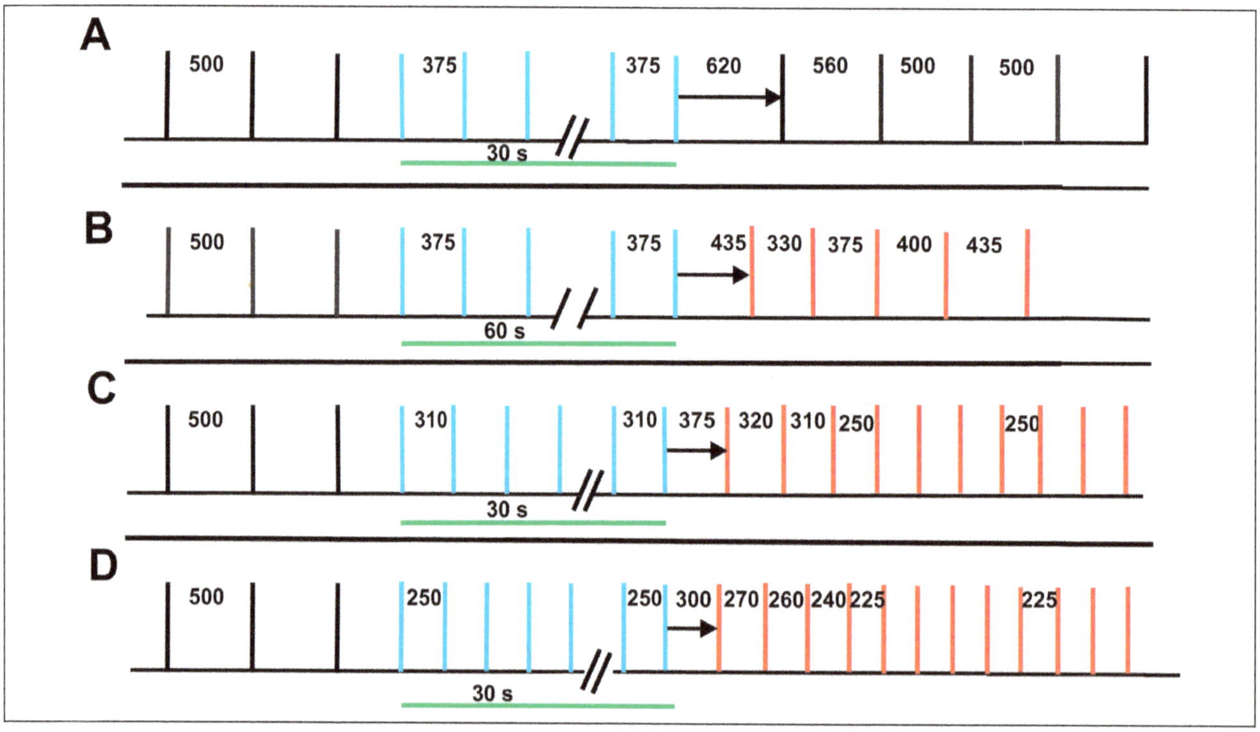

Figure 5-9 Initiation of a triggered arrhythmia by overdrive stimulation.

In Figure 5-9, Panel A, overdrive at a cycle length of 375 ms for 30 sec is followed by overdrive suppression of sinus node automaticity as described in Chapter 2. In Panel B, overdrive at the same cycle length, this time for 60 sec, is followed by an ectopic (triggered) rhythm (vertical red bars), the first impulse of which occurs at a coupling interval of 435 ms to the last stimulated impulse. The triggered rhythm is short lasting and shows a gradually lengthening of the cycle length prior to termination (cycle lengths indicated above). This illustrates that the duration of overdrive is related to the initiation of triggered activity. Therefore, a clinical overdrive protocol might consist of progressively increased duration of overdrive at a constant cycle length until an arrhythmia is initiated.

In Figure 5-9 Panel C, overdrive at a decreased cycle length of 310 ms (vertical blue bars) for the same duration (30 sec) as in Panel A is followed by an ectopic (triggered) rhythm (vertical red bars) of which the first impulse has a 375-ms coupling interval to the last stimulated impulse. The cycle length of the rhythm shows warm up, decreasing to 250 ms and the rhythm persists for the duration of the record. Termination may be preceded by a gradual lengthening of cycle length (not shown). In Panel D, the overdrive cycle length is 250 ms (vertical blue bars) for 30 sec and is followed by an ectopic (triggered) rhythm (vertical red bars) the first impulse of which has a 300-ms coupling interval. The rhythm also shows warm up to a shorter cycle length (225 ms) than in Panel C. The actual maximal rate of triggered arrhythmias depends on the clinical cause and may vary from 200 bpm (~315-ms cycle length) for right ventricular outflow tract tachycardia to less than 150 bpm (~400-ms cycle length) for arrhythmias related to ischemia and reperfusion.

Comparison of Panels A, C, and D illustrate that the initiation of triggered activity is dependent on the stimulus cycle length. Panels C and D show that the coupling interval between the first impulse of the triggered rhythm and the last stimulated impulse decreases with decreasing overdrive cycle length (direct relationship) and that the cycle length of the rhythm decreases as well. Arrhythmias caused by DAD-induced triggered activity are predicted to have these features: specifically, induction of arrhythmia at a critical pacing cycle length, a direct relationship between the coupling interval of the first impulse of the arrhythmia and the overdrive cycle length, and increased duration and rate of the arrhythmia with decreasing overdrive cycle length. These features are based on the characteristics of the DADs described in Figure 5-4 and Figure 5-5. They are a result of the mechanisms described for the effects of cycle length on diastolic Ca^{2+} levels.

Premature stimulation protocols can also initiate triggered activity because of the increase in Ca^{2+} entry as described in Figure 5-6. The same clinical protocol can be used as described in Chapter 1; with a premature stimulus applied every 10 to 15 basic impulses, either during sinus rhythm or during stimulation at a fixed basic cycle length as illustrated in **Figure 5-10**.

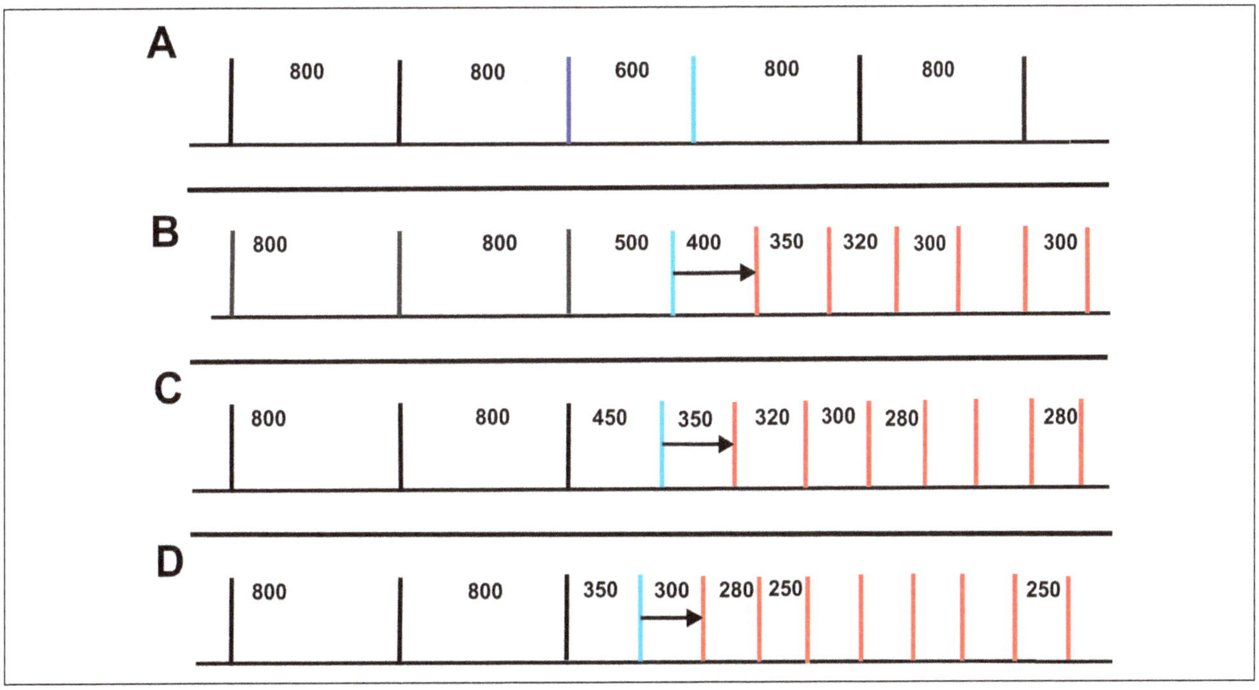

Figure 5-10 Initiation of a triggered arrhythmia by premature stimulation.

In Figure 5-10, the basic cycle length of 800 ms in each panel is indicated by the black vertical bars and the prematurely stimulated impulse by the blue vertical bar. In Panel A, after the premature stimulus with a 600-ms coupling interval, the basic (sinus) rhythm is reset. In Panel B, an ectopic (triggered) rhythm (vertical red bars) is initiated by the prematurely stimulated impulse with a coupling interval of 500 ms. The triggered rhythm begins with a coupling interval of 400 ms and accelerates to a cycle length of 300 ms. In Panels C and D the ectopic (triggered) rhythms that are initiated by premature stimuli begin with shorter coupling intervals (350 and 300 ms), as the coupling interval of the premature stimuli decreases (450 and 350 ms) and the cycle length of the induced rhythm also decreases with an initial warm-up phase. Therefore, similar to the characteristics of initiation by overdrive, in this example there is a direct relationship between the coupling interval of the first triggered impulse with the coupling interval of the premature impulse—and the cycle length of the tachycardia is related to the premature coupling interval. The duration of triggered activity might also increase when initiated by shorter premature cycle lengths.

In clinical studies, initiation of triggered activity by overdrive stimulation should occur more readily than after premature stimulation. Overdrive more effectively increases Ca^{2+} movement into the cell. Sometimes, overdrive may induce an arrhythmia while premature stimulation does not; however, the opposite usually does not occur. This is an important feature distinguishing triggered activity from reentry, which can also be induced by electrical stimulation. Reentry is often more readily initiated by premature stimulation than overdrive (Chapter 9). Also, premature stimulation may be more effective in initiating triggered activity at shorter basic cycle lengths because of the elevated basal Ca^{2+} levels that may be opposite to initiation of reentry, which is often more easily accomplished at longer basic cycle lengths which increases heterogeneities in repolarization (Chapter 9, Figure 9-14). Another feature suggestive of triggered activity is difficulty in reinitiation of the arrhythmia shortly after it stops because of persistent activity of the Na^+–K^+ pump as described in Figure 5-7.

All of the characteristics described in Figure 5-9 and Figure 5-10 may not be observed when studying initiation of a clinical arrhythmia, although initiation of triggered activity by overdrive or premature stimulation at critical cycle lengths is a general feature that is expected to occur. Characteristics such as the direct relationship between coupling interval of the triggering impulse(s) to the first triggered impulse, the cycle length of triggered activity and the duration of triggered activity may not be seen for reasons described above that are related to the amount of Ca^{2+} overload. Conduction delay of stimulated impulses into the site of triggered activity and conduction delay out of this site can also distort some of these relationships, as described in Figure 2-10. For example, conduction delay out of the triggered site may negate the shortening of the coupling interval between the last stimulated impulse and the first triggered impulse and may even lengthen it. If this delay progressively increases as triggering cycle length shortens, the coupling interval to the first triggered impulse may continue to increase, giving an inverse relationship that would then not be helpful in identifying the mechanism as triggered activity.

Overdrive and Premature Stimulation; Termination of Triggered Arrhythmias

Triggered tachycardias can be terminated by electrical stimulation, in contrast to automatic tachycardias, which cannot. **Figure 5-11** diagrams the effects of overdrive stimulation during a tachycardia. The organization of each panel is the same as for Figure 5-9.

In Figure 5-11, the vertical red lines at the left in each pane indicate an ongoing tachycardia with a cycle length of 300 ms. The horizontal green line is the period of overdrive, the double black bars indicate a break in the time scale during which most of the overdrive occurs. Overdrive is initiated for 60 sec at a cycle length of 280 ms in Panel A, as indicated by the vertical blue lines. Following the period of overdrive, there is a short period of acceleration of the tachycardia rate (decrease in cycle length to 180–200 ms) before it slows back to the pre-overdrive rate. In Panel B, overdrive for the same duration at a shorter cycle length of 250 ms (vertical blue lines) is also followed by overdrive acceleration at a shorter cycle length (170–200 ms), a gradual prolongation in the cycle length, and then a return to the pre-overdrive cycle length. In Panel C, overdrive at a still shorter cycle length of 200 ms is followed by even further acceleration (cycle length 150–180 ms), then slowing and termination (vertical black bar at the right is a sinus impulse). In Panel D, following overdrive at a cycle length of 180 ms, there is immediate termination and restoration of sinus rhythm (vertical black bars). The relationship of the effects of overdrive to intracellular Ca^{2+} and Na^+, which is responsible for this behavior, is described in conjunction with Figure 5-7.

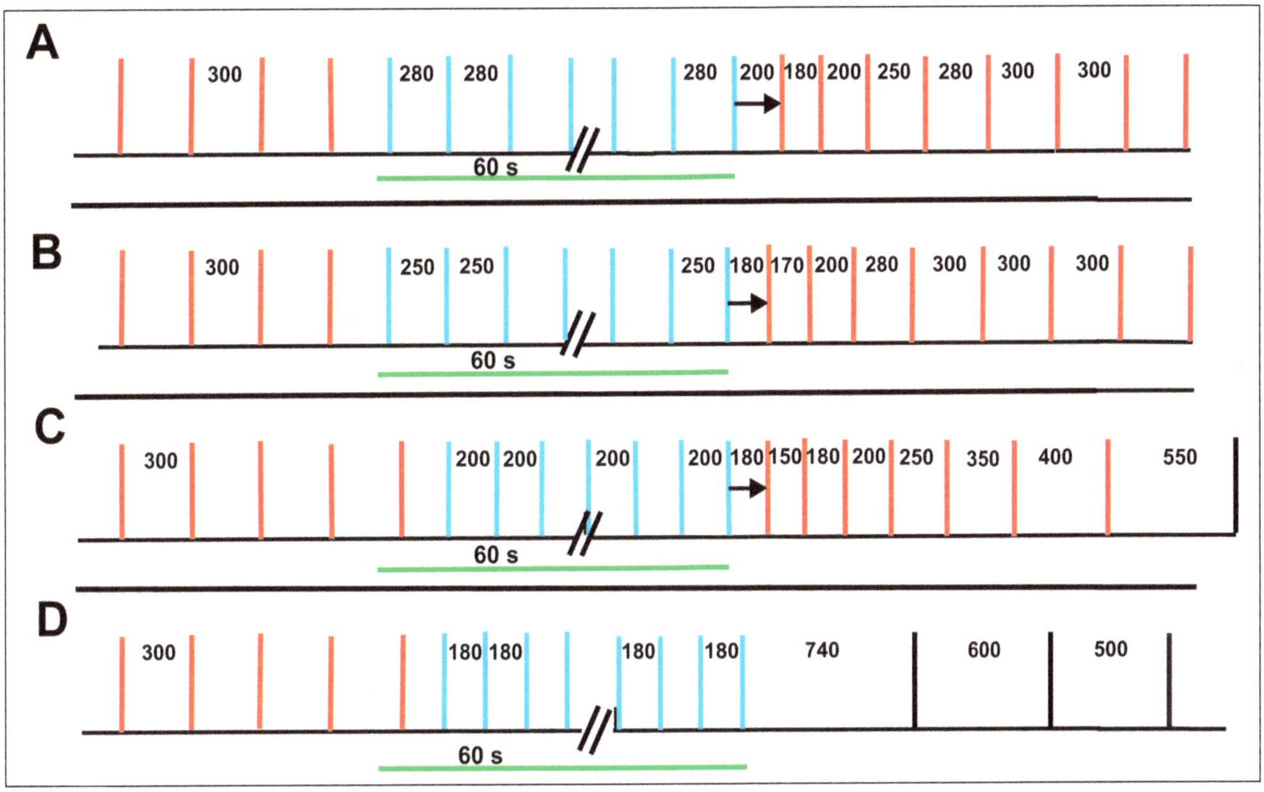

Figure 5-11 Effects of overdrive stimulation on a triggered arrhythmia.

Appropriately timed stimulated premature impulses might also terminate triggered tachycardia, but termination is much more unpredictable compared to termination by overdrive. The mechanism for termination is not certain. Sometimes hyperpolarization of the membrane potential follows an early premature action potential (membrane potential becomes more negative than prior to stimulation), resulting in failure of the DAD of the premature action potential to reach threshold. Effects of premature impulses that do not terminate tachycardia cause resetting; prematurely stimulated impulses might be followed by the same or a decreased return cycle length because of increased Ca^{2+} entry decreasing the DAD coupling interval.

Use of Pharmacological Agents to Identify DAD-Induced Triggered Arrhythmias

The effects of some representative drugs on DADs has already been described earlier in this chapter. In general, most drugs that terminate triggered activity also affect other arrhythmogenic mechanisms and are not useful for identifying triggered activity. Termination by L-type Ca^{2+}-channel blockers may help confirm a triggered mechanism when other features of the arrhythmia, such as ECG characteristics and response to electrical stimulation, are consistent with the expected characteristics of triggered activity. Adenosine may sometimes specifically identify triggered activity both in the atria and ventricles, particularly when it is catecholamine-dependent, by preventing catecholamine-induced increase in cAMP and I_{CaL}. Clinical examples are shown in the next chapter.

SUMMARY

Delayed afterdepolarizations (DADs) are oscillations in membrane potential following repolarization of the action potential. When their amplitude is large enough to reach threshold potential, triggered action potentials occur. DADs are caused by Ca^{2+} release from the SR during diastole, often related to SR Ca^{2+} overload. Elevated diastolic Ca^{2+} causes the inward current generated by the Na^{+}–Ca^{2+} exchanger (I_{NCX} or I_{TI}) that results in DADs.

Table 5-1 summarizes properties of DAD-induced triggered activity based on the descriptions in this chapter and descriptions in Chapter 6, and compares them to the properties of normal and abnormal automaticity from Chapters 1–4. These properties are translated into the expected behavior of clinical arrhythmias caused by DAD-triggered activity described in Chapter 6. An asterisk (*) is used to indicate a difference between triggered activity and both automatic mechanisms.

Table 5-1 Comparison of DAD-Triggered Activity and Automaticity

	DAD-Triggered Activity	Normal Automaticity	Abnormal Automaticity
A) Spontaneous initiation	Initiated by acceleration of heart rate or by premature impulse that originates in a sinus or ectopic pacemaker (*)	Not initiated by acceleration of heart rate or by a premature impulse	Not initiated by acceleration of heart rate or by a premature impulse
B) Onset and termination	Starts with a premature impulse that can be early (*)	Starts with premature impulse late in the cycle length or an impulse that is not premature during a long cycle length	Starts with premature impulse mid or late in the cycle length or during an impulse that is not premature during a long cycle length
	Direct relationship of first tachycardia cycle length to previous heart rate or coupling interval of initiating premature impulse (triggering cycle length) (*)	No relationship between previous heart rate and first tachycardia cycle length, or rate and duration of tachycardia	No relationship between previous heart rate and first tachycardia cycle length, or rate and duration of tachycardia
	Direct relationship of tachycardia duration and rate to triggering cycle length (*)		
	Sometimes shows warm up	Sometimes shows warm up	Sometimes shows warm up
	Sometimes slowing of rate prior to termination	Sometimes slowing of rate prior to termination	Sometimes slowing of rate prior to termination
	Conduction delay not required	Conduction delay not required	Conduction delay not required
	PR interval directly related to atrial tachycardia rate	PR interval directly related to atrial tachycardia rate	PR interval directly related to atrial tachycardia rate
C) Origin	Focal origin, can arise in most regions.	Focal origin, arises in special regions	Focal origin, but can arise in most regions
a = atrial j = junctional v = ventricular	P wave (a) or QRS (j, v) characteristic of site of origin	P wave (a) or QRS (j, v) characteristic of site of origin	P wave (a) or QRS (j, v) characteristic of site of origin
D) Autonomic nervous system	Initiated and accelerated by sympathetics and β_1-agonists	Initiated and accelerated by sympathetics and β_1-agonists	Initiated and accelerated by sympathetics and β_1-agonists
	Slowed and terminated by parasympathetics (carotid massage) and cholinergic agonists (a, ++, *)	Slowed but not terminated by parasympathetics (carotid massage) and cholinergic agonists (a)	Slowed but not terminated by parasympathetics (carotid massage) and cholinergic agonists (a)
	Slowing and termination not related to A-V conduction delay or block	Slowing not related to A-V conduction delay or block	Slowing not related to A-V conduction delay or block
E) Pharmacology			
Adenosine	Slowed and terminated; not related to A-V nodal delay or block (a, ++,*)	Transient slowing; not related to A-V nodal delay or block (a)	Transient slowing; not related to A-V nodal delay or block (a)
Verapamil	Prevented, slowed or terminated not related to A-V nodal delay or block (#)	Little effect, minor slowing (‡)	Slowed or terminated not related to A-V nodal delay or block (#)
Na⁺-channel blockers	Sometimes slows and terminates	Sometimes slows and terminates	Little or no effect

(continued)

	DAD-Triggered Activity	Normal Automaticity	Abnormal Automaticity
F) Electrical stimulation	Initiated by overdrive and premature stimulation (*)	Not initiated by overdrive nor premature stimulation	Not initiated by overdrive nor premature stimulation
	First coupling interval of tachycardia directly related to overdrive or premature cycle length (*)	Not initiated by electrical stimulation	Not initiated by electrical stimulation
	Duration directly related to overdrive cycle length (*)	Not initiated by electrical stimulation	Not initiated by electrical stimulation
	Terminated by overdrive and premature stimulation (*)	Not terminated by overdrive, nor premature stimulation	Not terminated by overdrive, nor premature stimulation
	Overdrive stimulation causes transient acceleration (#)	Overdrive stimulation causes transient suppression	Overdrive stimulation causes transient acceleration (#)
	Reset by premature stimulation	Reset by premature stimulation	Reset by premature stimulation
	Cycle length following premature impulse is directly related to premature coupling interval	Cycle length following premature impulse is same as spontaneous cycle length	Cycle length following premature impulse is same or shorter than spontaneous cycle length

(*) Difference between triggered and both automatic mechanisms.
(‡) Junctional automaticity arising in the A-V node is stopped by verapamil, but not in the His bundle.
(#) Similar between triggered and abnormal automaticity.
(++) Only applies to DAD exercise-induced ventricular tachycardia.
Arrhythmia location: (a) atrial arrhythmias, (v) ventricular arrhythmias, (j) junctional arrhythmias.

SOURCES

Blaustein MP, Lederer J. Sodium/calcium exchange: Its physiological implications. *Physiol Rev.* 1999;79:764–830.

Boyden PA, Hirose M, Dun W. Cardiac Purkinje cells. *Heart Rhythm.* 2010;7:127–135.

Boyden PA, Pu J, Pinto J, ter Keurs HEDJ. Ca^{2+} transients and Ca^{2+} waves in Purkinje cells. Role in action potential initiation. *Circ Res.* 2000;86:448–455.

Cranefield PF. Action potentials, afterpotentials, and arrhythmias. *Circ Res.* 1977;41:415-423

Dangman KH, Dresdner KP, Zaim S. Automatic and triggered impulse initiation in canine subepicardial ventricular muscle. cells from border zones of 24-hour transmural infarcts. New mechanisms for malignant cardiac arrhythmias? *Circulation.* 1988;78:1020–1030.

Fagioni M, Knollmann BC. Calsequestrin 2 and arrhythmias. *Am J Physiol Heart Circ Physiol.* 2012;302:H1250–H126.

Gorgols APM, Beenkman HDM, Brugada P, et al. Extrastimulus-related shortening of the first postpacing interval in digitalis-induced ventricular tachycardia: Observations during programmed electrical stimulation in the conscious dog. *J Am Coll Cardiol.* 1983;1(3):840–857.

Gorgols APM, De Wit B, Beekman HDM, et al. Effects of different modes of stimulation on the morphology of the first QRS complex following pacing during digitalis-induced ventricular tachycardia: Observations in the conscious dog with chronic complete atrioventricular block. *Pacing Clin Electrophysiol.* 1986;9:842–859.

Hirose M, Stuyvers BD, Dun W, et al. Function of Ca^{2+} release channels in Purkinje cells that survive in the infarcted canine heart. A mechanism for triggered Purkinje ectopy. *Circ Arrhythmia Electrophysiol.* 2008;1:387–395.

Eisner DA, Lederer WJ. Na-Ca exchange: stoichiometry and electrogenicity. *Am J Physiol.* 1985;2248(3 Pt 1):C189–C202.

Faber GM, Rudy Y. Calsequestrin mutation and catecholaminergic polymorphic ventricular tachycardia: A simulation study of cellular mechanism. *Cardiovasc Res.* 2007;75:79–88.

Fernández-Velasco M, Rueda A, Rizzi N, et al. Increased Ca^{2+} sensitivity of the ryanodine receptor mutant RyR2 underlies catecholaminergic polymorphic ventricular tachycardia. *Circ Res.* 2009;104:201–209.

Fill M, Copello JA. Ryanodine receptor calcium release channels. *Physiol Rev.* 2002;82:894–914.

Herron TJ, Milstein ML, Anumonwo J, Priori SG, Jalife J. Purkinje cell calcium dysregulation is the cellular mechanism that underlies catecholaminergic polymorphic ventricular tachycardia. *Heart Rhythm.* 2010;7:1122–1128.

Kang G, Giovannone SF, Liu N, et al. Purkinje cells from RyR2 mutant mice are highly arrhythmogenic but responsive to targeted therapy. *Circ Res.* 2010;107:512–519.

Katra RP, Oya T, Hoeker GS, Laurita KR. Ryanodine receptor dysfunction and triggered activity in the heart. *Am J Physiol Heart Circ Physiol.* 2007;292:H2144–H2151.

Kjeldsen K, Nørgaard A, Gheorghiade M. Myocardial Na,K-ATPase: The molecular basis for the hemodynamic effect of digoxin therapy in congestive heart failure. *Cardiovasc Res.* 2002;55: 710–713.

Levi AJ, Boyett, Lee CO. The cellular actions of digitalis glycosides on the heart. *Prog Biophys Mol Biol.* 1994;62:1–54.

Li P, Rudy Y. A model of canine Purkinje cell electrophysiology and Ca^{2+} cycling. Rate dependence, triggered Activity, and comparison to ventricular myocytes. *Circ Res.* 2011;109:71–79.

Liu N, Priori SG. Disruption of calcium homeostasis and arrhythmogenesis induced by mutations in the cardiac ryanodine receptor and calsequestrin. *Cardiovasc Res.* 2008;77:293–301.

Malfatto G, Rosen TS, Rosen MR. The response to overdrive pacing of triggered atrial and ventricular arrhythmias in the canine heart. *Circulation.* 1988;77:1139–1148.

Priori SG, Chen W. Inherited dysfunction of sarcoplasmic reticulum Ca^{2+} handling and arrhythmogenesis. *Circ Res.* 2011;108:871–883.

Priori S, Mantica M, Schwartz PJ. Delayed afterdepolarizations elicited in vivo by left stellate ganglion stimulation. *Circulation.* 1988;78:178–185.

Rosen MR, Gelband H, Merker C, Hoffman BF. Mechanisms of digitalis toxicity. Effects of ouabain on phase four of canine Purkinje fiber transmembrane potentials. *Circulation.*1973;57;681–689.

Scoote M, Williams AJ. The cardiac ryanodine receptor (calcium release channel): Emerging role in heart failure and arrhythmia pathogenesis. *Cardiovasc Res.* 2002;56:359–372.

Song Y, Shryock JC, Belardinelli L. An increase of late sodium current induces delayed afterdepolarizations and sustained triggered activity in atrial myocytes. *Am J Physiol Heart Circ Physiol.* 2008;294:H2031–H2039.

Song Y, Shryock JC, Knot HJ, Belardinelli L. Selective attenuation by adenosine of arrhythmogenic action of isoproterenol on ventricular myocytes. *Am J Physiol Heart Circ Physiol.* 2001;281: H2789–H2795.

Song Y, Thedford S, Lerman BB, Belardinelli L. Adenosine-sensitive afterdepolarizations and triggered activity in guinea pig ventricular myocytes. *Circ Res.* 1992;70:743–753.

Sung RJ, Lo C-P, Hsiao PY, Tien H-C. Targeting intracellular calcium cycling in catecholaminergic polymorphic ventricular tachycardia: a theoretical investigation. *Am J Physiol Heart Circ Physiol.* 2011;301:H1625–H1638.

Ter Keurs HDJ, Boyden PA. Calcium and arrhythmogenesis. *Physiol Rev.* 2007;87:457–506.

Venetucci LA, Trafford AW, O'Neill SC, Eisner DA. The sarcoplasmic reticulum and arrhythmogenic calcium release. *Cardiovasc Res.* 2008;77:285–292.

Wasserstrom JA. Are we ready for a new mechanism of action underlying digitalis toxicity? *J Physiol.* 2011;589:21;5015.

Wasserstrom JA, Aistrup GL. Digitalis: new actions for an old drug *Am J Physiol Heart Circ Physiol.* 2005;289:H1781–H1793.

Wit AL, Cranefield PF. Triggered and automatic activity in the canine coronary sinus. *Circ Res.* 1977;41:434–445.

CHAPTER

6

Delayed Afterdepolarizations: Triggered Arrhythmias

SECTION

6A Atrial Delayed Afterdepolarizations and Triggered Arrhythmias

This section describes examples of arrhythmias that are likely caused by delayed afterdepolarization (DAD)-induced triggered activity. In general, each of the triggered arrhythmia examples fulfills only a subset of the characteristics described in Table 5-1, in part because detailed clinical electrophysiological data are not available for all the criteria in the table.

Basic Electrophysiological Mechanisms

LOCATION AND ELECTROPHYSIOLOGY OF DADS AND TRIGGERED ACTIVITY IN THE ATRIA

DADs and triggered activity occur at ectopic atrial sites to cause atrial arrhythmias. Cells capable of generating DADs and triggered activity (triggerable cells) are located throughout the atria. These regions overlap location of cells with normal automaticity, as shown in Figure 3-1. The same cells may sometimes be capable of both normal automaticity and DADs. The most prominent locations for cells that can generate triggered activity include in and around the superior and inferior crista terminalis, around the mitral and tricuspid annuli and in the mitral and tricuspid valves, in the pulmonary veins, and in the coronary sinus. **Figure 6-1** shows DADs and triggered activity from an atrial cell in the coronary sinus.

In addition to regions that overlap with cells capable of automaticity, atrial muscle cells scattered throughout the right and left atria have the capability for generating DADs. In many of these regions, action potentials with Na^+-dependent phase 0 arise from highly negative membrane potentials (~ –70 to –80 mV). The action potentials of muscle fibers extending into the valves are similar to those in the A-V node with low membrane potentials and slow Ca^{2+}-dependent depolarization phases (0). Diseased atrial muscle in which membrane potential is reduced (< –70 mV) can also generate DADs and triggered action potentials.

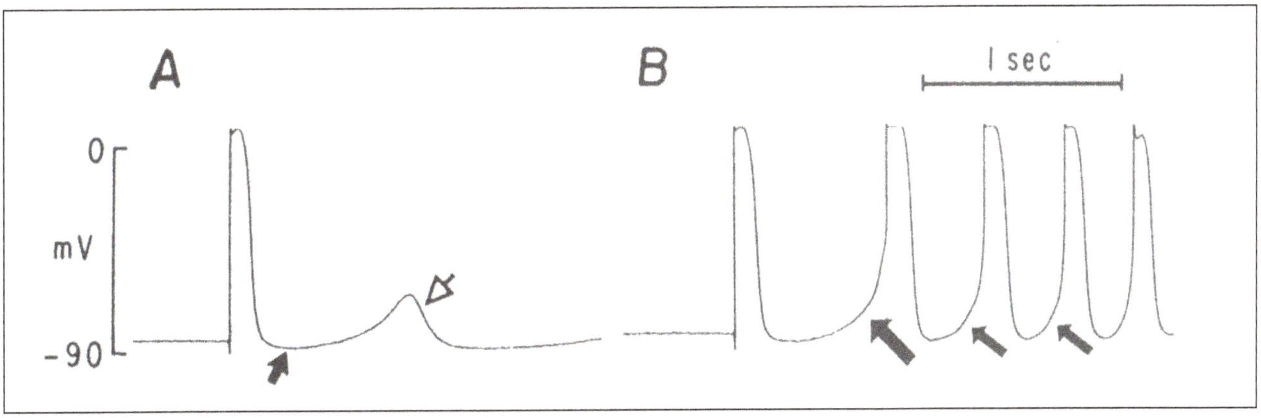

Figure 6-1 Action potentials recorded from an atrial cell in the canine coronary sinus in the presence of norepinephrine. **Panel A** is an action potential followed by an after-hyperpolarization (**first upward black arrow**) and a DAD (**downward unfilled arrow**). At right (**Panel B**), the DAD reaches the threshold to trigger a series of action potentials shown by the **arrows**.

Electrophysiological Foundations of Cardiac Arrhythmias: A Bridge Between Basic Mechanisms and Clinical Electrophysiology, Second Edition.

The basic cellular mechanisms of the DADs in the different atrial locations are described in Chapter 5. DADs result mostly from elevated diastolic Ca^{2+} that leads to the generation of the transient inward current (I_{TI}) caused by I_{NCX}. Elevated Ca^{2+} often results from sympathetic stimulation. DADs can occur in the absence of catecholamines as well, such as in digitalis toxicity, steady-state depolarization of the membrane potential, or dysfunction of the sarcoplasmic reticulum (SR), all of which can increase diastolic Ca^{2+} release from the SR. The properties of DADs and triggered activity in atrial cells with regard to effects of rate and rhythm, autonomics, and pharmacology are consistent with the general properties described in Chapter 5 and will be related to clinical arrhythmias in the next section.

Examples of Arrhythmias Caused by DAD-Triggered Activity in the Atria

TRIGGERED ATRIAL TACHYCARDIA

Paroxysmal Atrial Tachycardia

The ECG in **Figure 6-2** shows a paroxysmal atrial tachycardia caused by triggered activity in a patient without structural heart disease. Tachycardia begins after an increase of the heart rate (shortening of the second and third cycles at the left) caused by acceleration of a sinus or high right atrial ectopic pacemaker, not caused by exercise. This acceleration of rate initiates tachycardia, which begins with a premature impulse (fifth impulse) characterized by a change in P-wave morphology with no change in QRS. Tachycardia does not show a "warm-up" phase but immediately assumes a cycle length of 400–450 ms. Tachycardia terminates abruptly at the right.

Electrophysiological Characteristics of Triggered Atrial Tachycardia

The electrophysiological characteristics of triggered atrial tachycardia are included in the left column (DAD-Triggered Activity) of Table 5-1. The subheadings below describe these characteristics and also point out comparisons to tachycardias caused by automaticity (Table 5-1 middle and right columns) and to tachycardias caused by reentry (not included in the table; see Chapter 5).

Onset and Termination

Triggered atrial tachycardia often begins after an acceleration of the heart rate as shown in Figure 6-2. An increase in heart rate increases DAD amplitude until it reaches threshold to trigger action potentials. This arrhythmia can also be initiated after a premature impulse (which is not triggered) that also increases DAD amplitude (Table 5-1, rows A and B). The timing of the first impulse of tachycardia is dependent on the coupling interval of the first DAD, which in turn is dependent on the triggering cycle length (Figure 5-4). The first triggered tachycardia impulse can occur early in the cycle length when the coupling interval of the DAD is short (Figure 6-2) but also can occur in mid or late cycle with longer-coupled DADs. Automaticity, on the other hand, often occurs late in the sinus cycle or during a long cycle that allows phase 4 depolarization to reach threshold potential.

Prior to termination, the rate of triggered tachycardia often slows (see below) although this did not occur in Figure 6-2.

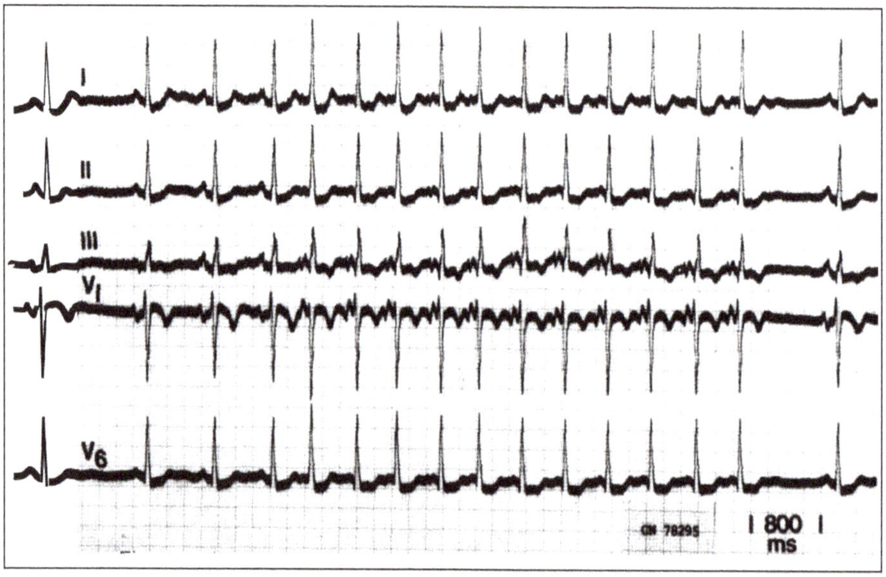

Figure 6-2 ECG leads I–III, V_1, and V_6 from a patient with periods of atrial tachycardia and no evidence of structural heart disease (Wellens' ECG collection).

Relationship to A-V Nodal Conduction

Triggered atrial tachycardia onset is not dependent on slowed conduction in the A-V node, as would be the case for the onset of supraventricular tachycardia caused by A-V nodal reentry (see Figure 11-3). Note that in Figure 6-2, the PR interval does not prolong prior to the onset of tachycardia indicating that A-V nodal conduction does not slow. The PR interval during tachycardia is governed by the tachycardia rate and shows the normal rate dependent slowing of atrial impulses in the A-V node (faster rate leads to longer PR). In contrast, in A-V nodal reentrant tachycardia (Chapter 11), AV nodal conduction determines the tachycardia rate; a longer PR is associated with a slower rate because the A-V node is part of the reentrant circuit (Figure 11-3). Automatic tachycardia has the same relationships to the PR interval as triggered tachycardia (Table 5-1, row B).

Warm Up

Triggered atrial tachycardia onset may be associated with a "warm-up" phase due to the effects of cycle length on DAD coupling described in Figure 5-4. However, this is not always evident, as in Figure 6-2. Tachycardia may also slow before terminating because of the increase in I_P that occurs at rapid rates (Figure 5-4) also not evident in Figure 6-2. Possible reasons for the absence of warm up and gradual slowing are described in Chapter 5. Warm up and slowing prior to termination are also sometimes features of automaticity (Table 5-1). In general, triggered atrial tachycardias have cycle lengths similar to automatic tachycardias, in the range from about 250 ms to 650 ms.

Focal Origin

Triggered atrial tachycardia originates in small circumscribed foci in the atria and therefore, like automatic tachycardias, are focal tachycardias (Table 5-1, row C). The location of the focus can be determined by the morphology of the P waves and electrophysiological mapping. P-wave morphology is usually the same for all tachycardia impulses, including the first tachycardia impulse that is premature and subsequent tachycardia impulses indicating the same site of origin. Localization by P-wave morphology is not always precise (see Figure 3-6, Figure 3-7, and Figure 3-8). In Figure 6-2, based on P-wave morphology, the location of tachycardia origin is in the low right atrium. The sites of origin of focal atrial tachycardias are described in Chapter 3 (Figure 3-1). These sites likely reflect the origin of triggered as well as automatic tachycardias, but might also include focal reentry (see Chapter 10).

Autonomic Nervous System Influences

Triggered atrial tachycardia is influenced by the autonomic nervous system (ANS) (Table 5-1, row D). It can be initiated by sympathetic activation such as during exercise or administration of a β-adrenergic agonist such as isoproterenol (β_1 stimulation). Acceleration of the sinus rate increases DAD amplitude in the ectopic triggerable focus (Figure 5-4). Catecholamines also directly increase DAD amplitude independent of rate by increasing intracellular Ca^{2+} (Figure 5-2). The rate of tachycardia is accelerated by sympathetic stimulation because of the decreased coupling interval of DADs. Automatic tachycardias can also be initiated and accelerated by the sympathetic nervous system and β-adrenergic agonists.

Triggered atrial tachycardia is slowed and terminated by cholinergic stimulation independent of its effects on the A-V node. In **Figure 6-3**, Panel B, edrophonium (10 mg IV), a drug that prevents breakdown of acetylcholine released from the vagus and therefore increases its concentration at its target (the M_2 receptor), is shown to terminate a triggered atrial tachycardia (asterisk) independent of any effects on the A-V node. Acetylcholine (vagal stimulation) decreases DAD amplitude by increasing an outward K^+ current (I_{ACh}) and by inhibiting the effects of β-adrenergic stimulation as described in Chapter 5.

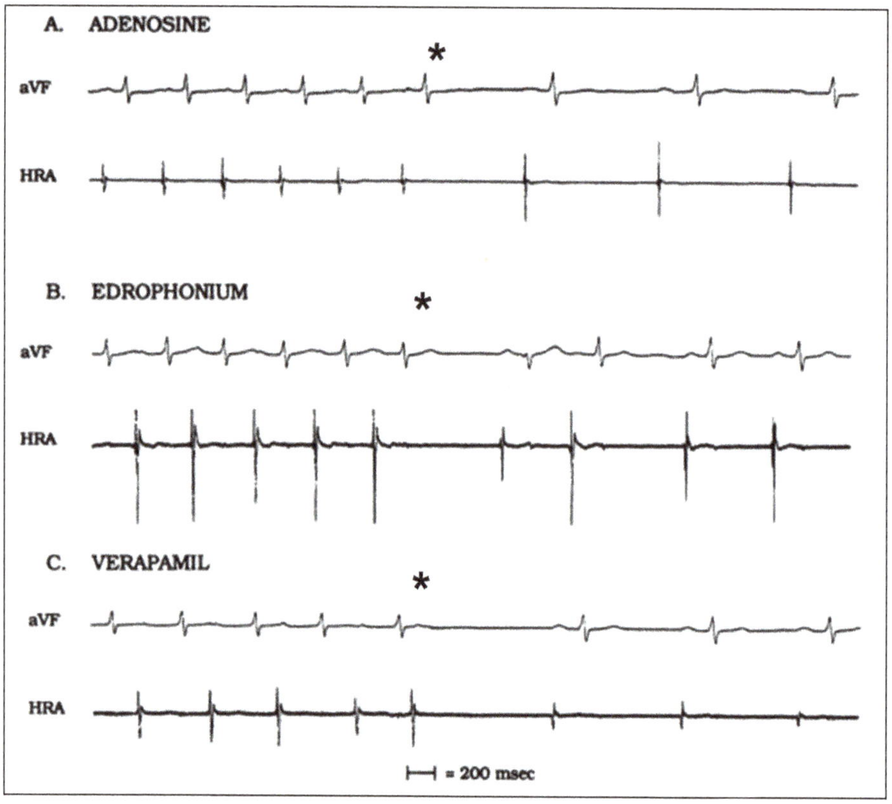

Figure 6-3 Pharmacological responses of atrial tachycardia due to triggered activity. Surface ECG lead aVF and intracardiac recordings from the high right atrium (HRA) are shown. (Reproduced from Engelstein ED, Lippman M, et al. Mechanism-specific effects of adenosine on atrial tachycardia. *Circulation.* 1994;89:2645–2654.)

Pharmacological Effects

Triggered atrial tachycardia is stopped by adenosine and verapamil (Table 5-2, row E). Figure 6-3, Panel A shows a triggered atrial tachycardia which terminates 6 sec after 6 mg IV adenosine administration (asterisk). Adenosine decreases DAD amplitude to terminate the tachycardia by increasing an outward K^+ current or by blocking the effects of adrenergic stimulation independent of its effects on A-V nodal conduction, whereas it only transiently slows automatic tachycardia. In Figure 6-3, Panel A, the ventricular rate slows both because of atrial slowing and transient A-V block.

In Figure 6-3, Panel C, the termination of triggered atrial tachycardia after 10 mg IV verapamil is illustrated (asterisk). Verapamil decreases DAD amplitude by decreasing diastolic Ca^{2+}. Verapamil has little effect on automatic atrial tachycardia.

Electrical Stimulation

DAD-Triggered Tachycardias Can Be Induced by Electrical Stimulation

An important feature of DAD-induced triggered atrial tachycardia that distinguishes it from automatic atrial tachycardia is that it can be induced by overdrive or premature electrical stimulation (Table 5-1, row F). Overdrive is usually more effective. The mechanisms by which stimulation causes triggered activity are described in detail in Chapter 5, Figure 5-4; DAD amplitude increases with a decrease in stimulus cycle length. Automatic tachycardia cannot be initiated by electrical stimulation. The site of pacing is not a determinant as long as the rate is increased at the site of the triggerable focus. Ventricular stimulation is as effective as atrial stimulation for triggering an atrial focus, when all the ventricular impulses pass through the AV junction to the atria.

In **Figure 6-4**, overdrive pacing from the right ventricular apex (bottom recording) initiates an atrial tachycardia.

Overdrive at a cycle length of 400 ms at the left (last 3 stimulated impulses of a 15-sec overdrive period) activates the atria 1:1 (upward arrow shows ventricular activation preceding coronary sinus (Cs) electrograms) and initiates triggered atrial tachycardia originating in the infero lateral tricuspid annular region (note that downward arrow shows Cs electrogram activated prior to the ventricular electrogram).

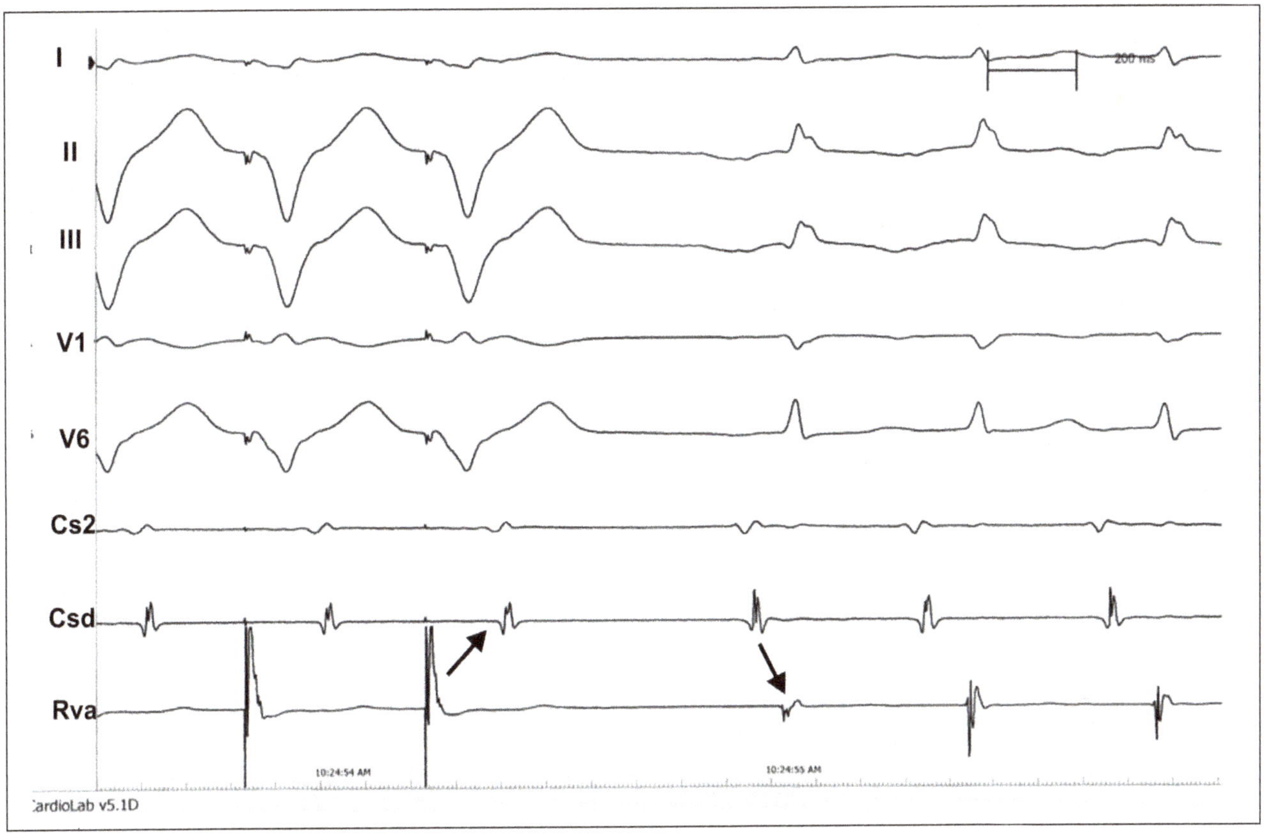

Figure 6-4 Initiation of triggered atrial tachycardia by ventricular stimulation. ECG leads I, II, III, V_1, and V_6, and electrograms from the coronary sinus (Cs2 [proximal] and Csd [distal]) and the right ventricular apex (RVa).

Direct Relationship between Triggering Stimulus Cycle Length and Coupling Interval to First Tachycardia Impulse

Another important feature of initiation of triggered tachycardia by stimulation is a direct relationship between triggering (overdrive or premature stimulus) cycle length and coupling interval between the last stimulated impulse and the first tachycardia impulse. The cause is a decrease in DAD coupling interval as stimulation cycle length decreases (Figures 5-4, 5-5, and 5-6). This feature helps distinguish triggered activity from reentry, which often has an inverse relationship (see Chapter 9). **Figure 6-5** shows this direct relationship.

In Panel A, during pacing from the coronary sinus region at a cycle length of 665 ms (A1-A1), a stimulated premature impulse at a coupling interval of 420 ms (A1-A2) is followed by the first tachycardia impulse (A') with a coupling interval (A2-A') of 420 ms. In Panels B–E, as A1-A2 is decreased to 390, 380, 320, and 290 ms, the coupling interval to the first tachycardia impulse (A2-A') also decreases to 415, 410, 380, and 290 ms. This relationship is the same as plotted for DAD coupling interval to initiating cyce length in Figure 5-5.

Other features of triggered tachycardia initiation by electrical stimulation can include warm-up at the onset of tachycardia and shorter tachycardia cycle length and longer duration of tachycardia with shorter initiating cycle lengths, similar to initiation of triggered activity by spontaneous increases in heart rate or spontaneous premature impulses (Table 5-1, row B). These features, including the direct relationship at the initiation of tachycardia (Figure 6-5), are not always present for reasons described in Chapter 5 and their absence does not negate the diagnosis of triggered tachycardia.

Transient Acceleration with Overdrive

Overdrive stimulation during a triggered tachycardia may transiently accelerate it. The first and following cycle lengths of tachycardia following overdrive are directly related to the overdrive cycle length as illustrated in **Figure 6-6**.

Panel A shows the atrial tachycardia at a cycle length of 430 ms. Panels B–D show records during progressively shorter overdrive pacing cycle lengths (PCL). The last stimulated impulse of a period of overdrive is shown by the arrows above the LA electrogram in each panel.

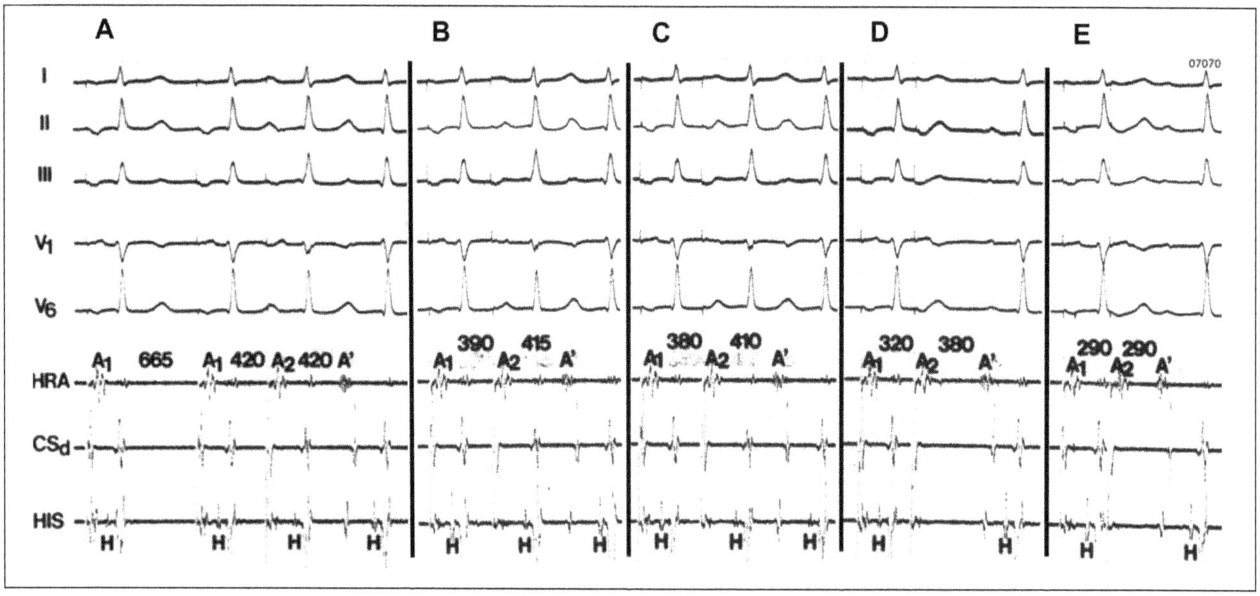

Figure 6-5 ECG leads I, II, III, V_1, and V_6, and electrograms from high right atrium (HRA), distal coronary sinus (CSd), and His bundle region (HIS) (H is His bundle deflection) during initiation of atrial tachycardia (Wellens' ECG collection).

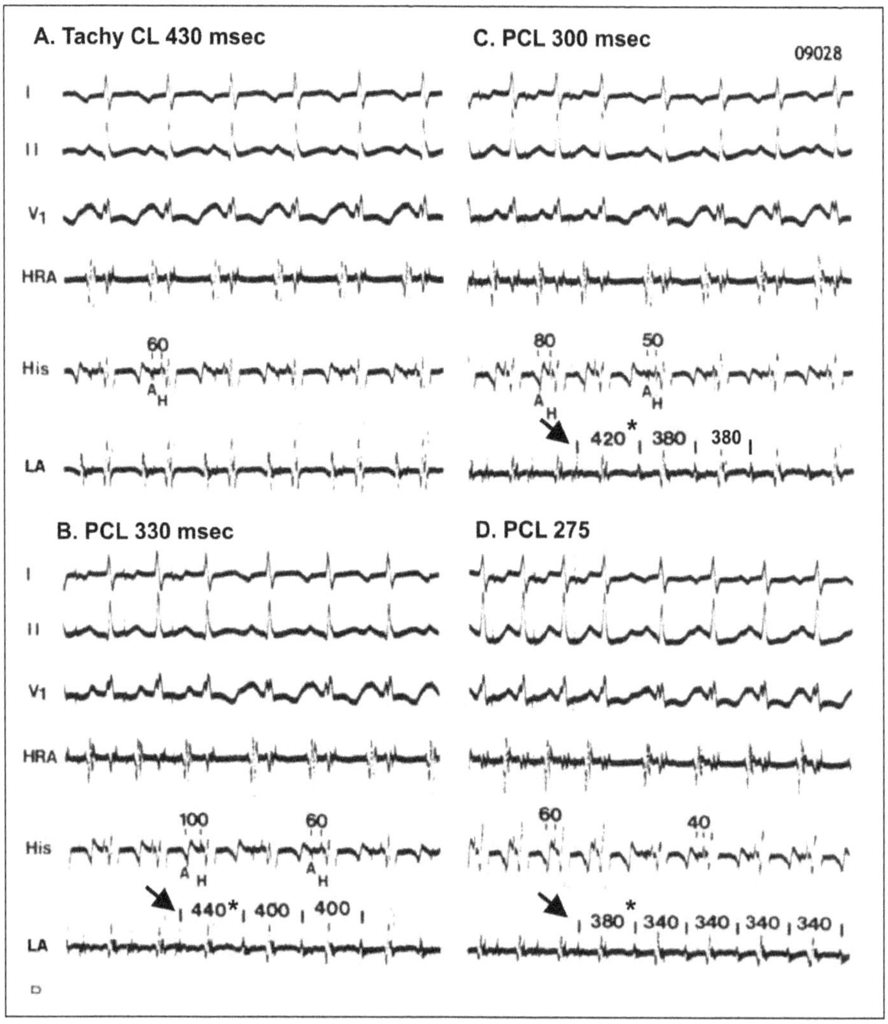

Figure 6-6 Overdrive acceleration. Each panel displays ECG leads I, II, and V_1, and electrograms from the high right atrium (HRA), His bundle region (His), and left atrium (LA) (Wellens' ECG collection).

The first post-pacing (asterisk) and subsequent tachycardia cycle lengths are indicated (ms). The post-pacing cycle lengths become shorter as the pacing cycle length decreases from Panels B–D, thus illustrating overdrive acceleration of the tachycardia. A much shorter-lasting acceleration occurs after a single premature stimulus (not shown), often confined to the first one or two cycle lengths, thus resetting the tachycardia. The mechanism for post overdrive acceleration is based on rate-dependent increases in SR Ca^{2+} that increase DAD amplitude and decreases its coupling interval as described in Figure 5-4.

Termination After Overdrive

At a critically short overdrive pacing cycle length, triggered tachycardia can be terminated. In **Figure 6-7** at the top left, a triggered atrial tachycardia is shown with a cycle length (TC CL) of 460 ms. The tachycardia is overdriven by stimulation at a rate of 200 impulses/min for 10/sec from an electrode catheter in the coronary sinus (CS PACE).

Following pacing ('off' in the bottom panel), the tachycardia resumes at a shorter CL of 360 ms, then slows and terminates. Acceleration of the tachycardia is caused by increased Ca^{2+} entry during overdrive and the subsequent slowing and termination from increased I_P (explained in Figure 5-7). Overdrive acceleration followed by slowing and then termination does not always occur. Tachycardia may sometimes terminate almost immediately after overdrive. Tachycardia can sometimes be terminated by a premature stimulated impulse, which is not as effective as overdrive stimulation.

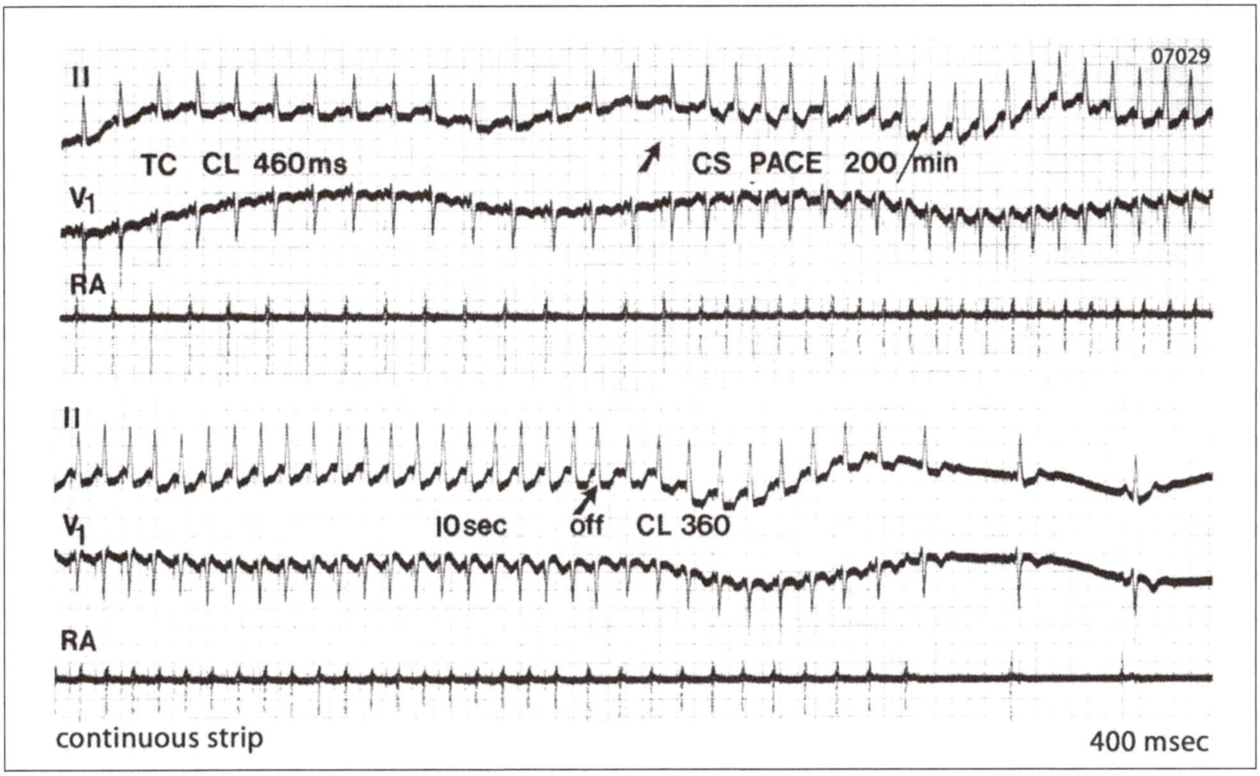

Figure 6-7 Overdrive termination of atrial tachycardia. ECG leads II, V_1, and a right atrial (RA) electrogram (Wellens' ECG collection).

ATRIAL TACHYCARDIA ASSOCIATED WITH DIGITALIS TOXICITY

The ECG in **Figure 6-8**, Panel A, shows atrial tachycardia with 2:1 A-V block. This atrial arrhythmia is most commonly associated with digitalis toxicity, although it can also occur in its absence. It is more likely to occur in patients with atrial disease than with normal atria and sometimes may be paroxysmal. The accompanying A-V block is due to the concomitant effect of digitalis to depress A-V nodal conduction. Figure 6-8, Panel A illustrates the features of this arrhythmia which are: (1) an atrial rate between 140–250 bpm, (2) 2:1 A-V block or A-V Wenckebach, (3) inferior directed P axis (P wave positive in leads II, III, and aVF) indicating an origin in the high right atrium, and (4) ventriculophasic PP alternation (the PP interval that includes a QRS is shorter than the PP without a QRS). Figure 6-8, Panel B shows sinus rhythm after digitalis administration was stopped.

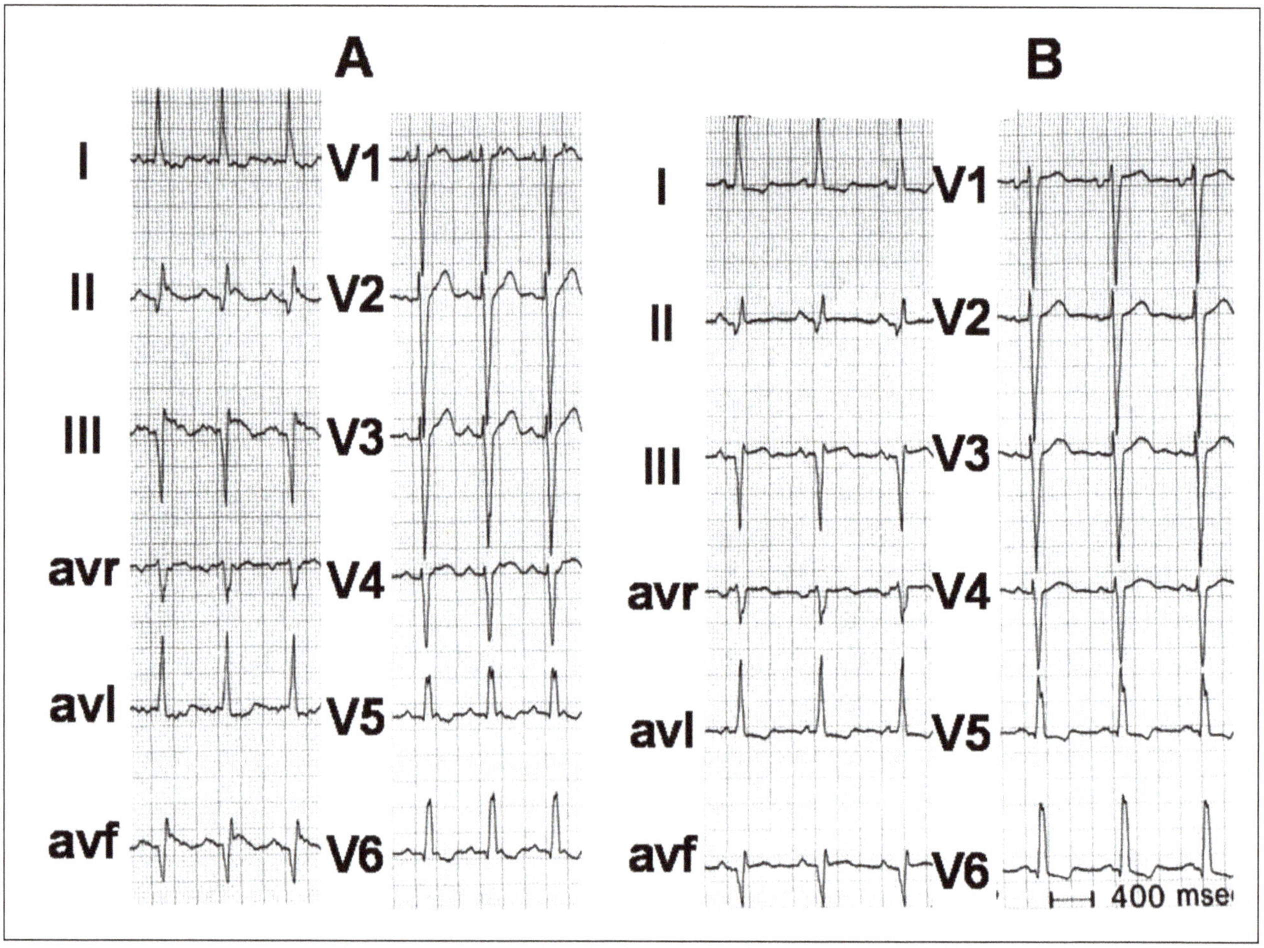

Figure 6-8 **Panel A:** 12-lead ECG showing atrial tachycardia, recorded from a patient with systolic heart failure taking digitalis along with quinapril and furosemide. **Panel B:** ECG showing sinus rhythm from the same patient after digitalis was stopped. (Reproduced from Wellens HJJ, Conover, M. *The ECG in Emergency Decision Making*. St. Louis, MO: Saunders Elsevier; 2006.)

Mechanism of Digitalis-Induced Atrial Tachycardia with Block

In addition to automaticity (see Chapter 3), digitalis-induced arrhythmias are also caused by DADs as a result of Ca^{2+} overload resulting from inhibition of the Na^+–K^+ pump (Figure 5-8). In normal atria, DADs occur mostly in cells in and around the crista terminalis that are characterized by action potentials with a plateau phase 2 of repolarization (see Chapter 3). Ordinary working atrial muscle action potentials that do not have a prominent phase 2 usually do not develop DADs. In diseased atrial myocardium in which cells have a low (less negative) resting membrane potential, the occurrence of DADs is not confined to atrial cells with prominent phase 2 (plateaus) but can occur most anywhere in the atria.

Clinical Electrophysiology of Atrial Tachycardia with Block

The supposition that atrial tachycardia with block is triggered is based on the known effects of digitalis to cause DADs in atrial cells in the experimental laboratory. The clinical evidence necessary to attribute atrial tachycardia associated with digitalis to triggered activity is lacking. Evidence that A-V junctional and ventricular arrhythmias associated with digitalis toxicity are caused by triggered activity is more extensive (described later in this chapter).

RELATIONSHIP OF TRIGGERED ACTIVITY TO ATRIAL FIBRILLATION

It has been proposed that DAD-induced-triggered activity might sometimes be a mechanism underlying the initiation and/or maintenance of atrial fibrillation (see Chapter 10). Atrial fibrillation (AF) under some circumstances is initiated after the sudden appearance of rapid activity in atrial muscle extending into pulmonary veins or, less often, into the vena cavae or coronary sinus. *In vitro* studies of these tissues have demonstrated DADs under special laboratory conditions. Sometimes the rapid activity in these regions prior to the onset of AF in patients can be initiated by rapid pacing. Elevated diastolic Ca^{2+} resulting from abnormal Ca^{2+} release from the SR has also been observed in experimental laboratory models, particularly in animals with mutations in Ca^{2+} handling proteins such as the RYR2 protein. Although consistent with properties of DAD-induced triggered activity, additional evidence that would make this more conclusive such as cycle length dependence of initiation, effects of stimulation on the rapid activity and actions of pharmacological agents is not available.

SUMMARY

DADs in atrial cells result from elevated diastolic Ca^{2+} that leads to the generation of the transient inward current (I_{TI}) that is based on I_{NCX}. Elevated Ca^{2+} often results from sympathetic stimulation that enhances I_{CaL}. DADs also accompany digitalis toxicity that can increase diastolic Ca^{2+} by reducing Ca^{2+} extrusion from the cell as a consequence of inhibition of the Na^+–K^+ exchange pump. The properties of DADs and triggered activity in atrial cells caused by sympathetic stimulation, with regards to effects of rate and rhythm, are consistent with the general properties detailed in Chapter 5.

DAD-triggered paroxysmal atrial tachycardia begins after acceleration of sinus rate or an ectopic premature impulse early or late in the cycle length. Both increase DAD amplitude that reaches the threshold for triggered action potentials. Tachycardia has a focal origin with a P wave preceding a normal QRS in the absence of conducting system disease. P-wave morphology depends on the location of the focus as described for focal tachycardias caused by automaticity in Chapter 3. As tachycardia rate increases, PR interval also increases due to rate-dependent conduction delay in the A-V node. Tachycardia may show a warm-up phase and can terminate either after gradual slowing or abruptly.

DAD-triggered atrial tachycardia can be initiated by overdrive or programmed premature stimulation. The coupling interval of the first tachycardia impulse decreases with a decrease in the initiating cycle length (direct relationship). This characteristic is specific for DAD-triggered arrhythmias. The duration of tachycardia also may also last longer when initiated by faster overdrive rates. Tachycardia can be terminated by overdrive and premature stimulation. After overdrive, there may be transient acceleration.

Tachycardia rate is increased by sympathetic stimulation and slowed and stopped by adenosine, verapamil, and parasympathetic stimulation unrelated to their effects on the A-V node. Termination distinguishes triggered from automatic tachycardia. Na^+-channel blockers can also decrease DADs and prevent triggered tachycardia although normal automaticity can also be terminated.

Atrial tachycardia caused by digitalis toxicity is identified by an atrial rate between 140–250 bpm; 2:1 A-V block or A-V Wenckebach related to increased vagal activity; inferior directed P axis (P wave positive in leads II, III, and aVF) indicating an origin in the high right atrium; and ventriculophasic P-P alternation (the P-P interval encompassing the QRS is shorter than the PP without a QRS). Once identified as caused by digitalis, a DAD-triggered mechanism is likely although not proven.

SECTION 6B

Atrioventricular (A-V) Junctional Delayed Afterdepolarizations and Triggered Arrhythmias

Basic Electrophysiologic Mechanisms

ELECTROPHYSIOLOGY OF DADS AND TRIGGERED ACTIVITY IN THE A-V JUNCTION

In Chapter 3, the anatomy and cellular electrophysiology of A-V junctional cells with normal automaticity are described (Figure 3-12 and Figure 3-13). Comparable detailed information from cellular electrophysiological studies, on the location and electrophysiology of DADs in the A-V junction is lacking, DADs have not been recorded with microelectrodes. The occurrence of DADs is supported by the properties of the junctional arrhythmias described below. It is likely that triggered junctional rhythms can arise in any region of the A-V junction, including the A-V node and His bundle. Automaticity and DADs may even occur in the same cell under different circumstances, but cells that are not normally automatic may also be capable of generating DADs. The mechanism for DADs in A-V junctional cells is likely to be similar to the general description of DAD mechanisms in Chapter 5. In general, the events that incite DADs, such as catecholamines or digitalis excess, can cause Ca^{2+} overload and enhanced intracellular Ca^{2+} releases that result in DAD generation irrespective of whether or not a cell has the normal intrinsic properties of automaticity. Similarly, the properties of DADs in A-V junction (e.g., response to cycle length, autonomics, pharmacological agents) are likely to be the same as indicated in the general description of DADs in Chapter 5.

The coupling through gap junctions of upper nodal (AN) cells to the atria and the gap junction coupling between mid nodal (compact node, CN) cells and upper (AN) and lower nodal (NH) cells tend to suppress DAD formation as it does for automaticity, due to electrotonic current flow (see Figure 1-3). However, since DADs result from Ca^{2+} overload, which also can decrease gap junction coupling, this suppressive effect of cell coupling may be reduced in situations that cause triggered activity.

Examples of Arrhythmias Caused by DAD-Triggered Activity

ACCELERATED JUNCTIONAL RHYTHMS AND NONPAROXYSMAL JUNCTIONAL TACHYCARDIA

Figure 6-9 shows an ECG from a patient with a junctional rhythm at a rate of 110 bpm caused by digitalis toxicity. The QRS is identical to that during sinus rhythm (not shown). The rate of junctional rhythms caused by digitalis toxicity can range from about 70–140 bpm. Junctional impulse initiation at rates of between 70 and 100 bpm are considered to be accelerated junctional rhythms since they are more rapid than the intrinsic automatic rate of the normal A-V junction (see Chapter 3). At rates above 100 bpm, they are classified as nonparoxysmal junctional tachycardias, as is the case in this patient. Accelerated junctional rhythms can occur in patients treated with digitalis, after open-heart surgery, in the presence of electrolyte disturbances, and during or after myocardial ischemia and infarction. All these factors can act as stimuli to increase normal automaticity or cause DADs in the A-V junction. Many of the properties of accelerated junctional arrhythmias including nonparoxysmal junctional tachycardia, no matter what their cause, conform to the characteristics of DAD-triggered activity and are distinguishable from normal automaticity as described in Table 5-1.

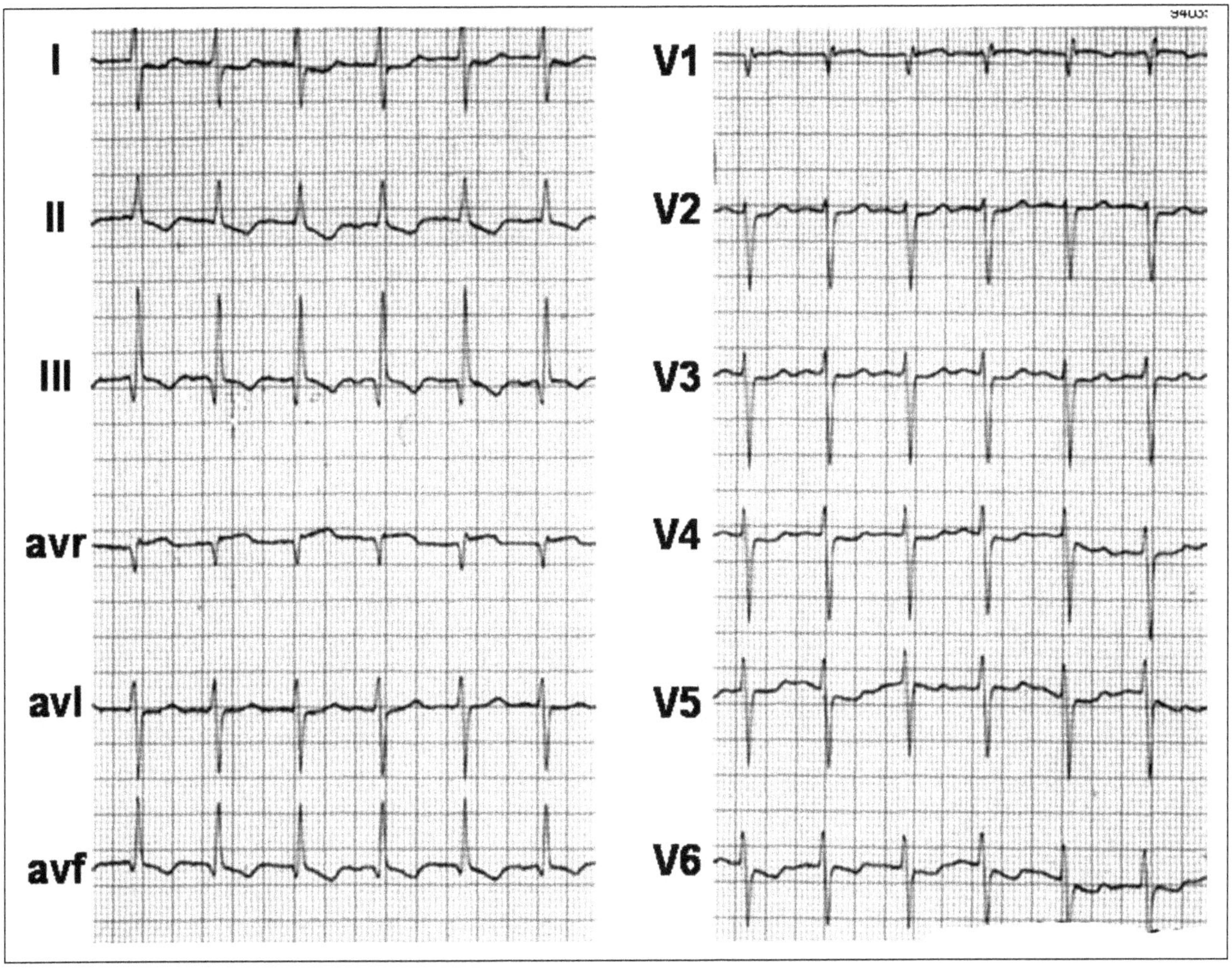

Figure 6-9 12-lead ECG recorded from a patient with nonparoxysmal junctional tachycardia, who was treated for heart failure with quinapril, furosemide, and digoxin (Wellens' ECG collection).

Electrophysiological Properties of Triggered Accelerated Junctional Arrhythmias

Initiated by Acceleration of Heart Rate

Triggered accelerated junctional rhythms often interrupt periods of sinus rhythm. The likelihood of their occurrence is related to the dominant (sinus) rate; they are more likely to occur during faster rather than slower sinus rates (Table 5-1, row A).

Figure 6-10 top panels shows bar graphs of the dominant (sinus) heart rate distribution calculated as cycle length (Dominant R-R) in a study of 55 patients with accelerated junctional rhythms.

Panel A (top) shows the entire arrhythmia population with a variety of causes (n = 55), and Panel B (top) shows the smaller subset of those who were taking digitalis (n = 27). In Panel A, the number of patients who had this arrhythmia over a range of cycle lengths, increased with a decrease in cycle length of the dominant sinus rhythm (Dominant R-R, CL) to a peak at a dominant cycle length between 600–700 ms, beyond which it declined. In the patients receiving digitalis, the dominant (sinus) cycle length at which accelerated junctional rhythm was most prevalent is between 500 and 600 ms (Figure 6-10, Panel B).

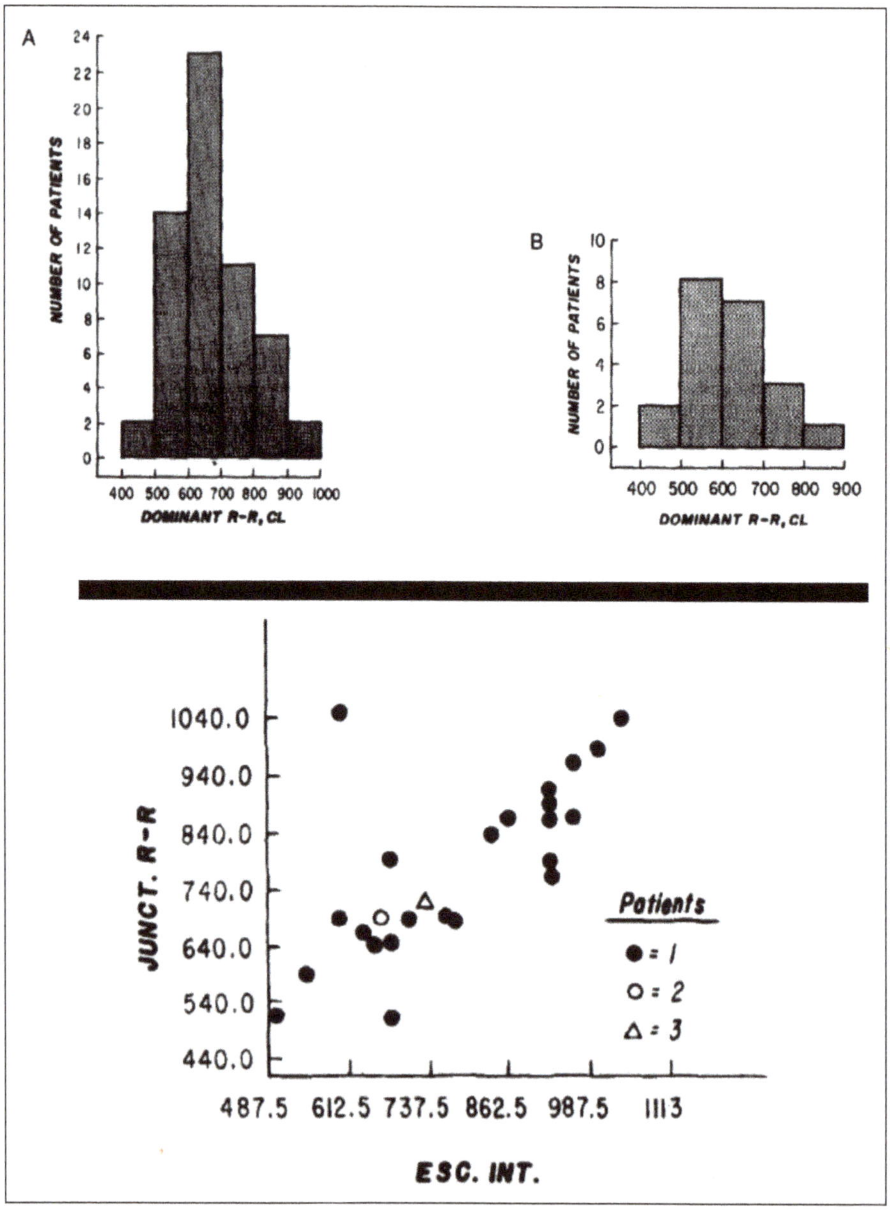

Figure 6-10 **Top** (**Panel A** and **Panel B**): Bar graphs showing relationship of dominant (sinus) R-R intervals to occurrence of accelerated junctional rhythm. **Bottom:** Relationship between R-R interval of junctional rhythm to escape interval (ESC.INT.) of the first impulse of the junctional rhythm. (Reproduced from Rosen MR, Fisch C, et al. Can accelerated atrioventricular junctional escape rhythms be explained by delayed afterdepolarizations? *Am J Cardiol.* 1980;45:1272–1284.)

The effects of decreasing sinus cycle length to increase the occurrence of the arrhythmia is explained by the effects of decreased cycle length to increase DAD amplitude and trigger impulse initiation by increasing Ca^{2+} entry, subsequent SR Ca^{2+} loading and diastolic Ca^{2+} release (see Figure 5-2). The decrease in incidence of arrhythmias at the most rapid rates may result from suppression of DADs by outward pump current (I_p) that is expected to increase at faster stimulus rates, eventually leading to a decreased net inward I_{TI}. On the other hand, the likelihood of arrhythmias caused by normal or abnormal automaticity is not enhanced by an acceleration in heart rate, and is likely decreased.

Coupling Interval Directly Related to Triggering Cycle Length

The coupling interval of the first impulse of an accelerated junctional rhythm to the previous impulse, whether it is a sinus impulse or an ectopic (nonjunctional) premature impulse, is shorter than the expected escape interval of an A-V junctional automatic pacemaker. The coupling interval of the first junctional impulse is also directly related to the previous cycle length, becoming shorter as the triggering cycle length decreases (Table 5-1, row B). This direct dependence of the first coupling interval on the triggering cycle length is shown in **Figure 6-11** that displays the onset of a junctional rhythm following atrial pacing in a patient with an acute myocardial infarction. In addition to showing this relationship, Figure 6-11 shows that accelerated junctional rhythms can be initiated by overdrive stimulation, unlike automaticity (Table 5-1, row F).

From bottom to top, going from slower (64 bpm) to faster (94 bpm) pacing (heart) rate (Hr), the coupling interval from the last paced impulse (arrow) to the first junctional impulse (asterisk) decreases from 1100 ms (In the bottom strip, the fourth pacemaker impulse failed to capture the atria, permitting emergence of the junctional escape beat.) to 960 ms to 800 ms, showing the direct relationship characteristic of triggered impulses (Figure 5-5).

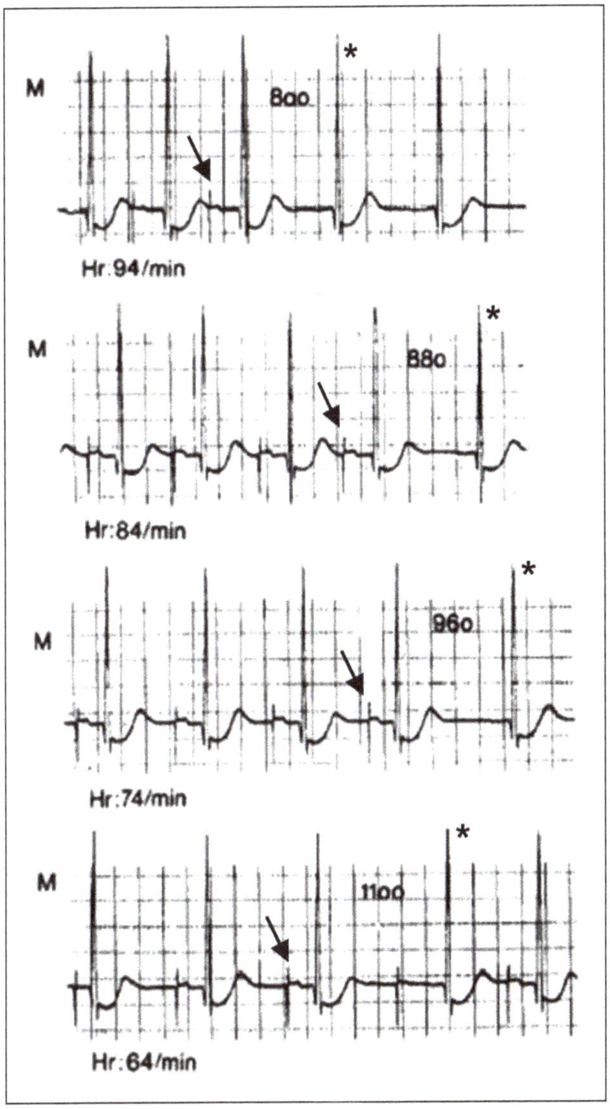

Figure 6-11 Junctional rhythm triggered by atrial pacing. Hr =heart rate; M = monitor lead. (Reproduced from Tenczer J, Littman L, et al. Atrioventricular junctional rhythm induced by atrial stimulation: A suspected clinical manifestation of "triggered" activity. *Am J Cardiol.* 1984;53:631–632.)

Rate of Junctional Rhythm Is Directly Related to Triggering Heart Rate

The cycle length of a triggered accelerated junctional rhythm or nonparoxysmal tachycardia is directly related to the cycle length of the triggering impulses (sinus or paced) (Table 5-1, row B). This is an expected property of a triggered rhythm where the triggering cycle length determines the coupling interval of the first triggered impulse, which in turn determines the cycle length of the triggered rhythm (described in Figure 5-4 and Figure 5-6). Figure 6-10 (bottom graph) shows this direct relationship between the coupling interval of the first triggered impulse (ESC. INT.) and the cycle length of a junctional rhythm (Junct R-R). As the coupling interval of the first triggered impulse decreases the R-R interval of the triggered rhythm also decreases. The cycle length of an automatic accelerated junctional rhythm (normal or abnormal) is unrelated to either the previous dominant cycle length or the coupling interval of the first junctional impulse.

Warm Up

As described in Table 5-1, row B, accelerated junctional rhythms may show warm up after initiation and gradual slowing prior to termination, although these characteristics are not always observed. Arrhythmias caused by normal automaticity also have these characteristics. The description in Chapter 3 of the relationship of the site of origin of an automatic junctional focus to the P-R or R-P interval and P-wave morphology also applies to a triggered focus. Triggered activity is not dependent on A-V junctional conduction delay (increased P-R interval) as is A-V junctional reentrant rhythms (Chapter 11).

Autonomic Nervous System Effects

Triggered accelerated junctional rhythms can occur in response to catecholamines or β1-adrenergic stimulation in addition to digitalis. Digitalis-induced triggered A-V junctional rhythm accelerates with exercise. Catecholamines exert these effects by increasing Ca^{2+} entry into A-V junctional cells through L-type Ca^{2+} channels. Since catecholamines also accelerate automatic rhythms, the effects of sympathetic activation do not distinguish triggered from automatic junctional rhythms (Table 5-1, row D). The rate of triggered activity arising in both A-V nodal and His bundle cells is expected to increase so the response to sympathetic stimulation cannot distinguish between these sites of origin.

The effects of parasympathetic stimulation are variable but do provide a clue to the site of the triggered arrhythmogenic focus within the A-V junction. For example, **Figure 6-12** shows the effects of carotid sinus massage (CSM) on an accelerated junctional rhythm (nonparoxysmal tachycardia) caused by digitalis toxicity with a cycle length of 480 ms that is likely caused by triggered activity. With CSM, the cycle length prolongs to 960 ms, which is twice the junctional rate, suggesting 2:1 block between the junctional focus and the ventricles. Since the upper (AN) and mid-nodal (CN) regions are more sensitive to conduction block by acetylcholine (CSM-induced), than lower nodal-His bundle (LN-HB), the triggered focus is likely in the mid node, or proximal to it. Parasympathetic stimulation might also stop a triggered rhythm arising in the upper or mid node.

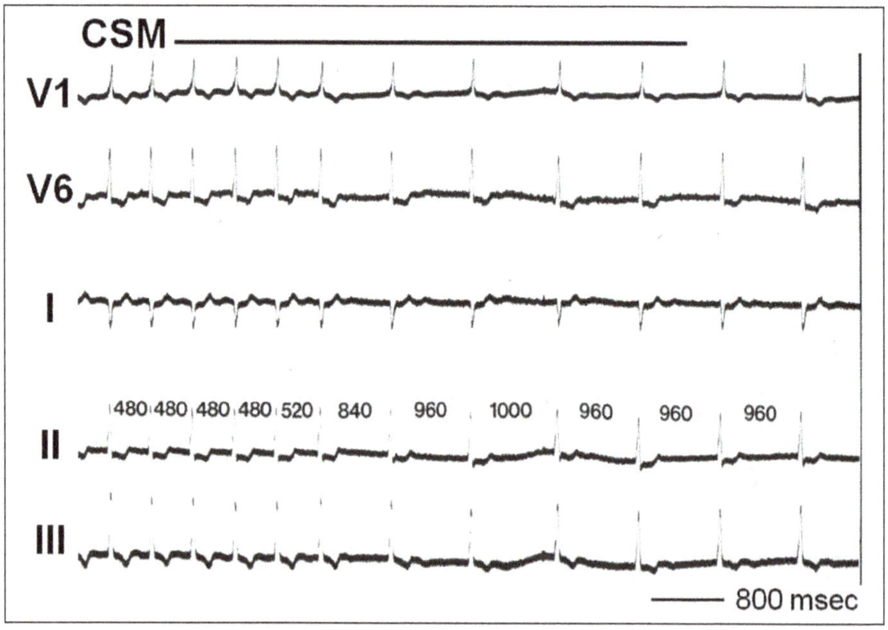

Figure 6-12 ECG leads V_1, V_6, I, II, and III in a patient with a junctional arrhythmia caused by digitalis toxicity. **Horizontal line** above shows a period of carotid sinus massage (CSM). Cycle lengths are shown above the lead II recording (Wellens' ECG collection).

In other cases, CSM has no effect on digitalis-induced accelerated junctional rhythms, a likely scenario when the focus is in the lower node or His bundle which are less sensitive to acetylcholine. However, triggered foci caused by sympathetic stimulation in these regions might be slowed or inhibited owing to accentuated antagonism, whereby parasympathetic activation overcomes sympathetic activation. Similar responses can also happen with an automatic junctional pacemaker.

Response to Adenosine and Other Pharmacological Agents

The response to adenosine can distinguish between an automatic and triggered junctional focus (Table 5-1, row E). The junctional arrhythmia in **Figure 6-13**, which was initiated by isoproterenol, was terminated by adenosine (administered just before the start of the recording). This is the expected response of a triggered rhythm caused by β-adrenergic stimulation in the A-V node or His bundle. Automatic arrhythmias are transiently suppressed but not terminated.

L-type Ca^{2+}-channel block, by verapamil, is also predicted to terminate and prevent accelerated A-V junctional rhythms in contrast to automatic rhythms (Table 3-1, row E) although clinical data are not available. The response to Na^{+} channel-blocking drugs is unknown.

Effects of Electrical Stimulation

Accelerated junctional rhythms caused by DAD-triggered activity can be initiated by overdrive stimulation, and possibly by premature stimulation, as already explained in Figure 6-11. This contrasts with automaticity in the A-V junction that is not initiated by stimulation. Clinical data are not available to support the other characteristic responses of triggered activity to clinical stimulation protocols shown in Table 5-1, row F. It is predicted that overdrive stimulation might terminate triggered junctional rhythms, whereas it does not terminate automatic junctional rhythms.

JUNCTIONAL ECTOPIC TACHYCARDIA

Figure 6-14 shows a junctional rhythm with a rate of 190 bpm. The first two impulses are of sinus origin, sinus cycle length 840 ms. A rapid rhythm begins with a premature junctional impulse with a coupling interval of 420 ms that is conducted to the ventricles but not the atria (the HBEd recording of the premature impulse (unfilled arrowhead) shows a His bundle electrogram (H) followed by a ventricular electrogram but the absence of an atrial electrogram). The arrhythmia is classified as a junctional ectopic tachycardia (JET) (also see Chapter 3, Section 3B). Typical features of the ECG of JET include a rapid, sometimes irregular rate that is faster than a nonparoxysmal junctional tachycardia (about 100–250 bpm in adults; 150–275 bpm in infants), a narrow QRS identical to the sinus QRS, and A-V dissociation, all of which are evident in Figure 6-14. JET occurs in infancy in association with congenital cardiac defects or postoperatively after surgery near the A-V junction, when it is often incessant. In adults, JET can occur with either congenital heart defects or in the absence of heart disease. Here it is usually not incessant but can last from several seconds to hours.

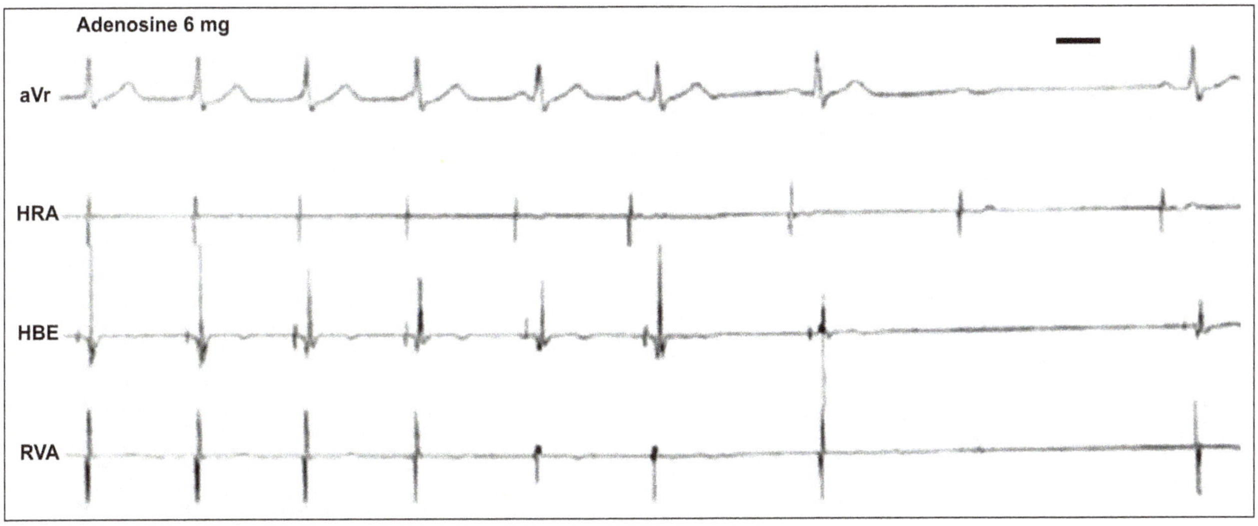

Figure 6-13 ECG lead aVR and electrograms from the high right atrium (HRA), His bundle (HBE), and right ventricular apex (RVA) during accelerated junctional rhythm resulting from isoproterenol administration and its termination by adenosine. (Lee KL, Chun HM, et al. Effect of adenosine and verapamil in catecholamine-induced accelerated atrioventricular junctional rhythm: Insights into the underlying mechanism. *Pacing Clin Electrophysiol.* 1999;22:866–870.)

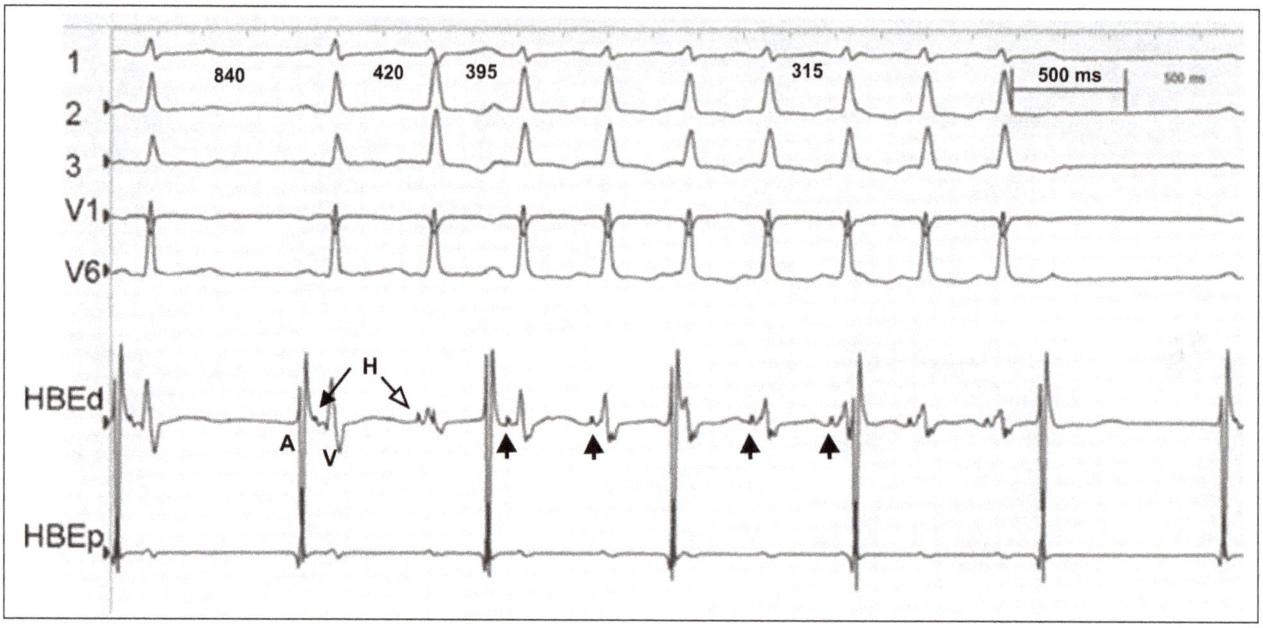

Figure 6-14 ECG leads I, II, III, V_1, and V_6, and intracardiac recordings from distal (HBEd) and proximal His bundle (HBEp) in a patient with JET after aortic valve replacement for aortic stenosis. Cycle lengths indicated above lead II recording. **H** and **arrows** indicates His bundle deflection. (Reproduced from Josephson ME. *Josephson's Clinical Cardiac Electrophysiology: Techniques and Interpretations* (5th ed.). Philadelphia, PA: Wolters Kluwer; 2016.)

This arrhythmia can be caused by automaticity of A-V junctional cells either in the A-V node or His bundle (Figure 3-23), but also by triggered activity arising in the same regions. Triggered junctional tachycardias have different electrophysiological properties than automatic junctional tachycardias as described in Table 5-1. They do have some features that overlap with characteristics of A-V nodal reentry (see Chapter 11).

Properties of Junctional Ectopic Tachycardias (JET) Caused by Triggered Activity

Initiation

Triggered JET begins with a junctional premature impulse with a similar QRS morphology as the sinus QRS (Figure 6-14). Junctional automaticity is not initiated by a decrease in the previous cycle length (Table 5-1, row A). Onset of triggered tachycardia is not associated with conduction slowing in the A-V node (Table 5-1, rows A and B) eliminating A-V nodal reentry as a cause (Chapter 11). Similar to automatic tachycardia, A-V dissociation, a characteristic of JET, eliminates an atrial origin. Information is not available on JET properties such as the relationship of triggering coupling interval to tachycardia rate and duration and to first tachycardia impulse coupling interval.

Focal Origin

Triggered JET originates in a focus (Table 5-1, row C) either in the A-V node or His bundle. Suggestions as to the site of origin come from characteristics of His bundle electrograms as described for junctional automatic tachycardias in Chapter 3, Section 3B. In Figure 6-14, the His bundle electrograms (upward black arrows) associated with junctional impulses are followed by ventricular depolarizations with an H-V interval that is shorter than the H-V interval of the sinus impulses (at left, downward black arrow), suggesting a distal His bundle origin with retrograde His bundle activation and antegrade ventricular activation.

Autonomic Nervous System Effects

Triggered JET can be initiated by β-adrenergic stimulation (sympathetic activation or isoproterenol administration) and suppressed by a β-blocking drug irrespective of the location of the junctional focus, similar to automatic tachycardia (Table 5-1, row D). It can be terminated by vagal activation, such as by carotid sinus massage, when the tachycardia origin is in the upper or mid node, unlike automatic tachycardia, which is only transiently slowed. Effects of vagal activation on JET arising in the His bundle is uncertain. It may slow or stop it by inhibiting sympathetic stimulation but is not expected to have much of an effect in the absence of sympathetic stimulation.

Response to Adenosine and Pharmacological Agents

Triggered JET can be terminated by adenosine. It is likely that junctional tachycardias that originate in the AN or CN regions of the A-V junction are terminated by adenosine because of the marked effects of adenosine in this region (Table 5-1, row E). Tachycardias originating in the His bundle may not be as sensitive to adenosine unless they are caused by catecholamine-induced DADs (see Section 6C). Automatic tachycardias are transiently suppressed but not terminated (Chapter 3, Section 3B).

Because of the suppressant effects of L-type Ca^{2+} channel-blocking drugs such as verapamil and diltiazem on DADs, it is expected that they should terminate triggered JET arising in either the A-V node or His bundle, although clinical data is lacking. They also terminate automaticity arising in the A-V node but not the His bundle (see Chapter 3).

Electrical Stimulation

Triggered JET can be initiated and terminated by electrical stimulation (Table 5-1, row F). In **Figure 6-15**, the junctional tachycardia was initiated by an atrial prematurely stimulated depolarization (arrow, APC) at a coupling interval of 470 ms during a sinus cycle length of 650 ms. The initiation of tachycardia is not associated with slow conduction through the A-V node (as would be the case with A-V nodal reentry, Chapter 11), since the time interval from atrial depolarization to His bundle depolarization (A-H interval) of the His bundle electrogram is not prolonged by the APC. The first few cycle lengths of tachycardia show warm up to 470 ms as sometimes occurs with a triggered rhythm.

This tachycardia was also initiated by ventricular pacing (not shown). Data have not been published on initiation over a wide range of overdrive cycle lengths or premature coupling intervals to document a direct relationship between triggering coupling intervals and coupling intervals of the first tachycardia cycle length as sometimes occurs for other triggered arrhythmias. Automatic tachycardias are not initiated by electrical stimulation (Table 5-1, row F).

The JET in **Figure 6-16** was terminated by a ventricular prematurely stimulated impulse (arrow above lead I and HBE 2 recording). Note that following the premature impulse, the sequence of activation on the His bundle electrogram (HBE 2) is from atrium (A) to His bundle (H) to ventricles (V), whereas during JET, atrial and ventricular depolarization were almost simultaneous. Termination by a premature impulse is a property of triggered tachycardia, in contrast to automatic tachycardia, which cannot be terminated by stimulation (Table 5-1, row F). Resetting characteristics over a wide range of coupling intervals are not available, nor are responses to overdrive stimulation.

In Figure 6-16, the conduction time from His bundle (H) to ventricle (horizontal black bar at the left) during JET is the same as during sinus rhythm (horizontal black bar at the far right), indicating that the likely site of origin of tachycardia was above the His bundle in the A-V node.

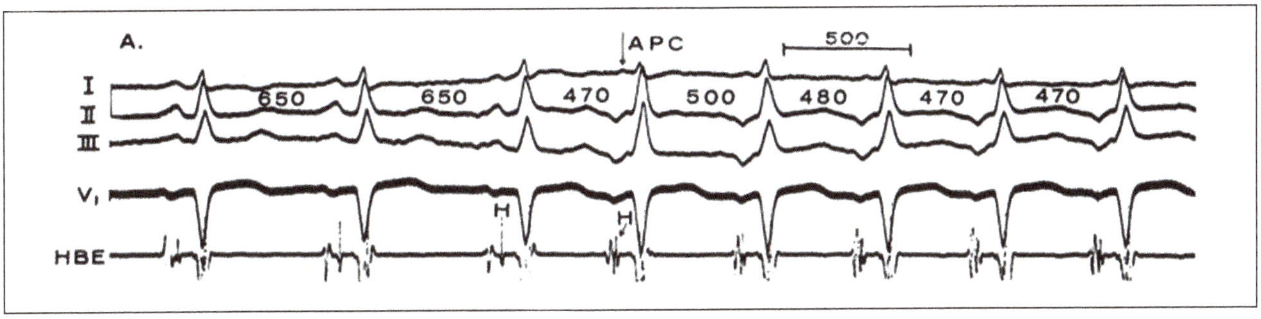

Figure 6-15 ECG leads I, II, III, V_1, and an electrogram from the His bundle region (HBE), His bundle electrogram (H). **Arrow** shows an atrial premature impulse (APC). (Reproduced from Rosen KM. Junctional tachycardia: mechanisms, diagnosis, differential diagnosis, and management. *Circulation.* 1973;47:654–664.)

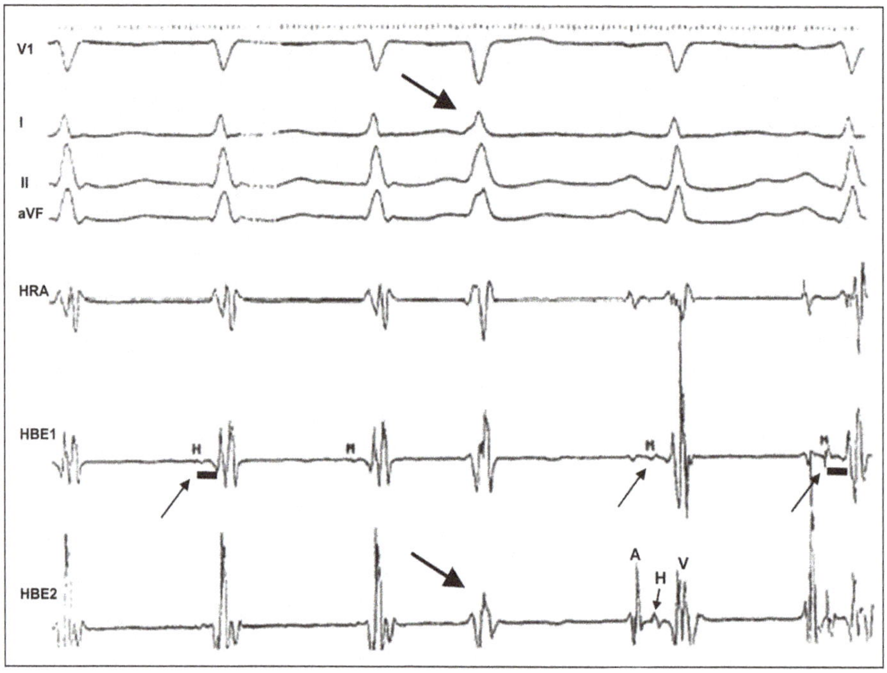

Figure 6-16 ECG leads V_1, I, II, and aVF, and electrograms from the high right atrium (HRA) and His bundle region (HBE1 and HBE2). **Small arrows** show His bundle electrogram (H). A, atrial depolarization; V, ventricular depolarization. (Reproduced from Scheinman MM, Gonzalez RP, et al. Clinical and electrophysiologic features and role of catheter ablation techniques in adult patients with automatic atrioventricular junctional tachycardia. *Am J Cardiol.* 1994;74:565–572.)

SUMMARY

Catecholamines and digitalis excess are predicted to cause Ca^{2+} overload and DADs in the A-V node and His bundle. The properties of the DADs and response to electrical stimulation (cycle length dependent) and pharmacological agents (enhanced by β_1-adrenergic stimulation, suppressed by parasympathetics, L-type Ca^{2+}-channel blockers, and adenosine) are consistent with the general properties described in Chapter 5.

Accelerated junctional rhythms (70–100 bpm) and nonparoxysmal junctional tachycardias (>100 bpm) are examples of triggered arrhythmias. They have electrophysiological characteristics congruent with those expected of a DAD-causal mechanism, including: (1) they are more likely to occur during faster than slower sinus rates; (2) the coupling interval of the first triggered impulse is directly related to the previous cycle length; (3) the cycle length of the arrhythmia is directly related to the cycle length of the triggering impulses (sinus or paced); (4) they can be initiated by electrical stimulation; and (5) sympathetic stimulation increases the rate of the arrhythmia and parasympathetic stimulation and adenosine, suppress the triggered rhythms.

JET is another example of a triggered arrhythmia. It has a rapid and sometimes irregular rate of 100–250 bpm in adults and 150–275 bpm in infants; A-V dissociation; and a narrow QRS identical to the sinus QRS. Triggered JET has different electrophysiological properties than automatic junctional tachycardias. Triggered JET can be initiated and terminated by atrial or ventricular overdrive or premature stimulation not associated with slow conduction through the A-V node. A direct relationship between triggering coupling intervals and coupling intervals of the first tachycardia cycle length has not been documented. These arrhythmias can also be terminated by stimulation. Triggered JET can be initiated by β-adrenergic stimulation and,depending on the site of origin, terminated by vagal activation and adenosine; unlike automatic tachycardia, which is transiently slowed but not terminated. Tachycardias originating in the His bundle may not be as sensitive to vagal stimulation and adenosine as those originating in the A-V node unless they are caused by catecholamine-induced DADs.

SECTION

6C Ventricular Delayed Afterdepolarizations and Triggered Arrhythmias

Basic Electrophysiological Mechanisms

LOCATIONS, MECHANISMS, AND PROPERTIES OF TRIGGERED ARRHYTHMIAS IN THE VENTRICLES

Both Purkinje cells in the specialized conducting system and ventricular muscle cells generate DADs under appropriate conditions. Purkinje cells are more prone to develop DADs than ventricular muscle, as described in Chapter 5. Whether a triggered arrhythmia arises in Purkinje or ventricular muscle cells may sometimes depend on the inciting cause as described in the sections below on specific arrhythmias. The underlying mechanisms causing DADs and their properties are described in Chapter 5 (Figure 5-2 and Figure 5-8). In the following description of the example arrhythmias, additional details relating to the different causes of DADs are explained.

Examples of Arrhythmias Caused by DAD-Triggered Activity in the Ventricle

DIGITALIS-INDUCED VENTRICULAR TACHYCARDIA

The arrhythmia in **Figure 6-17** is a bidirectional ventricular tachycardia caused by digitalis toxicity, which is a triggered arrhythmia. Note the relatively narrow QRS (0.12 sec) with a RBBB pattern in V_1, indicating that all impulses are arising from the left bundle branch, and alternating left- and right-axis deviation in leads I, II, and III, indicating alternating triggered impulses in the left posterior and anterior fascicle.

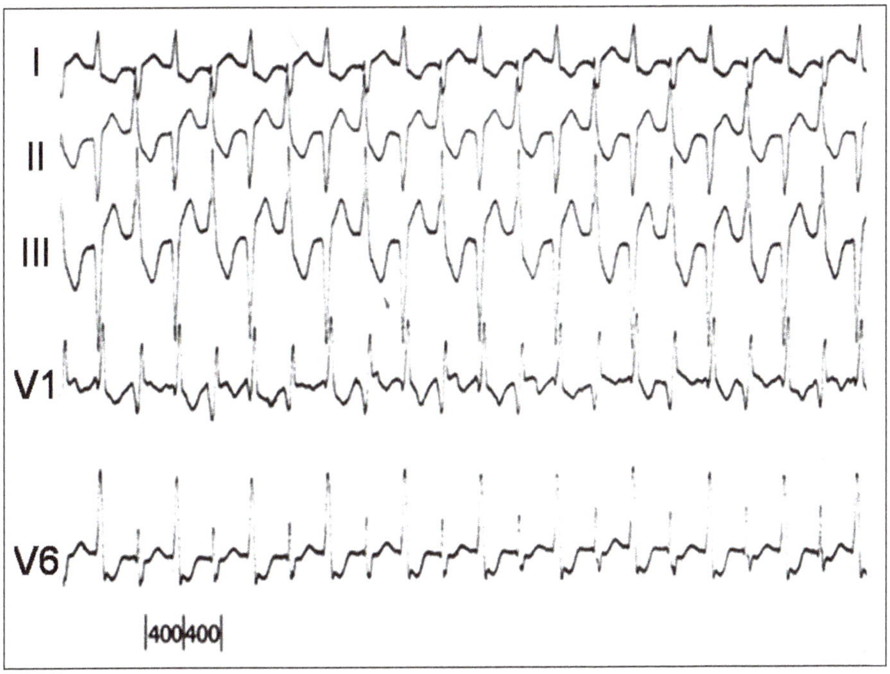

Figure 6-17 ECG leads I, II, III, V_1, and V_6 recorded during bidirectional ventricular tachycardia caused by digitalis toxicity. (Reproduced with permission from Wellens HJJ, Conover M. *The ECG in Emergency Decision Making.* St. Louis, MO: Saunders Elsevier; 2006.)

Properties of Digitalis-Induced DADs Causing Ventricular Arrhythmias

Arrhythmia Initiation

In Chapter 5 and Figure 5-8, the mechanism by which digitalis toxicity causes DADs and triggered activity is described. DADs result from intracellular Ca^{2+} loading as a consequence of inhibition of the Na^+–K^+ pump leading to a decrease in Ca^{2+} extrusion from the cell. Although digitalis-induced ventricular tachycardia (VT) is caused by triggered activity, digitalis sometimes increases normal automaticity that can cause ventricular premature impulses (see Chapter 3, Section 3C).

DADs associated with digitalis toxicity are more prevalent in Purkinje cells than in ventricular muscle and occur preferentially in Purkinje cells of the left conducting system over the right. Although speculative, the longer plateau phase (phase 2) and duration of L-type Ca^{2+} current on the left side of the conducting system may lead to more rapid Ca^{2+} overload in the face of Na^+–K^+ pump inhibition.

Digitalis-induced DADs can also occur as two or more oscillations following the action potential as shown in **Figure 6-18**. In this experiment, a canine Purkinje bundle exposed to toxic amounts of digitalis was stimulated at a regular cycle length (left). After stimulation was stopped, the last stimulated action potential (black arrow) is followed by three DADs (1, 2, 3) with diminishing amplitude. Stimulation is started again at right (unfilled arrowhead).

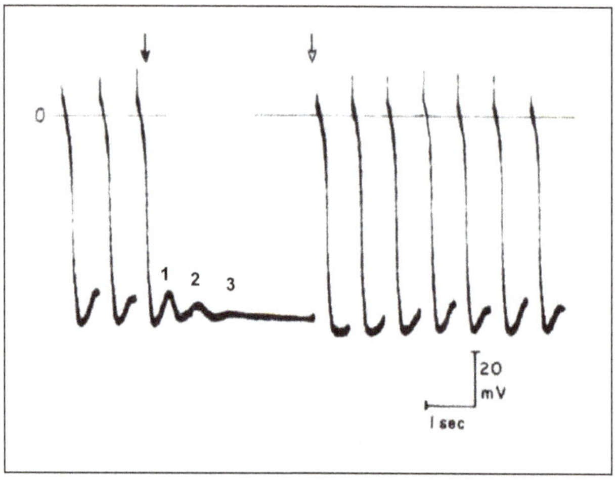

Figure 6-18 Action potentials from a canine Purkinje cell in the presence of digitalis. (Reproduced with permission from Rosen MR, Reder RF. Does triggered activity have a role in the genesis of cardiac arrhythmias. *Annals of Intern Med.* 1981;94:794.)

When two oscillations are present, the relationship of their amplitude and coupling interval to the stimulation cycle length is complex. This complexity can lead to characteristics of initiation of digitalis-induced triggered arrhythmias that do not always coincide with catecholamine-induced triggered activity. For example, as stimulation cycle length is decreased, DAD 1 first reaches threshold to trigger action potentials while DAD 2 is still subthreshold. A further decrease in stimulation cycle length causes DAD 2 to reach threshold to trigger action potentials while the amplitude of DAD 1 declines. The switch of the triggered action potential arising from DAD 1 to DAD 2 causes a sudden increase in coupling interval of the first triggered impulse and cycle length of the triggered tachycardia.

Despite this complex behavior, the effect of drive cycle length on DADs predicts that digitalis-induced ventricular arrhythmias should be more prevalent at more rapid heart rates (Table 5-1, row A), as is described for digitalis-induced junctional rhythms in the previous section, although the same kind of detailed clinical data is not available. An example of the initiation of VT by an increase in heart rate in a clinical case is shown in **Figure 6-19**. The onset of atrial tachycardia with 2:1 A-V block (atrial cycle length 260 ms, P waves pointed out by downward arrows) decreases the ventricular cycle length (R-R) to 500 ms (upward arrows) from the longer cycle length during sinus rhythm (not shown). The decreased ventricular cycle length (R-R) then triggers a VT (at the asterisk) with a 480-ms cycle length (note the change in QRS morphology).

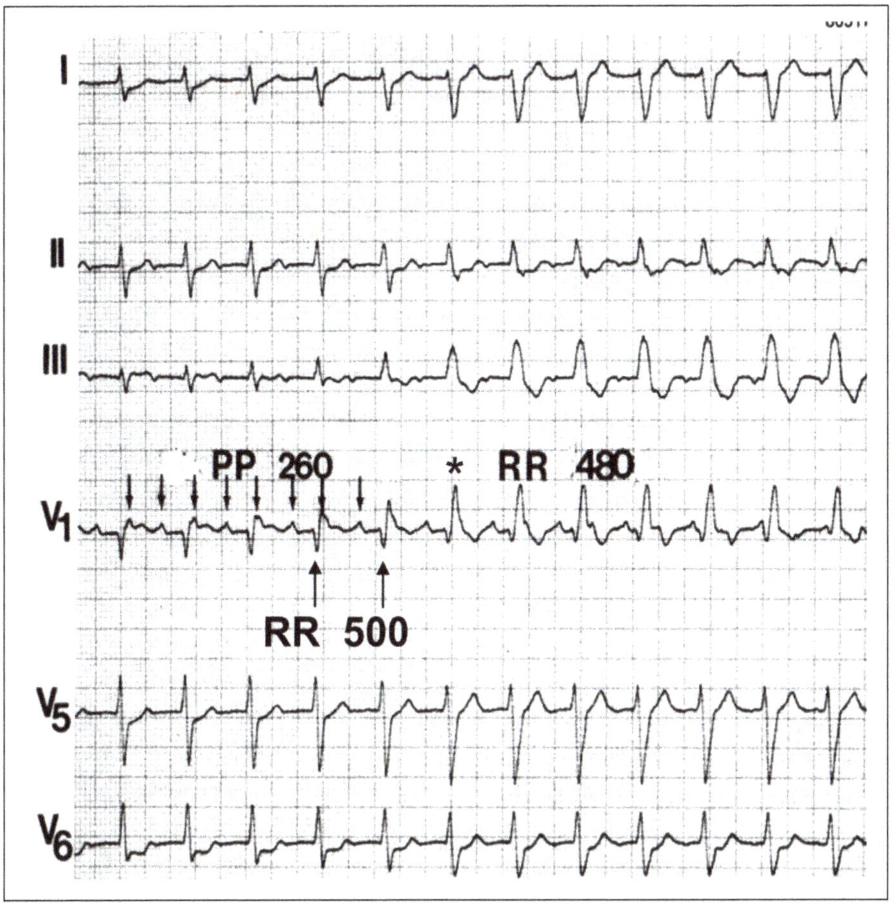

Figure 6-19 Triggerd VT initiated by increase in heart rate. ECG leads I, II, III, V_1, V_5, and V_6 recorded from a patient with digitalis toxicity (Wellens' ECG collection).

Origin

The site of origin of VT caused by digitalis-induced DADs is usually in one or more foci on the left side of the ventricular conducting system. Purkinje cells (particularly in the left bundle) have greater sensitivity to the DAD-causing effects of digitalis than ventricular muscle (Table 5-1, row C). Fascicular tachycardias with rates of between 90–160 bpm, with a relatively narrow QRS and right or left QRS axis deviation is usually present (right axis indicating origin in the anterior fascicle and left axis indicating origin in the posterior fascicle of the left bundle branch). During tachycardia, changes may occur in the QRS morphology from one impulse to the next when there is competition among multiple sites in the conducting system with triggered activity. A common occurrence is the alternating focus between the anterior and posterior fascicles (bidirectional tachycardia) as shown in Figure 6-17.

Effects of Electrical Stimulation

Stimulation of the ventricles during the administration of digitalis to patients was undertaken in the 1960s in an attempt to develop a test that would indicate impending toxicity. From those studies, it was shown that VT caused by digitalis could be initiated by stimulation, a characteristic of triggered activity (Table 5-1, row F). A more detailed analysis of the effects of stimulation rate on coupling intervals of the first tachycardia impulse and cycle length of VT is not available for clinical cases, although in experimental animals, the expected direct relationship has been documented.

Overdrive stimulation of an ongoing VT caused by digitalis results in the characteristic response of overdrive acceleration that is characteristic of a triggered mechanism (**Figure 6-20**).

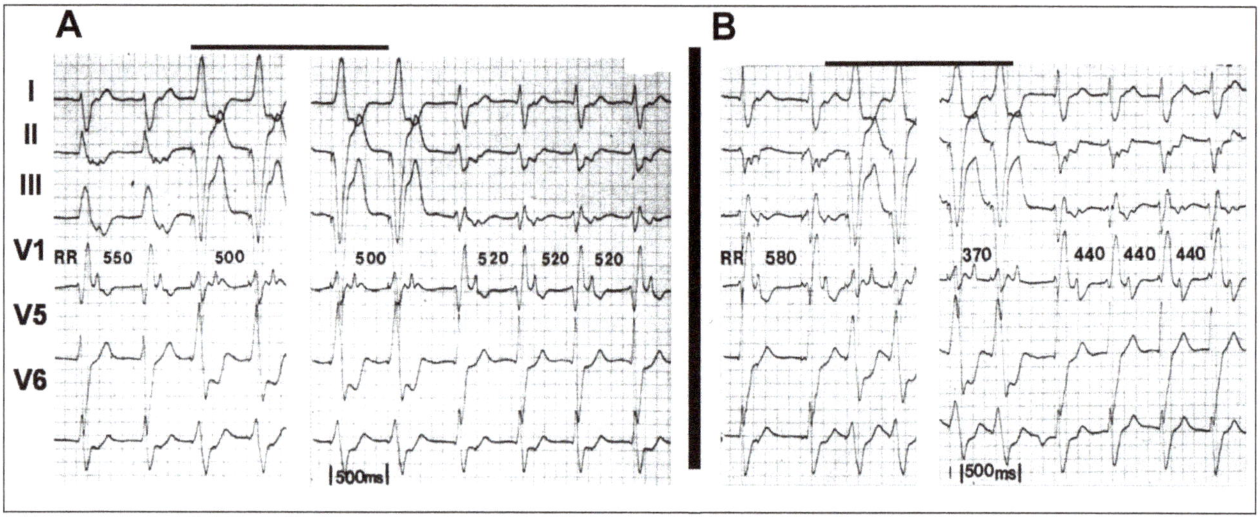

Figure 6-20 Effects of overdrive on ventricular tachycardia caused by digitalis toxicity. ECG leads I, II, III, V_1, V_5, and V_6 are shown (Wellens' ECG collection).

In Figure 6-20, Panel A, shows a VT with a cycle length of 550 ms (left) in a patient with digitalis toxicity. Overdrive from the right ventricle is indicated by horizontal line above (at a cycle length of 500 ms for 1 min). Following the period of overdrive, tachycardia cycle length transiently decreased to 520 ms (at the right in Panel A). In Panel B, at a more rapid rate of overdrive (cycle length of 370 ms for 1 min, horizontal line above), tachycardia cycle length decreased to 440 ms (at the far right). This example of overdrive acceleration is a property of triggered activity (Table 5-1). Note also the change in QRS after overdrive, indicating a change in the arrhythmogenic focus within the left bundle branch. This change occurs because digitalis is likely affecting many cells to cause DADs that are close to initiating triggered activity. Overdrive-induced enhancement of DADs occurs in a cell in a slightly different region, which is often near the site of stimulation. After a few impulses from the new triggered focus, the original focus regains dominance. Although in experimental studies digitalis-induced triggered activity can be terminated by overdrive, clinical data demonstrating termination is not available. The response of overdrive acceleration points out possible dangers of pacemakers in patients with digitalis-induced VT.

EXERCISE-INDUCED VENTRICULAR TACHYCARDIA

The ECG in **Figure 6-21** shows periods of VT induced by exercise. There is a QS complex in aVL, which suggests an origin towards the septum. A left bundle branch block (LBBB) pattern is evident with inferior frontal plane axis consistent with an origin of tachycardia in the outflow tract of the right ventricle (RVOT), a common site of origin of this kind of tachycardia (see below and Chapter 3, Figure 3-42).

Exercise-induced VT is an idiopathic focal VT that is also described in Chapter 3, Section 3C because it can be caused by automaticity in addition to triggered activity. To briefly reiterate, it often occurs in patients who have no evidence of structural heart disease, although it may sometimes be associated with disease. The arrhythmia is not usually associated with exercise-induced ischemia (absence of ST-segment changes). Clinical presentation can include frequent premature impulses and bouts of unsustained, repetitive, monomorphic tachycardia as well as sustained (usually monomorphic) tachycardia. The cycle length of VT is generally between 300–400 ms, somewhat longer than reentrant VT (Chapter 12).

Properties of (Triggered) Exercise-Induced VT

Basic Mechanisms of Catecholamine-Induced DADs

Chapter 3, Section 3C, points out that sympathetic-induced ventricular arrhythmias caused by normal automaticity arise in Purkinje cells of the specialized conducting system and probably not ventricular muscle. However, catecholamines can induce DADs and triggered activity in both Purkinje cells and ventricular muscle under special conditions. Catecholamines cause DADs by increasing Ca^{2+} entry into cells via the L-type Ca^{2+} channels and enhancing Ca^{2+} uptake into the SR to cause Ca^{2+} overload of the SR (Figure 5-2). In the experimental laboratory, although small DADs may be induced by catecholamines in both normal muscle and Purkinje cells, triggered activity does not readily occur without additional experimental interventions that enhance Ca^{2+} overload or decrease the outward currents that usually inhibit DADs.

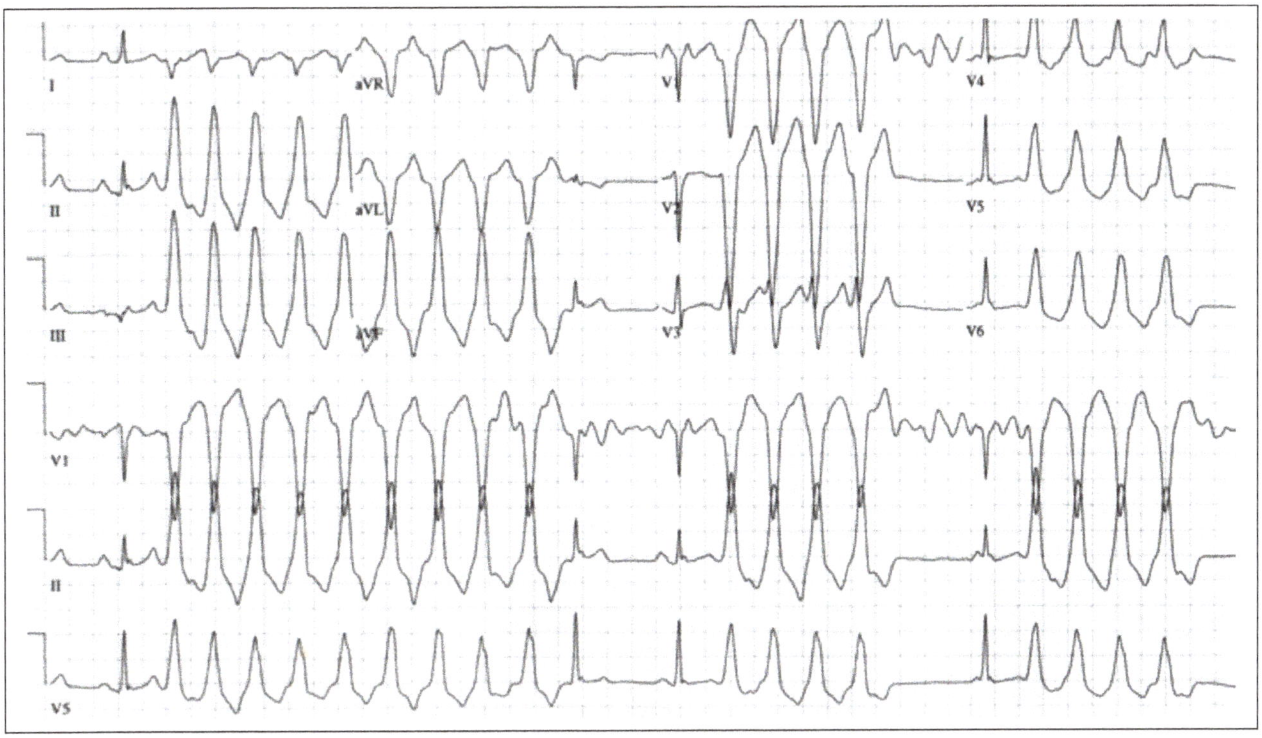

Figure 6-21 12-lead ECG showing exercise-induced VT in a patient with a structurally normal heart.

Sympathetic stimulation or β_1-adrenergic agonist administration alone does not cause triggered tachycardia in patients who do not have exercise-induced VT. This suggests that there must be additional, as yet unknown, abnormal properties of the sympathetic nervous system or cardiac cells in patients who have DAD-induced VT despite the absence of structural heart disease. As is the case for automatic tachycardias, this might be caused by increased numbers of sympathetic nerve terminals and an unusually high local release of norepinephrine or enhanced responsiveness of the β-adrenergic signaling cascade. Other possibilities include abnormalities in membrane currents, such as decreased outward I_{K1}, that normally opposes DAD occurrence or a reduction in gap-junction coupling that reduces the inhibitory effects of electrotonic current.

Onset of VT

Exercise-induced VT occurs during an increase in the sinus rate associated with exercise (Table 5-1, row A). **Figure 6-22** shows ECGs from a patient without structural heart disease who had spontaneous episodes of VT during exertion or exercise.

Panel A shows the resting ECG at rest a sinus cycle length of 0.84 sec. In Panel B, during handgrip exercise, sinus cycle length decreases to 0.53 sec, and then further decreases to 0.49 sec in Panel C and 0.47 sec in Panel D. The decreased sinus cycle length in Panels B and C is followed by the onset of triggered VT. The horizontal bar in Panels B and C indicates the coupling interval to the first beat of the VT (0.52 sec and 0.45 sec, respectively). Triggered activity did not occur at the shorter sinus cycle length of 0.47 sec in Panel D.

A DAD-triggered mechanism for the VT in Figure 6-22 is indicated by the direct relationship between sinus cycle length (first measurement) and the coupling interval between the last sinus impulse and first VT impulse (horizontal bar, second measurement in Panels B and C (Table 5-1, row B). The decreased sinus cycle length in Panels B and C contributes to the increased amplitude of DADs that leads to the onset of VT (see Figure 6-25), in addition to the direct effects of catecholamines to promote increased DAD amplitude independent of rate. The failure of the short sinus cycle length to trigger VT in Panel D probably results from the inhibitory effect of increased outward Na^+–K^+ pump current (I_p). Further evidence that the VT in Figure 6-22 is caused by triggered activity is its suppression by verapamil (shown in Panels E and F), even though the acceleration in heart rate was not prevented (Table 5-1, row E).

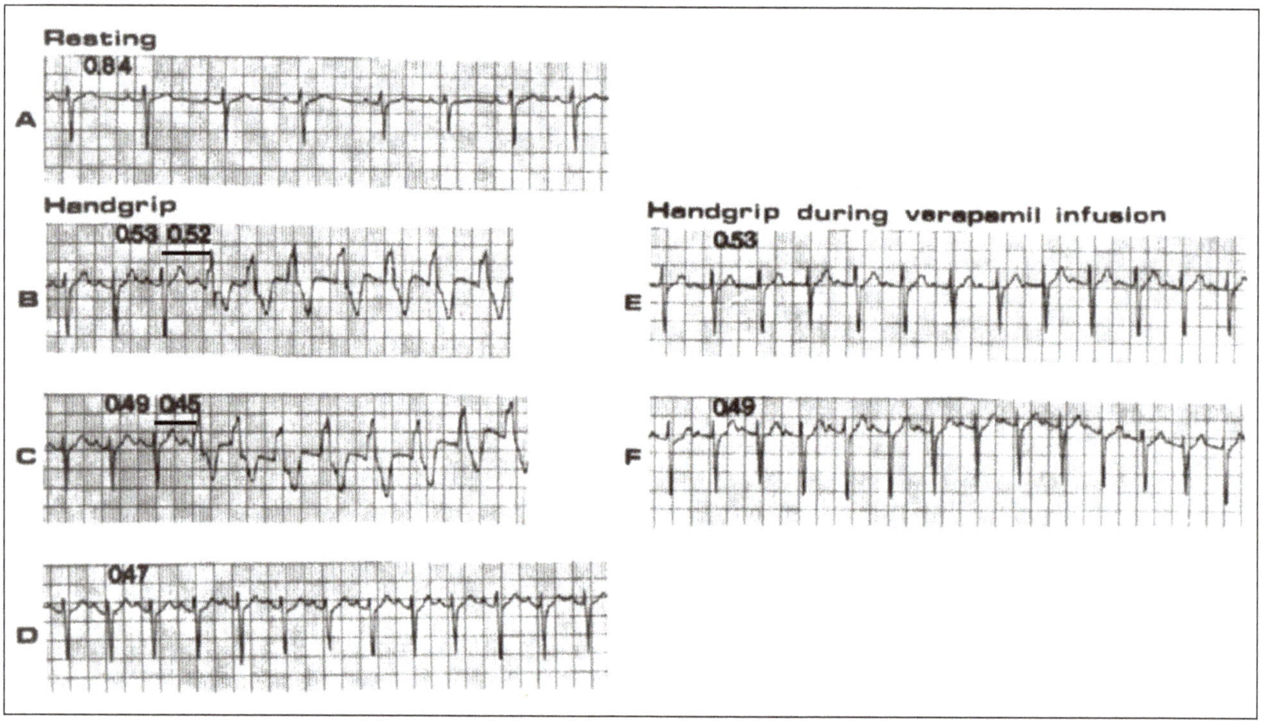

Figure 6-22 Cycle length dependency for the initiation of VT during sinus rhythm in a patient with no clinical evidence of organic heart disease and a history of exercise-induced VT. **Panel A:** Resting ECG. **Panels B, C,** and **D:** Effects of handgrip exercise. **Panels E** and **F:** Effects of verapamil. (Reproduced from Sung RJ, Shapiro WA, et al. Effects of verapamil on ventricular tachycardias possibly caused by reentry, automaticity, and triggered activity. *J Clin Invest.* 1983;72:350–360.)

In contrast, although sinus cycle also decreases prior to exercise-induced VT caused by automaticity, tachycardia is not initiated by the increase in sinus rate. As shown in Figure 3-39, the increased rate is not a cause for the onset of automatic VT, but is a concomitant effect of exercise. The automatic tachycardia in Figure 3-39 could not be started by pacing since automaticity is suppressed by overdrive.

Origin of VT

The origin of exercise-induced VT is focal (Table 5-1) and occurs most frequently in the right ventricular outflow tract (RVOT) (about 80% of the time) (see Figure 3-42). Most of the remainder originate in the left ventricular outflow tract (LVOT), including the superior basal region of the left interventricular septum, the aortomitral continuity, around the mitral annulus, and in the vicinity of the aortic coronary cusps. In addition, tachycardias can originate at epicardial sites in the region of the great cardiac and anterior interventricular veins. Occasionally, VT may arise at the other sites of origin of focal idiopathic tachycardia described in Chapter 3, Section 3C. The cell type of origin has not been defined. As described in Chapter 3, Section 3C, Purkinje cells have not been identified in all these regions although Purkinje or embryonic precursor remnants may exist there. Either Purkinje cells or ventricular muscle cells may be the origin of triggered tachycardias. No matter the cell type of origin, it must be postulated that in patients with this arrhythmia the cells of origin have special (unusual) properties since exercise-induced VT is not a common arrhythmia.

Autonomic Nervous System Effects

Triggered VT, like automatic tachycardia can be initiated by β-adrenergic stimulation, either during exercise or by administration of a β-agonist such as isoproterenol (Table 5-1, row D). The rate of triggered tachycardia is also increased by sympathetic stimulation. Triggered exercise-induced VT can also be terminated by enhanced parasympathetic activity unlike other types of VT, since acetylcholine decreases the amplitude of catecholamine-induced DADs even in the ventricles.

Figure 6-23 shows termination of an exercise-induced triggered VT by carotid sinus massage (CSP). While parasympathetic activation sometimes might slow automatic VT because of accentuated antagonism, it does not terminate tachycardia caused by automaticity (Table 5-1, row D).

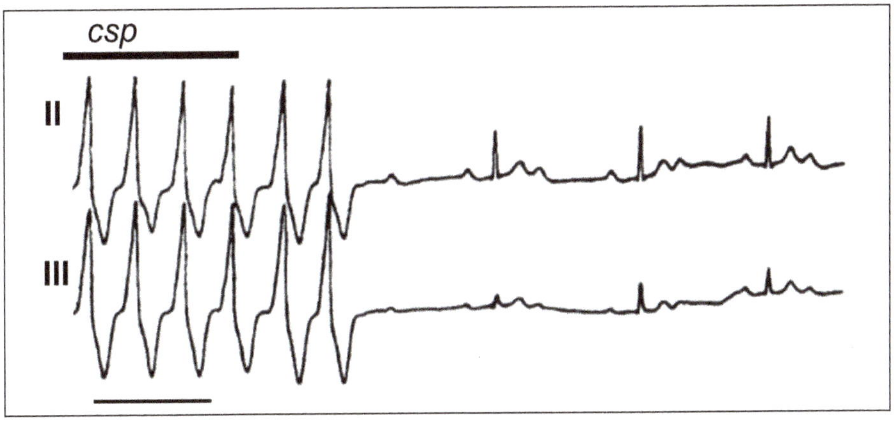

Figure 6-23 ECG leads II and III recorded during exercise-induced VT during carotid sinus massage. CSP = carotid sinus pressure.

Pharmacological Effects

Exercise-induced triggered VT is terminated by adenosine and L-type Ca^{2+} channel-blocking drugs (Table 5-1, row E). **Figure 6-24** shows termination of exercise-induced VT by adenosine (administered during the VT prior to the beginning of the recordings). Adenosine prevents β-adrenergic stimulation of DADs by inhibiting the formation of adenylyl cyclase. As a result, adenosine prevents triggered VT that results from sympathetic activation (Table 5-1, row E) but not other kinds of triggered VTs owing to only minor direct effects of adenosine on Purkinje and ventricular muscle cells.

It may slow automatic tachycardia caused by sympathetic stimulation but usually has little effect (Figure 3-41). Therefore, adenosine can be used to identify DADs as a cause of exercise-induced VT.

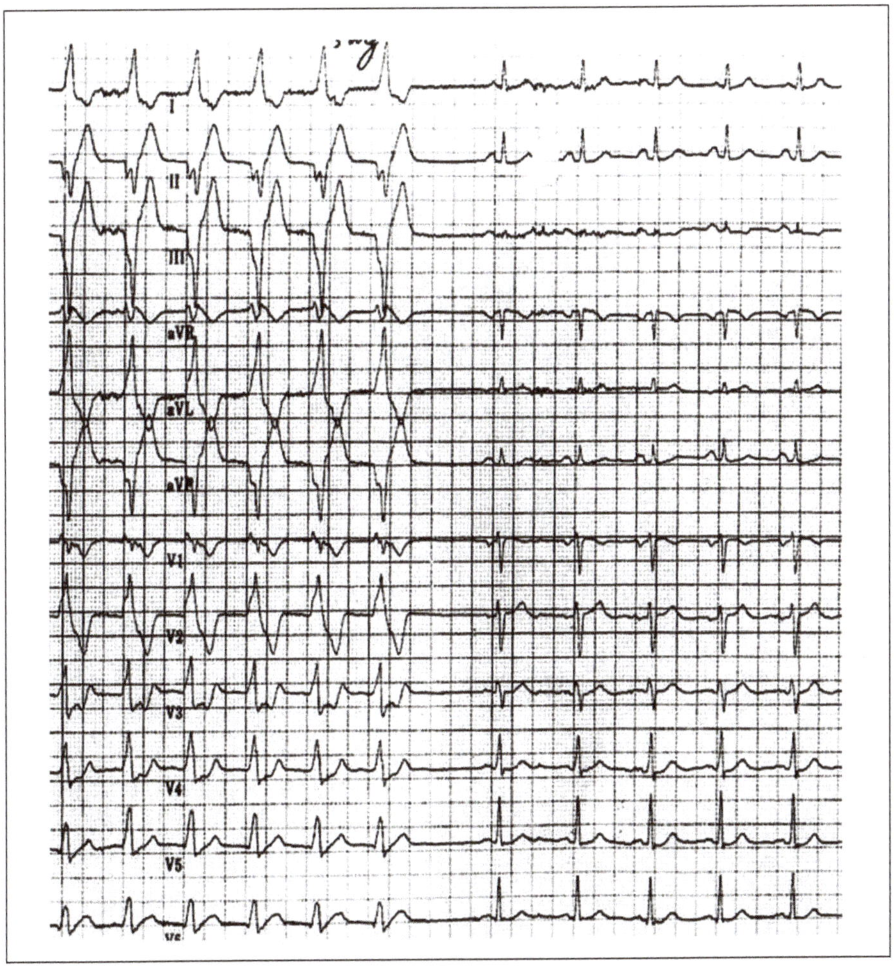

Figure 6-24 12-lead ECG recorded during VT (**left**). Just prior to the recording, 6 mg IV adenosine was administered that terminated VT (**right**) (Wellens' ECG collection).

L-type Ca^{2+} channel-blocking drugs prevent the occurrence of DADs and triggered exercise induced VT (Figure 6-22, Panels E and F) by decreasing Ca^{2+} influx while having little effect on VT caused by normal automaticity (Table 5-1, row E). However, these drugs can stop VT caused by abnormal automaticity.

Electrical Stimulation

Overdrive and programmed premature stimulation can start and stop triggered VT, in contrast to their inability to start and stop automatic VT (Table 5-1, row F). **Figure 6-25** shows ECGs and electrograms recorded from a patient with exercise-induced VT.

Each panel starts with the last three complexes of a period of overdrive at a cycle length indicated above lead V_1. In Panel A, stimulation at a 700-ms cycle length did not initiate an arrhythmia. In Panels B, C, and D, stimulation at cycle lengths of 690, 630, and 500 ms, respectively, initiated VT. The coupling interval between the last stimulated impulse (S) and the first tachycardia impulse (F) decreases with the decreasing stimulus cycle length (670 in B, 620 in C and 480 in D) as is characteristic of triggered activity (Table 5-1, row F).

The initiation of VT results from a cycle-length–dependent increase in DAD amplitude and the decrease in coupling interval of the first tachycardia impulse results from the cycle-length dependence of the DAD coupling interval (Figure 5-4). In Panel E, stimulation at a cycle length of 480 ms does not initiate VT, likely resulting either from an increase in I_P that inhibits DADs or conduction block preventing the stimulated impulse from reaching the triggerable focus. Similarly, programmed premature stimulation can initiate tachycardia with a direct relationship between premature coupling interval and coupling interval of first cycle of tachycardia (see Figure 5-6).

Also, unlike automatic tachycardias (Figure 3-40), triggered tachycardias can be terminated by overdrive or premature stimulation. In **Figure 6-26**, the triggered tachycardia with a cycle length of 385 ms is terminated by a short period of ventricular overdrive at a 340-ms cycle length. The mechanism for the effects of overdrive to suppress triggered activity is an increase in I_P as described in Figure 5-7.

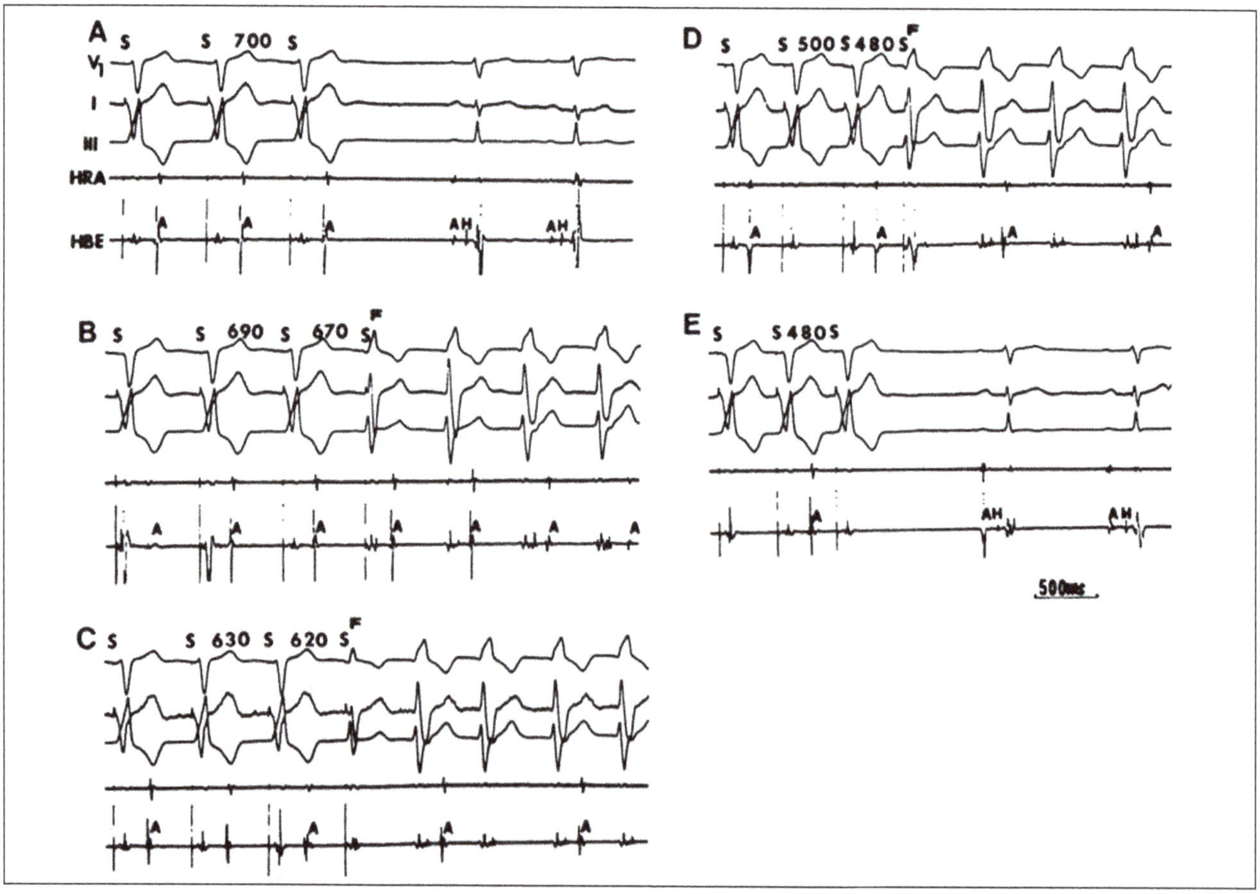

Figure 6-25 ECG leads I, III, and V_1, and electrograms from high right atrium (HRA) and His bundle region (HBE) recorded during pacing-induced VT in a patient with exercise-induced VT. A, atrial electrogram; H, His bundle electrogram; S, stimulated impulses; F, first impulse of VT. (Reproduced from Sung RJ, Shapiro WA, et al. Effects of verapamil on ventricular tachycardias possibly caused by reentry, automaticity, and triggered activity. *J Clin Invest.* 1983;72:350–360.)

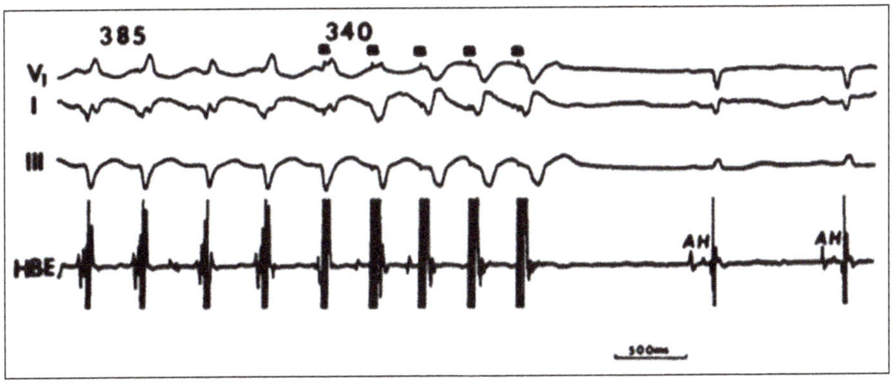

Figure 6-26 ECG leads I, III, V_1, and electrogram from His bundle region (HBE) recorded during VT with 385-ms cycle length. A period of overdrive stimulation at 340-ms cycle length that terminates VT is indicated above. (Reproduced with permission from Sung RJ, Shapiro WA, et al. Effects of verapamil on ventricular tachycardias possibly caused by reentry, automaticity, and triggered activity. *J Clin Invest.* 1983;72:350–360.)

CATECHOLAMINERGIC POLYMORPHIC VENTRICULAR TACHYCARDIA (CPVT)

CPVT is uncommon before the age of 2 years. It normally first manifests during early childhood, but sometimes first manifestation may extend into young adulthood. Typically, the clinical presentation is syncope triggered by exercise, emotion, or stress. Occasionally, initial presentation may be sudden death. Untreated, it is highly lethal. CPVT is usually associated with a normal resting ECG although occasionally there may be some arrhythmias at rest. The heart rate may be bradycardic. P-R interval, QRS duration, and axis are normal. Prominent U waves sometimes occur. Although it has been suggested that U waves are surface manifestations of DADs, it is uncertain if this interpretation is correct. U waves are described in more detail in Chapter 7, as they relate to early afterdepolarization. The QTc (QT interval corrected for heart rate) is within normal limits. Ventricular function, chest radiographs, and coronary arteries are usually normal.

The ECG in **Figure 6-27** shows a CPVT. There are no abnormalities in any ECG leads during sinus rhythm (Figure 6-27, Panel A). The exercise ECG (Figure 6-27, Panel B) is characterized by a rapid VT with a rate of about 250 bpm that has a polymorphic QRS in leads V_1–V_6.

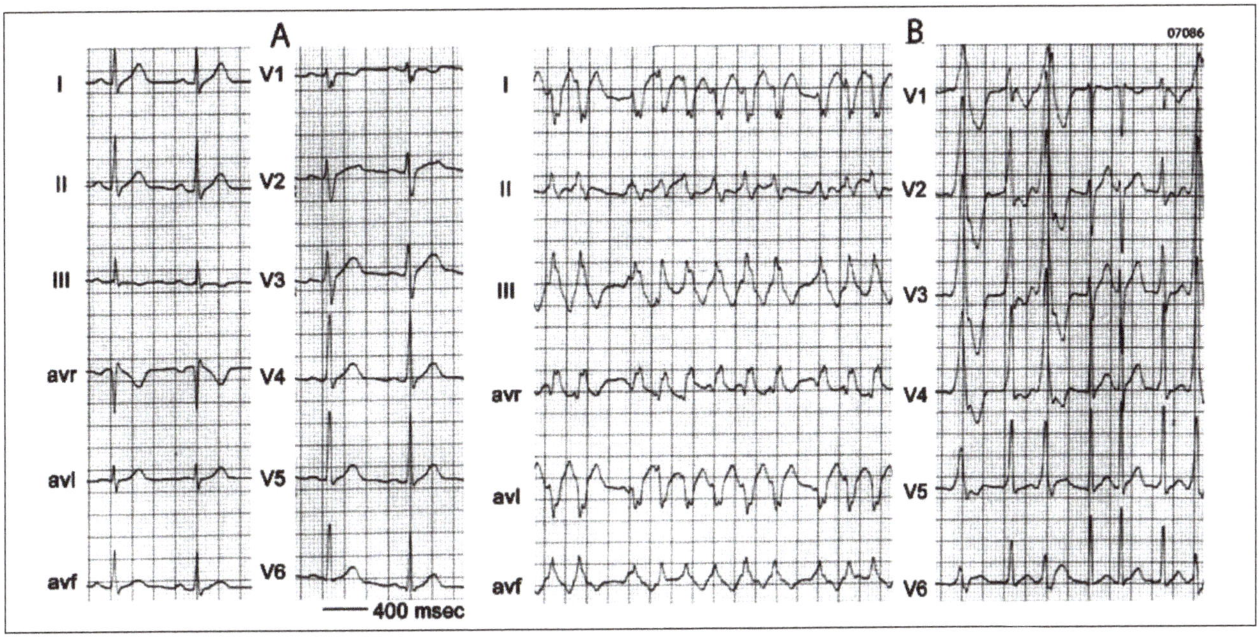

Figure 6-27 12-lead ECG of a patient with CPVT. **Panel A:** Sinus rhythm. **Panel B:** CPVT (Wellens' ECG collection).

Molecular Mechanisms of CPVT

CPVT is caused by DAD-induced triggered activity. Unlike the other examples of DAD-triggered activity described so far, most of the evidence linking CPVT to triggered activity comes from the elucidation of the genetic causes and not from electrophysiological characteristics of the arrhythmia. CPVT is associated with genetic alterations in the processes that control Ca^{2+} release from the SR (see Chapter 5 and Figure 5-2). The most common cause is an autosomal dominant mutation in the gene that encodes the ryanodine receptor (RyR2). More than 80 mutations have been identified, most of which are single base-pair substitutions resulting in the substitution of an amino acid. Although usually inherited, mutations can occur *de novo* in about 20% of cases. A different form of CPVT can also result from an autosomal recessive mutation in the gene that encodes calsequestrin (*CASQ2*), the function of which is also described in Chapter 5. Fourteen different mutations in the *CASQ2* gene have been detected. This form is infrequent, accounting for only about 2%–8% of cases. Heterozygous carriers are usually asymptomatic, while homozygous carries have all the features of CPVT.

Both mutations cause a "gain in function" of the RyR2-release channel, resulting in increased spontaneous SR Ca^{2+} release and Ca^{2+}-induced propagating Ca^{2+} waves during diastole that is responsible for DAD formation (Figure 5-3). RyR2-mutated channels have a reduced threshold for opening and open at low SR Ca^{2+} levels during diastole, instead of being closed as they normally would be. Whether or not RyR2 mutations also increase release channel sensitivity to myoplasmic Ca^{2+} is unclear. The SR Ca^{2+} load release threshold may also be reduced by mutations in *CASQ2*, which alter its interaction with RyR2 since *CASQ2* is instrumental in causing RyR2 channel closure in diastole (see Chapter 5). Some *CASQ2* mutations result in a reduction in SR Ca^{2+} buffering/storing capacity by reducing affinity of *CASQ2* for Ca^{2+} or by reducing the amount of protein from altered trafficking or increased protein degradation. In fact, in some mutations, *CASQ2* may be absent. The loss of Ca^{2+}-related buffering after systole in the SR may result in a more rapid rise of free Ca^{2+}, thereby triggering Ca^{2+} release channels to open during diastole.

Arrhythmias in CPVT usually do not occur in the absence of sympathetic stimulation. The diastolic leak of Ca^{2+} from the SR due to the change in function of RyR2 alone, caused by the mutation, may not be sufficient to generate DADs that reach threshold potential for triggered activity. Furthermore, the diastolic leak caused by the mutation may sometimes reduce SR Ca^{2+} below the RyR2 threshold for Ca^{2+} release. Threshold may only be reached when β-adrenergic stimulation increases SR Ca^{2+}. As for the other catecholamine-triggered arrhythmias such as exercise-induced VT (Figure 6-21), sympathetic stimulation increases Ca^{2+} entry into the cell through L-type Ca^{2+} channels and the uptake of Ca^{2+} by the SR. Even during sympathetic activation, SR Ca^{2+} levels in CPVT may be normal or even lower (as contrasted with catecholamine- and digitalis-induced triggered activity described previously), because of the increased diastolic Ca^{2+} release.

DADs in CPVT are generated by the same mechanism as described for the other examples of triggered arrhythmias. In the presence of increased diastolic Ca^{2+} as a consequence of SR Ca^{2+} release during sympathetic stimulation, an inward diastolic TI current (I_{TI}) is generated by Ca^{2+} extrusion and Na^+ entry via the Na^+–Ca^{2+} exchanger (I_{NCX}).

Properties of DAD-Induced CPVT

The evidence from genetic studies that CPVT is caused by DAD-triggered activity is supported by some of its clinical electrophysiological features, but a detailed analysis of electrophysiological studies that are used to show that RVOT or digitalis toxic arrhythmias are caused by triggered activity (Table 5-1) is not available.

Onset

The onset of arrhythmias is related to the increase in heart rate resulting from increased sympathetic activity during exercise that increases DAD amplitude (Table 5-1, rows A and D). The threshold is usually around 120–130 bpm as shown in **Figure 6-28**, where premature ventricular impulses begin to appear after 0.5 min of exercise (compare to resting sinus rate in top trace).

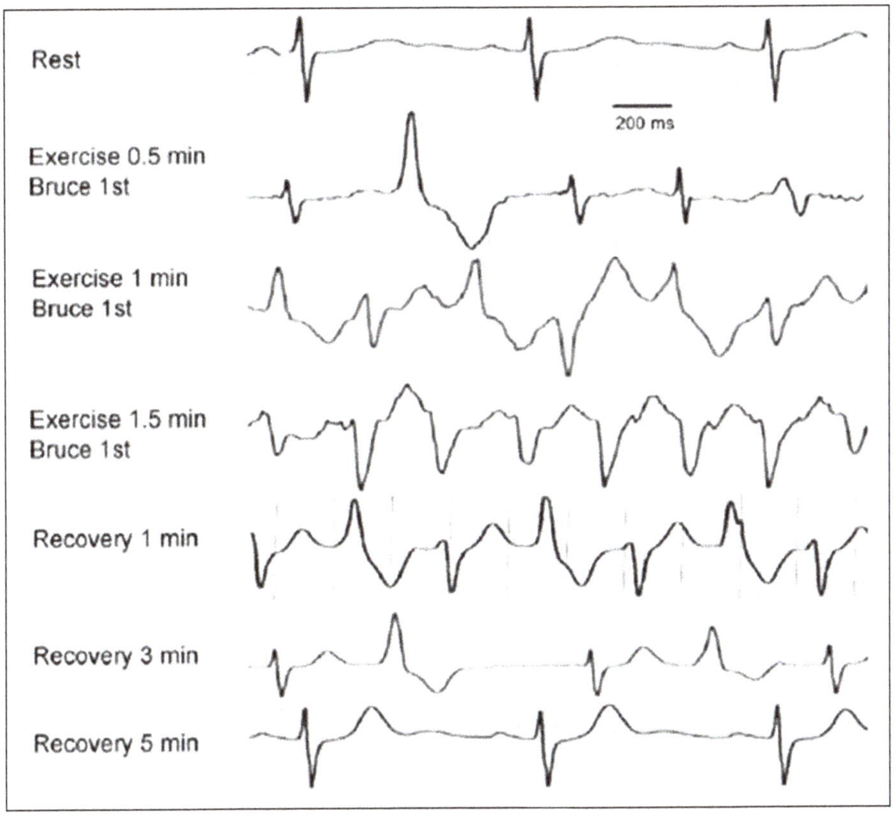

Figure 6-28 ECG recordings during exercise stress test in a patient with CPVT. (Reproduced from Liu N, Priori SG. Disruption of calcium homeostasis and arrhythmogenesis induced by mutations in the cardiac ryanodine receptor and calsequestrin. *Cardiovasc Res.* 2008;77:293–301.)

Frequency and Complexity of Ventricular Impulses

In Figure 6-28, the frequency and complexity of ventricular impulses increases as the heart rate increases related to increased duration and severity of exercise. The characteristic ECG pattern with increasing exercise is first quadrigeminy, trigeminy, and bigeminy (0.5 min in the second ECG recording), followed by salvoes of bidirectional tachycardia (1 min of exercise in the third ECG recording), and finally bursts of rapid, irregular, and polymorphic VT (1.5 min exercise, fourth recording). There are no data relating coupling intervals of triggered impulses to the sinus rate. However, the increased number of ventricular impulses with increasing sinus rate is an important feature of triggered activity (Table 5-1, row B). This sequence of events can also be provoked in the clinical laboratory with isoproterenol administration. There are no ST-T changes prior to the onset of polymorphic VT and VF eliminating an ischemic cause. When syncope occurs, it is associated with a very fast polymorphic VT resembling fibrillation that can spontaneously convert to sinus rhythm. Occasionally, VF may be the first arrhythmia manifested. At the end of the exercise, the arrhythmia disappears in the reverse order (Figure 6-28, recovery 1 min, 3 min, and 5 min).

Bidirectional tachycardia is characteristic of CPVT (Figure 6-28, exercise 1 min). Bidirectional tachycardia, (rate 150–250 bpm, unsustained or sustained) is characterized by RBBB with a 180-degree rotation of the QRS axis in the frontal plane from beat to beat with alternating right and left QRS axis deviation. Bidirectional tachycardia is occasionally characterized by alternating RBBB and LBBB patterns. The recording lead is important for demonstration of the QRS changes; tachycardia may appear to be bidirectional in some leads and polymorphic in others. This type of arrhythmia is also characteristic of VT caused by digitalis toxicity and may be related to the mechanism of DAD-triggered activity (see Figure 6-17). However, some patients have only polymorphic VT.

Site of Origin

CPVT has a focal origin that is likely to be in Purkinje cells of the conducting system (Table 5-1, row C). The RyR2 mutations have a greater effect on Purkinje cells than on ventricular muscle resulting in greater frequency, amplitude and duration of diastolic spontaneous Ca^{2+} release. The bidirectional and polymorphic tachycardias can be caused by shifts in the sites of the dominant triggered cells with beat-to-beat shifts in the axis during RBBB, indicating alternating triggered impulse origin between the posterior and inferior fascicles of the left bundle branch. Similar patterns might also be created by alternating sites of triggered activity in ventricular muscle or a single focus in a bundle branch with alternating sites of conduction block of impulses arising in that focus. No mapping data to locate the site(s) of origin are available from clinical studies.

Pharmacological Effects

The response of CPVT to selected pharmacological agents is not necessary to elucidate the mechanism of this arrhythmia, as it is for other types of tachycardia. No information is available on the effects of adenosine on CPVT. β-receptor blocking drugs decrease the severity of the arrhythmias but may not completely prevent them. This is an expected effect of β-blockers on sympathetic-induced arrhythmias irrespective of their mechanism. Acute verapamil administration reduces the incidence of ventricular arrhythmias during exercise stress testing but does not abolish them (Table 5-1). Its effects are additive to those of a β-blocker. This effect is supportive evidence for a DAD-triggered mechanism. In addition to decreasing Ca^{2+} entry into the cell, verapamil interacts with the RyR2 receptor in experimental studies but it is uncertain if the drug concentration that does this is reached during administration to patients.

The Class IC Na^{+} channel-blocking drug flecainide has been shown to be effective in a limited number of cases of CPVT refractory to β-blockers. Flecainide and also propafenone, in addition to their Na^{+} channel-blocking effect, block the open state of the RyR2-operated calcium-release channels, reducing diastolic Ca^{2+} release.

Electrical Stimulation

Overdrive stimulation in the absence of β-adrenergic stimulation does not induce CPVT, nor does programmed premature stimulation, unlike the other triggered arrhythmias described above that can be induced by pacing or premature stimulation (Table 5-1, row F). Information on stimulation in the presence of isoproterenol is not available. Diastolic Ca^{2+} release in the absence of sympathetic stimulation is probably small, and any increase in release caused by stimulation may not be sufficient to cause DADs to reach threshold for initiating action potentials. The effects of overdrive or premature stimulation during tachycardia are not known.

TRIGGERED ACTIVITY AND VENTRICULAR ARRHYTHMIAS IN THE SETTING OF HEART FAILURE AND/OR ISCHEMIA

Based on experimental laboratory experiments, it has been proposed that DAD-induced triggered activity may cause ventricular arrhythmias in additional clinical situations. However, the clinical characterization of these arrhythmias is not as complete as the examples discussed above. Additional data is necessary to demonstrate triggered activity. Two possible causes of triggered arrhythmias are heart failure and ischemia.

DAD-Induced Triggered Activity Caused by Systolic Heart Failure

Chronic heart failure and hypertrophy, irrespective of the underlying cause, is frequently accompanied by ventricular arrhythmias ranging from ventricular premature depolarizations to unsustained and sustained VT. Sudden cardiac death accompanying chronic heart failure can be caused by VT or fibrillation. In some instances, these arrhythmias may be caused by DAD-induced triggered activity.

Molecular Mechanisms Linked to Contractile Defects and Ion Channel Remodeling

Ventricular myocytes in hypertrophic and/or failed ventricles undergo electrical remodeling, during which there are multiple changes in the function of ion channels and membrane transporters, causing alteration in action potentials and changes in intercellular connections through gap junctions. Some of the electrical remodeling predisposes ventricular muscle to the development of DADs and triggered activity. The mechanisms causing DADs are linked to the contractile defects. One abnormality is in Ca^{2+} cycling between the SR and myoplasm (see Figure 5-2). Contractility is decreased because the SR has a decreased Ca^{2+} content resulting in decreased Ca^{2+} release during the action potential, and therefore decreased Ca^{2+} to activate contraction.

The reduced amount of SR Ca^{2+} is one of the main characteristics of heart failure that can lead to ventricular arrhythmias. It is partially caused by a decrease in SERCA pumping of Ca^{2+} from the myoplasm into the SR that may result from either decreased expression of pump molecules or changes in function of regulatory proteins. An increase in Na^{+}–Ca^{2+} exchanger expression that is part of the remodeling process also increases transport of Ca^{2+} out of the cell during diastole, another factor in the maintenance of low SR Ca^{2+}. The relative increased amount of Ca^{2+} removed from the cell and the decreased Ca^{2+} pumped back into the SR may differ in different patients depending on the cause and severity of failure. When the increased amount of Ca^{2+} extruded by the exchanger compensates for the reduced reuptake of Ca^{2+} into the SR, diastolic Ca^{2+} in the myoplasm is low and normal relaxation occurs. However, when the exchanger does not maintain diastolic Ca^{2+} at a sufficiently low level in the face of decreased SERCA activity, diastolic Ca^{2+} is elevated and relaxation is impaired. The elevation in diastolic Ca^{2+} may lead to DADs as described in Figure 5-2.

Continuous spontaneous SR Ca^{2+} leak through RyR2 channels is another factor that may contribute to the decreased SR Ca^{2+} content in heart failure. The exact mechanism is not known, but may be related to hyperphosphorylation and/or oxidation of RyR2 receptors or components of the RyR2 calcium-release channel complex. SR Ca^{2+} leak can occur during diastole because of defective regulation (recall that normally during diastole, RyR2 channels are closed because SR Ca^{2+} levels are below their opening threshold). Because of the increased Na^+–Ca^{2+} exchanger activity, a larger TI current (I_{TI}) caused by I_{NCX} can occur for any given level of diastolic Ca^{2+}, resulting from SR Ca^{2+} leak, thus generating DADs.

Even though total SR Ca^{2+} is reduced, β-adrenergic stimulation resulting from enhanced sympathetic activity—which is characteristic in patients with heart failure—can increase SR Ca^{2+} to a level sufficient to result in enough diastolic Ca^{2+} release to cause DADs. This sequence of events is similar to the events in CPVT in which the β-adrenergic stimulation enhances the leak caused by RyR2 mutations also in the setting of reduced SR Ca^{2+}.

Sarcolemmal ion channel remodeling also contributes to the occurrence of DAD-induced triggered activity. Prolongation of action potential duration caused by remodeling of the repolarizing membrane channels I_{to}, I_{Kr}, and I_{Ks} (decreasing these outward currents) results in an increased duration of the action potential plateau (phase 2) and increased inward I_{CaL} during the plateau. (Figure 7-2 describes the membrane currents involved in repolarization.) As a result, SR Ca^{2+} is maintained at a higher level than it would be in the absence of this remodeling, and SR Ca^{2+} release is enhanced. Remodeling of I_{K1} also decreases this membrane current that sets the resting potential, making the resting potential less negative. The reduced outward I_{K1} current that would oppose DAD development, enables smaller I_{TI} currents causing DADs to depolarize membrane potential to threshold potential. Decreased cellular coupling (the number of gap junctions decreases with heart failure) may also contribute by reducing electrotonic current flow that inhibits DADs (Figure 1-3).

Electrophysiological Properties

In heart failure, arrhythmias may or may not be inducible by typical stimulation protocols, depending on the clinical background. In cases in which arrhythmias have been initiated, the relationship of coupling intervals of the initial impulse to the initiating impulse have not been quantified. In addition, the other features that assist in identifying a triggered mechanism described in Table 5-1 have not been sought in clinical investigations. Thus, important electrophysiological evidence for triggered activity as a cause of these clinical arrhythmias is lacking. Nevertheless, because of the prominent abnormalities of Ca^{2+} cycling with heart failure, there is a possibility that some of these arrhythmias are triggered.

DAD-Triggered Activity in Ischemia and Infarction

Cardiac ischemia can occur acutely resulting in myocardial infarction or over a long period of time causing ischemic cardiomyopathy (see Chapter 12). The acute phase of myocardial ischemia and infarction refers to events occurring within the first several hours after a sudden reduction in blood flow through a coronary artery and is often caused by rupture of an atherosclerotic plaque. Acute ischemia can occur transiently with spontaneous reperfusion or can be persistent. Both persistent ischemia and ischemia followed by reperfusion incite ventricular arrhythmias. With persistent ischemia ventricular arrhythmias may occur over a period of several weeks. In hearts with coronary disease and myocardial infarcts, arrhythmias may also be chronic, persisting for many months as the infarcted ventricle heals and remodels. Arrhythmias may also occur years after the acute event in patients with healed infarcts.

Molecular Mechanisms

Multiple electrophysiological mechanisms cause the ventricular arrhythmias accompanying ischemia and infarction. The mechanisms depend on the severity of ischemia, and whether or not there is reperfusion. Mechanisms also change with time as the infarct remodels. Reentrant excitation is a primary cause of acute ischemic arrhythmias, and the arrhythmias in patients with healed myocardial infarcts and are described in Chapter 12. DAD-induced triggered activity may also play a role in acute arrhythmias and later on during chronic ischemia.

Ischemia decreases SR Ca^{2+} and spontaneous Ca^{2+} release from the SR by decreasing ATPase, which is necessary for Ca^{2+} pumping by SERCA, making generation of DADs unlikely in the ischemic core. However, DAD generation in less-ischemic regions adjacent to the core where

SERCA function is maintained, is a possibility owing to SR Ca^{2+} overload caused by ischemia in these regions, in combination with substances in the ischemic environment. Experimental studies on isolated, superfused ventricular muscle show DAD generation under conditions where cells are exposed to components of the ischemic environment, e.g., low pO_2, low pH, absence of glucose, and the presence of lysophosphoglycerides, oxygen free radicals, catecholamines, etc. Coupled to results of experimental mapping studies showing focal (nonreentrant) origin of some acute ischemic arrhythmias, these observations support an hypothesis of a triggered mechanism. However, clinical evidence of triggered activity during the acute ischemic phase is lacking.

Similarly, for subacute arrhythmias (several days to a few weeks), experimental data show that Purkinje and ventricular muscle cells surviving in border zones adjacent to myocardial infarcts can have DADs and cause triggered activity. Purkinje cells that form an endocardial border zone also have abnormal automaticity (see Figure 4-3). The occurrence of abnormal automaticity or DADs is dependent on the level of membrane potential (dependent on the severity of ischemia), the former occurring at membrane potentials < 65 mV where the I_{TI} current is not prominent. Catecholamines potentiate DAD occurrence. Subendocardial Purkinje cells that form the endocardial border zone have large cell-wide Ca^{2+} waves despite normal SR Ca^{2+} levels, due to increased sensitivity of Ca^{2+} release channels to SR luminal Ca^{2+}. Ca^{2+} waves lead to increased Ca^{2+} extrusion by the Na^+–Ca^{2+} exchanger, generating DADs. Subendocardial Purkinje fibers are also uncoupled from underlying necrotic ventricular muscle removing the inhibitory effects on DADs of electrotonic current flow from ventricular muscle to Purkinje fibers through gap junctions.

Electrophysiological Properties

Purkinje tissue can be the origin of clinical ventricular arrhythmias in subacute and chronic ischemia/infarction. When this occurs, a Purkinje electrogram precedes ventricular depolarization of a ventricular premature impulse that initiates the arrhythmia. Ventricular premature impulses arising in Purkinje tissue may initiate ventricular tachycardia and fibrillation. It is possible that DAD-triggered activity is the cause of impulse initiation by the Purkinje cells, but evidence such as that listed in Table 5-1 that supports this mechanism is lacking. In patients with chronic ischemia and healed myocardial infarction, VT can be initiated by electrical stimulation. However, there is strong evidence for a reentrant rather than a triggered mechanism (Chapter 12).

SUMMARY

Both Purkinje cells in the specialized conducting system and ventricular muscle cells generate DADs and triggered activity, although Purkinje cells are more prone to develop them. Factors that incite occurrence of triggered activity are digitalis toxicity, sympathetic activity, genetic alterations in SR function, and changes in Ca^{2+} cycling caused by pathology (heart failure, ischemia). Digitalis-induced DADs result from intracellular Ca^{2+} loading as a consequence of inhibition of the Na^+–K^+ pump that leads to a decrease in Ca^{2+} extrusion from cells. Catecholamines cause DADs by increasing Ca^{2+} entry into cells via the L-type Ca^{2+} current and enhancing Ca^{2+} uptake into the SR to cause Ca^{2+} overload of the SR. Genetic alterations in the processes that control Ca^{2+} release from the SR can cause DADs and heritable triggered arrhythmias.

Triggered tachycardia caused by digitalis can be initiated by stimulation. Overdrive stimulation of an ongoing VT caused by digitalis results in overdrive acceleration. Clinical data on termination of digitalis-triggered arrhythmias are not available, but they can be terminated in experimental laboratory studies by electrical stimulation.

A common site of origin of triggered exercise-induced VT is the RVOT. Overdrive and programmed premature stimulation can start and stop exercise-induced triggered VT. A direct relationship occurs between the initiating (triggering) cycle length and the first cycle length of tachycardia. Exercise-induced triggered VT is initiated by sympathetic stimulation or also β_1-adrenergic agonists that increase DAD amplitude. Tachycardia rate is also increased. VT is terminated by parasympathetic activation such as by carotid massage, which does not terminate tachycardia caused by automaticity. VT is terminated by adenosine and L-type Ca^{2+} channel-blocking drugs, both of which are specific for triggered VT.

CPVT has a rate of about 250 bpm and a polymorphic QRS in leads V_1–V_6. It is related to a genetic mutation in proteins that alter Ca^{2+} release from the SR. Another ECG characteristic that is suggestive of DAD-triggered activity is that the onset of arrhythmias is related to the increase in heart rate resulting from increased sympathetic activity during exercise. The frequency and complexity of ventricular impulses increases as the heart rate increases, including the occurrence of bidirectional tachycardia that is characteristic of a triggered arrhythmia.

SOURCES

Agarwal BL, Agarwal BV. Digitalis induced paroxysmal atrial tachycardia with AV block. *Brit Heart J.* 1972;34:330–335.

Castellanos A, Lemberg L, Centurion MJ, Berkovits BV. Concealed digitalis-induced arrhythmias unmasked by electrical stimulation of the heart. *Am Heart J.* 1967;73:484–490.

Iwai S, Markowitz SM, Stein KM, et al. Response to adenosine differentiates focal from macroreentrant atrial tachycardia. Validation using three-dimensional electroanatomic mapping. *Circulation.* 2002;106:2793–2799.

Kim RJ, Iwai S, Markowitz SM, et al. Clinical and electrophysiological spectrum of idiopathic ventricular outflow tract arrhythmias. *J Am Coll Cardiol.* 2007;49:2035–2043.

Kontula K, Laitinen PJ, Lehtonen A, et al. Catecholaminergic polymorphic ventricular tachycardia: Recent mechanistic insights. *Cardiovasc Res.* 2005;67:379–387.

Lerman BB. Mechanism of outflow tract tachycardia. *Heart Rhythm.* 2007;4:973–976.

Lerman BB. Response of nonreentrant catecholamine-mediated ventricular tachycardia to endogenous adenosine and acetycholine evidence for myocardial receptor-mediated effects. *Circulation.* 1993;87:382–390.

Marchlinski FE, Miller JM. Atrial arrhythmias exacerbated by theophylline. Response to verapamil and evidence for triggered activity in man. *Chest.* 1985;88:931–934.

Priori SG, Napolitano C, Memmi M, et al. Clinical and molecular characterization of patients with catecholaminergic polymorphic ventricular tachycardia. *Circulation.* 2002;106:69–74.

Sumitomo N, Harada K, Nagashima M, et al. Catecholaminergic polymorphic ventricular tachycardia: electrocardiographic characteristics and optimal therapeutic strategies to prevent sudden death. *Heart.* 2003;89:66–70.

Wyndham CRC, Arnsdorf MF, Levitsky, et al. Successful surgical excision of focal paroxysmal atrial tachycardia. Observations in vivo and in vitro. *Circulation.* 1980;62:1365–1372.

Basic Principles of Early Afterdepolarizations and Triggered Action Potentials

CHAPTER 7

Early afterdepolarizations (EADs) cause the second type of triggered arrhythmias. Both the cellular mechanism and the characteristics of these arrhythmias are different from DAD-induced triggered arrhythmias. Evidence for the role of automaticity and DAD-triggered activity as a cause of arrhythmias comes from characteristic responses to electrical stimulation and selected pharmacological agents in clinical electrophysiological studies. The evidence relating a clinical arrhythmia to an EAD mechanism is more problematic. Clinical electrophysiological studies are less suited for elucidating an EAD mechanism. Nevertheless, the clinical characteristics of certain arrhythmias strongly suggest that they are related to the occurrence of EADs.

CHARACTERISTICS OF EADS AND EAD-TRIGGERED ACTION POTENTIALS

Comparison of EADs and DADs

Whereas DADs are oscillations of the membrane potential that occur after repolarization of the action potential (Chapter 5), early afterdepolarizations (EADs) are oscillations that occur during repolarization. In **Figure 7-1**, Panel B, the first action potential (1) indicated in blue arises from a resting potential of –90 mV. The blue line and blue arrow show a normal, "smooth" time course of repolarization. An EAD occurs when repolarization is interrupted by a transient shift of membrane potential in a positive (depolarizing) direction, indicated by the red line and red arrow during repolarization of action potential 1. It occurs prior to complete repolarization (early), in contrast to DADs, which are delayed until after complete repolarization.

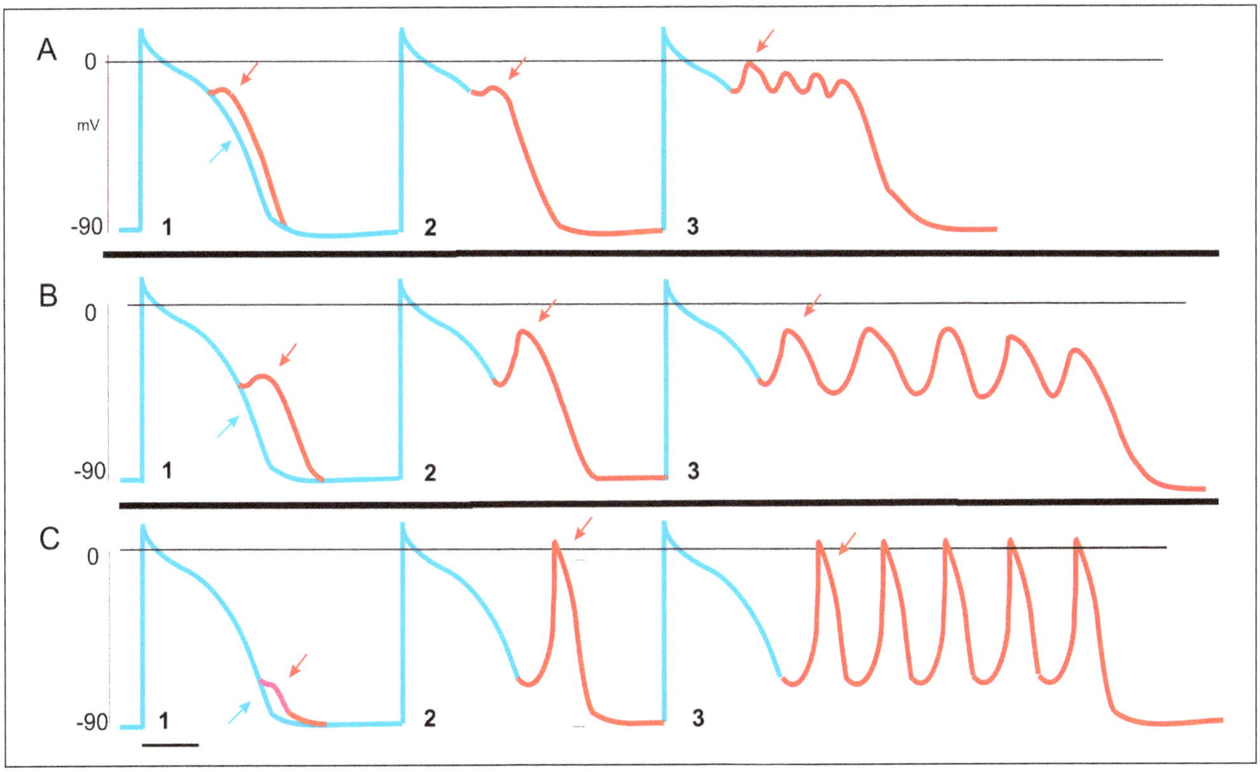

Figure 7-1 EADs and triggered activity at different times during repolarization. Short **black bar** below action potential 1 in **Panel C** is 150 ms.

Electrophysiological Foundations of Cardiac Arrhythmias: A Bridge Between Basic Mechanisms and Clinical Electrophysiology, Second Edition.
© 2020 Andrew L. Wit, Penelope A. Boyden, Mark E. Josephson, Hein J. Wellens. Cardiotext Publishing, ISBN: 978-1-942909-42-2.

Figure 7-1, Panel B shows that when an EAD is large enough, the positive shift in membrane potential leads to a nondriven action potential before complete repolarization (red arrow and tracing following action potential 2). This action potential is "triggered" in the sense that it is evoked by an EAD, the occurrence of which is dependent on the preceding action potential, described as the triggering action potential (action potential 2). If the membrane potential then repolarizes back to the resting level, only one triggered action potential occurs as follows action potential 2. However, the first triggered action potential (red arrow following action potential 3) may also be followed by additional action potentials (red tracing), all occurring at the less negative, depolarized level of membrane potential characteristic of incomplete repolarization. This triggered activity may continue for a variable number of impulses and terminates when the membrane potential repolarizes back to the negative normal resting level of membrane potential characteristic of the triggering action potential (at the far right in Panel B). The return of the membrane potential to the initial level results from "turning on" repolarizing membrane currents that are described below. Triggered activity stops because the inward currents that cause the triggered action potentials only occur at the reduced (less negative) membrane potential associated with the EADs.

Properties of EAD-Induced Triggered Action Potentials

The example shown in Figure 7-1, Panel B is an EAD occurring early during phase 3 of repolarization. EADs can also occur earlier or later; the time of their occurrence influences the properties of the triggered action potentials that they cause. In Figure 7-1, Panel A, the normal time course of repolarization is shown by the blue tracing and blue arrow; the EAD of action potential 1 occurs earlier in phase 2 (red arrow following action potential 1). It is small and does not lead to a triggered action potential (red arrow following action potential 2), only a series of low amplitude nonconducting oscillations in membrane potential (red arrow and red tracing following action potential 3). In Panel C, the EAD arises from the more negative membrane potential characteristic of late phase 3 (red arrow following action potential 1) (blue arrow shows normal repolarization). When late phase 3 EADs become large enough, they can give rise to triggered action potentials (red arrow following action potential 2 in Panel C) that have a larger amplitude than the triggered action potential arising earlier in phase 3 (red arrow following action potential 2 in Panel B). A series of triggered action potentials can also occur during late phase 3 (red action potentials after action potential 3 in Panel C).

As described in Chapter 4 and Figure 4-5, Na^+ channels are inactivated at membrane potentials of around −60 mV and inactivation is removed (more channels are available for excitation) as membrane potential becomes more negative during repolarization, accounting for the increased amplitude and rate of phase 0 depolarization of the triggered action potential after action potential 2, in Panel C compared to Panel B, and in Panel B compared to Panel A.

Propagation of Triggered Action Potentials to Cause Arrhythmias

The amplitude and rate of depolarization of phase 0 of the triggered action potentials determines their ability to propagate and cause arrhythmias. The EADs in Figure 7-1, Panel A cannot generate an action potential or cause arrhythmias because they occur at the very low (less negative) membrane potential characteristic of phase 2, and therefore action potential 3 is followed by only low-amplitude, nonpropagating local oscillations in membrane potential (in red following action potential 3). In Panels B and C, after action potential 3, the EAD-triggered activity occurs in the form of action potentials with a larger amplitude (red action potentials) because they arise from more negative membrane potentials (action potentials in Panel C are larger than in Panel B) that can propagate away from their site of origin to cause arrhythmias (see Chapter 8).

CELLULAR MECHANISMS OF EADS AND EAD-TRIGGERED ACTIVITY

There are several components of EAD-triggered activity described in this section:

- A critical lengthening of the time for action potential repolarization (prolongation of action potential duration [APD]) that leads to EAD occurrence
- The EAD itself
- The depolarization phase 0 of the (first) triggered action potential that arises from the EAD
- The propagation of subsequent triggered action potentials causing triggered arrhythmias

Alterations in Membrane Channels and Currents That Prolong Action Potential Repolarization

EADs are often (but not always) associated with a critical prolongation of the time course of action potential repolarization (prolongation of APD).

EADs Are Associated with Lengthening of QT Interval on the ECG; Long QT Syndromes

Most of the time course of repolarization of ventricular muscle occurs during the time interval from the end of the QRS to the end of the T wave, which is included in measurements of the QT interval of the ECG. Therefore, prolongation of ventricular repolarization that causes EADs is associated with lengthening of the QT interval and alterations in the characteristics of the T wave. This leads to long QT interval (LQT) syndromes that are the most common clinical abnormalities likely to be associated with EAD-triggered arrhythmias. These clinical arrhythmias are described in Chapter 8. The basic mechanisms of the triggered activity causing the arrhythmias are described in this chapter.

Repolarization of the ventricular muscle action potential involves several different inward and outward currents, the properties of which change to cause LQT syndromes. **Table 7-1** summarizes the changes in these repolarizing membrane currents associated with LQT syndromes and triggered activity. The table also includes the specific gene mutation and clinical syndrome associated with each membrane current. More details regarding the membrane currents are provided in subsequent figures.

Although mutations in a large number of different genes encoding channel complexes have been found associated with LQT syndromes, only a few representative ones are shown in the Table 7-1 as an introduction. In addition, remodeling of ion channels caused by pathology such as heart failure or block of ion channels caused by drugs, also not included in Table 7-1, can prolong APD.

The specific membrane currents during repolarization that contribute to the LQT syndromes are described in detail in the next few paragraphs. First, however, a brief overview of the repolarization process. During repolarization there is a net flow of positive charges from inside the cell to outside (outward current flow) that increases with time after the action potential phase 0 and returns the membrane potential back to its original negative diastolic value. This net outward current flow actually consists of both outward currents and inward currents during the phases (1, 2, and 3) of repolarization. A reduction in outward current, an increase in inward current, or a combination of both slows repolarization and can lead to EAD-induced triggered activity. As Table 7-1 shows, an increase in inward membrane currents (referred to as a gain in function) prolongs APD by increasing depolarizing current. A decrease in outward currents (referred to as a loss of function), decreases repolarizing currents to prolong APD.

Membrane Currents Involved in Repolarization

Repolarization of the action potential involves several different inward and outward currents, the properties of which change to cause LQT syndromes. These currents are shown in **Figure 7-2**. The major inward or depolarizing currents are I_{Na}, and I_{CaL} (downward shaded areas under the action potential waveforms) and the major outward or repolarizing currents (upward shaded areas), which are K^+ currents. Each of these currents is described in more detail below.

Table 7-1 Membrane Current Changes Causing Action Potential Prolongation and Associated LQT Syndromes

INWARD MEMBRANE CURRENT	CHANGE INCREASING APD	GENE	CLINICAL SYNDROME
Sodium current, I_{Na}	Increase (gain of function)	*SCN5A*	LQT3
L-type Ca^{2+}-current, I_{CaL}	Increase (gain of function)	*CACNA1C*	LQT8 (Timothy syndrome)
OUTWARD MEMBRANE CURRENT	**CHANGE INCREASING APD**	**GENE**	**CLINICAL SYNDROME**
Slow delayed rectifier, I_{Ks}	Decrease (loss of function)	*KCNQ1*	LQT1
		KCNE1	LQT5
Rapid delayed rectifier, I_{Kr}	Decrease (loss of function)	*KCNH2*	LQT2
Ultra rapid delayed rectifier, I_{Kur}	Decrease (loss of function)	*KCNA5*	Familial AF
Inward rectifier, I_{K1}	Decrease (loss of function)	*KCNJ2*	LQT7 (Andersen-Tawil syndrome)
Transient outward current, I_{to}	Decrease	*KCNA4*	Ischemia, heart failure

APD = action potential duration.

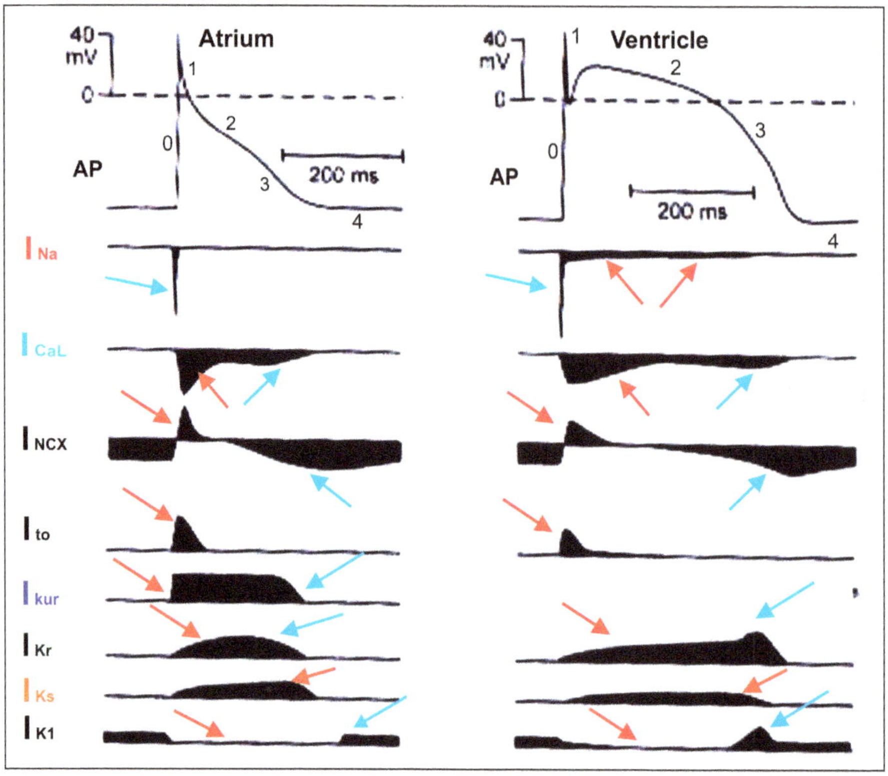

Figure 7-2 Main ionic currents involved in repolarization of the action potential (AP). The relative time courses of the currents are shown. The amplitudes are not drawn to scale and the scale varies for the different currents so the relative magnitude of each current is not indicated, i.e., a large size of a current only indicates the phase where the size of that particular current is large. (Modified from Figure IV.36 in Carmeliet E, Vereecke J. *Cardiac Electrophysiology.* Boston, MA: Kluwer Academic Publishers; 2002).

Alterations in Inward Currents That Prolong APD to Cause EADs

Inward fast Na$^+$ current; I_{Na}. The voltage-dependent Na$^+$ channel provides the inward current (I_{Na}) responsible for the upstroke (Phase 0) and conduction of the action potential in atrial, ventricular and Purkinje tissue (I_{Na}, blue arrow, in Figure 7-2). The gene that encodes the protein subunit that forms the channel pore through which Na$^+$ ions flow (designated as the alpha subunit, Nav 1.5) is called *SCN5A*. The channel is also composed of other protein (b) subunits that modify channel function. The Na$^+$ current activation has a threshold of about −60 to −55 mV, which is reached when a cell is excited by a propagating impulse. After I_{Na} quickly depolarizes the cell to levels positive to around −10 mV, the magnitude of the current decreases rapidly, causing the membrane potential to stop moving in a positive direction to begin the repolarization process. I_{Na} decreases because of the decrease in the electrochemical force driving Na$^+$ ions into the cell and rapid voltage-dependent inactivation (within 1–10 ms) of the channel protein. A small fraction of the total I_{Na}, however, persists during the plateau phase 2 (called late Na$^+$ current, $I_{Na\ late}$), primarily in ventricular muscle and Purkinje fibers (red arrows under I_{Na}, ventricular trace in Figure 7-2) providing extended depolarizing current that retards repolarization.

Mutations in the gene SCN5A, which alter the alpha protein subunit of the Na$^+$ channel pore to destabilize channel inactivation, are associated with one of the forms of the congenital LQT syndrome, designated LQT3 (clinical aspects are discussed in Chapter 8). **Figure 7-3** shows the effects of this gain of function mutation on the action potential (Panel A) and I_{Na} (Panel B) in the ventricles.

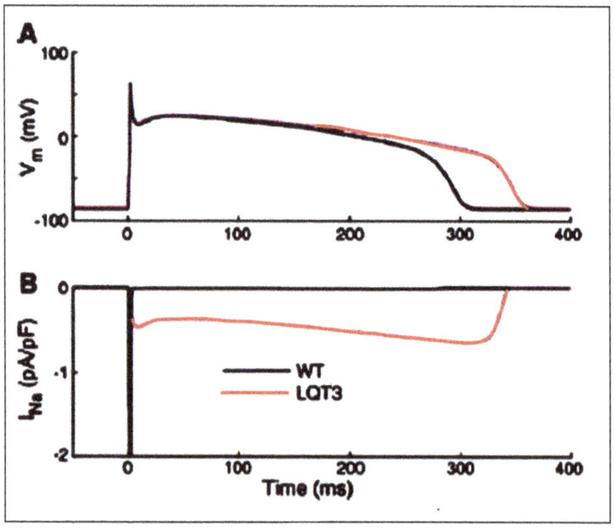

Figure 7-3 Computer simulation of a ventricular muscle cell showing action potential waveforms in **Panel A** and inward Na$^+$ current in **Panel B**. (Reproduced from Nerbonne JM, Kass RS.. Molecular physiology of cardiac repolarization. *Physiol Rev.* 2005;85:1205–1253.)

In Panel A, the ventricular muscle action potential with normal channel function is shown in black. The effect of the mutation is a transient failure of inactivation of Na^+ channels. This results in prolongation of the plateau phase of the action potential indicated by the red trace in Panel A.

Panel B shows the time course of activation and inactivation of I_{Na} of the cell. The black tracing shows I_{Na} with normal channel function (the black spike (WT or wild type) at time zero). The normal persistence of a small inward I_{Na} described in Figure 7-2 is too small to be shown. The red trace in Panel B (LQT3) shows the effect of the mutation on I_{Na}, resulting in increased persistent (late) inward Na^+ current during the plateau. This is called a "gain of function" mutation because current is increased through the Na^+ channel. Under certain conditions, this prolongation of repolarization leads to EADs (described below).

The amount of action potential prolongation caused by the increase in late I_{Na} varies in different regions of the ventricles because there is regional variation in the amount of net inward current that late I_{Na} contributes during repolarization. Prolongation of repolarization may be more severe in myocardial muscle cells toward the midmyocardial wall (sometimes designated as "M" cells) than in epicardial or endocardial cells because late I_{Na} contributes more inward current to repolarization of midmyocardial cells. The different amount of action potential prolongation in different regions of the ventricle can increase the heterogeneity of repolarization time (i.e., the difference in repolarization time among different regions) and heterogeneity of refractoriness that is dependent on recovery of Na^+ channel function during repolarization. This heterogeneity can be arrhythmogenic (described later). However, any increase in heterogeneity is limited by the effects of electrotonic current flow through gap junction connections between cells with different APDs. An increase in the late I_{Na} also prolongs APD in Purkinje cells and possibly atrial cells.

The increased persistent I_{Na} also causes an increased amount of Na^+ in the cell. This in turn can result in an increase in intracellular (SR) Ca^{2+} via the Na^+–Ca^{2+} exchanger that extrudes the excess Na^+ in exchange for Ca^{2+} at the membrane potential of the plateau phase (see Figure 5-2). This raises the possibility that gain-of-function mutations in *SCN5A* or other conditions that prolong APD may increase SR Ca^{2+} to cause DADs.

An acquired increase in late Na^+ current can also be a result of ion-channel remodeling secondary to events such as heart failure, which leads to prolongation of repolarization and EADs.

Parenthetically, a loss of function of the I_{Na} channel caused by a different mutation in *SCN5A* occurs in the Brugada syndrome. This may contribute to conduction changes that underlie reentrant arrhythmias.

Inward L-type Ca^{2+} current (I_{CaL}). I_{CaL} is a second inward current that is involved in the process of repolarization. The gene *CACNA1C* encodes the Ca^{2+} channel pore-forming alpha subunit. This current plays an important role in maintaining the plateau phase (phase 2) of the action potential in atrial, ventricular, and Purkinje cells (Figure 7-2, I_{CaL}). As described in Chapter 5 (Figure 5-2), it also triggers Ca^{2+} release from the SR resulting in forward mode excitation-contraction coupling. The channel activates after depolarization of the membrane potential by the Na^+ current to levels positive to about –30 to –25 mV (membrane potential may vary in the different cell types). Activation is maximal at around 0 mV. Inactivation of the channel is dependent on both intracellular Ca^{2+} and membrane voltage. Ca^{2+}-dependent inactivation is rapid, albeit not as rapid as the Na^+ current just described (Figure 7-2, I_{CaL}, red arrow), and is caused by increased Ca^{2+} in the subsarcolemmal space that occurs during the plateau. During the remainder of the action potential, I_{CaL} inactivates via a voltage-dependent mechanism as membrane potential repolarizes to more negative levels (Figure 7-2, I_{CaL}, blue arrow).

Mutations in *CACNA1C* characterized by reduced voltage-dependent inactivation of the channel underlie Timothy syndrome (LQT8). The result is a persistent inward I_{CaL} (another gain-of-function mutation) that prolongs the APD in the ventricles and prolongs the QT interval, which can lead to EADs and triggered ventricular arrhythmias. Increased intracellular Ca^{2+} as a consequence of this mutation might also lead to DAD-triggered activity. L-type calcium channels are widely expressed, and LQT8 patients may have extracardiac manifestations of the mutations such as syndactyly.

Alterations in Outward I_K Currents That Prolong APD to Cause EADs

I_K designates K^+ currents flowing through membrane channel proteins from the inside of the cell to the outside. I_K flowing through voltage gated delayed rectifier K^+ channels mediates repolarization during late phase 2 and all of phase 3 of the action potential. It is called the delayed rectifier current because significant current flow is delayed after the channels are initially activated during phase 0. Maximum current flow occurs during phase 3. The channels close (deactivate) during membrane repolarization because of the negative voltage. "Rectifier" refers to the channel's preference to pass current in only one direction:

outward. EADs and triggered activity are associated with reduction of current flow (loss of function) through one of the ion channel components of I_K controlled by separate genes. Loss of function of any component prolongs APD. On the basis of electrophysiological properties, three delayed currents can be distinguished, I_{Ks}, I_{Kr}, and I_{Kur}. Another K^+ current, I_{K1}, called the inward rectifier, sets the resting potential and can also influence repolarization.

Outward K^+ current; I_{Ks}. The I_{Ks} channel pore-forming (alpha) protein is K_v7-1 and the gene encoding it is designated *KCNQ1*. I_{Ks} channels are formed by coassembly of this protein with a small protein called minK (a small "minimal" K^+ channel protein, encoded by gene *KCNE1*). Alterations of either component can cause LQT. I_{Ks} activates slowly following phase 0 depolarization and increases gradually during the plateau phase of the action potential (hence the "s" designation) (Figure 7-2, red arrow). It persists throughout phase 3 of repolarization when it slowly deactivates. I_{Ks} is small and may even be absent in normal human ventricular myocardium particularly at long cycle lengths. It assumes more importance as heart rate increases and/or during sympathetic stimulation, both of which increase the magnitude of this current and cause acceleration of repolarization (see Figure 7-6). It also provides important repolarizing current when I_{Kr} (the other component of I_K described below) is reduced by genetic alterations or drugs. Therefore, it provides a *repolarization reserve* under these circumstances. I_{Ks} varies quantitatively in different regions of the ventricle, being expressed more in epicardial and endocardial muscle than in mid-ventricular regions (M cells). As a result of the lack of I_{Ks}, the intrinsic APD is longer in the midmyocardial cells. This characteristic is only minimally expressed under normal conditions when they are tightly coupled to epicardial and endocardial cells that have shorter time courses of repolarization because of repolarizing electrotonic current flow from cells with shorter APDs to cells with longer APDs. The longer APD of midmyocardial cells may manifest itself under conditions of poor gap junctional coupling such as fibrosis. I_{Ks} is also weakly expressed in Purkinje cells, which have a long APD and are poorly coupled to myocardial cells except in regions of Purkinje–muscle junctions.

The congenital LQT syndromes LQT1 and LQT5 have been linked to inherited loss of function mutations in *KCNQ1* and *KCNE1* respectively. These mutations alter the protein makeup of the I_{Ks} channel and cause a reduction in the I_{Ks} repolarizing current. **Figure 7-4**, shows the theoretical effect of loss of function of I_{Ks} expected under baseline conditions in which I_{Ks} has assumed a more prominent role in repolarization—e.g., rapid heart rate, sympathetic stimulation, or some loss of I_{Kr}.

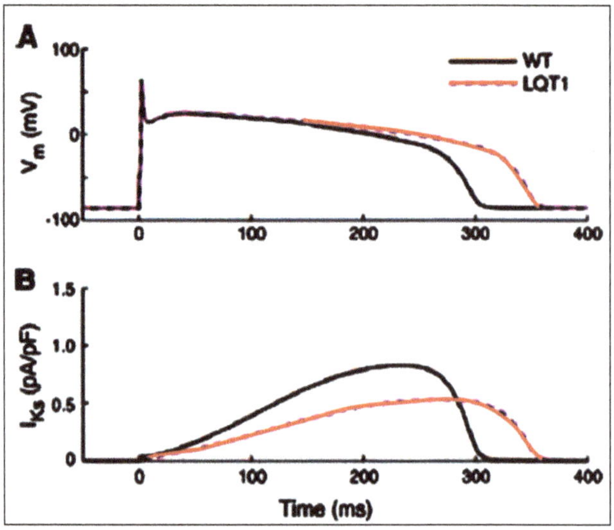

Figure 7-4 Effects of loss of function of I_{Ks} on a ventricular muscle action potential (**Panel A**) and membrane current (**Panel B**) from a computer simulation. (Reproduced from Nerbonne JM, Kass RS. Molecular physiology of cardiac repolarization. *Physiol Rev.* 2005;85:1205–1253.)

In Panel A, a normal (wild type (WT)) ventricular action potential is shown by the solid black line. The solid black line in Panel B shows the time course of activation and inactivation of I_{Ks} associated with this normal action potential. Also shown in Panel A is the action potential after a loss of function of I_{Ks} (LQT1, red line). In Panel B, the red line shows the time course of I_{Ks} after the loss of function (LQT1). EADs and triggered ventricular arrhythmias are associated with the action potential prolongation (not shown). APD is also expected to be prolonged in Purkinje cells, which may be a source of some triggered arrhythmias. The effects in the atria are not prominent although there may be some prolongation of the APD.

Outward K^+ current; I_{Kr}. Outward I_{Kr} is responsible for termination of the action potential plateau and initiation of action potential repolarization (Figure 7-2). I_{Kr} activates relatively rapidly for depolarizations positive to −40 mV (hence the designation "r") (red arrow) and maintains significant outward current during phase 3 repolarization (blue arrow). Deactivation can be slower than for I_{Ks}. The gene *KCNH2* encodes the I_{Kr} channel formed by a protein designated hERG (human ether-a-go-go-related gene). Small peptides designated MiRP, the expression of which are controlled by the gene family *KCNE* (*KCNE2*), may function as accessory subunits of the channel but their role is uncertain. Inherited loss of function mutations in *KCNH2*, causing a decrease in I_{Kr} are associated with prolongation of the action potential repolarization and congenital LQT2. The loss of function may have a greater effect in midmyocardial (M) cells than epicardial or endocardial muscle cells because of the weak I_{Ks} in these cells. I_{Ks} may provide some repolarization reserve in epicardial and endocardial muscle cells, damping the effects of loss of I_{Kr}. Similarly, loss of function of I_{Kr} in Purkinje cells may have a marked effect to prolong APD because I_{Ks} is weakly expressed in Purkinje cells. EADs associated with the action potential prolongation causes ventricular arrhythmias associated with LQT2 (see Chapter 8). The effects in the atria are not prominent although there may be some prolongation of the atrial APD.

I_{Kr} channels are also blocked by certain drugs causing a similar loss of function as the genetically induced effect. The result is acquired long QT and EADs (Chapter 8).

Opposite to the effects of loss of function mutations described above, gain in function mutations in the genes controlling I_{Ks} and I_{Kr} accelerate ventricular repolarization and are associated with short QT syndromes (QTc < 350 ms). These syndromes are associated with atrial and ventricular fibrillation of uncertain mechanism (see *Josephson's Clinical Cardiac Electrophysiology*, Chapter 11).

Outward K⁺ current; I_{Kur}. Outward I_{Kur} is an ultra rapid activating current (almost instantaneous compared to I_{Ks} and I_{Kr}) (Figure 7-2, red arrow) with slow inactivation taking several seconds (blue arrow). The alpha pore-forming subunit of the channels is encoded by the gene *KCNA5*. This current contributes to phase 2 repolarization in atrial cells and is an important reason for the short duration of the atrial action potential. I_{Kur} is less important in ventricular cells but does exist in Purkinje cells. Loss of function mutations have been documented in cases of familial atrial fibrillation but an association with EADs is not established.

The inward rectifier K⁺ current; I_{K1}. The inward rectifier current I_{K1} provides substantial outward current and sets the resting potential at –75 to –90 mV in atrial, ventricular, and Purkinje cells. It also is involved in terminal repolarization (Figure 7-2, blue arrow). The I_{K1} channel (protein Kir 2.1) is encoded by the gene *KCNJ2*. The channel does not allow much outward current flow during depolarization to potentials more positive than about –40 mV (Figure 7-2, red arrow) (hence the term "inward rectifier"), thus preventing excessive repolarizing current during the plateau of the action potential. Outward current begins to flow again during late phase 3 and contributes to the final rapid repolarization (blue arrow). An inherited loss-of-function mutation in *KCNJ2*, decreases I_{K1} current, resulting in prolongation of APD and congenital LQT7 (Andersen-Tawil syndrome). LQT7 is associated with bidirectional ventricular tachycardia rather than the arrhythmia, torsades de pointes, commonly associated with EADs (see Chapter 8). The occurrence of this bidirectional arrhythmia suggests that DADs may be an inciting mechanism, since bidirectional tachycardia is associated with digitalis toxicity and catecholaminergic polymorphic ventricular tachycardia, both caused by DADs (Chapter 6). As described in Chapter 5, DADs may result when prolonged APD causes Ca^{2+} overload. *KCNJ2* is expressed in tissues other than the heart. Neuromuscular symptoms can accompany LQT7.

The transient outward K⁺ current (I_{to}). I_{to} is a short-lasting outward K⁺ current that is rapidly activated upon depolarization of the action potential to between –10 and +20 mV and then rapidly inactivates (Figure 7-2, red arrow). The channel is composed of multiple protein subunits, including an alpha subunit that forms the channel pore and is encoded by gene *KCND3*. The major effect is to cause rapid phase 1 repolarization of the action potential both in atrial and ventricular muscle cells, particularly midmyocardial and epicardial ventricular muscle cells, as well as Purkinje cells. It can influence the membrane potential at which the plateau phase 2 begins and influence the time course of repolarization; e.g., a prominent phase 1 results in the plateau starting at a more negative membrane potential than in the absence of a prominent phase 1 and a shorter APD. There are several components to this current with different properties, only the fast component is shown in Figure 7-2. While rare genetic mutations have been described, loss of I_{to} in chronic ischemia and heart failure is associated with some prolongation of the APD.

Alterations in Pump and Exchanger Currents That Prolong APD to Cause EADs

The Na⁺–K⁺ (ATPase) pump. The Na⁺–K⁺ (ATPase) pump is described in Chapter 1, Figure 1-6 in relation to its effects on spontaneous diastolic depolarization and automaticity and in Chapter 5, Figure 5-7 in relation to DADs and triggered activity. To reiterate, the pump generates an outward current (I_p) owing to the exchange ratio of 3 Na⁺ moving out of the cell in exchange for 2 K⁺ ions moving into the cell. This outward current (not shown in Figure 7-2) is generated throughout the action potential (as well as during diastole) and contributes outward current to repolarization. A decrease in pump current can cause prolongation of APD, although QT usually does not lengthen significantly. An increase in pump current that occurs at rapid rates accelerates repolarization, and may be involved in preventing EADs (see Figure 7-6).

The Na⁺–Ca^{2+} exchanger. The Na⁺–Ca^{2+} exchanger is described in Chapter 2, Figure 2-6 and Chapter 3, Figure 3-3, in relation to its role in automaticity and in Chapter 5, Figure 5-2 in relation to its role in DAD-triggered activity. Three Na⁺ are exchanged for 1 Ca^{2+}, generating a current carried by Na⁺, the direction of which is dependent on the membrane potential. This current can be outward during the positive membrane potential of early repolarization (Figure 7-2, I_{NCX}, red arrow) and inward as membrane potential becomes more negative during later repolarization and diastole (blue arrow). Increases in inward exchanger current during later repolarization can prolong APD and contribute to EAD formation both in ventricles and atria (see Figure 7-5).

Mechanisms for EAD Formation and Triggered Activity Caused by Prolonged Action Potential Repolarization

Prolonging the time course for repolarization as a consequence of increased inward or decreased outward membrane currents during phases 2 and 3 as described in the previous section, can lead to the occurrence of EADs. This change in repolarization that leads to EADs is sometimes called a *conditioning phase.* When it is caused specifically by a decrease in a component of I_K (I_{Kr} or I_{Ks}), it is also referred to as *reduced repolarization* reserve. The concept of repolarization reserve is described in more detail in Chapter 8 on acquired LQT syndrome.

Ionic Mechanism of EADs–Increased Net Inward Current During Repolarization

EADs are caused by a period of increased net inward current as a consequence of the delayed repolarization, which itself is caused by a decrease in net outward current. The inward current can be I_{CaL}, I_{NCX}, $I_{Na\ late}$, or a combination of these currents.

L-type Ca^{2+} current (I_{CaL}). I_{CaL} is important for the generation of EADs in addition to sometimes being involved in action potential prolongation through gain of function mutation in the channel (Table 7-1). **Figure 7-5** diagrams the ionic mechanism of EADs occurring during late phase 2 and early phase 3 of repolarization.

The normal time course and magnitude of I_{CaL} are described in Figure 7-5, Panel A. I_{CaL} normally inactivates through Ca^{2+}-dependent (red arrow on I_{CaL} trace, bottom half of figure) and voltage-dependent (blue arrow on I_{CaL} trace) mechanisms during phases 2 and 3 of repolarization respectively (see previous description). In the top half of the figure, the length of the downward purple arrows superimposed on the action potential show qualitatively the decrease in I_{CaL} during repolarization, which coincides with this inactivation. Panel B shows changes in I_{CaL} when repolarization time is prolonged. In this situation, I_{CaL} can partly recover from inactivation, and continue to generate an inward current. This is diagrammed in Panel B as an increase in the downward purple arrow designated with an asterisk superimposed on the action potential during the EAD. Recovery from inactivation resulting in this increased I_{CaL} results when the Ca^{2+}-mediated inactivation of I_{CaL} is reduced during prolonged repolarization shown by the red curved line and second red arrow (asterisk) on the I_{CaL} trace. The reason for the reduction of Ca^{2+}-mediated inactivation is that the level of intracellular Ca^{2+} in the subsarcolemmal space declines during prolonged repolarization owing to both its uptake by the SR and extrusion from the cell by I_{NCX}. The maintenance of the membrane in the depolarized state during the prolonged APD and EAD also retards the voltage-dependent inactivation of I_{CaL} (blue curve and arrow on I_{CaL} trace). As a result, there are open L-type Ca^{2+} channels as well as inactivated channels during the prolonged plateau. The reactivated inward I_{CaL} flowing through the open channels late in the plateau phase can depolarize the membrane potential, causing an EAD (vertical dashed line). In the case of loss of function in one of the I_K channels as previously described, the reduction of I_K outward current at the depolarized level of phase 2 and early phase 3 amplifies the depolarizing effects of the inward current I_{CaL}, since I_K does not strongly oppose it. The I_{CaL} current causing the EAD is transient. As membrane potential repolarizes during the EAD, I_{CaL} decreases (shorter downward purple arrow indicated by the + sign), and time-dependent outward currents such as I_{Kr} and/or I_{Ks} are further activated. If the outward currents predominate, the EAD is followed by repolarization back to the resting membrane potential. However, if I_{CaL} depolarization reaches a threshold for it to become regenerative, I_{CaL} causes or contributes to phase 0 of the triggered action potential during phase 2 and early phase 3 EADs (see Figure 7-1, Panel B).

The Na^+–Ca^{2+} exchanger (I_{NCX}). I_{NCX} is the source of another inward current that can be involved in both the conditioning phase (prolongation of APD) and EAD formation. As shown in Figure 7-5, Panel A (bottom trace labeled I_{NCX}), the exchanger generates an inward current I_{NCX} (blue arrow) when intracellular Ca^{2+} is elevated during late phase 2 and early phase 3. (Early in repolarization I_{NCX} is outward (red arrow) as described in Chapter 5). In Figure 7-5, Panel A at the top, inward I_{NCX} is shown by the green arrows superimposed on the action potential. Increased I_{NCX} can result (Panel B), if myoplasmic Ca^{2+} is elevated during the prolonged plateau phase of repolarization, perhaps as a result of either SR Ca^{2+} release caused by reactivation of I_{CaL} or another cause of SR Ca^{2+} release, e.g., heart failure (described in Chapter 8).

Panel B shows that in this situation, I_{NCX} may be large enough (green curve and green arrow on I_{NCX} trace) to contribute to the EAD depolarization (top trace, downward green arrows superimposed on the EAD).

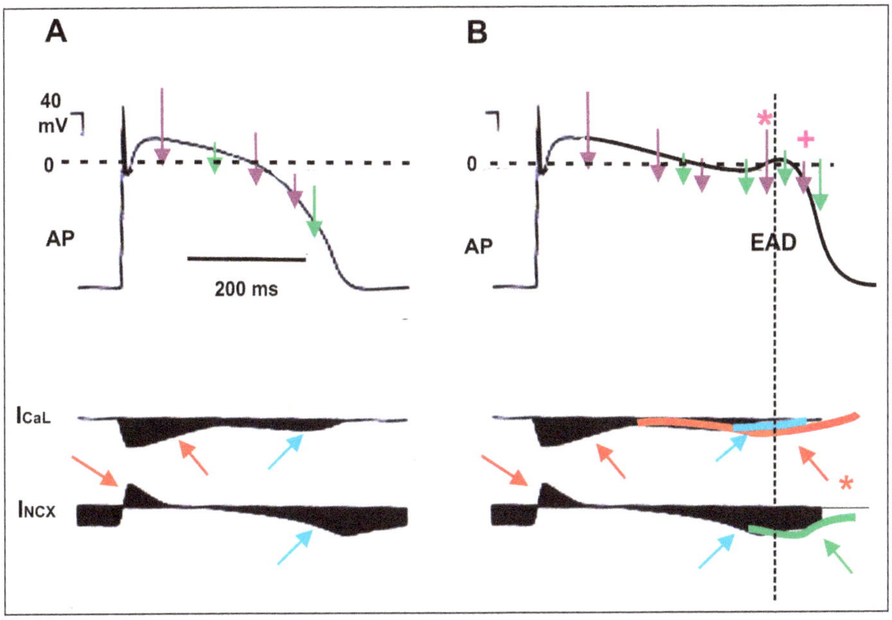

Figure 7-5 The top trace shows a normal ventricular muscle action potential (AP) in **Panel A** and an AP with prolonged repolarization and EAD in **Panel B**. Below are diagrams of membrane currents associated with EAD formation.

EADs can occur without the increased Ca^{2+} loading that is often associated with DADs although under certain circumstances Ca^{2+} loading may play a role. Thus, I_{NCX} and I_{CaL} can act synergistically to cause phase 2 and early phase 3 EADs. I_{NCX} may play a more dominant role in EADs in late phase 3 where the membrane potential is more negative since it becomes larger at more negative potentials (Panel B, top, green arrow during phase 3). At the more negative membrane potentials there is less reactivation of L-type Ca^{2+} channels. By this later stage of repolarization, some Na^+ channels are also reactivated and I_{Na} may contribute to EADs. I_{NCX} may also assume an important role in generating EADs during sympathetic stimulation, when SR Ca^{2+} uptake and release is enhanced.

Prolonged repolarization does not always result in EADs. EADs do not occur if the prolonged plateau phase remains more positive than 0 mV. The reactivation of I_{CaL} shown in Figure 7-5, (I_{CaL} red and blue current traces in Panel B) occurs at a restricted range of membrane potentials between approximately 0 and −40 mV.

There are some exceptions where prolongation of action potential repolarization is not required for EADs to occur. In the presence of simultaneous sympathetic and parasympathetic activation, atrial cells in pulmonary veins can generate phase 3 EADs during acceleration of repolarization. These EADs result from I_{NCX}, enhanced by sympathetic stimulation in the presence of a highly negative membrane potential caused by the acceleration of repolarization, which increases the inward driving force on the current.

EAD-Triggered Action Potentials

The first triggered action potential occurs when an EAD depolarizes the membrane potential to activate a regenerative inward Ca^{2+} or Na^+ current (Figure 7-1, Panels B and C, action potential 2, red arrows). Once it occurs, membrane potential can either repolarize back to its normal resting negative level because of the repolarizing effects of I_K or a train of additional triggered action potentials can occur (Figure 7-1, Panels B and C, action potential 3, red arrows). When they propagate to surrounding myocardium, an arrhythmia results.

Characteristics of triggered action potentials. The triggered action potentials occurring from late phase 2 or early phase 3 EADs (Figure 7-1, Panel B) have a slow depolarization phase (0) dependent on I_{CaL}, since most of I_{Na} is still inactivated at membrane potentials positive to ~ −60 mV (see Figure 4-5). Na^+ channels begin to reactivate at membrane potentials more negative than −60 mV; the triggered action potentials occurring from later phase 3 EADs (Figure 7-1, Panel C) have a faster phase 0 dependent on either a mixture of I_{Na} and I_{CaL}, or I_{Na} alone.

Continuation of triggered action potentials. A question that still remains is, what is the mechanism causing the continuation of triggered action potentials following the first one triggered by the EAD? In a focus generating triggered action potentials, each triggered action potential during a period of triggered activity may be caused by EADs occurring during repolarization of the preceding action potential. Triggered activity following the first triggered action potential may also result from the same mechanism as abnormal automaticity, which likewise occurs at less negative levels of membrane potential (see Chapter 4). Abnormal automaticity would occur because the conditions leading to an EAD maintain the membrane potential at a depolarized level (during the prolonged time course for repolarization). Another possibility is that triggered activity is maintained by a DAD occurring after each triggered action potential. This might occur in situations where there is dysfunction of the SR leading to spontaneous diastolic elevation of Ca^{2+}, such as in cells in the failing heart.

Continued triggered activity after the first EAD-induced triggered action potential might also be caused by reentrant excitation involving more of the heart than just the focus of EADs. An example is the tachycardia called *torsades de pointes*, loosely translated from the French as "twisting of the points" (of the QRS complex). Torsades de pointes is characterized by a rapid rate (170 bpm) and a polymorphic QRS morphology with gradual shifting of R waves from positive to negative, which is often unsustained but can progress into ventricular fibrillation. It is associated with ventricular action potential prolongation and congenital and acquired LQT syndromes (see Chapter 8).

Torsades de pointes may be initiated by an EAD-triggered impulse but perpetuated by reentry. The reentry mechanism would be facilitated by the heterogeneity of action potential repolarization caused by the unequal effects of ion channel changes in LQT that occur over a larger area than just a focus. Mechanisms for reentry related to heterogeneity are described in Chapter 9. Briefly, the model involves the initial EAD causing a short-coupled, premature, triggered impulse that propagates from its site of origin and forms reentrant circuits due to block in regions with longer action potential and refractory period durations, while continuing to propagate slowly through regions of shorter APDs and refractory periods (see Figure 9-14 for details on reentry caused by action potential heterogeneity). If this is the mechanism for clinical EAD-triggered tachycardia, the origin of tachycardia is not focal, unlike DAD-triggered tachycardia. As usually evident in at least one ECG lead (but a 12-lead ECG should be recorded), the QRS complexes during tachycardia gradually change from upright to downward, which is the typical morphology of EAD-triggered torsades de pointes. These changes result from a changing sequence of ventricular activation that might be caused by changing exit routes from a stable reentrant circuit or by a reentrant circuit that changes its location (see Figure 8-1).

Propagation of EAD-triggered action potentials. In order for action potentials caused by EADs to cause arrhythmias, no matter whether it is only the first triggered action potential or a number of triggered action potentials, they must propagate from their site of origin to surrounding myocardium. The level of membrane potential at which triggered action potentials occur has an important influence on the ability to propagate. In Figure 7-1, Panel A, the triggered action potentials (actually just oscillations in membrane potential) arising at the low (less negative) level of membrane potentials characteristic of phase 2 EADs, have very low amplitudes dependent on I_{CaL}. They cannot propagate, since the weak current is not able to depolarize surrounding myocardium to its threshold for generating action potentials. EADs arising later in phase 2 or in phase 3 of repolarization (Figure 7-1, Panels B and C) occur at more negative membrane potentials and have a larger and stronger depolarization phase 0 caused by I_{CaL} (Panel B) and I_{Na} (Panel C), thus making propagation more likely (for a description of the mechanism of propagation, see Figure 9-4). The current arising from both late phase 2 and phase 3 triggered action potentials that spreads from this EAD focus to depolarize cells in the pathway of propagation (axial current) is enhanced to ensure propagation when the triggered action potentials of a critical number of cells are synchronized to occur simultaneously, thus summating the current from each cell. Synchronization is achieved by gap junction coupling among cells. If the cells in the focus were not coupled to each other, EADs would occur at random in each cell and propagation of an impulse away from the focus might not occur.

Gap junction coupling also plays an additional role in influencing the propagation of action potentials from a triggered focus. EADs can be inhibited by coupling to adjacent myocytes with normal repolarization. Normal repolarization of adjacent sites occurs more rapidly than in the region generating EADs. When this occurs, the EAD focus is surrounded by a region with a more negative membrane potential at the time of EAD generation. Then electrotonic current flows through gap junctions in the repolarizing direction from the surrounding regions to the focus of EADs that would inhibit EAD formation, in the same way it can inhibit automaticity (see Figure 1-3). It is therefore unlikely that EAD-triggered arrhythmias could arise in small regions with normal coupling to surrounding normal myocardium. Under situations in which EAD-triggered arrhythmias occur, there is usually reduced repolarization reserve of surrounding myocytes prolonging their repolarization or reduced gap junction coupling both of which reduce the inhibiting electrotonic current flow. The increased susceptibility of Purkinje cells to generate EADs may be at least partly be due to gap junction coupling to fewer surrounding myocardial cells at Purkinje–muscle junctions.

ELECTROPHYSIOLOGICAL PROPERTIES OF EADS AND TRIGGERED ACTIVITY

Prolongation of the time course for repolarization leading to an increase in APD is one of the main causes of EADs. This prolongation of repolarization is, in turn, affected by a number of factors, including the location of cells in the ventricles (epicardial, midmyocardial, endocardial), the type of myocardial cell (atrial vs. ventricular vs. Purkinje), and the heart rate (slow vs. rapid) and rhythm (regular vs. premature impulses).

Action Potential Duration (APD) Varies by Location and Influences Occurrence of EADs

The occurrence of EADs is dependent on action potential characteristics that vary among different anatomic locations in the heart. Myocardial cells with intrinsically long APDs due to a well-defined plateau phase, such as ventricular muscle and Purkinje fibers, are more prone to develop EADs than cells with intrinsically short APDs such as atrial muscle (Figure 7-2). Within the ventricle and Purkinje system, there is variability (heterogeneity) of the time for repolarization in different regions. Endocardial and epicardial muscle cells have shorter intrinsic APDs than midmyocardial (M) cells in the ventricular walls, although in the presence of normal gap junction coupling, this difference is not prominent because of electrotonic interactions. APD in the Purkinje system lengthens from the His bundle through the bundle branches and then shortens prior to making contact with ventricular muscle—the "gate" phenomenon. Purkinje and muscle cells with longer APDs are more prone to develop either phase 2 or phase 3 EADs under appropriate circumstances. Atrial muscle, lacking a well-defined plateau phase, can develop phase 3 EADs, but because of the short APDs, this is less likely than in the ventricles.

EADs have not been recorded from A-V nodal cells, which have a less negative level of membrane potential (≤ −60 mV) and are unlikely to be a cause of A-V nodal arrhythmias.

Rate-Dependent Changes in Repolarization Influences Occurrence of EADs

EADs are more likely to occur at long cycle lengths, which slow repolarization and prolong APD and EADs can disappear at short cycle lengths that accelerate repolarization and shorten APD.

The effects of cycle length on ventricular muscle APD are illustrated in **Figure 7-6**, which shows recordings of monophasic action potentials from the endocardial surface of the human right ventricle. This technique does not involve an intracellular microelectrode but can record extracellular current flow with a specially designed electrode catheter.

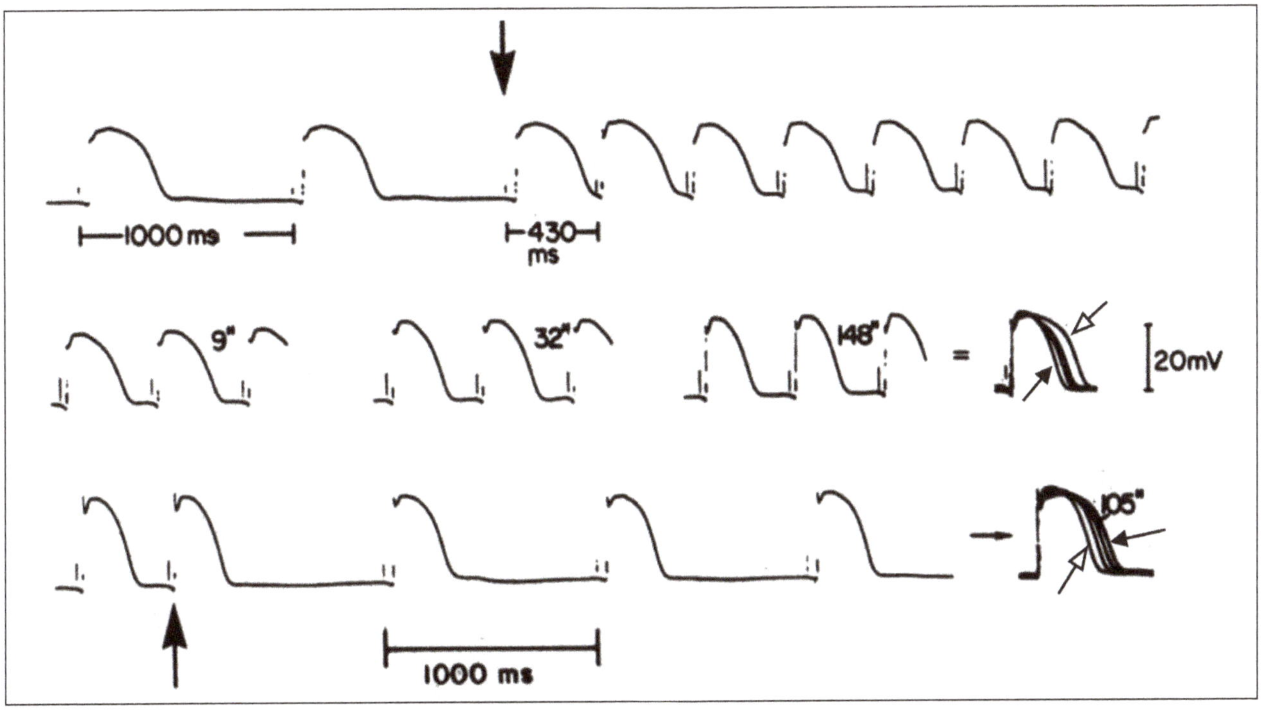

Figure 7-6 Monophasic action potentials recorded from the endocardial surface of the right ventricle during changes in the pacing cycle length. (Reproduced from Franz MR, Swerdlow CD. Cycle length dependence of human action potential duration *in vivo*. Effects of single extrastimuli, sudden sustained rate acceleration and deceleration, and different steady-state frequencies. *J Clin Invest*. 1988;82:972–979.)

In Figure 7-6, at the left of the top trace, action potential waveforms are shown at a pacing cycle length of 1000 ms. At the arrow, the cycle length is suddenly reduced to 430 ms. This results in an acceleration of repolarization, rapidly shortening the APD. This initial shortening is called *rate-dependent adaptation*.

In the second row, the action potential continues to shorten but at a slower time course as the pacing continues at cycle length 430 ms. This phase is called *accommodation*. The slower phase of continued shortening is shown at 9, 32, and 148 seconds. At the far right of the middle recordings, the action potentials at these different times are superimposed, emphasizing the decrease in APD that occurred with the decreased cycle length. The unfilled arrow head points to the first action potential before the change in cycle length, the black arrow points to the last shortened action potential. In the bottom row at the arrow, the cycle length is suddenly restored to 1000 ms resulting in slowing of repolarization and lengthening of APD that required several hundred impulses (105 sec total) to recover. The lengthening of APD at the slower heart rate is emphasized by the superimposed action potentials at the far right of the bottom recordings. The unfilled arrow head indicates the last action potential at the short cycle length, the black arrow indicates the APD at the long cycle length.

Figure 7-7 summarizes the effects of decreased cycle length on repolarization. In this figure, the monophasic APD (on the ordinate) is plotted vs. time in seconds (s on the abscissa). It shows that shortening of the cycle length from 750 to 480 ms (downward pointing arrow at the left at time zero) results in an initial rapid shortening of the APD caused by acceleration of repolarization during the first 30 sec (upper curve; rate-dependent adaptation).

In Figure 7-7, the amount of rapid shortening is directly related to the cycle length; note that APD is shorter at a cycle length of 410 ms (lower curve) than at 480 ms (upper curve). Since repolarization is associated with diastolic relaxation, this property allows time for adequate diastolic filling of the ventricles as heart rate increases. This rapid phase of shortening is then followed by a further gradual shortening over a few minutes (the phase of *accommodation*), also characterized by greater shortening at a shorter cycle length (compare CL of 410 ms lower curve with CL 480 ms upper curve). At the second arrow (180 ms), the pacing cycle length returns to 750 ms for both curves and APD lengthens back toward initial values.

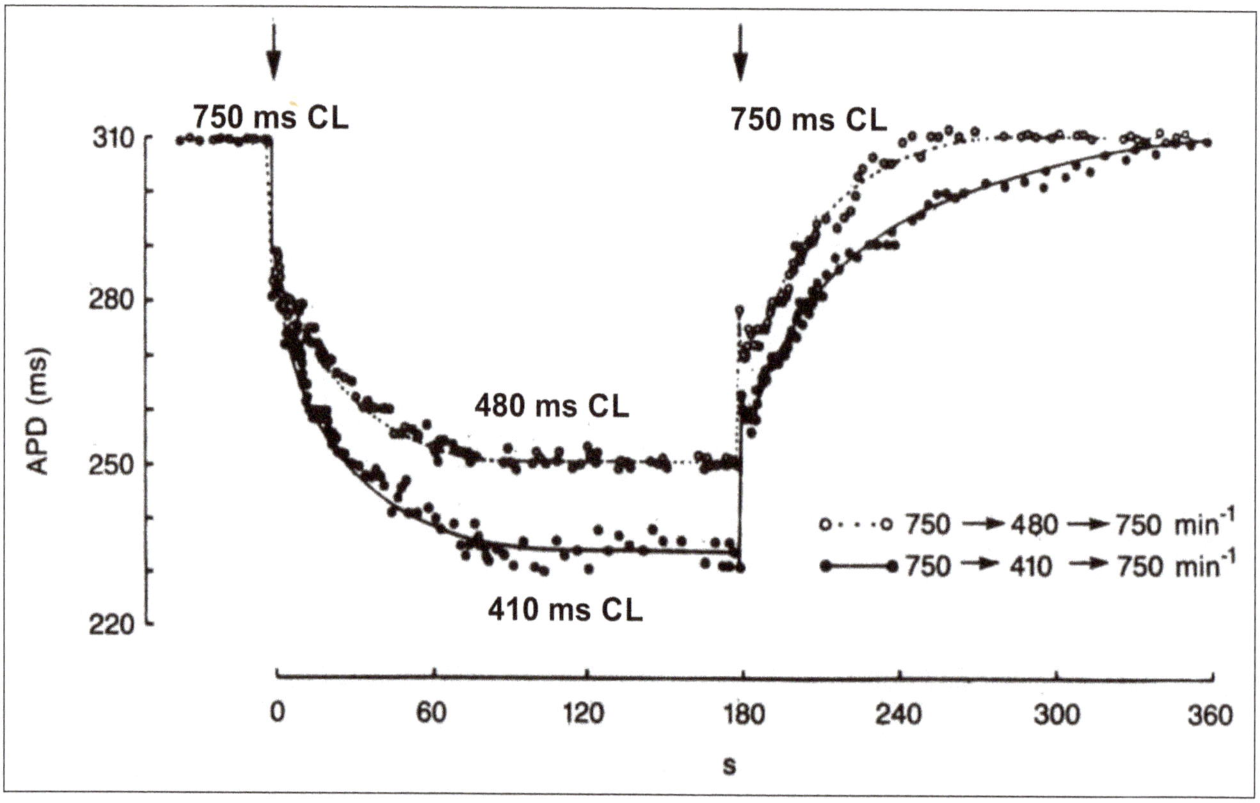

Figure 7-7 Changes in APD with decreased cycle length. Monophasic action potential duration (APD in milliseconds = ms) of human right ventricle is plotted vs. time (seconds = s). (Reproduced from Franz MR, Swerdlow CD, et al. Cycle length dependence of human action potential duration *in vivo*. Effects of single extrastimuli, sudden sustained rate acceleration and deceleration, and different steady-state frequencies. *J Clin Invest.* 1988;82:972–979.)

The relationship between cycle length and APD varies in different regions. In general, Purkinje cells have a greater sensitivity to changes in cycle length than ventricular muscle cells, which in turn have a greater sensitivity than atrial cells. Within the ventricles and Purkinje system, cells with the longer APDs show more shortening with decreased cycle length than cells with short APD. For this reason, heterogeneity of repolarization and refractoriness is reduced at short cycle lengths and increased at long cycle lengths.

Initial Rapid Shortening of APD Due to Intracellular Ca^{2+} and I_{Ks}

The rapid initial shortening of the repolarization phase (shown in Figure 7-6 and Figure 7-7) results primarily from decreased I_{CaL}. As previously explained, initial inactivation of the L-type Ca^{2+} channel is caused by interaction of intracellular Ca^{2+} with the channel protein (Figure 7-2). More Ca^{2+} enters the cell when cycle length is decreased and intracellular Ca^{2+} initially increases since the Na^+–Ca^{2+} exchanger does not have time to extrude the Ca^{2+} from the cell. Accumulated Ca^{2+} enhances inactivation and slows recovery from inactivation of I_{CaL}, resulting in fewer available L-type Ca^{2+} channels with each subsequent action potential. Since I_{CaL} is a primary cause of the plateau phase of repolarization, a decrease in I_{CaL} shortens the plateau and APD.

Although I_{Ks} makes only a small contribution to ventricular repolarization in human hearts at normal heart rates, I_{Ks} increases at short cycle lengths because these channels open more quickly contributing more repolarizing current to acceleration of repolarization at fast rates. I_{Ks} also assumes a greater role in repolarization in the presence of sympathetic (β-adrenergic) stimulation which enhances this current. During sympathetic stimulation, I_{Ks} contributes significantly to rate-dependent shortening. During β-adrenergic stimulation, there is an accumulation of open I_{Ks} channels over time through which repolarizing current continues to flow, because at these short cycle lengths channel inactivation is slowed.

Slower Phase of APD Shortening (Accommodation) and Na^+–K^+ Pump

Accomodation (the slower phase of shortening of APD to a new steady state as cycle length is decreased) requires several minutes (Figure 7-6 and Figure 7-7). This phase has a different mechanism than the initial rapid phase of shortening. During activation at the decreased cycle length, increased Na^+ enters the cell via I_{Na} because of the increased frequency of action potential upstrokes. In addition, as Ca^{2+} accumulates it is removed from the cell in exchange for Na^+ by the Na^+–Ca^{2+} exchanger, further contributing to an increase in intracellular Na^+. The increase in intracellular Na^+ stimulates the Na^+–K^+ pump to remove the Na^+, generating increased outward I_p during repolarization that shortens APD.

Additional Mechanisms

Superimposed on these normal mechanisms controlling rate-dependent changes in APD are the effects of clinical (heritable) conditions leading to EADs and the associated alteration of the ion channels. Compared to normal, LQT1 (with loss of function of I_{Ks}) results in decreased shortening of APD (QT interval) during cycle length shortening because the normal role of I_{Ks} in acceleration of repolarization is absent. On the other hand, in LQT3 (with gain in function of late I_{Na}) action potentials shorten more than normal with decreased cycle length because of increased Na^+ stimulated I_p, resulting in a steeper QT-RR relationship.

EAD Potentiation at Long Cycle Lengths

Slowing of rate (lengthening cycle length), by prolonging APD, potentiates the occurrence of EADs by allowing more time for activation of the inward currents that cause them (Figure 7-5). Likewise, increase in rate (shortening cycle length) can prevent EADs by shortening APD, preventing these currents. **Figure 7-8** illustrates these rate effects under conditions favoring the occurrence of EADs such as a loss of function of a component of I_K or gain of function of I_{Na}.

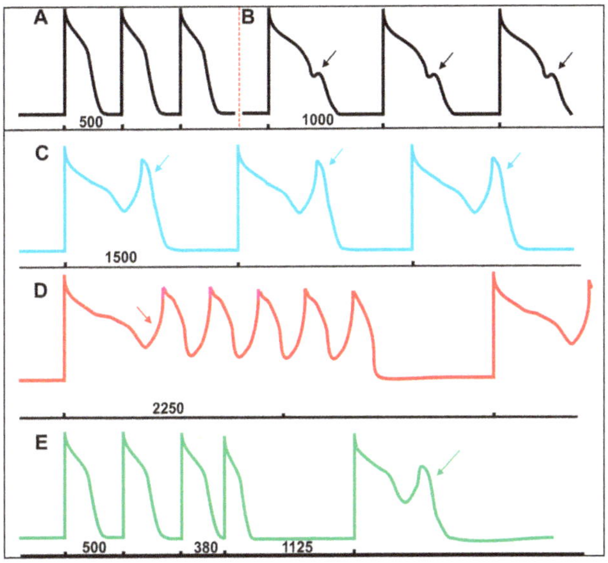

Figure 7-8 Effects of cycle length on action potential duration (APD) and EADs. Cycle length is indicated by time marks on abscissa under each trace, in ms.

Figure 7-8, Panel A (first three impulses at the left) diagrams Purkinje cell action potentials occurring at a cycle length of 500 ms. At this cycle length, APD is not long enough to generate EADs. EADs appear in Panel B (indicated by the arrows), when APD prolongs because of the increased cycle length to 1000 ms. In Panel C, after further increase of the cycle length to 1500 ms and the resultant prolongation of APD, the EADs give rise to single triggered action potentials (blue arrows). In Panel D, when cycle length is increased further, a number of triggered action potentials (triggered activity, red arrow) occur because of additional prolongation of the APD.

Even a single long cycle length can lead to prolongation of APD of the subsequent action potential and EADs and triggered activity under appropriate conditions such as genetic or drug-induced ion-channel alterations. For example, as shown in Figure 7-8, Panel E, when action potentials occur at a cycle length at which EADs are not occurring (500 ms at the left), a premature impulse (380-ms coupling interval) is followed by a long cycle length (1125 ms). This is possibly caused by a compensatory pause and can lead to prolongation of the action potential and an EAD (green arrow). This phenomenon is the basis for the use of "short-long" stimulus patterns in clinical studies in an attempt to initiate EAD-triggered arrhythmias (see section on electrical stimulation).

Effects of Premature Impulses on APD and EADs

APD is affected by a single premature impulse. The effects are relevant to the effects of programmed premature stimulation on EAD-triggered activity described later in this chapter. The APD of premature action potentials is shortened, and therefore, typical programmed premature stimulation protocols neither cause EADs nor induce EAD-dependent triggered activity, contrary to the effects of premature stimulation to induce DAD-triggered activity (see Chapter 6).

Figure 7-9 shows the relationship of premature cycle length to ventricular muscle APD in the human heart (7 different subjects represented by the 7 curves). APD of the premature impulse (from monophasic action potential recordings described above) is plotted against premature (extrastimulus) cycle length.

At the shortest premature coupling interval (extrastimulus cycle length of 200 ms) the APD has substantially shorter duration than the steady-state action potentials at the basic drive cycle length of 600 ms. As premature coupling interval (extrastimulus cycle length) increases, a sharp increase in APD occurs, followed by a slower increase. The recovery of APD with increasing premature coupling interval is referred to as *restitution*.

The cause of the shortening of APD with premature excitation is accounted for by the effects of premature stimulation on both inward and outward currents. A decrease in I_{CaL} recovery from inactivation during the premature cycle length results in fewer channels available to carry inward current during the premature action potential plateau phase 2. An increased outward current through I_{Ks} channels also occurs due to both increased speed of activation and accumulation of channels in the open state. Other channels such as I_{to} and I_{Kr} are also involved. The functions of these channels return toward normal as premature cycle length increases. Owing to the different ion channel properties in different regions of the heart, the details concerning patterns and mechanisms of restitution vary for different regions and pathologies, although in all regions repolarization is accelerated after premature activation.

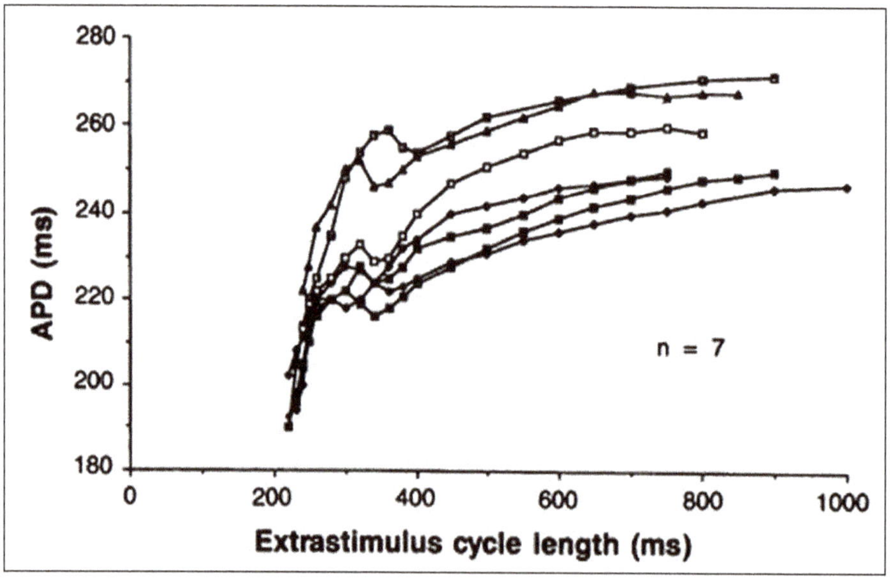

Figure 7-9 Electrical restitution curves of right ventricular myocardium at a basic drive cycle length of 600 ms in 7 different subjects. APD = action potential duration, extrastimulus cycle length refers to premature cycle length. (Reproduced from Franz MR, Swerdlow CD, et al. Cycle length dependence of human action potential duration in vivo. Effects of single extrastimuli, sudden sustained rate acceleration and deceleration,and different steady-state frequencies. *J Clin Invest.* 1988;82:972–979.)

Rate of EAD-Triggered Activity

The rate of EAD-induced triggered activity, if perpetuated by EADs or abnormal automaticity, is expected to be related to the level of membrane potential at which this triggered activity occurs. As described in Figure 4-1, the rate of abnormal automaticity increases as membrane potential becomes less negative. This means that phase 2- and early phase 3-generated triggered activity would be more rapid than later phase 3-generated triggered activity since they occur at a less negative membrane potential. Even so, based on experimental laboratory studies, the maximum rate generated by abnormal automaticity or DAD-triggered activity is probably not rapid enough to explain the rapid rate of > 170 bpm of the polymorphic ventricular tachycardia (torsades de pointes)—this being the hallmark triggered arrhythmia accompanying congenital and acquired LQT syndromes. The more rapid rate of torsades de pointes might be explained by competing foci of multiple simultaneously triggered cells as proposed in one experimental model (multifocal origin).

Simultaneously, a multifocal model might also explain the peculiar polymorphic characteristic of this arrhythmia's "twisting of the points." Competing foci of triggered cells with slightly different rates, alternating control of ventricular activation (multifocal origin) to produce changes in the activation pattern of the ventricles might result in the twisting pattern. This model presumes that the generation of EADs is widespread, but certain sites have a higher tendency to generate triggered action potentials due to intrinsically long APDs—e.g., midmyocardial cells or Purkinje cells—greater adrenergic sensitivity, or other factors. Other models for torsades de pointes that could result in the rapid rate involve reentry initiated by a premature EAD because of heterogeneous APD as mentioned previously, with the location of reentrant circuits shifting across the heart or shifting exit routes from a single circuit.

Autonomic Nervous System Effects on EADs and EAD-Triggered Activity

Sympathetic Nervous System

Sympathetic effects in the ventricles that are expressed as alterations in the QT interval and T-wave morphology are the result of both the actions of norepinephrine (β_1-adrenergic stimulation) on repolarization and the heterogeneous distribution of the sympathetic nerve endings. Both of these properties also influence EADs and EAD-triggered activity.

Acceleration of repolarization. The sympathetic nervous system has important actions on ion channels that affect repolarization of Purkinje and ventricular muscle cells, thereby influencing EADs by altering APD. Norepinephrine accelerates repolarization, independent of its effects on cycle length. It does this by acting on 3 membrane currents involved in repolarization: I_{CaL}, I_{Ks}, and I_P. Norepinephrine increases the magnitude of I_{CaL}, elevating the plateau phase 2 to more positive levels while increasing Ca^{2+} entry into the cell and uptake of Ca^{2+} by the SR. Increased intracellular Ca^{2+} inactivates I_{CaL} more rapidly through Ca^{2+}-induced inactivation described in Figure 7-2, and shortens the duration of the plateau phase 2 (even though it is more positive). Norepinephrine stimulation also increases activation of I_{Ks} that provides outward current accelerating phase 3 repolarization (Figure 7-2). Another contributing factor to shortening of APD is an increase in outward I_P owing to stimulation of the Na^+–K^+ pump by norepinephrine. The effects that accelerate repolarization as described above are amplified by the concomitant increase in heart rate that may occur with sympathetic activation (but does not always; see heterogeneous effects, below). On the basis of these effects on repolarization alone, it might be predicted that sympathetic activity suppresses EADs and the initiation of EAD-triggered activity.

However, sympathetic stimulation also has direct effects on EADs and triggered activity independent of effects on repolarization. The increased intracellular Ca^{2+} increases I_{NCX}. The increase in both I_{CaL} and I_{NCX} that underlie EADs (Figure 7-5) can increase their amplitude, enhancing their ability to cause triggered activity despite the acceleration of repolarization.

Increased rate and duration of triggered arrhythmias. Once a triggered arrhythmia has been induced, if EADs are the cause of its perpetuation, the increase in I_{CaL} and I_{NCX} caused by sympathetic stimulation would increase its rate and possibly its duration. If abnormal automaticity is the cause of its perpetuation, sympathetic stimulation would accelerate rate by increasing I_{CaL} and I_{NCX} that cause SDD at reduced levels of membrane potential (see Figure 4-4). If perpetuation of triggered activity is dependent on DADs (see Chapter 5), rate and duration would also be increased as a result of increased intracellular Ca^{2+} that increases DAD amplitude. The effects of sympathetic stimulation on rate and duration if perpetuation is caused by a reentrant mechanism are described in the next section.

Heterogeneous effects. The differential effects of sympathetic stimulation on ventricular muscle cells in different regions of the ventricular wall, caused by both the regional difference in importance of I_{Ks} on repolarization and the heterogeneous distribution of sympathetic nerve endings, might also have an effect on EAD-triggered activity. The effects of sympathetic stimulation on repolarization are not uniform throughout the ventricular walls. Since an important mechanism of acceleration of repolarization is an increase in I_{Ks}, midmyocardial (M) cells are little affected because they have a weak I_{Ks} compared to a stronger manifestation of this current in epicardial and endocardial muscle. Therefore, the direct and rate-dependent effects of sympathetic stimulation on accelerating repolarization are greater in epicardial and endocardial muscle than in the midmyocardial regions. The differential effects tend to increase the differences (heterogeneity) in action potential repolarization and heterogeneity of refractoriness, since APD and refractoriness in epicardial and endocardial regions become shorter while midmyocardial APD and refractoriness remain the same. The increased heterogeneity is expected to facilitate initiation and perpetuation of EAD-triggered activity when it is caused by reentry. A short-coupled, premature impulse initiated by an EAD blocks in a region of long APD and conducts through regions with shorter APDs more easily when heterogeneity is increased, according to the model for reentry described in Figure 9-14

The heterogeneous distribution of the sympathetic nerve endings in the heart also underlies increased differences of effects on repolarization in different regions resulting from sympathetic stimulation that might perpetuate EAD-triggered arrhythmias by the model for reentry described in Figure 9-14. The right side of the sympathetic nervous system innervates mainly the sinus and A-V nodes, the right ventricles, and the anterior left ventricle. The left side influences the posterior left ventricle more than the anterior and lateral and has little chronotropic effect. According to the model of increased heterogeneity based on sympathetic nerve distribution, excision of the source of the sympathetics on the left side to the heart (cervical sympathetic ganglion), which is sometimes effective therapy for the LQT syndrome (see Chapter 8), would lengthen repolarization on the posterior ventricular surface, reduce the heterogeneity of repolarization and refractory period, and reduce perpetuation of triggered activity caused by reentry. While this is a possible mechanism for the antiarrhythmic effect of cervical sympathectemy, it requires additional verification.

Parasympathetic Nervous System

Parasympathetic activation might cause EAD-triggered activity in the ventricles in situations where occurrence of EADs is dependent on bradycardia. The parasympathetics slow the heart rate that prolongs APD (Figure 7-8) without directly affecting ion channels that cause EADs. On the other hand, parasympathetic stimulation might inhibit EADs when they are caused by sympathetic activation through parasympathetic accentuated antagonism of the sympathetic release of norepinephrine. This same accentuated antagonism should also slow the rate of EAD-triggered arrhythmias when perpetuation is caused by EADs, abnormal automaticity, and DAD-triggered activity.

In atrial myocardium, parasympathetic stimulation should slow EAD-triggered activity in the atria by increasing outward I_{KACh}. Vagal stimulation might terminate triggered activity in the atria by repolarizing the membrane potential back to a highly negative level through the increased outward K^+ current (I_{KACh}).

Pharmacological Effects on Mechanisms of EADs and Triggered Activity

The pharmacology of EADs and triggered activity as determined from laboratory experiments mostly on isolated tissues is complicated and is not described in detail here. In the sections on automaticity (Part I) and DADs (Chapters 5 and 6) emphasis is placed on effects of drugs that can assist in determining the arrhythmogenic mechanisms because of a unique response of the mechanism to the drug. With regard to EAD-dependent triggered activity, there is no unique drug response that would assist in identifying this mechanism as the cause of a clinical arrhythmia. Sometimes, however, the response of an arrhythmia helps to confirm an EAD mechanism in conjunction with other features of the arrhythmia.

EAD-induced triggered activity is prevented in experimental models by drugs that alter many of the factors that lead to EADs. Further information on drugs that have been used in clinical studies on EADs is included in Chapter 8. Briefly, drugs that have been effective in experimental models include drugs that shorten APD in ventricular muscle and Purkinje fibers, such as Vaughan Williams Class IB Na^+ channel-blocking drugs (lidocaine); drugs that interfere with inward currents, for example, L-type Ca^{2+} channel-blocking drugs (verapamil), and late Na^+ current-blocking drugs (mexilitene, flecainide, and ranolazine in LQT3); and drugs that interfere with the effects of the sympathetic nervous system (β-blockers).

Some of these drugs have had effectiveness in limited clinical studies. These drugs also affect other arrhythmogenic mechanisms so they cannot be used to identify EAD-induced triggered arrhythmias. It is unlikely that adenosine, a drug used to identify other mechanisms of arrhythmias, would have a direct effect in the ventricle to stop EAD-induced triggered arrhythmias owing to its lack of direct effects on ventricular ion channels, although it might interfere with the actions of the sympathetic nervous system. Bradycardia caused by adenosine might exacerbate EADs.

Certain chemically diverse drugs can cause the appearance of EADs and triggered activity. Many of them block I_{Kr} (*KCNH2* channel), which may be the mechanism. Drugs with this effect prolong the time course of repolarization of ventricular muscle and Purkinje cells and lead to a prolongation of the QT interval on the ECG, designated as "acquired LQT." Included in this group of drugs are class IA antiarrhythmic drugs, such as disopyramide and quinidine, and class III antiarrhythmic drugs, such as sotalol and dofetilide.

Another more recently discovered effect of drugs that prolong the QT is an inhibition of a tyrosine kinase enzyme (designated as phosphoinositide 3-kinases (PI3Ks)). This enzyme helps to control repolarization by playing a role in the inactivation process of the persistent Na^+ current, $I_{Na\ late}$. Therefore, its inhibition prolongs APD by increasing this persistent current. The time course of this effect is prolonged compared to the rapid inhibition of I_{Kr} accounting for the long-time course of dofetilide to prolong the QT.

Drug-induced triggered activity associated with the acquired LQT syndrome is described in Chapter 8.

IDENTIFYING EAD-TRIGGERED ACTIVITY AS A CAUSE OF CLINICAL ARRHYTHMIAS

ECG Characteristics of Triggered Arrhythmias

The features of the ECG are the best indicators to suggest EADs and EAD-triggered activity, taking precedence over effects of electrical stimulation that are important in identifying other arrhythmogenic mechanisms. Some of the key features are: prolongation of the QT interval, U waves, premature ventricular depolarizations during the T wave, and a short/long cycle length pattern of arrhythmia initiation.

An important ECG characteristic that is associated with EAD-triggered activity is the prolongation of the QT interval resulting from lengthening of ventricular muscle APD associated with genetic or acquired LQT syndrome. Changes in T-wave morphology may also occur. These changes are illustrated in more detail in Chapter 8.

There also may be prominent U waves associated with EADs. U waves can occur on the normal ECG, manifested as a low amplitude (< 0.1 mV) wave following the T wave with the same polarity as the T wave. In patients with LQT syndrome, one hypothesis is that exaggerated U waves may be caused by EADs in Purkinje or muscle cells. Theoretically, prominent EADs in a sufficiently large area of the ventricles would lead to enough extracellular current flow to cause the U-wave deflection on the ECG. Sometimes, U waves are not observed on the ECG until shortly before the onset of torsades de pointes, the arrhythmia commonly associated with LQT and hypothesized to be initiated by EADs (Chapter 8).

LQT syndromes are also sometimes associated with premature ventricular depolarizations that occur shortly after the peak of the T wave and possibly during the end of a U wave, consistent with the occurrence of EADs at the end of phase 2 or during phase 3 of the prolonged action potential. Torsades de pointes begins with a premature ventricular depolarization that also occurs shortly after the peak of the T wave or U wave, consistent with a triggered impulse (Figure 8-1).

In many cases (but not all), particularly in congenital LQT2 and LQT3 and acquired LQT, a long cycle length following a short cycle length precedes the first tachycardia impulse. For example, a spontaneously occurring premature impulse (short cycle length) may be followed by a long cycle length owing to resetting of the dominant pacemaker. The long cycle length potentiates action potential prolongation of the associated impulse (Figure 7-8, Panel E), which is expected to increase the amplitude of the EAD and the U wave. If this gives rise to a triggered impulse that starts tachycardia, the triggered impulse would have a short coupling interval to the phase 0 of the action potential occurring after the long cycle length (Chapter 8).

The characteristics of the ECG just described, while highly suggestive of EADs and EAD-triggered arrhythmias, are not completely specific. Prolonged QT interval and torsades de pointes can occur in clinical situations in which other mechanisms of arrhythmogenesis predominate. Despite the association of U waves with EAD-triggered activity, they are not entirely a specific identifier. Theoretically, U waves might be caused by DADs, which can result in depolarization after the end of the T wave. U waves are also caused by other factors not associated with triggered arrhythmias, such as hypokalemia.

Electrical Stimulation and Characteristics of EAD-Dependent Triggered Activity

The expected clinical effects of electrical stimulation on EAD-triggered activity are based on the property that the time course of repolarization is cycle-length dependent (see Figures 7-7 and 7-8). Overdrive pacing or premature stimulation-induced shortening of the cycle length (as done in clinical protocols), accelerates repolarization and suppresses EADs, while prolongation of the cycle length lengthens repolarization and enhances EADs. This property underlies the response of patients with LQT to these standard protocols, described in the next chapter.

Limited Use of Pharmacological Agents to Identify EAD-Induced Triggered Arrhythmias

In general, most drugs that prevent or terminate EAD-triggered activity also affect other arrhythmogenic mechanisms and are not very useful for identifying an EAD mechanism. Some drugs are described with the arrhythmia examples in Chapter 8.

SUMMARY

Early afterdepolarizations (EADs) occur during phase 2 or 3 of repolarization, characterized by a transient shift of membrane potential in a positive (depolarizing) direction. The shift in membrane potential can lead to regenerative inward (depolarizing) current that causes triggered action potentials.

EADs and triggered activity are often associated with a critical prolongation of APD manifested as a long QT interval and are associated with long QT syndromes (LQTS). Gene mutations of repolarizing ion channels leading to a reduction in outward current (loss of function of I_{Kr}, I_{Ks}, or I_{K1}) or an increase in inward current (gain of function of I_{Na} or I_{CaL}) prolongs APD. EADs during phase 2 or early phase 3 result from decreased inactivation of I_{CaL}. Increased I_{NCX} causes EADs during phase 3 repolarization.

Slowing of heart rate by prolonging APD potentiates the occurrence of EADs and triggered arrhythmias. An increase in rate can prevent EADs by shortening APD. Therefore, programmed stimulation protocols do not initiate EAD-triggered activity but might prevent it.

Once initiated by an EAD, triggered activity may be perpetuated by additional EADs, abnormal automaticity or DAD-triggered activity. Another model for torsades de pointes, an arrhythmia associated with EADs, involve reentry initiated by a premature impulse caused by an EAD with the location of reentrant circuits shifting across the heart or shifting exit routes from a single circuit.

Sympathetic stimulation can initiate triggered arrhythmias by increasing both I_{CaL} and I_{NCX} that underlie EADs. Once a triggered arrhythmia has been induced, sympathetic stimulation would increase its rate and duration. Parasympathetic activation can cause EAD-triggered activity in the ventricles by slowing the heart rate that prolongs APD. On the other hand, parasympathetic stimulation might inhibit EADs when they are caused by sympathetic activation by antagonizing the sympathetic effects.

The features of the ECG are the best indicators that are suggestive of EADs and EAD-triggered activity. Prolongation of the QT interval is associated with EAD-triggered activity. Exaggerated U waves may also occur that are caused by EADs in Purkinje or muscle cells. Torsades de pointes often begins with a premature ventricular depolarization shortly after the peak of the T wave or U wave. In congenital LQT2 and LQT3 and acquired LQT, a long cycle length following a short cycle length precedes the first tachycardia impulse. The long cycle length potentiates action potential prolongation that in turn should enhance EADs.

SOURCES

Clancy CE, Tateyama M, Kass RS. Insights into the molecular mechanisms of bradycardia-triggered arrhythmias in long QT-3 syndrome. *J Clin Invest.* 2002;110:1251–1262.

Decker KF, Heijman J, Silva JR, et al. Properties and ionic mechanisms of action potential adaptation, restitution, and accommodation in canine epicardium. *Am J Physiol Heart Circ Physiol.* 2009;296:H1017–H1026.

Roden DM. Long-QT syndrome. *N Engl J Med.* 2008;358:169–176.

Roden DM, Yang T. Protecting the heart against arrhythmias: Potassium current physiology and repolarization reserve. *Circulation.* 2005;112;1376–1378.

Silva J, Rudy Y. Subunit interaction determines IKs participation in cardiac repolarization and repolarization reserve. *Circulation.* 2005;112:1384–1391.

Viswanathan PC, Yoram R. Cellular arrhythmogenic effects of congenital and acquired long-QT syndrome in the heterogeneous myocardium. *Circulation.* 2000;101:1192–1198.

Viswanathan PC, Yoram R. Pause induced early afterdepolarizations in the long QT syndrome: a simulation study. *Cardiovasc Res.* 1999;42:530–542.

Volders PGA, Vos MA, Szabo B, et al. Progress in the understanding of cardiac early afterdepolarizations and torsades de pointes: Time to revise current concepts. *Cardiovasc Res.* 2000;46:376–339.

Weiss JN, Garfinkel A, Karagueuzian HS. Early afterdepolarizations and cardiac arrhythmias. *Heart Rhythm.* 2010;7:1891–1899.

CHAPTER

8

Early Afterdepolarizations: Triggered Arrhythmias

The previous chapter describes the basic electrophysiology of early afterdepolarizations (EADs) and how they cause triggered activity. In this chapter, examples of clinical arrhythmias are described that demonstrate properties of triggered activity caused by EADs.

Congenital Long QT (LQT) Syndromes

ARRHYTHMIAS DUE TO CONGENITAL LQT SYNDROMES

Figure 8-1 shows an ECG from a patient with LQT2. A genetic alteration in the ion channel I_{Kr} involved in action potential repolarization is responsible for a prolonged QT interval corrected for heart rate (QTc) measuring greater than 500 ms (Figure 8-1, Panel A). The alterations in membrane currents and how they affect action potential duration (APD) are described in Chapter 7 and Table 7-1. An abnormally long QTc in general is greater than approximately 460 ms in women and 440 ms in men. A QTc interval of more than 500 ms is indicative of a particularly high risk for sudden death. The ECG in Figure 8-1, Panel B shows the polymorphic ventricular tachycardia called torsades de pointes (black arrow) (rate > 170 bpm, undulating QRS, sometimes referred to as torsade or torsades). When the tachycardia is self-terminating, presyncope and syncope can occur—and when it progresses to VF, sudden death can occur. No structural evidence of heart disease is present in these patients. In this case tachycardia terminated, the termination is not shown.

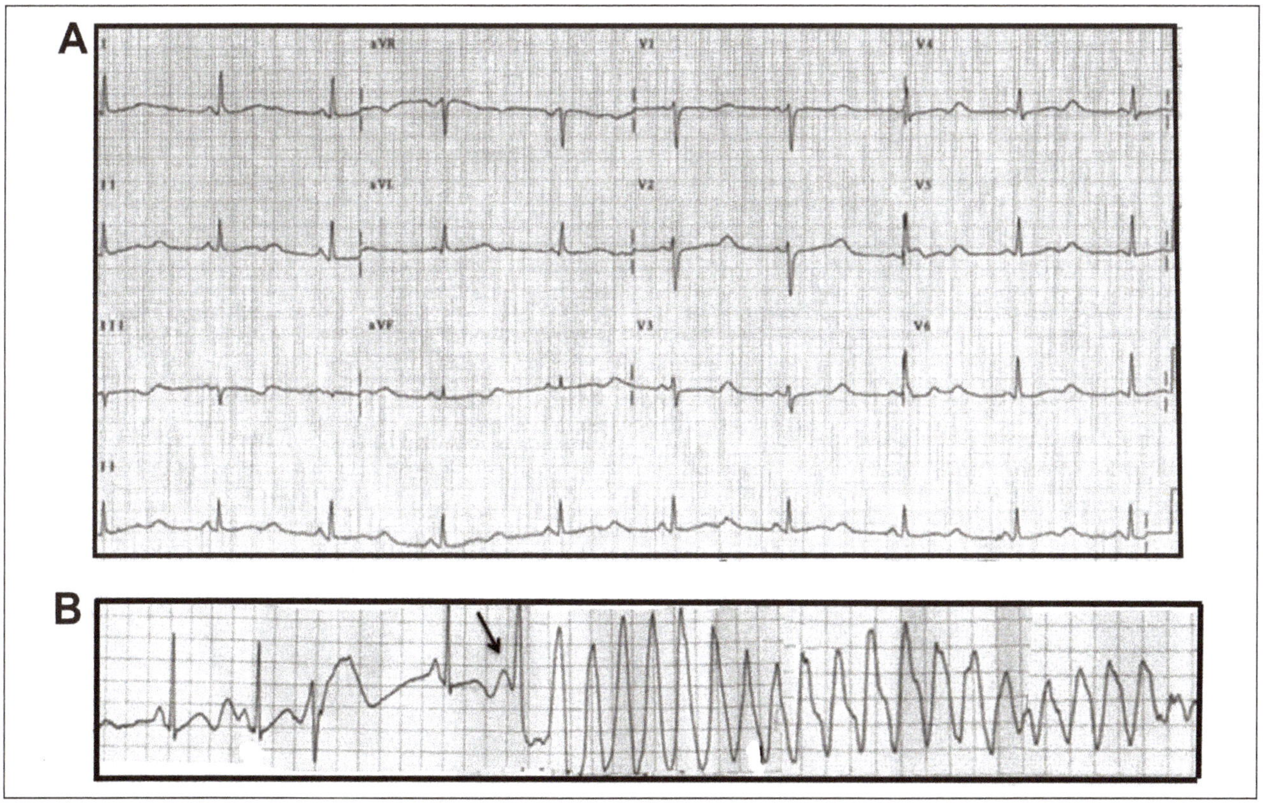

Figure 8-1 **Panel A:** 12-lead ECG recorded during sinus rhythm from a patient with a history of syncope. **Panel B:** Lead II rhythm strip recorded during syncopal episode caused by torsades de pointes.

Electrophysiological Foundations of Cardiac Arrhythmias: A Bridge Between Basic Mechanisms and Clinical Electrophysiology, Second Edition.
© 2020 Andrew L. Wit, Penelope A. Boyden, Mark E. Josephson, Hein J. Wellens. Cardiotext Publishing, ISBN: 978-1-942909-42-2.

GENETIC MUTATIONS IN CONGENITAL LONG QT SYNDROME

Hundreds of mutations in more than a dozen genes can cause congenital long QT (LQT) syndrome. Only a brief introductory description is provided here. These syndromes have been designated LQT1–LQT13, depending on the location of the mutation. Low penetrance of these mutations in some patients can result in the absence of a LQT phenotype on the ECG. They are still at risk for life-threatening arrhythmias and may be at particular risk if they are administered QT interval-prolonging drugs (see section below on acquired LQT syndrome). The two most common forms of congenital LQT syndrome, LQT1 and LQT2, are autosomal dominant forms with a pure cardiac phenotype that result from loss-of-function mutations in genes designated *KCNQ1* (LQT1; Romano Ward syndrome) and *KCNH2* (LQT2), that underlie the outward currents I_{Ks} and I_{Kr} (see Table 7-1). Along with the gain of function mutation in *SCN5A* (LQT3) (Table 7-1) the mutations in these three genes, account for approximately 75% of clinically defined LQT syndrome. Other genes contribute an additional 5% collectively. The genes responsible for an estimated 20% of congenital LQT syndrome have not been defined.

ELECTROPHYSIOLOGY OF CONGENITAL LQT SYNDROMES; RELATIONSHIP TO EADS AND TRIGGERED ACTIVITY

Table 8-1 summarizes the clinical electrophysiological characteristics of the three most common forms of the LQT syndrome. These characteristics are used to formulate the hypothesis that LQT arrhythmias accompanying these syndromes are related to the occurrence of EADs. However, there is a lack of clinical tools that would help to identify an EAD mechanism more precisely, such as the response to electrical stimulation and drugs that have been used to demonstrate automaticity or DAD-triggered activity. Some clinical studies have used monophasic action potential recordings to show EADs, which have provided some confirmation of their occurrence despite the problems associated with this method, mainly distinguishing valid recordings from artifacts.

Resting ECG

The resting ECG is often characterized by sinus bradycardia. The QRS morphology is normal. Despite the fact that congenital LQT syndromes are all related to prolongation of repolarization, after 2 years of age the characteristics of the ST segment and the T waves differ among the different syndromes (Table 8-1, row 1). These differences are diagrammed in **Figure 8-2**, which shows the typical patterns. Exceptions and variants occur. The reason for the different patterns is not entirely certain.

Table 8-1 Clinical Electrophysiology of Common Congenital LQT Syndromes

Characteristics	LQT1 (decreased I_{Ks})	LQT2 (decreased I_{Kr})	LQT3 (increased I_{Na})
1) T wave of the sinus rhythm ECG	Broad T wave	Low-amplitude T wave with notching	Long isoelectric ST segment
2) Environmental triggers	Exercise, emotional or physical stress	Emotional or physical stress, sudden loud noise	Rest, sleep
3) ECG at onset of arrhythmia	Sinus rate acceleration, no pause	Pause	Bradycardia?
4) Cycle length dependence of QT	Failure to shorten	Normal	Shortens more than normal
5) Clinical response to β-blockers	Yes	Yes, but less than LQT1	Uncertain

(Modified from Roden DM, Long QT syndrome. *N Engl J Med.* 2008;358:169–176.)

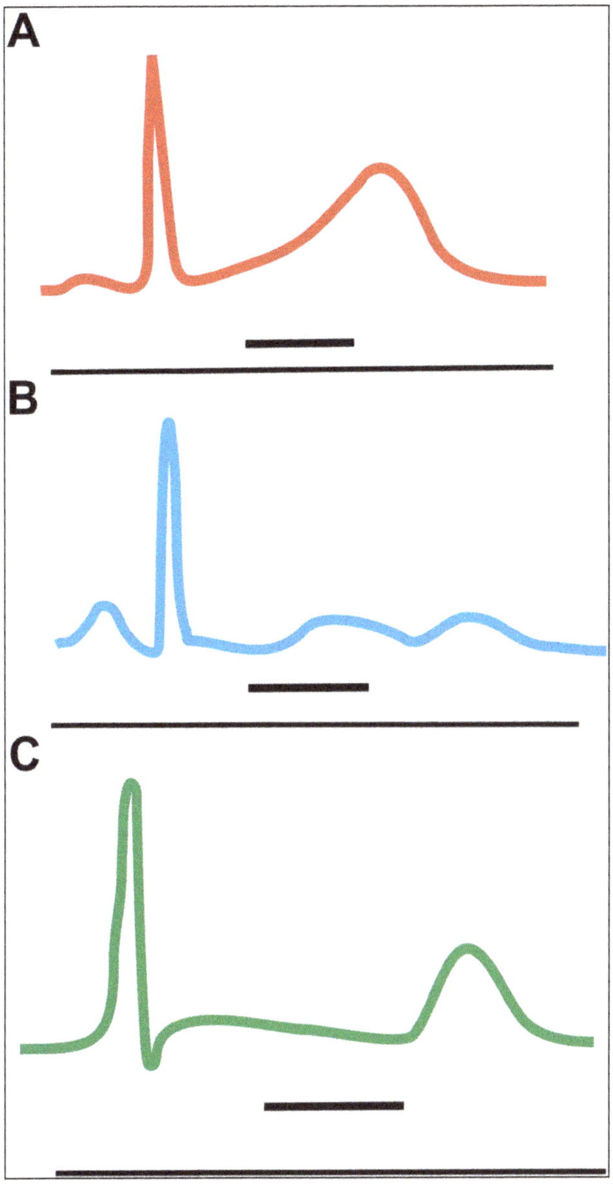

Figure 8-2 Diagrams of ST segment and T-wave morphologies in lead II in LQT1 (**Panel A**), LQT2 (**Panel B**), and LQT3 (**Panel C**). **Horizontal bar** below T wave in each panel represents 200 ms.

LQT1 (Figure 8-2, Panel A) is associated with a long QT interval and smooth, broad T wave. This characteristic of the QT might result if the loss of function of I_{Ks} (which underlies LQT1), prolongs repolarization relatively equally throughout the ventricular wall without increasing the differences (dispersion) of repolarization that exists in the normal heart.

LQT2 is associated with a low-amplitude, often bifid, T wave in most leads (Figure 8-2, Panel B). This feature is also evident in Figure 8-1, Panel A. A theoretical model to explain this characteristic is that the loss of function of I_{Kr} in LQT2 produces more action potential prolongation in midmyocardial (M) cells than in epicardial or endocardial muscle cells. This occurs because the epicardial and endocardial cells also have I_{Ks}, which assumes a greater role in repolarization after removal of I_{Kr} (repolarization reserve), while midmyocardial cells lack a significant I_{Ks} to assume this role. If there is a greater prolongation of midmyocardial cell APDs, increased heterogeneity of APD might account for the bifid T waves. However, differential changes in APD in different layers of the ventricular wall are tempered by electrotonic current flow between the regions, through gap junctions. Another possibility is that the second component of the T wave is actually a U wave.

LQT3 is associated with a long isoelectric ST segment and a narrow, tall, peaked T wave (Figure 8-2, Panel C). A proposed mechanism is that the gain in function of late I_{Na} associated with LQT3 (Table 7-1) prolongs action potential phase 2 duration in epicardial and endocardial cells as well as in midmyocardial (M) cells. Prolongation of repolarization in epicardial cells, which are responsible for the peak of the T wave, produces a long ST segment with the late-onset T wave possibly related to greater prolongation in midmyocardial cells because of the greater contribution of late I_{Na} to repolarization in this region.

Mode of Onset and Site of Origin of Triggered Ventricular Arrhythmias

Conditions Leading to Onset

A distinguishing feature among the different congenital LQT syndromes are the types of events (triggers) that initiate the occurrence of torsades de pointes (Table 8-1, row 2).

LQT1. The primary initiator of torsades de pointes in LQT1 patients is enhanced sympathetic activity, which can accompany exercise or an emotional or stressful event. Torsades de pointes in LQT1 often follows an acceleration in sinus rate and usually is not associated with pauses, which are prevalent in LQT2 and LQT3 (Table 8-1, row 3). **Figure 8-3** shows the effects of β-adrenergic stimulation in a patient with LQT1.

In Figure 8-3, the ECG at the top left shows a prolonged QTU interval (QT plus U wave) with a prominent late component (small unfilled arrow) at baseline. Epinephrine (5 mg/kg) is administered at the time indicated by the large downward black arrow. Toward the end of the second row, the late component of the TU complex or U wave begins to increase in amplitude, which may indicate occurrence of EADs. In the third row, the U wave continues to increase leading to ventricular premature beats and torsades de pointes which quickly degenerates into ventricular fibrillation (bottom row).

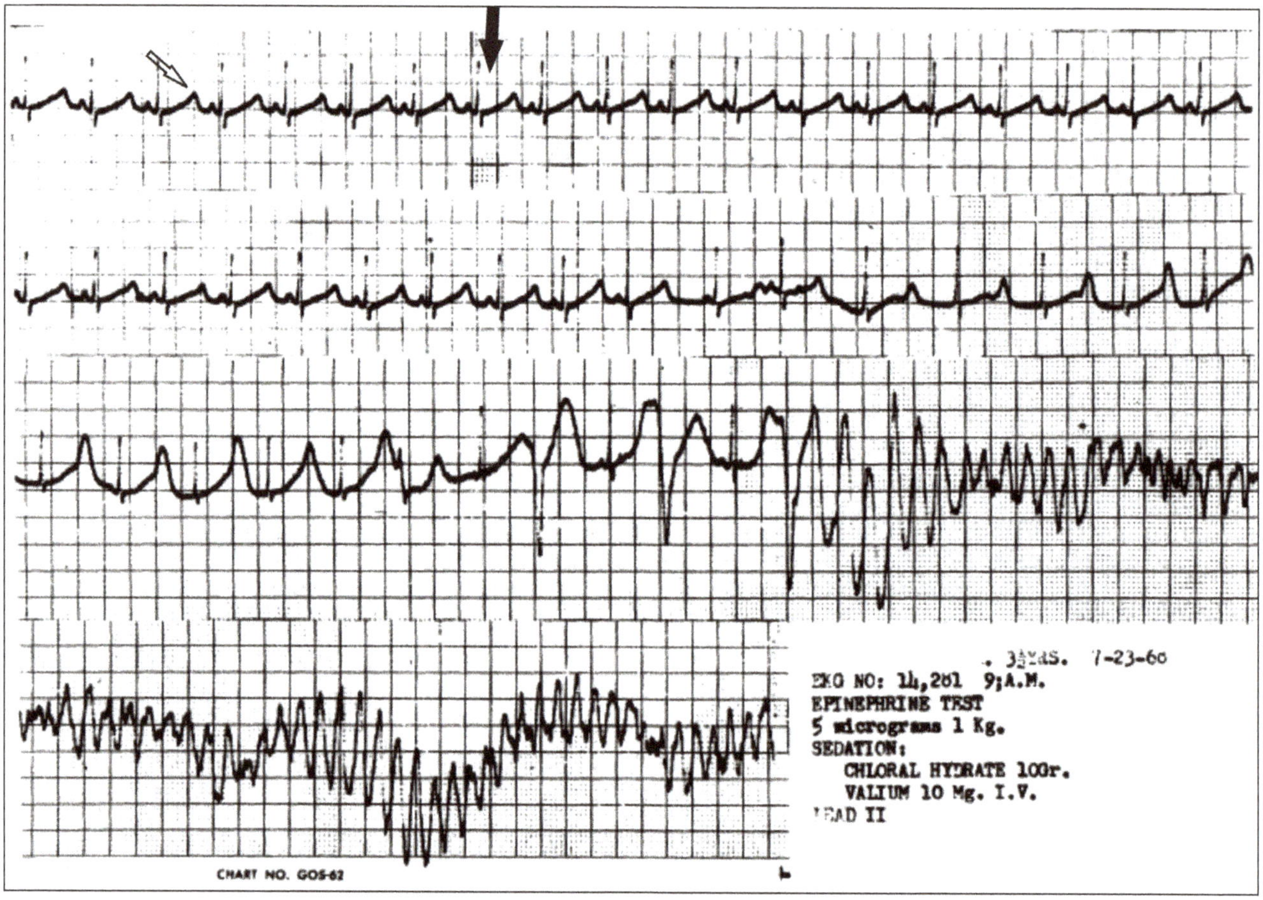

Figure 8-3 Epinephrine-induced torsades de pointes in a patient with congenital LQTS. (Reproduced from Garza LA, Vick RL, et al. Heritable QT prolongation without deafness. *Circulation.* 1970;41:39–48.)

In LQT1, there is an underlying deficiency of I_{Ks}, which normally participates in acceleration of repolarization during sympathetic stimulation. Therefore, the expected acceleration of repolarization (and shortening of the APD) due to an increase in sinus rate accompanying sympathetic stimulation, which normally would tend to inhibit EADs, does not occur in LQT1 (Table 8-1, row 4). Instead, there is a lengthening of the QTc. There also is decreased coupling of β-adrenergic receptors, with I_{Ks} channels contributing to the failure of cycle length-dependent shortening of APD.

T-wave alternans in amplitude or polarity is another feature sometimes seen on the ECG. This is another marker of electrical instability indicating the stress of increased heart rate on repolarization.

β-adrenergic stimulation also increases I_{CaL} and I_{NCX}, which play roles in EAD formation (see Figure 7-5). The combination of failure of shortening of repolarization and increased I_{CaL} and I_{NCX} can lead to EAD initiation and triggered activity. Enhanced EADs could account for the increase in U-wave amplitude preceding the onset of torsades de pointes in Figure 8-3.

If perpetuation of triggered activity is dependent on abnormal automaticity or on DADs (see Chapter 7), these two mechanisms would also be enhanced by increased sympathetic stimulation. If it is caused by reentry (Chapter 7), the dispersion of refractoriness that perpetuates reentry may be increased because of the differential distribution of sympathetic nerves throughout the ventricles or a greater increase in I_{Ks} and acceleration of repolarization in epicardial and endocardial muscle rather than in midmyocardium, which lacks significant I_{Ks}.

Because of the important role of sympathetic activity in the initiation and perpetuation of torsades de pointes in LQT1, β-receptor blockade or left cervical sympathectomy can be effective in reducing syncope or sudden death, although residual events still occur (Table 8-1, row 5).

LQT2. Torsades de pointes can be initiated in LQT2 patients (loss of function of I_{Kr}) by either emotion or stress, but it can also occur at rest. Another relatively specific trigger is a sudden, loud noise. Although emotion and stress are associated with an increase in sympathetic activity, there is often a lack of a significant heart rate increase before onset of torsades de pointes. This possibly might indicate a role for the left sympathetics, which do not have a prominent effect on the sinus node (Chapter 7) while exerting all the other arrhythmogenic effects of the sympathetic nervous system (increased EADs, triggered rate, or heterogeneity of refractoriness).

Exercise is not an important initiator of torsades de pointes in LQT2, possibly because of normal I_{Ks} function. I_{Ks} can accelerate repolarization in the presence of the heart rate increase with exercise; hence, the QT interval shortens during acceleration of the heart rate accompanying exercise which would prevent the occurrence of EADs (Table 8-1, row 4).

In LQT2, torsades de pointes often begins after a short-long-short cycle length sequence, as illustrated in Figure 8-1, Panel B. In this figure, in the sequence leading to onset of the arrhythmia, a premature ventricular depolarization (short cycle) follows the second sinus impulse. The premature impulse is followed by the long cycle length of a compensatory pause. The sinus impulse after the long cycle length is followed by another premature ventricular depolarization shortly after the U wave (short cycle, arrow) followed by torsades de pointes. The long cycle length is likely to potentiate EAD amplitude, leading to triggered activity.

β-blocking drugs reduce arrhythmias and sudden death in patients with LQT2 but less so than in LQT1 (Table 8-1, row 5). Arrhythmias are also reduced by left cardiac sympathectomy. The efficacy of antisympathetic therapy may be increased by using a pacemaker to prevent pauses.

LQT3. Clinically, LQT3 is usually associated with arrhythmias occurring at slow heart rates during rest or sleep (Table 8-1, row 2), a situation that prolongs action potential repolarization and enhances EADs. Rate responsiveness of repolarization is still present (Figure 7-6) and cycle length dependence of the QT interval may even be exaggerated (Table 8-1, row 4). At the slow heart rates characteristic of rest or sleep, increased late I_{Na} caused by a gain of function of the Na^+ channel, results in a larger-than-normal increase in the plateau duration and QT interval, and possibly EADs. The prolongation of repolarization is accentuated by pauses, which often occur in these patients.

β-blockers are less effective in patients with LQT3 than in LQT1 and LQT2 (Table 8-1, row 5), suggesting less of an arrhythmogenic role of the sympathetic nervous system. Preventing the pauses with a pacemaker can enhance the efficacy of β-blocker therapies.

Site of Origin

The site or sites of origin of torsades de pointes in patients with congenital LQT syndromes are unknown. Similarly, the mechanism(s) that underlies the characteristic changes of the QRS axis have not been elucidated from clinical studies, although several theoretical models have been proposed (see Chapter 7).

EFFECTS OF ELECTRICAL STIMULATION ON CLINICAL EAD-TRIGGERED ARRHYTHMIAS

As explained in Chapter 7, the EAD mechanism for triggering torsades de pointes may be different than the mechanism for sustaining the arrhythmia (abnormal automaticity, DADs, and reentry have all been postulated). Therefore, interpretation of the effects of stimulation are complicated by the lack of information on the mechanism for perpetuation of the tachycardia following the first triggered impulse that is likely to be caused by an EAD (see Chapter 7).

Failure to Initiate by Overdrive or Premature Stimulation

In general, torsades de pointes mimicking the spontaneously occurring arrhythmia cannot be initiated by either overdrive pacing or premature stimulation in congenital LQT patients. Although rapid pacing does not initiate the arrhythmia in patients with congenital LQT1, pharmacological β-adrenergic stimulation, which increases the heart rate, sometimes does initiate it (see Figure 8-3). Very aggressive stimulation protocols in LQT patients, such as three premature stimuli, can initiate episodes of polymorphic ventricular tachycardia that nevertheless do not meet the criteria for torsades de pointes. They appear different from the spontaneous tachycardias in both rate (faster) and QRS contour (absence of twisting of the points). These tachycardias are similar to those that can be induced by aggressive stimulation protocols in normal hearts and are likely due to reentry (Chapter 12).

Failure to initiate the clinical arrhythmia at the time of electrophysiological study may possibly be explained by the absence of transient surges in adrenergic discharge or some other undefined neural factors that are necessary for occurrence of the arrhythmia in LQT1 and LQT2. Failure to initiate is consistent with an EAD mechanism for onset and perpetuation since overdrive or premature stimulation are not expected to cause EAD-triggered impulses. Short cycle lengths from overdrive or premature stimulation typically accelerate repolarization and suppress EADs (Figure 7-6). Failure to initiate by stimulation is also consistent with an abnormal automatic mechanism for perpetuation of the arrhythmia, since abnormal automaticity also cannot be initiated by stimulation. The failure to initiate torsades de pointes is not consistent with models of reentry or DAD-triggered activity perpetuating this arrhythmia, since arrhythmias caused by either of these mechanisms can be initiated by electrical stimulation (Chapter 7).

Patients with structural heart disease can have polymorphic ventricular tachycardia similar to torsades de pointes, but unrelated to long QT. Polymorphic ventricular tachycardia in these patients can often be initiated with programmed premature stimulation because a substrate for reentry from the structural disease is present (for further discussion, see Chapter 12).

Because in congenital LQT2 and LQT3, torsades de pointes often occurs after a pause that potentiates EADs (Figure 8-1), clinical stimulation protocols mimicking such pauses might provide evidence for an EAD mechanism. However, in most clinical studies, imposition of stimulation protocols to cause short-long intervals (a pause after overdrive or a premature stimulus) has not been successful in initiating the arrhythmia. Whether this would be more effective in the presence of β-adrenergic stimulation in LQT1 and LQT2 has not been tested although in LQT3, the sympathetic nervous system does not appear to be involved in arrhythmia initiation. Even in instances when this protocol induces torsades de pointes, it would not be specific for EAD-induced arrhythmias since long pauses can prolong refractoriness, which can increase the likelihood of developing conduction block required for reentrant ventricular arrhythmias (Figure 9-1).

Therapeutic Effect of Overdrive Pacing for Arrhythmia Prevention

Overdrive pacing at appropriate rates prevents the pauses that are often associated with onset of torsades de pointes in congenital LQT2 and LQT3. This explains the therapeutic effect of pacing in these patients (often in combination with β-blockers, which sometimes may accentuate bradycardia or pauses). Overdrive pacing not only accelerates repolarization and shortens APD, but it also can reduce the dispersion of APDs (the difference in repolarization time in different regions) because action potentials with long APDs often show a greater degree of shortening than those with short APDs. This effect is more prominent during atrial pacing, when the ventricles are activated in normal sequence, than during ventricular pacing, when APD dispersion might actually increase because of the abnormal sequence of ventricular activation. The reduction of APD dispersion could account for prevention of the arrhythmia, if dispersion is a cause of perpetuation of torsades de pointes.

It has not been possible to test the effects of electrical stimulation on the ongoing triggered arrhythmia in LQT syndromes to determine if it can be terminated or shows overdrive suppression or acceleration, which would provide clues to the mechanism for perpetuation.

TRIGGERED ATRIAL ARRHYTHMIAS IN CONGENITAL LQT SYNDROME

Some patients with congenital LQT syndrome have atrial arrhythmias ranging from short-lasting tachycardias and atrial fibrillation to persistent atrial fibrillation. These arrhythmias occur in the absence of the typical atrial remodeling that accompanies atrial fibrillation in structural heart disease (see Chapter 10). Early-onset atrial fibrillation (e.g., in patients < 20 years old) has been documented in patients with congenital LQT syndrome.

Many of the same ion channels that are involved in ventricular repolarization also participate in atrial repolarization (Figure 7-2). These channels can undergo the same changes in function that occur in the ventricles in patients with congenital LQT syndrome. Atrial APD is prolonged and can sometimes lead to EADs. However, clinical evidence linking EADs to these atrial arrhythmias is lacking. Although the mechanism for atrial fibrillation in structural heart disease involves shortening of APD (Chapter 10), in the case of LQT syndrome it may involve EADs and triggered activity associated with action potential lengthening. The mechanism for perpetuation of the triggered activity might involve reentry, abnormal automaticity or DAD-triggered activity as in the ventricles.

EAD-induced triggered activity has been shown to occur in pulmonary veins in experimental animal studies, leaving open the possibility that it might initiate clinical atrial fibrillation (described further in Chapter 10).

Long QT Caused by Structural Heart Disease and/or Ischemia

LONG QT AND EAD-TRIGGERED ARRHYTHMIAS IN STRUCTURAL HEART DISEASE

In patients with coronary artery disease, myocardial infarction, and heart failure, a prolonged QTc interval greater than approximately 440 ms resulting from pathology-induced remodeling of repolarizing ion channels, particularly loss of function of I_K, is associated with a greater propensity for ventricular arrhythmias and an increased risk for sudden cardiac death. In dilated and hypertrophic cardiomyopathy, a decrease in repolarization reserve, e.g., cycle length–dependent acceleration of repolarization (Chapter 7), and an increase in dispersion in APD may also predispose to triggered arrhythmias. These properties, as described above, are related to EADs and triggered activity, but as yet, this particular mechanism for these arrhythmias has not been confirmed in clinical studies.

Ventricular pacing may be helpful in some specific cases of structural heart disease associated with torsades de pointes. Some patients (usually women) with disease of the conducting system, and possibly some disease of the ventricles, who develop heart block may manifest a long QT interval. These patients have a normal QT before heart block and an idioventricular rate of 40 bpm or less during heart block. The long QT during heart block is associated with episodes of polymorphic ventricular tachycardia resembling torsades de pointes. Overdrive pacing can prevent the occurrence of torsades de pointes as it does in congenital LQT. Similarly, after A-V junctional ablation in patients with atrial fibrillation (a procedure used to control ventricular rate), ventricular pacing can prevent the occurrence of torsades de pointes, consistent with, but not proof of, an EAD mechanism.

EADS ASSOCIATED WITH ACUTE ISCHEMIA

In experimental laboratory studies lowering the oxygen in the perfusate causes single action potentials or repetitive activity to arise from EADs during the plateau of Purkinje cell action potentials. The combination of hypoxia and acidosis with or without catecholamines to mimic the acute ischemic environment, also induces EADs. If these effects occur *in vivo*, they might cause triggered arrhythmias early after a coronary artery occlusion, although it has not as yet been demonstrated in patients.

Acquired Long QT Syndrome

ARRHYTHMIAS DUE TO ACQUIRED LQT SYNDROME

The ECG in **Figure 8-4** was recorded from a patient who was administered disopyramide for the treatment of atrial fibrillation. A lead II rhythm strip at the bottom shows a sinus impulse at the left with a long QT followed by a ventricular premature depolarization with a coupling interval of 600 ms, followed by a second sinus impulse after a prolonged cycle length of 1000 ms. The second sinus impulse is followed by an episode of polymorphic unsustained ventricular tachycardia. The first impulse of tachycardia arises at a coupling interval of 600 ms from the exaggerated TU wave of the sinus impulse that occurred after the long 1000-ms cycle length. Tachycardia occurred after a sequence of short-long-short cycle lengths. The long cycle length increased APD and potentiated the EAD. The latter short cycle length is the first tachycardia impulse, which is premature. The changing QRS morphology during tachycardia (negative R waves progressing to positive R waves) identifies the arrhythmia as torsades de pointes. The patient has acquired LQT syndrome; the administration of disopyramide caused a long QT interval and torsades de pointes.

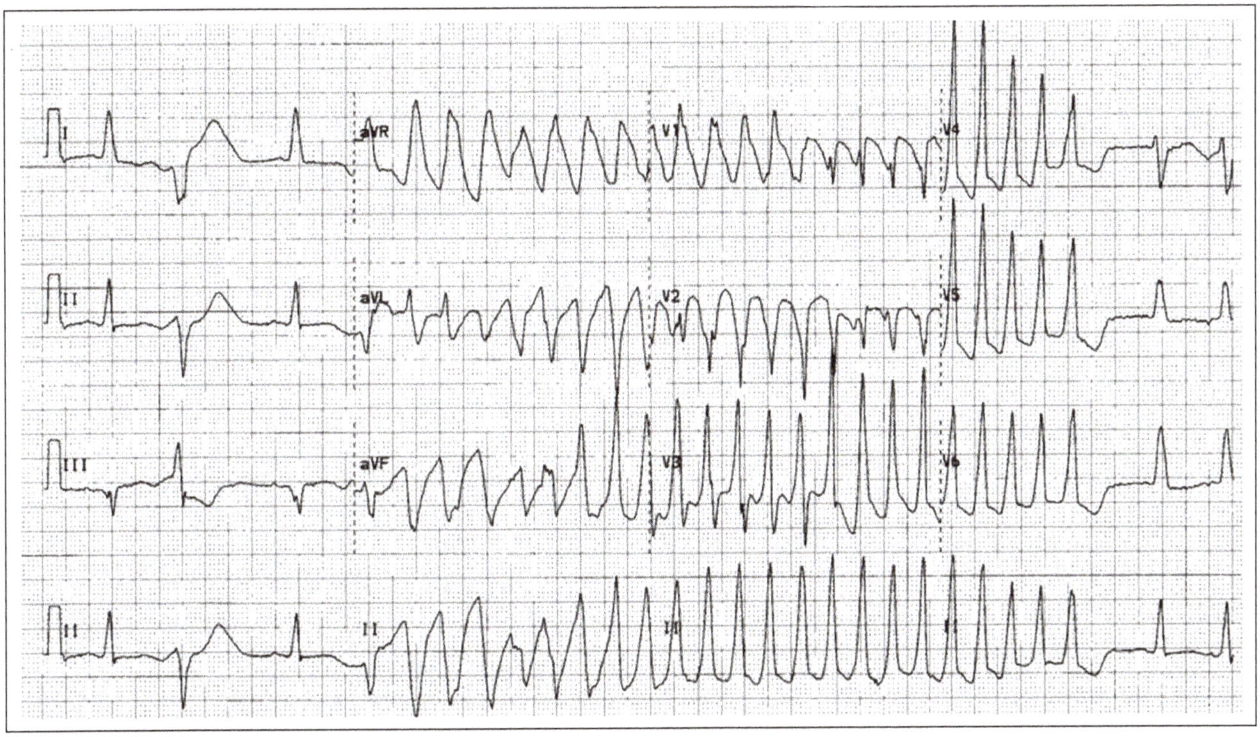

Figure 8-4 12-lead ECG and lead II rhythm strip (**bottom**) recorded after atrial fibrillation was terminated by the Class IA antiarrhythmic drug, disopyramide (Wellens' ECG collection).

BASIC ELECTROPHYSIOLOGICAL MECHANISMS UNDERLYING ACQUIRED LQT SYNDROME

Drug-Induced Block of I_{Kr}

Acquired LQT syndrome and torsades de pointes can occur after administration of drugs used as therapy for cardiac arrhythmias as well as a diverse group of agents used for treatment of noncardiac diseases. One common effect of these drugs is that they prolong the QT interval by blocking I_{Kr} in ventricular muscle cells (*KCNH2* channel). Prolongation of the absolute QT interval beyond 500 ms is commonly regarded as conferring an increased risk for torsades de pointes. Blocking I_{Kr} also prolongs APD in Purkinje cells of the conducting system. EADs and triggered activity might therefore occur in either muscle of Purkinje cells.

As mentioned in Chapter 7, another more recently discovered effect of drugs that prolong the QT is an inhibition of tyrosine kinase enzymes, phosphoinositide 3-kinases (PI3Ks). These enzymes play a role in controlling repolarization by participating in the inactivation of the persistent (long lasting) Na^+ current. Therefore, inhibition prolongs APD by increasing this persistent current. The time course of this effect is prolonged compared to the rapid inhibition of I_{Kr} accounting for the long-time course it takes dofetilide to prolong the QT. Its role in the QT prolonging effects of other drugs is under investigation.

The drug administered in Figure 8-4, disopyramide, is a Class IA antiarrhythmic drug. This class of drugs, which also includes quinidine and procainamide, has a primary effect to block the fast Na^+ channel and reduces I_{Na} responsible for phase 0 of the action potential. It also prolongs repolarization by blocking the I_{Kr} channel, decreasing I_{Kr} (loss of function) and possibly PI3Ks. Since disopyramide can also have a vagolytic effect, the speeding of the sinus rate may offset some of the QT prolongation. Class III antiarrhythmic drugs, including amiodarone, sotalol, and dofetilide also reduce I_{Kr} and can cause torsades de pointes, although the incidence with amiodarone is much less than with the other drugs in this class. In addition to the loss of function of I_{Kr}, it is proposed that a rapid ventricular rate during atrial fibrillation prior to conversion to sinus rhythm as in Figure 8-4 causes excess Ca^{2+} to enter ventricular cells through L-type Ca^{2+} channels. The Ca^{2+} is then extruded by the Na^+–Ca^{2+} exchanger after conversion in the presence of the delayed repolarization caused by the drug, contributing to the occurrence of EADs.

Additional Drug Effects in Acquired LQT

Reverse Use-Dependence

Class III antiarrhythmic drugs have a property, referred to as *reverse use-dependent effects*, that also potentiates the occurrence of torsades de pointes. Reverse use-dependence means that the drug's effects to prolong APD is greater at long cycle lengths than at short cycle lengths. Therefore, EADs and triggered activity are more likely to occur during bradycardia, which is a common occurrence in patients with acquired LQT syndrome.

Drug Dose-Dependence

With the exception of quinidine, torsades de pointes in acquired LQT is usually drug dose or blood concentration-dependent. Higher than therapeutic plasma levels occur either because of administration of too much drug or because of defects in drug metabolism. Quinidine-induced torsades de pointes can occur at low plasma levels particularly in the presence of hypokalemia which potentiates the effects of all QT-prolonging drugs. Low plasma K^+ accelerates inactivation of the I_{Kr} channel, reducing the current, and also potentiates drug blockade of residual current. Hypomagnesemia also increases the risk of torsades de pointes, possibly because of an interaction with the L-type Ca^{2+} channel to increase I_{CaL}, which participates in EAD formation. This interaction may underlie the antiarrhythmic effects of intravenous magnesium, which is sometimes effective in the therapy of drug-induced torsades de pointes.

Individual Response to Drugs Varies

Although I_{Kr} block by a drug is likely to be a major causative mechanism of acquired LQT syndrome, not every patient receiving drugs that block I_{Kr} develops marked QT prolongation and ventricular arrhythmias. Some drugs that prolong the QT by blocking I_{Kr}, also reduce inward currents necessary for EADs to trigger action potentials. Amiodarone blocks membrane channels associated with I_{CaL} and late I_{Na} in addition to I_{Kr}, possibly explaining the low incidence of torsades de pointes after amiodarone administration even in the face of a marked prolongation of the QT interval (> 500 ms). It also may decrease heterogeneity of repolarization by blocking I_{Ks} reducing the possibility of reentry. Verapamil blocks I_{Kr} channels, but its concomitant block of I_{CaL} that suppress EADs is the likely reason that it does not cause torsades de pointes. Ranolazine blocks the late I_{Na} in addition to I_{Kr}, with preliminary data suggesting it might prevent triggered activity in LQT3 that is related to increased late I_{Na}.

Patients may respond differently to QT prolonging drugs, some having greater QT prolongation and a higher incidence of torsades de pointes than others. Drug-induced torsades de pointes occurs more frequently in female than male patients, possibly because testosterone increases I_{Kr} in males to maintain a short QT in the face of drug-blocking effects. Some patients in whom torsades de pointes develops on exposure to drugs that prolong the QT interval harbor mutations associated with the congenital long-QT syndrome and can therefore be viewed as having a subclinical form of the congenital syndrome. In particular, mutations of the gene *KCNQ1* that controls I_{Ks} (Table 7-1), with incomplete penetrance so there is no overt LQT2 syndrome, can potentiate the effects of I_{Kr} block by a drug. Other polymorphisms in ion channel genes, particularly those associated with I_{Ks} that have minor functional effects at baseline, may increase risk for torsades de pointes in the presence of a QT-prolonging drug. The significance of subclinical LQT syndrome is that these patients have reduced repolarization reserve (Chapter 7). Some patients who develop torsades de pointes on Class IA drugs exhibit an increase in QTc interval on exercise indicating the absence of normal action potential shortening with increased heart rate. Since cycle length-dependent acceleration of repolarization is partly dependent on I_{Ks}, these patients may have some loss of function of I_{Ks} indicating a form of LQT1, which is not apparent in the absence of drug effects.

IDENTIFYING EAD-TRIGGERED ACTIVITY IN ACQUIRED LQT SYNDROMES

ECG Characteristics and Onset of Torsades de Pointes

Characteristic ECG patterns are the best evidence linking ventricular arrhythmias in acquired LQT syndrome to EAD-triggered activity, similar to the argument that congenital LQT is related to EADs. Progressive lengthening of the QT interval to values greater than 500 ms and development of prominent U waves after drug administration are markers of EAD occurrence, and these ECG features increase the risk of syncope or death from torsades de pointes. **Figure 8-5** shows these features after the administration of sotalol to a patient for therapy of ventricular tachycardia. The U waves are most prominent in leads V_3–V_6, where they have a larger amplitude on alternating beats (arrows).

An additional similarity to congenital LQT2 and LQT3 is the occurrence of torsades de pointes after a short-long cycle length that markedly prolongs APD and favors the occurrence of EADs. The first tachycardia impulse has a short coupling interval because it occurs during the U wave (short-long-short sequence) (Figure 8-4).

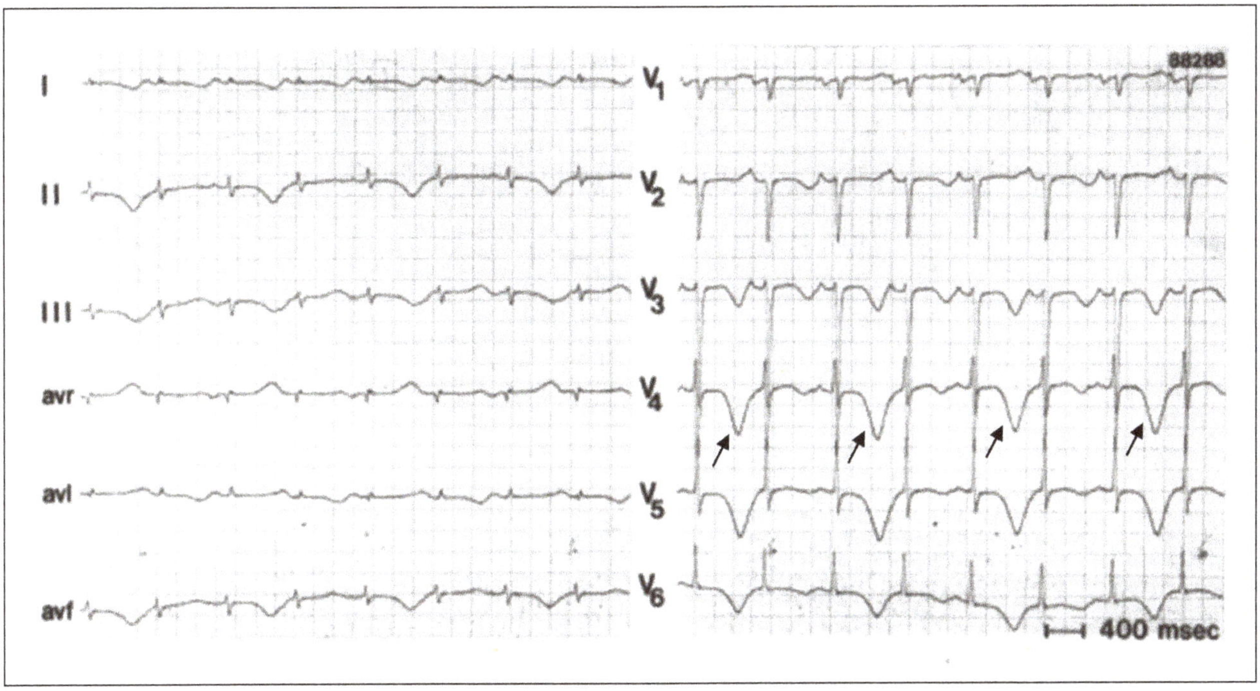

Figure 8-5 ECG recorded from a patient who was administered sotalol for the treatment of ventricular arrhythmias. **Arrows** point out alternating U waves (Wellens' ECG collection).

Effects of Electrical Stimulation

Failure to Initiate

Similar to congenital LQT syndrome, in acquired LQT syndrome the effects of electrical stimulation do not provide evidence for EAD-triggered arrhythmias. With drugs that have a primary effect of blocking I_{Kr}, such as sotalol and dofetilide, torsades de pointes resembling spontaneously occurring arrhythmias cannot usually be induced by overdrive or premature stimulation. In general, both overdrive and premature stimulation should suppress EADs because they usually accelerate action potential repolarization. The failure to initiate the arrhythmia also argues against a reentrant mechanism for perpetuation of the triggered arrhythmia, since reentry caused by dispersion of refractoriness can be induced by premature stimulation (see Figure 9-14). Interpretation of results of programmed stimulation in patients with torsades de pointes related to administration of Class IA antiarrhythmic drugs is more problematic since these drugs also have significant Na^+ channel-blocking effects. The reduction of I_{Na} enables reentrant arrhythmias to be induced by programmed stimulation (Chapter 12). When induced, these tachycardias usually do not have the features of torsades de pointes; rather, they are monomorphic and sustained. Protocols using short-long stimulus cycle lengths is not usually successful in initiating torsades de pointes in patients with acquired LQT, similar to its lack of efficacy for initiating torsades de pointes in congenital LQT syndrome.

Therapeutic Effect of Overdrive Pacing

Overdrive stimulation is effective in preventing the occurrence of drug-induced torsades de pointes. This effect is consistent with it being caused by EAD-triggered activity, since pacing eliminates the pauses associated with arrhythmia onset and APD decreases as pacing cycle length decreases, which suppresses EADs. In **Figure 8-6** spontaneous episodes of drug-induced torsades de pointes occurs in the top two recordings after long pauses in the sinus cycle length, with rates of 250/min and 230/min. Black arrows indicate a U wave at the terminal part of the long QT interval preceding the onset of torsades de pointes. The bottom recording shows overdrive ventricular pacing that prevented the pauses and shortened the QT, eliminating the U wave and preventing the occurrence of the arrhythmia.

Isoproterenol-induced acceleration of heart rate can have a similar effect even though β-adrenerigic stimulation might also increase EADs. As is the case with congenital LQT, no information is available describing electrical stimulation during tachycardia to help determine its mechanism.

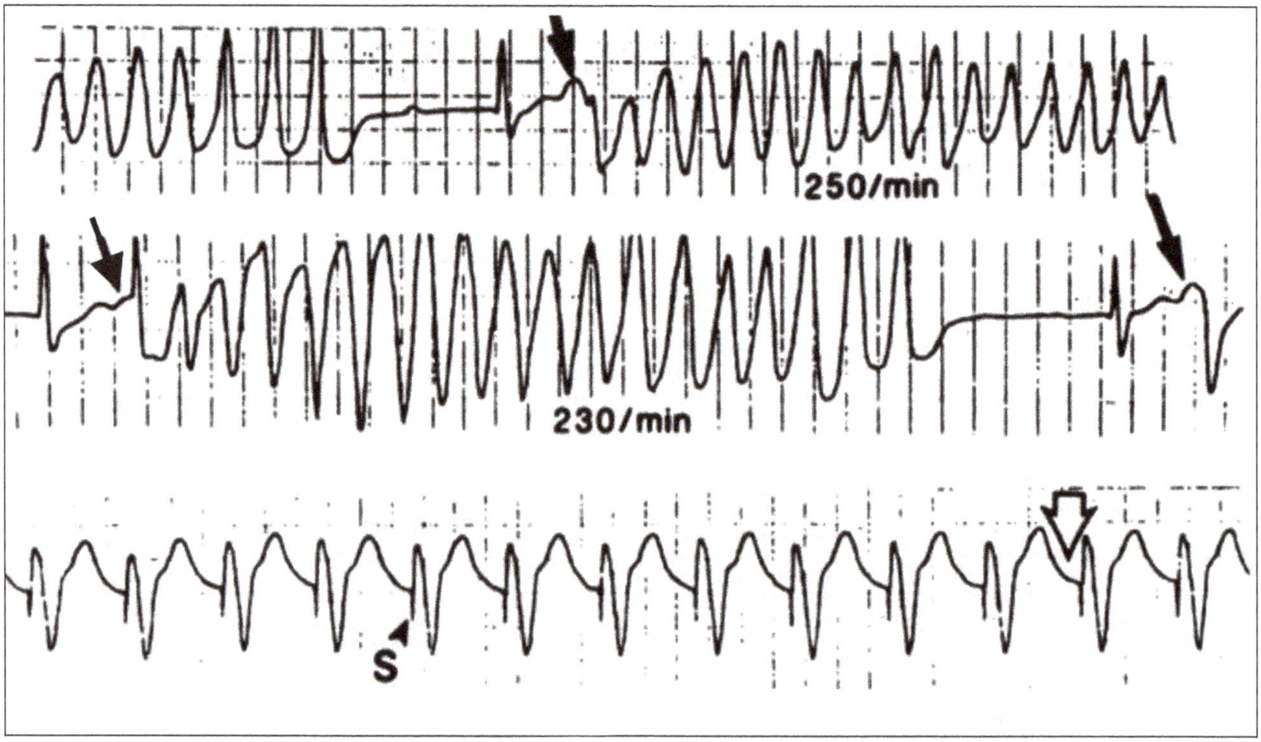

Figure 8-6 Prevention of drug-induced torsades de pointes by overdrive ventricular pacing. (Reproduced from Josephson ME. *Josephson's Clinical Cardiac Electrophysiology: Techniques and Interpretations* (5th ed.). Philadelphia, PA: Wolters Kluwer; 2016.)

SUMMARY

Long QT interval (LQT) syndromes are associated with APD prolongation. The most common forms of congenital LQT syndrome are LQT1 and LQT2, which result from loss-of-function mutations in genes that underlie the outward repolarizing currents I_{Ks} and I_{Kr}, and LQT3, which results from the gain-of-function mutation that increases persistence of inward depolarizing current, I_{Na}.

Polymorphic ventricular tachycardia, torsades de pointes, is associated with EAD-triggered activity. The primary initiator of torsades de pointes in LQT1 patients is enhanced sympathetic activity, which can accompany exercise or an emotional or stressful event. The QT fails to shorten with acceleration of heart rate at onset because of the I_{Ks} deficiency. β-receptor blockade or left cervical sympathectomy can be effective in reducing syncope or the risk of sudden death. Torsades de pointes occurs in LQT2 patients (loss of function of I_{Kr}) with either emotion, stress (but usually not with exercise), or at rest. I_{Ks} is able to accelerate repolarization in the presence of an increased heart rate; hence, the QT interval shortens. Onset is sometimes characterized by a short-long-short sequence of cycle lengths. LQT3 is usually associated with arrhythmias occurring at slow heart rates during rest or sleep, a situation that prolongs APD and enhances EADs. β-blockers are much less effective in patients with LQT3 than in LQT1 and LQT2, suggesting less of an arrhythmogenic role of the sympathetic nervous system. The efficacy of β-blocker therapy can be enhanced if any associated pauses are prevented by a pacemaker.

In general, in congenital LQT patients, torsades de pointes cannot be initiated by either overdrive pacing or premature stimulation. This failure to initiate is consistent with either an EAD mechanism for onset and perpetuation or an abnormal automatic mechanism for perpetuation after EAD initiation. The failure to initiate the arrhythmia is not consistent with models of reentry or DAD-triggered activity perpetuating it. Overdrive pacing at appropriate rates prevents the pauses that are often associated with onset of torsades de pointes in congenital LQT2 and LQT3.

Acquired LQT syndrome and torsades de pointes can occur after administration of drugs used as therapy for cardiac arrhythmias as well as agents used for treatment of noncardiac diseases. These drugs prolong the QT interval by blocking I_{Kr}. QT interval prolongation can also be caused by inhibition of phosphoinositide 3-kinases (PI3Ks) that play a role in controlling repolarization by participating in the inactivation of the persistent Na^+ current.

With the exception of quinidine, torsades de pointes in acquired LQT is usually drug dose- or blood concentration-dependent. Quinidine-induced torsades de pointes can occur at low plasma levels, particularly in the presence of hypokalemia, which potentiates the effects of all QT-prolonging drugs. The failure to initiate the arrhythmia by programmed stimulation protocols also argues against a reentrant mechanism for perpetuation of the triggered arrhythmia. Overdrive stimulation is effective in preventing the occurrence of drug-induced torsades de pointes consistent with it being caused by EAD-triggered activity since pacing eliminates the pauses (long cycle lengths) that potentiate EADs.

SOURCES

Jacobs A, Knight BP, McDonald KT, Burke MC. Verapamil decreases ventricular tachyarrhythmias in a patient with Timothy syndrome (LQT8). *Heart Rhythm.* 2006;3:967–970.

Moss AJ, Liu JE, Gottlieb S, et al. Efficacy of permanent pacing in the management of high-risk patients with long QT syndrome. *Circulation.* 1991;84:1524-1529.

Moss AJ, Zareba W, Benhorin J, et al. ECG T-wave patterns in genetically distinct forms of the hereditary long QT syndrome. *Circulation.* 1995;92:2929–2934.

Napolitano C, Bloise R, Priori SG. Gene-specific therapy for inherited arrhythmogenic diseases. *Pharmacol Therap.* 2006;110:1–13.

Opthof, T, Coronel R, Janse MJ. Is there a significant transmural gradient in repolarization time in the intact heart? *Circ Arrhythm Electrophysiol.* 2009;2:89–96.

Priori SG, Barhanin J, Hauer RNW, et al. Genetic and molecular basis of cardiac arrhythmias: impact on clinical management: Parts I and II. *Circulation.* 1999;99:518–528.

Sauer AJ, Moss AJ, McNitt S, et al. Long QT syndrome in adults. *J Am Coll Cardiol.* 2007;49:329–337.

Schwartz PJ, Priori SG, Cerrone M, et al. Left cardiac sympathetic denervation in the management of high-risk patients affected by the long-QT syndrome. *Circulation.* 2004;109:1826–1833.

Schwartz PJ, Crotti L. QTc behavior during exercise and genetic testing for the long-QT syndrome. *Circulation.* 2011;124:2181–2184.

Tan HL, MD, Bardai A, Shimizu W, et al. Genotype-specific onset of arrhythmias in congenital long-QT syndrome. Possible therapy implications. *Circulation.* 2006;114:2096–2103.

Zareba W, Moss AJ, Schwartz PJ. Influence of the genotype on the clinical course of the long QT syndrome. *N Engl J Med.* 1998;339:960–965.

Zellerhoff S, Pistulli R, Monnig G, et al. Atrial arrhythmias in long-QT syndrome under daily life conditions: A nested case control study. *J Cardiovasc Electrophysiol.* 2009;20: 401–407.

Zhang L, MD, Timothy KW, Vincent M, et al. Spectrum of ST-T-wave patterns and repolarization parameters in congenital long-QT syndrome. ECG findings identify genotypes. *Circulation.* 2000;102:2849–2855.

CHAPTER 9

Basic Principles of Reentry: Altered Conduction and Reentrant Excitation

Overview and General Principles

Altered impulse conduction represents the second major category of arrhythmia mechanisms (Introduction, Table i-1). One means whereby altered impulse conduction results in the occurrence of arrhythmias is the manifestation of latent pacemakers that occurs when sinoatrial (S-A) or atrioventricular (A-V) block is present (described in Chapters 1-4. Altered impulse conduction also causes reentrant excitation (reentry), a mechanism for arrhythmias that does not depend on the generation of *de novo* impulses, as occurs with the mechanisms of automaticity and triggered activity.

REQUIREMENTS FOR REENTRY

While the underlying detailed mechanisms of clinical reentrant arrhythmias are more complicated, a simple ring model of reentry describing impulse movement in a circular pathway (circus movement) provides the foundation for these more complicated concepts.

The Ring Model

The basic principles underlying reentrant excitation are shown in a schematic diagram of a ring of excitable cardiac muscle with a central inexcitable region (in black) in **Figure 9-1**. The ring is a model of an anatomical reentrant circuit—an anatomically fixed pathway around an anatomical obstacle. Conducting impulses are indicated by the blue arrows, with the arrowhead showing the leading edge or head of the propagating impulse (the wave front), and the blue segment of the tail of the arrow indicating inexcitable myocardium (the effective refractory period) that the impulse has just excited. In Figure 9-1, the red segment of the tail indicates partially recovered myocardium during the relative refractory period. (Note that in other figures, e.g., Figure 9-14, the length of the arrow tail does not indicate the inexcitable or partially recovered myocardium as it does in Figure 9-1. Where not otherwise indicated, the entire arrow simply represents the direction of impulse propagation.)

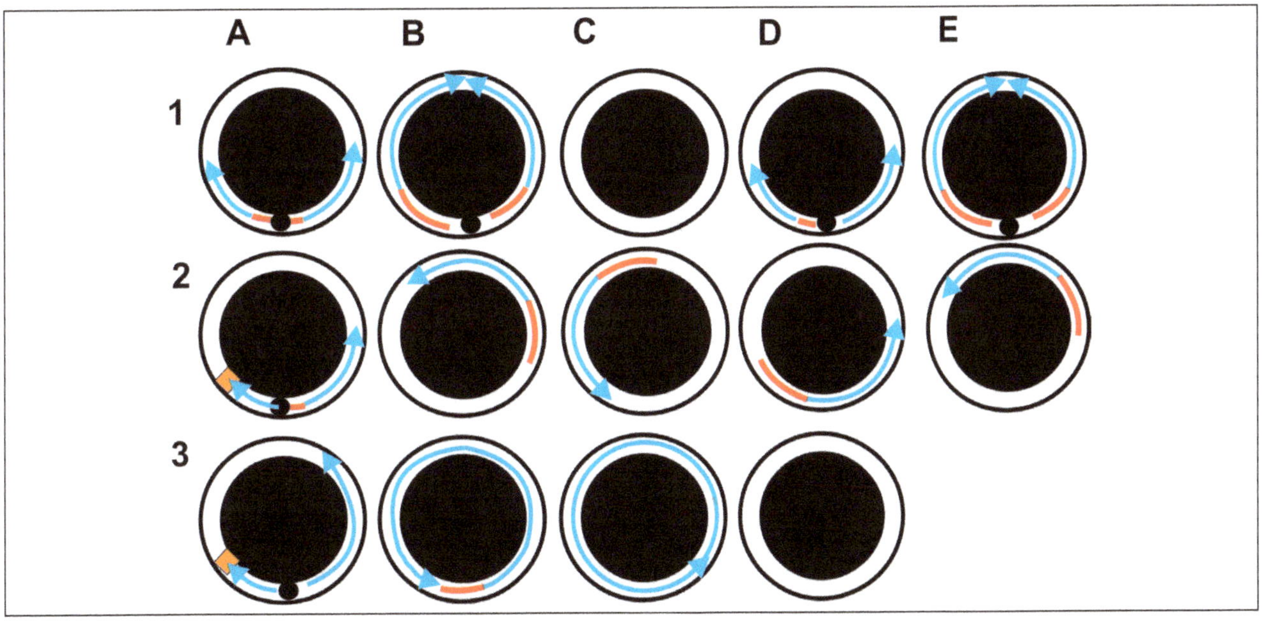

Figure 9-1 Model of reentry in an anatomical circular pathway. The diagrams show snapshots of the sequence of impulse propagation (**arrows**) over a period of time (across the row from **A–E**) after initiation at the **black dot in Column A1–A3**.

Electrophysiological Foundations of Cardiac Arrhythmias: A Bridge Between Basic Mechanisms and Clinical Electrophysiology, Second Edition.
 Cardiotext Publishing, ISBN: 978-1-942909-42-2.

Figure 9-1, row 1 diagrams bidirectional impulse conduction. Snapshot A1 illustrates impulses initiated at a point (black dot), propagating away from the site of origin in opposite directions in the ring. During the time period between A1 and B1, the two impulses reach the distal side of the ring where they collide (blue arrows in snapshot B1). The impulses die out because they are surrounded by tissue that has just been excited and that remains refractory for a period of time that outlasts the time for propagation. This pattern is somewhat analogous to an impulse originating in the sinus node (black dot) that dies out after exciting atria and ventricles because it is surrounded by effectively refractory myocardium and runs into the inexcitable fibrous annulus after depolarization of the ventricles. After a period of quiescence, (C1), a new impulse must be initiated for subsequent activation (at the black dot) (D1 and E1), analogous to the next sinus impulse.

Unidirectional Conduction Block Under Special Conditions

Diagrams in row 2, A2–E2, show how the propagating impulse can persist to reexcite, i.e., reenter, regions it has already excited.

In snapshot A2, excitation again is initiated at the black dot. By temporarily causing conduction block in the right-to-left (clockwise) direction near the site of stimulation (at the brown rectangle), excitation is induced to progress in only one direction, to the right (counterclockwise), around the ring (blue arrow). Mechanisms for transient block in the *in situ* heart that cause clinical arrhythmias are described in Figures 9-14, 9-15, and 9-16. After an impulse is conducting in one direction around the ring (B2–E2 show snap shots of the impulse at progressive time periods), if conduction is restored in the region of the block, the impulse can then return to its site of origin and reexcite (reenter) tissue it previously has excited (D2 and E2). Thus, the block is unidirectional (only clockwise) and the impulse can conduct counterclockwise. The ring forms a reentrant pathway or circuit. The impulse can also continue to circulate, repeating the pattern of snapshots B2–E2. This simple model demonstrates that for reentry to occur, a region of block must be present, even if only transiently (the brown rectangle in Panel A2). The block is necessary to launch propagation of the impulse in one direction and to prevent early excitation of the pathway (at the left side of the ring) that eventually becomes the return pathway that the impulse then uses to reenter the region it reexcites. In the ring model shown in Figure 9-1, identical circular movement would occur if, instead of transient block, permanent conduction block occurred in the clockwise direction (brown-shaded area of Panel A2), also known as unidirectional block. Electrophysiological mechanisms for permanent unidirectional conduction block are described later in Figures 9-15 and 9-16.

Importance of the Wavelength of the Conducting Impulse in Reentry

In addition to unidirectional conduction block, for reentry to occur, the impulse that is conducting around the circuit must always find excitable tissue in the direction in which it is propagating, i.e., the tissue that was excited in the previous transit around the ring must have recovered excitability. In order for this requirement to be fulfilled, the conduction time around the ring must be longer than the effective refractory period of the myocardium that comprises the ring. For purposes of describing the mechanism for reentry, the concept of wavelength of the conducting impulse can be used.

A definition of "wavelength" (λ is the distance traveled by the depolarization wave during the time the tissue restores its excitability sufficiently to propagate another impulse. Thus, wavelength (λ) = conduction velocity (θ) × effective refractory period (ERP). In Figure 9-1, A2–E2, the length of the blue arrow (from arrowhead to the end of blue tail) is the wavelength of the conducting impulse, the time between the head of the wavefront and recovery of excitability, even though recovery is not complete. The end of the blue tail signifies the functional refractory period, which is the earliest time that an impulse can propagate following a prior excitation. The myocardium in front of the arrowhead in Panels C2 to E2 has recovered as indicated by the unshaded region. This requirement that conduction around the circuit must take long enough to allow recovery from the effective refractory period can be expressed in terms of the relationship between the wavelength (λ) of the conducting impulse (the length from blue arrowhead to end of blue tail) and the length of the reentrant pathway (path length, l). In other words, the wavelength (λ) of the reentrant impulse must be shorter than the length of the pathway ($\lambda < l$). In Figure 9-1, A2–E2, the wavelength is significantly less than the path length, leaving a large part of the circuit excitable, enabling it to be reexcited by a propagating wavefront.

Spatial and temporal excitable gaps. The excitable region of the circuit forms the spatial excitable gap which is the distance occupied by the excitable region at any moment in time. The spatial excitable gap is comprised of a partially excitable gap where myocardium is still relatively refractory (curved red line), and a fully excitable gap where myocardium has completely recovered excitability (unshaded region).

In clinical studies to evaluate the excitable gap during a reentrant tachycardia, only a temporal excitable gap or excitable period can be identified, which is the time interval of excitability between the head of activation of one impulse and the tail of refractoriness of the prior impulse. This will be described in detail in Chapters 10, 11, and 12 on clinical reentrant arrhythmias. The temporal excitable gap is measured by stimulating premature impulses, usually outside the circuit, and observing the resetting response that results from the premature impulse entering and conducting around the circuit (described in detail in Figure 9-27, and Figure 9-28). The spatial excitable gap cannot usually be evaluated, since it would require stimulating at multiple sites within the circuit to evaluate how much of the circuit is excitable, which cannot usually be done in clinical studies.

Figure 9-1, row 3 A3–D3, diagrams a situation where the wavelength is longer than the path length ($\theta > l$), precluding reentry, since there is no excitable gap. Snapshot A3 shows initiation of conduction in one direction (counterclockwise) because of the region of transient block in the clockwise direction (brown-shaded region). Conduction velocity is much more rapid so that by Snapshot B3, the impulse has almost completed its transit around the circuit without providing enough time for recovery of excitability, indicated by the long length of the blue arrow. In C3, the wavefront (arrowhead) collides with its refractory tail and blocks. The reentering impulse dies out (D3).

In general, for reentrant circuits of the same length, the excitable gap decreases as the wavelength increases, either because of an increased conduction velocity or an increased effective refractory period. This is one reason that reentrant circuits causing fast tachycardias usually have small excitable gaps when the increase in the wavelength is caused by a faster conduction velocity.

Relation of wavelength to the propagating action potential. **Figure 9-2** pictures the wavelength of the conducting impulse as it relates to a propagating normal ventricular muscle action potential with typical voltage-dependent recovery of excitability. Panel A shows the time course of a ventricular muscle action potential. The voltage scale is on the ordinate. Time is indicated by the red arrow below it on the abscissa, beginning at 0 and ending at 400 ms. The depolarization phase 0 occurs first at time 0, followed by repolarization phases 1, 2, and 3, which end at time 400 ms. The effective refractory period ends at the vertical dashed green line (300 ms) followed by the relative refractory period. The conduction velocity of the action potential is not displayed in this kind of representation, and changes in velocity do not influence the appearance of the action potential as long as phase 0 and repolarization time are not altered.

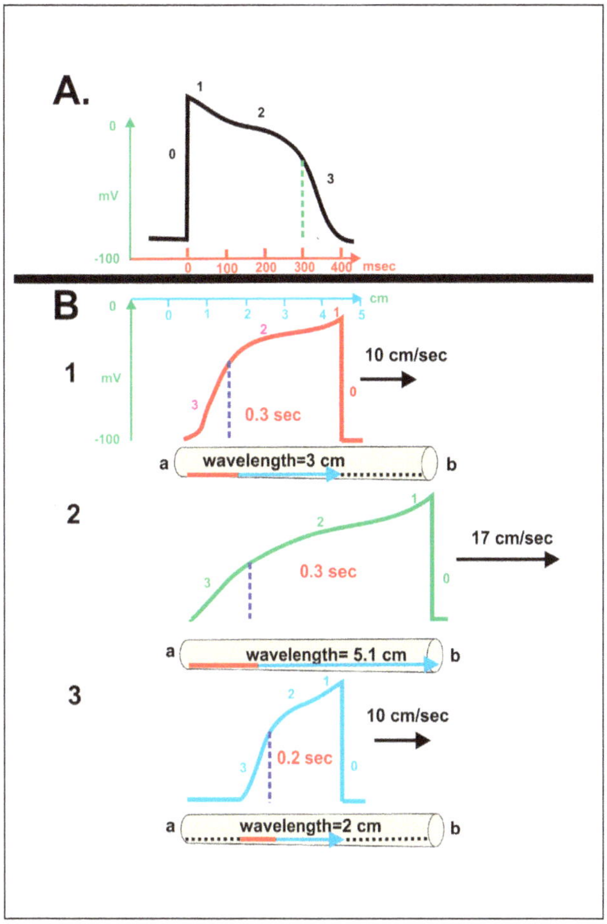

Figure 9-2 **Panel A** shows an action potential as it is traditionally displayed. **Panel B (1, 2, 3)** shows how much space the action potential waveform occupies (the wavelength).

Figure 9-2, Panel B shows a different way of depicting the action potential; it shows the action potential in space as it propagates along a 7-cm long muscle bundle from left to right. The muscle bundle depicted here represents a circular reentrant pathway that has been cut through and laid out in a straight line—the two ends, a and b, were attached before cutting. In this representation, the voltage scale is still on the ordinate, but the abscissa represents distance or space in cm (in blue at the top of the panel). The initial phase 0 of the action potential is now at the right, leading the movement of the depolarizing wavefront (blue arrowhead) as it conducts over the bundle.

At the time shown in Panel B1, action potential 1 has propagated for about 4.5 cm along the bundle. Action potential repolarization phases 1–3 trail the leading phase 0. The effective refractory period is between phase 0 and the vertical dashed purple line, showing the spatial extent of the tissue that is refractory in the muscle bundle. Repolarization to the end of the effective refractory period takes 0.3 sec. The wavelength of the action potential is the space occupied by the action potential between phase 0 and the end of the effective refractory period. It is dependent on both the conduction velocity (10 cm/sec in B1) and time for repolarization to the end of the effective refractory period (0.3 sec in B1) and is the product of these two values (wavelength = 3 cm). The extent of the wavelength is also shown by the blue arrowhead to end of blue arrow tail that corresponds with phase 0 of the action potential to the end of the effective refractory period. In muscle cells in diseased regions, the effective refractory period may extend further, beyond complete repolarization, called "postrepolarization refractoriness" (see Figure 9-7). Nevertheless, the concept of wavelength is still the same.

The impulse as represented by the wavelength does not occupy the entire muscle bundle, there is a region in front of it (dashed line in front of arrowhead) which has not yet been excited and is still completely excitable. This represents the fully excitable gap of the reentrant circuit. There is also a relatively refractory region between the end of the effective refractory period and complete repolarization at the left of the bundle, which represents a partially excitable gap (red segment of arrow tail).

In Panel B2, action potential 2 shows what happens to the wavelength when conduction velocity of the impulse increases to 17 cm/sec but the time for repolarization remains at 0.3 sec (factors that control conduction velocity are described later in this chapter). Phase 0 depolarization moves more rapidly from left to right down the length of the muscle bundle, propagating about 7 cm at the time shown. The impulse propagates a longer distance during the 0.3 sec required for repolarization to the end of the effective refractory period. As a result, the wavelength of the impulse expands to approximately 5 cm; conduction velocity of 17 cm/sec × 0.3 sec = 5.1 cm. There is no fully excitable gap (no dashed line ahead of the impulse). (Remember that the fiber bundle in the figure represents a circular reentrant pathway: the end of the bundle "b" connects to the beginning of the bundle "a".) The extent of the wavelength is also shown by the blue arrowhead to blue arrow tail which coincides with the action potential from phase 0 to the end of the effective refractory period. Part of the bundle indicated by the red line, is relatively refractory forming a partially excitable gap. The impulse can still conduct around the circuit in this partially excitable gap.

Panel B3, action potential 3 shows the effects of reducing the duration of the action potential by accelerating repolarization to 0.2 sec. The conduction velocity is 10 cm/sec, the same as in B1. Now, as the impulse moves over the same distance as in B1, the more rapid repolarization shortens the wavelength of the impulse to 2 cm so that it occupies less of the bundle (blue arrowhead to end of blue tail), leaving an extensive region of the bundle that is fully excitable. There is a large fully excitable gap (dashed line) as well as a partially excitable gap (red line).

Effect of variable conduction velocity and repolarization. At the beginning of the chapter, Figure 9-1 represents a simple model of a reentrant circuit where the wavelength remains constant during transit of the impulse around the circuit because conduction velocity and repolarization remain constant. If conduction velocity and refractory period vary from site to site in a circuit, the wavelength will change during propagation of the reentrant impulse, as diagrammed in **Figure 9-3**. Specific examples of clinical arrhythmias that show these features are described in subsequent chapters.

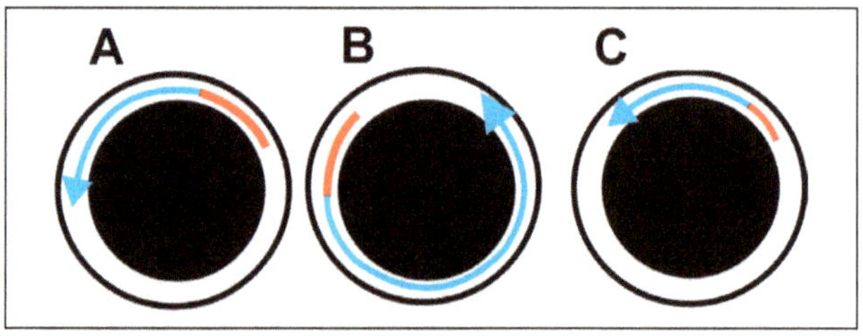

Figure 9-3 Reentry in a circuit in which wavelength changes in different regions of the reentrant pathway.

Figure 9-3 diagrams the propagating wavefront (blue arrowheads) and the effectively refractory (blue) and partially refractory (red) tail, at three different positions (A, B, and C) in a reentrant circuit. Conduction velocity is slower in the segments of the circuit in Snapshots A and C, resulting in a shorter wavelength (blue arrowhead to blue tail) than in Snapshot B, where conduction velocity is rapid causing a long wavelength (blue arrowhead to blue tail). Therefore, the spatial duration of the fully excitable gap when the propagating impulse is at the position in B, is much smaller than when the impulse is at the positions in A and C. However, the average wavelength must still be less than the path length.

Location and Form of Reentrant Circuits

Reentrant circuits can be located almost anywhere in the heart and can assume a variety of sizes and shapes. The size and location of an anatomically defined reentrant circuit remains fixed and results in what may be called "ordered reentry." Anatomical circuits have a central anatomical obstacle (Figures 9-1) that prevents the impulse from taking a "short cut" that would preexcite a segment of the pathway and stop reentry. The circuit may also be functional and its existence, size and shape determined by electrophysiological properties of the cardiac cells rather than an anatomically defined pathway. The size and location of reentrant circuits dependent on functional properties can be ordered but also may change with time leading to random reentry. Nevertheless, the relationship between path length and wavelength still apply. Reentrant circuits can also be a combination of anatomical and functional components. The different kinds of reentry are described in Figures 9-17 to 9-21.

The model of the reentrant circuit diagrammed in Figure 9-1 is modified for the description of clinical arrhythmias, the modification being dependent on the location of the reentrant circuit.

NECESSARY ELECTROPHYSIOLOGICAL PROPERTIES FOR REENTRY

The basic electrophysiological properties that facilitate reentry are slow conduction, unidirectional conduction block, and time for recovery of excitability.

Slow Conduction of the Propagating Wavefront

For reentry to occur, the conducting impulse must be delayed sufficiently in its transit through the reentrant pathway to allow regions in front of it to recover excitability (delayed until the effective refractory period ends). In other words, the wavelength must be shorter than the path length. If, for example, the impulse conducted at a normal velocity of 50 cm/sec in a reentrant pathway in the atrium, with an effective refractory period of 150 ms, it would have to conduct for at least 150 ms before it could return and reexcite a region it had previously excited. This means the conduction pathway must be at least 7.5 cm long (the value of the wavelength, $\lambda = \theta$ (50 cm/sec) $\times$ ERP (0.15 sec) for reentry to occur. Such long reentrant pathways, functionally isolated from the rest of the heart, are not likely to occur.

According to the concepts described in Figures 9-1 and 9-2, the length of the pathway necessary for reentry can be shortened if the conduction velocity is slowed. For example, if conduction velocity is slowed to 0.05 cm/sec, as can occur in diseased cardiac muscle, the reentrant circuit need be no more than 7.5 mm in length, which can readily exist. A slow conduction velocity can be a consequence of changes in active membrane properties determining the characteristics of inward currents depolarizing the membrane (phase 0) during the action potential or it can be a consequence of changes in passive properties governing the flow of current between cardiac cells through gap junctional channels; the axial current. Both often participate simultaneously. The factors that affect conduction velocity are described in the next section.

Effects of the Depolarization Phase (0) of the Action Potential on Conduction

Important features of transmembrane action potentials that govern the speed of propagation are (1) the amplitude of the action potential (positivity of phase 0) which reflects the magnitude of the inward depolarizing current, and (2) the rate at which phase 0 depolarizes the cell (dv/dt_{max} of phase 0 in volts/s, also expressed as $\dot{V}_{max}$), which indicates the speed at which the inward current reaches maximum intensity. Reduction of these parameters slows conduction. Figure 9-4, Panels A–C show the mechanism for normal rapid conduction and the effects of reducing the amplitude and dv/dt_{max} ($\dot{V}_{max}$) of phase 0, in a simple model of linear conduction through a strand of three myocardial cells (labeled 1, 2, and 3) with phase 0 of the action potentials dependent on I_{Na}. The cells are physically connected by the intercalated disks and electrically connected internally by channels in gap junctions that reside in the disks (in yellow). The model does not take into account microscopic discontinuities formed by the gap junctions that have an additional influence on conduction properties.

Panel A shows the three cells in the strand at rest with a resting potential of inside –90 mV negative with respect to the outside (red line above cells), within the normal range for atrial and ventricular cells. In Panel B, cell A is excited and inward I_{Na} (red arrows) generates an action potential (above the cell in red), with the inside of the cell becoming +30 mV with respect to the outside (also within the normal range). The juxtaposition of the excited cell (1) and the adjacent unexcited cells (2 and 3) results in flow of positive charges intracellularly (referred to as the axial current) between excited (cell 1) and unexcited cells (2 and 3) (from positive to negative) through the gap junction connections, indicated by the curved blue arrows (Panel B). The current, when large enough, can flow for several cells (from cell 1 to cells 2 and 3) as shown in the diagram. Some of the axial current (capacitive current) supplies positive charges to the inside of the membranes of the downstream cells (2 and 3), depolarizing their membrane potential to the threshold potential (~ –70 mV) so that they generate action potentials (red action potentials above cells 2 and 3 in Panel C).

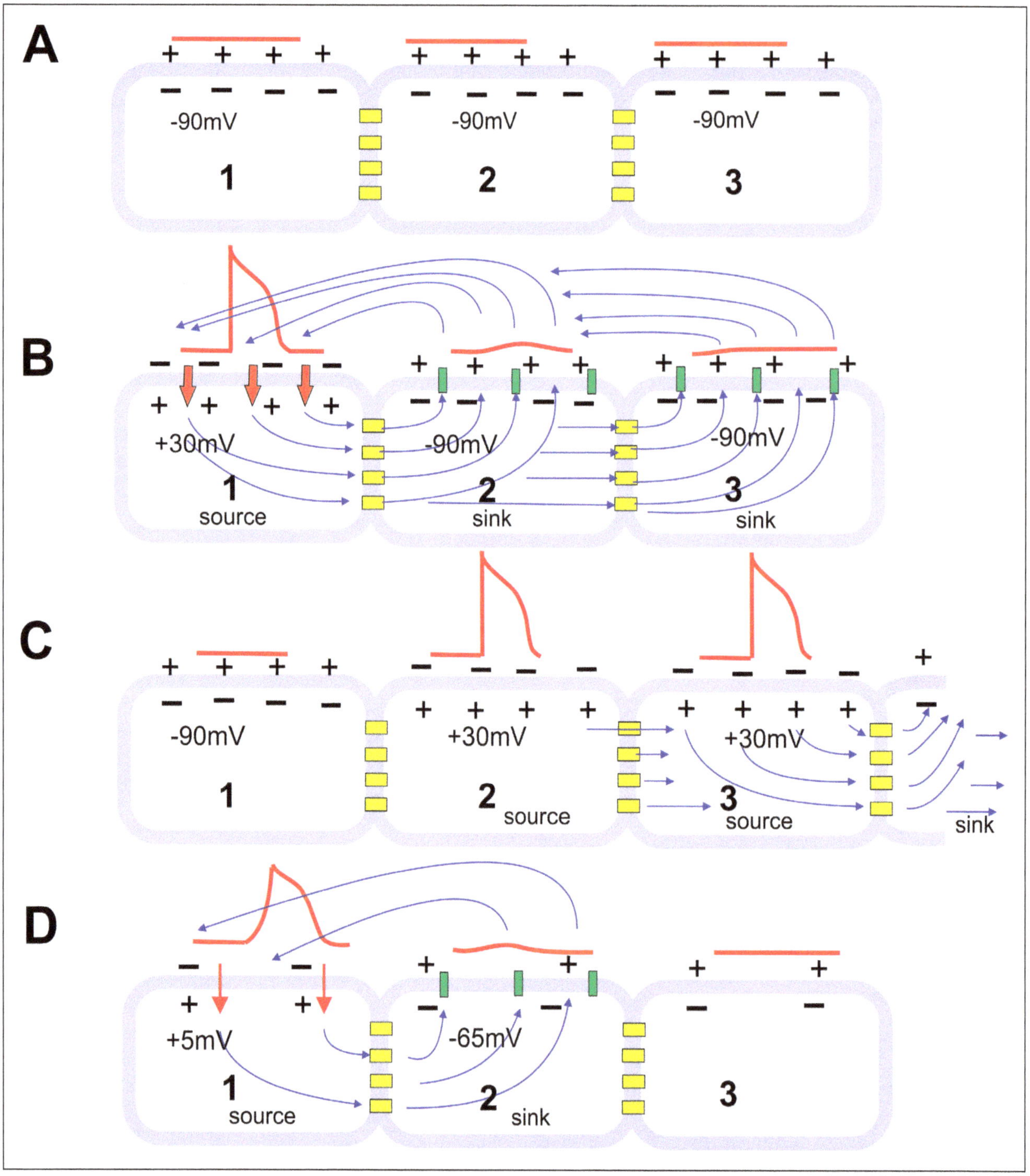

Figure 9-4 Diagram of conduction in a linear strand of three cells (**rectangles 1–3**) connected by gap junctional channels (**yellow**).

In Panel B, ionic current also flows out of cells 2 and 3 through the I_{K1} channel (green rectangles). In extracellular space, current generated by the transmembrane current flow in cells 2 and 3, flows from these cells back to the excited cell, from positive to negative (blue arrows right to left), completing the circuit. This is the current detected in electrogram and ECG recordings. The excited cell (1) generating the current in Panel B is the "source," the unexcited cell(s) (2 and 3) are the "sink." The action potential has conducted from cell 1 to cells 2 and 3 in Panel C (cell 1 has repolarized to reestablish its resting membrane potential of −90 mV, red line above cell). Once threshold is reached and an action potential is generated in cells 2 and 3, the newly excited cells switch from being a sink to being a source, generating axial current to depolarize downstream cells, perpetuating the process of action potential (impulse) propagation (Panel C).

Safety factor. For normal conduction to occur, the number of positive charges delivered by the source to the sink (Figure 9-4, Panel B cell 1) should be greater than the number of positive charges leaving the cells at the sink (cells 2 and 3). This property is responsible for depolarization of the membrane potential to threshold for generation of the action potential in cells of the sink. There is an "impedance match" between the source and the sink, meaning that the resistance to axial current flow (impedance) allows sufficient axial current that "matches" the requirements for depolarization of the sink to threshold potential. The ability to conduct from one cell to the next can be expressed in terms of the "safety factor" for conduction. This is a measurement of reliability (robustness) of conduction expressed as the ratio of the amount of net current generated by the source (cell 1) to the minimal amount of current required to excite the neighboring sink cells (2 and 3). A safety factor greater than 1 indicates more than sufficient current generated by the source for propagation, while a safety factor less than 1 causes propagation to fail because the sink is not depolarized to threshold potential. In myocardial cells with phase 0 caused by I_{Na} the safety factor is about 1.5 whereas it is smaller in the SA and A-V nodes (but still sufficient for propagation) that have depolarization phases dependent on the relatively weak I_{CaL}.

Determinants of Conduction Velocity

The conduction velocity depends on (1) the properties of the ionic current generated by the source (magnitude and speed to reach maximum intensity (dv/dt_{max}), (2) the resistance to intracellular and intercellular current flow between source and sink, which is the axial resistance or impedance, provided by myoplasm and gap junctions, and (3) the membrane properties of the sink. These properties influence how much axial current flows to unexcited sites ahead of the propagating wavefront, the distance at which the current can depolarize the membrane potential to threshold, and the amount of current needed to depolarize the sink to threshold.

An additional factor that must be kept in mind, but that is usually not emphasized, is the resistance to current flow in the extracellular space, which is part of the local electrical circuit. The extracellular space is actually compartmentalized into the microvascular tree and interstitial space. Only the resistance (impedance) of the interstitial space affects current flow. The microvascular tree is insulated from the interstitial space. Therefore, changes in extracellular resistance will also affect conduction velocity. However, the influence of changes in extracellular space with disease on conduction is uncertain. One example might be that an increase in interstitial fluid could decrease extracellular resistance to enhance velocity but this effect might be offset by changes in the other factors that affect conduction.

Na^+ channel properties. Figure 9-4, Panel D shows the effects of a reduction in the inward current at the source, in a cell with a reduced resting potential of −65 mV (0 potential not shown for measurement of resting potential) that inactivates a fraction of Na^+ channels, decreasing the net inward I_{Na} (see Chapter 4, Figure 4-5 for a description of the effects of resting membrane depolarization on the Na^+ channel). In cell 1, the decreased rate (dv/dt_{max}) and amount of current during phase 0 depolarizes the membrane potential only to +5 mV (red action potential), reducing the amount of source and axial current (blue arrows). This in turn decreases the rapidity at which cells in the pathway of propagation are depolarized to threshold potential and the distance in front of the propagating action potential that is depolarized (axial current flows only to cell 2 in the diagram), slowing conduction. A further reduction in axial current caused by inactivation of more Na^+ channels would lead to conduction block when source current is insufficient to depolarize the sink to threshold.

The relationship of I_{Na} to conduction velocity, determined in a computer model, is shown in **Figure 9-5.** I_{Na} is expressed on the abscissa as membrane excitability or the percent of maximum Na^+ conductance (%$\bar{g}$Na), a measurement of the ease at which ions flow through the channel. Conduction velocity on the left (ordinate) slows by about two-thirds to 17 cm/sec as %$\bar{g}$Na decreases before block occurs (horizontal bar at end of solid curved line), although in studies on tissue, velocity may be slower. The safety factor for conduction (dashed line, right ordinate) also decreases in parallel until conduction blocks when the safety factor falls below 1.

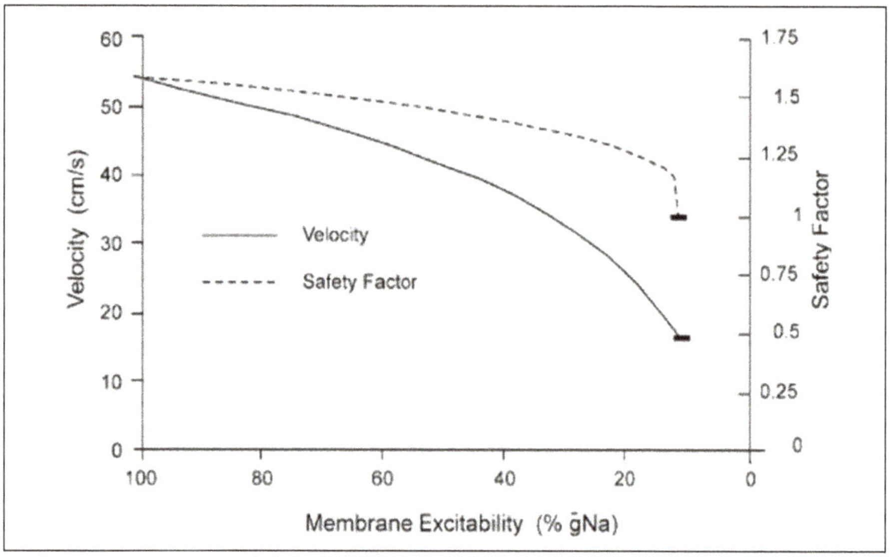

Figure 9-5 Conduction during reduced membrane excitability in a computer model. (Reproduced from Shaw RM, Rudy Y. Ionic mechanisms of propagation in cardiac tissue. Roles of the sodium and L-type calcium currents during reduced excitability and decreased gap junction coupling. *Circ Res.* 1997;81:727–741.)

Slow conduction and block caused by inactivation of Na^+ channels and reduction of I_{Na} can occur under several circumstances, such as cell activation during the relative refractory period or by inactivation of Na^+ channels by reduction in membrane potential in diseased tissues. Slow conduction caused by activation of a cell during phase 3 repolarization (during the relative refractory period) that can occur after a premature impulse or during activation at short cycle lengths is diagrammed in **Figure 9-6**.

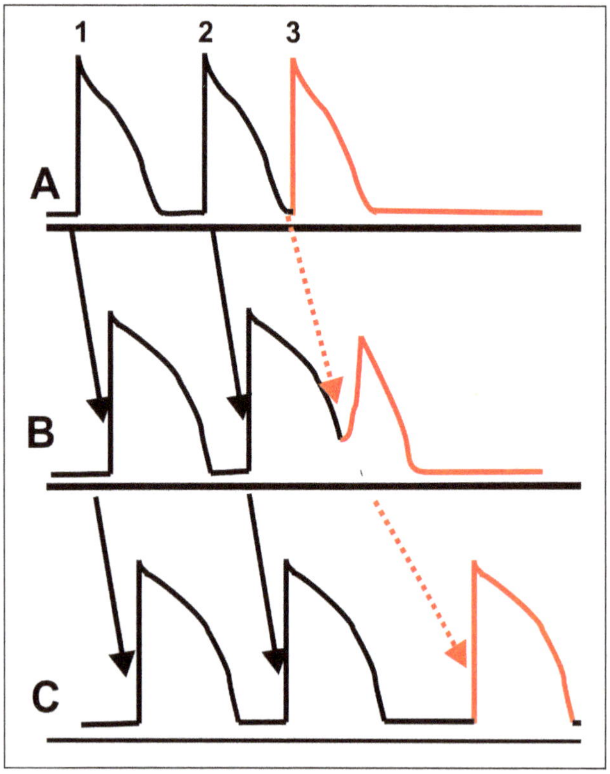

Figure 9-6 Conduction of an action potential occurring at a short cycle length.

The figure shows drawings of action potential recordings at three different sites in the His-Purkinje system. Site A in the His bundle has a shorter action potential duration than sites B and C in a distal bundle branch. Impulse conduction is from sites A to B to C, indicated by the arrows. At a relatively long cycle length, action potentials 1 and 2 have a rapid phase 0 and conduct rapidly from site A to sites B and C (black arrows). Action potential 3 (in red) occurs at a short cycle length (it is premature) at site A and reaches site B (dashed red arrow) before action potential repolarization is complete (during the phase 3 relative refractory period). The action potential arising during phase 3 at site B (red) has a slow phase 0 and low amplitude, because Na^+ channels that were inactivated during phase 0 of action potential 2 have not completely recovered at the less negative membrane potential of phase 3. As a result, action potential 3 in site B conducts slowly to site C (dashed red arrow). At a still shorter cycle length, during activation earlier in phase 3 (not shown), conduction block can occur. Slow conduction and block during phase 3 is one of the causes of reentry as described in Figure 9-14.

Slow conduction and block caused by inactivation of Na^+ channels also occurs in cells in diseased regions where resting membrane potential is decreased to less than normal negative values (Chapter 4, Figure 4-3 and Figure 4-10). Figure 9-7 diagrams conduction from site A, which has a normal resting potential, through a region with a decreased resting membrane potential (site B), to a distal site C with a normal resting potential (arrows).

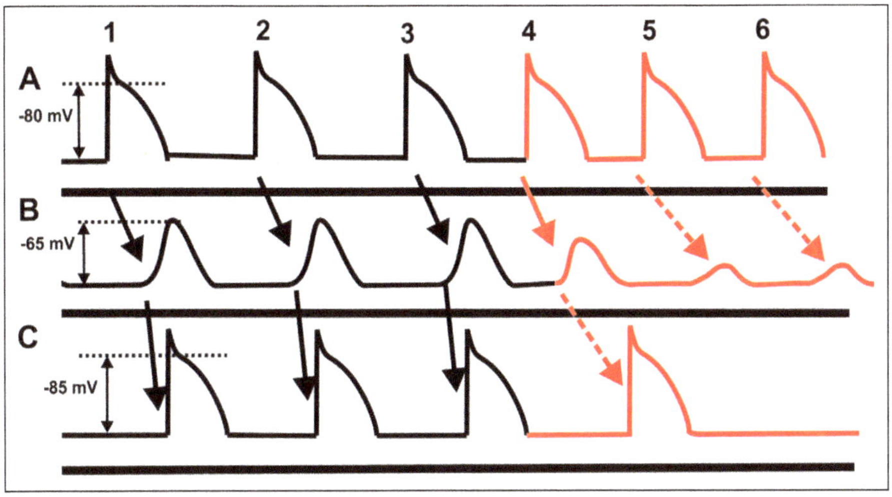

Figure 9-7 Postrepolarization refractoriness causes block at short cycle lengths.

In Figure 9-7, action potentials 1, 2, and 3 in site A (top row) conduct slowly through site B because of the inactivation of Na^+ channels at this site, reflected by the slow phase 0 and reduced action potential amplitude. When membrane potential is reduced, partially inactivating Na^+ channels (site B, membrane potential is −65 mV), refractory periods can even outlast complete repolarization, a phenomenon called "postrepolarization refractoriness." In Figure 9-7, the fourth action potential at site A (red) occurs at a shorter cycle length and arrives earlier at site B than the previous action potentials. Because of postrepolarization refractoriness, the amplitude of the early action potential (action potential 4) at site B is further reduced, reflecting incomplete recovery of Na^+ channels, and slowing conduction to site C (bottom row) even further (dashed red arrow). At this short cycle length, conduction of subsequent action potentials (5 and 6) from site A block at site B, even though they arrive well after complete repolarization (dashed red arrows), because of the postrepolarization refractoriness.

Slow response action potentials due to I_{CaL}. In Figure 9-5, slow conduction based on reduced I_{Na} alone has a velocity limit of around 17 cm/sec before conduction block occurs. However, much slower conduction, as slow as 1.0 to 0.05 cm/sec, sometimes occurs in diseased myocardium. Action potentials with phase 0 depolarization due to I_{CaL} can conduct this slowly. As explained in Chapter 4 (Figure 4-5 and Figure 4-6), under certain conditions in cells with resting potentials less than −60mV that completely inactivates I_{Na}, the normally weak I_{CaL} may give rise to phase 0 of conducting action potentials. Action potentials dependent on I_{CaL} (sometimes referred to as "slow responses") can occur in diseased cardiac cells with reduced resting potentials but also occur in the normal SA and A-V nodes (Figure 2-5 and Figure 3-13), where the maximum diastolic or resting potential is normally less than about −70 mV and there is a deficiency of functioning Na^+ channels. The L-type Ca^{2+} current can also assume an important role in conduction when gap junction coupling between myocardial cells is reduced, which also reduces conduction velocities below those that occur because of reduction of I_{Na} alone (explained in Figure 9-8).

Membrane properties of the sink. Conduction velocity also depends on the properties of the sink. For example, a reduction in resting potential that decreases I_{Na} source current (Figure 9-4, Panel D) also shifts the threshold potential more positively in the sink requiring more depolarization to excite an action potential (decreases its excitability). The current distribution in the sink, which influences the ability of axial current to depolarize it, is also influenced by its geometry. In Figure 9-4, in a linear strand, all the axial current is focused toward depolarizing the sink membranes. If the area of membrane of the sink is too large for the available source current to depolarize to threshold potential, which can be caused by an increase in the number of cells, conduction will fail. This situation is called "source-sink impedance mismatch" and is described in more detail in Figure 9-16.

The continuous model of conduction described in Figure 9-4 is an oversimplified model of heart muscle that does not show the macroscopic and microscopic discontinuities that interact with and affect current flow. Action potential propagation may transiently slow at the disks and then speed up distal to a disk, making propagation discontinuous on a microscopic scale that is not reflected in conduction on a macroscopic scale.

Effects of Gap Junction Coupling on Conduction

During conduction of the impulse, axial current flows from one myocardial cell (the source) to the adjacent cell(s) (the sink) through the gap junction channels as shown in Figure 9-4. In addition to the properties of phase

0 of the action potential previously described, the amount of axial current is dependent on the gap junctional conductance, which is determined by the permeability of gap junction channels to ions carrying current. The channels offer a resistance or impedance to the current flow in addition to the resistance of the myoplasm. Sometimes, the reciprocal value of the gap junctional impedance, gap junction conductance, is used to describe the "ease" of current flow through gap junctions. One factor determining gap junction conductance is the connexin protein isoform forming the channel. (High- and low-conductance channels are described in Chapters 2 and 3.) Other features that affect gap junction conductance are the total surface area of the gap junctions, the number of junctional channels per unit area of gap junction, and the proportion of these channels in the open state that allows current to flow. A decrease in current flowing through gap junctions caused by alterations in any of these determinants, expressed as a decrease in gap junction conductance or an increase in gap junction resistance, slows or blocks conduction. The decrease in conductance or increased resistance is also referred to as "cell or gap junction uncoupling." A number of different cardiac pathologies cause reentrant arrhythmias by causing uncoupling.

The relationship between gap junction (intercellular) coupling expressed in terms of coupling conductance, and conduction velocity is shown in **Figure 9-8**. As coupling (conductance) decreases (left to right on the abscissa), conduction velocity (ordinate) declines to a very low value of 0.26 cm/sec (solid line) before block occurs. At these very low conductance values, I_{CaL} assumes an important role in conduction by providing additional inward source current to that provided by I_{Na}, to depolarize the sink. The minimum conduction velocity that can be attained before block occurs is much slower than that associated with a reduction of I_{Na} alone (see Figure 9-5). At the same time, there is a transient rise in the safety factor (dashed line) meaning that despite the very slow conduction, there is less of a possibility of conduction block until conduction becomes very slow (block occurs when the safety factor reaches 1). This property is opposite from what one would intuitively expect, that is, as coupling decreases the likelihood of conduction block increases. It is also different from the continuous decline in safety factor with reduction of I_{Na} (Figure 9-5). Increased gap junctional resistance results in more current confined within a cell and less current shunted to downstream cells. Therefore, there is more current available for local excitation.

Anisotropic Slow Conduction

Conduction in cardiac muscle is anisotropic, meaning that conduction velocity varies depending on the direction in which impulse propagation occurs. The directional difference is caused by the structure of the myocardium. Anisotropic conduction is exemplified by the conduction properties of normal septal ventricular muscle diagrammed in **Figure 9-9**. It also occurs in the atria, other regions of the ventricles, and SA and A-V nodes.

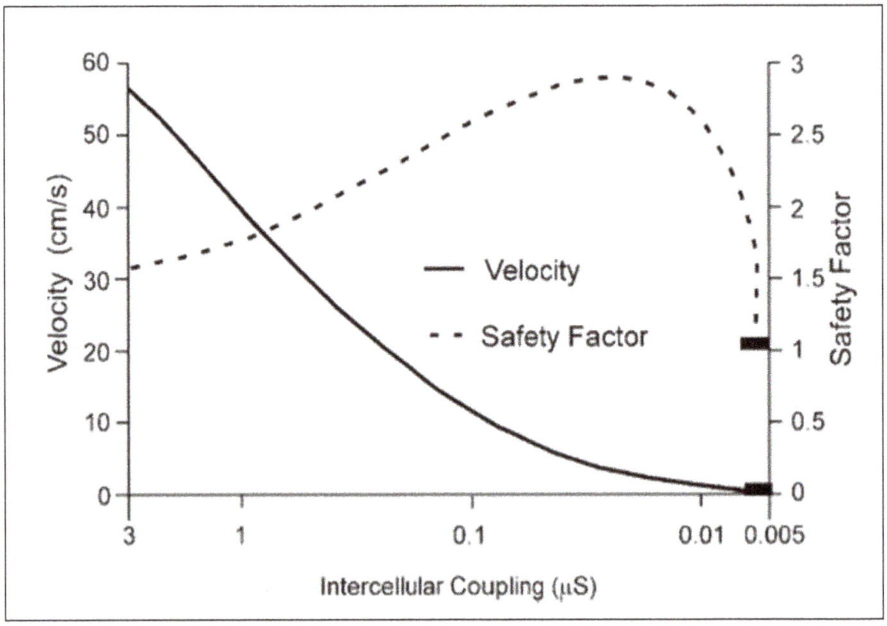

Figure 9-8 Conduction during reduced intercellular gap junctional coupling in a computer model. Conduction velocity (**solid line**) and safety factor (SF) for conduction (**dashed line**) versus gap junction conductance (intercellular coupling (μS) where S = siemens, which is a unit of electrical conductance). (Reproduced from Shaw RM, Rudy Y. Ionic mechanisms of propagation in cardiac tissue. Roles of the sodium and L-type calcium currents during reduced excitability and decreased gap junction coupling. *Circ Res.* 1997;81:727–741.)

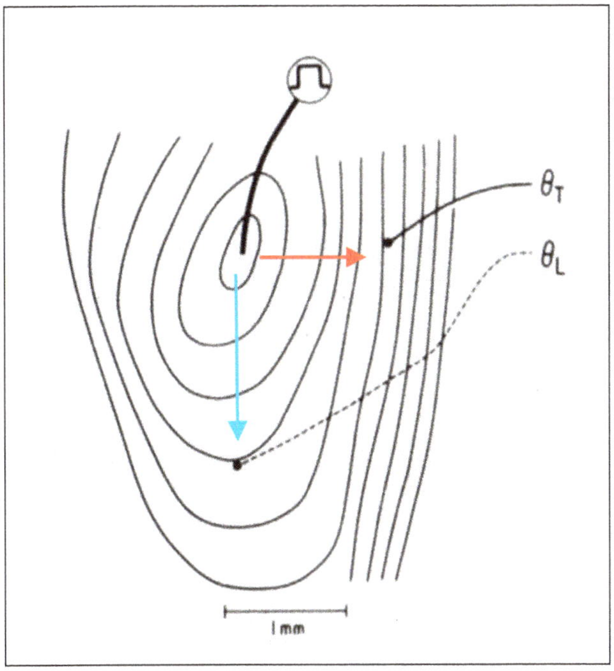

Figure 9-9 Properties of uniform anisotropic conduction. (Modified from Spach MS, Heidlage J. The stochastic nature of cardiac propagation at a microscopic level: Electrical description of myocardial architecture and its application to conduction. *Circ Res.* 1995;76(3):366–380.)

In Figure 9-9, the muscle in the diagram is stimulated in the center at the pulse symbol, and activation spreads away from this site in all directions, forming elliptical isochrones. In the direction of the long axis of the ellipse (from top to bottom) (blue arrow), the isochrones are widely spaced, indicating rapid conduction with a velocity (θ_L) of 51 cm/sec. In the direction transverse to the long axis (to the right) (red arrow) the isochrones are spaced closely together indicating a slower velocity (θ_T) of 17 cm/sec. The anisotropic ratio of fast to slow conduction, θ_L/θ_T, is 3.0. As the direction of propagation changes between these two axes, the conduction velocity changes monotonically from fast to slow (also note the curvature of the wavefront between the axes of longitudinal and transverse conduction which has an additional slowing effect on conduction, see Figure 9-13). The anisotropy illustrated here is considered to be uniform because it is characterized by an advancing macroscopic wavefront that has smooth isochrones in all directions relative to the orientation of the long axis.

The anisotropic propagation in normal ventricular myocardium illustrated in Figure 9-9 is related to the tissue architecture, that is, the size and shape of the myocardial cells and bundles and the distribution of their gap junction interconnections. **Figure 9-10** diagrams some of these relationships in a simplified form.

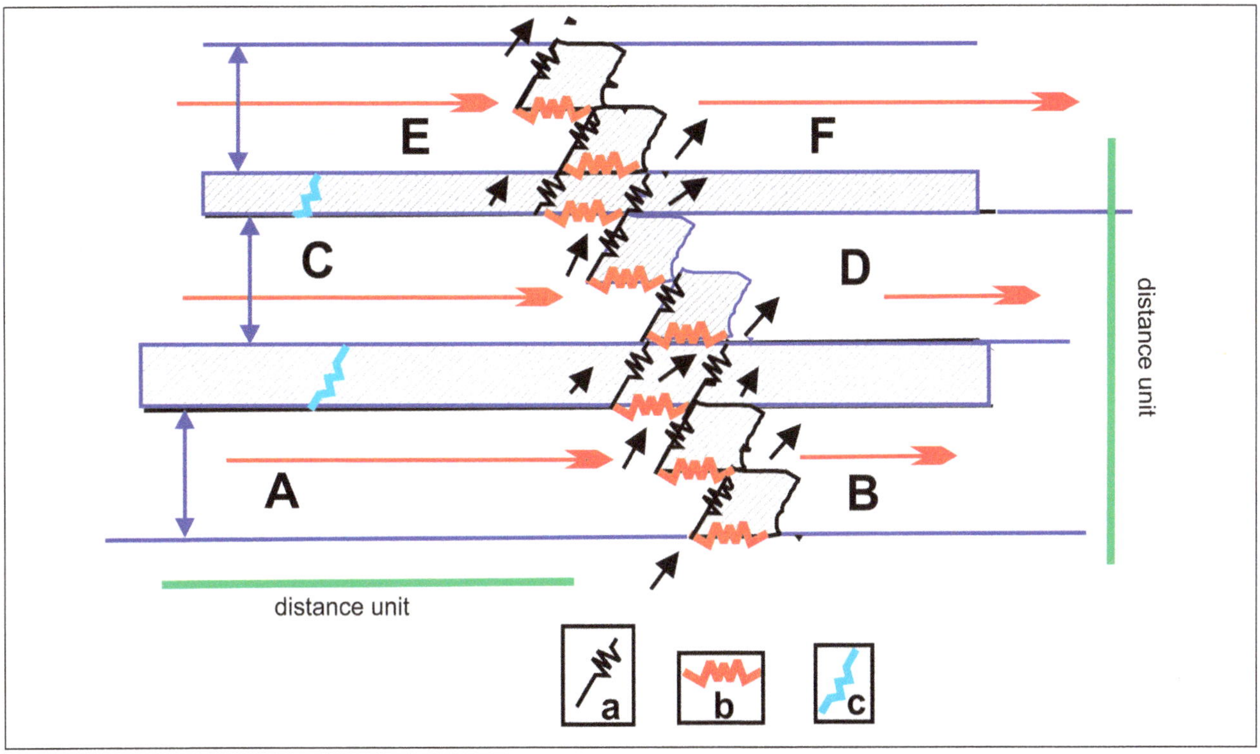

Figure 9-10 Diagram of anisotropic conduction in 6 interconnected myocardial cells, **A, B, C, D, E,** and **F**. (Based on Figure 2 in Spach MS, Heidlage JF. The stochastic nature of cardiac propagation at a microscopic level: Electrical description of myocardial architecture and its application to conduction. *Circ Res.* 1995;76(3):366-380. We assume responsibility for any errors in our interpretation of that figure.)

It shows the gap junctional coupling of six muscle cells (labeled A, B, C, D, E, and F) that have a normal, elongated shape, with their long axis from left to right, and their transverse axis perpendicular to the long axis (double-headed arrow at the left). The location of gap junctions is indicated by resistor symbols, indicating their resistive properties. They are located in the intercalated disks that step back and forth across the ends of the cells, alternating between longitudinal and transverse orientations with respect to the long axis of the myocytes (shaded regions). Most gap junctions are in the segments of the disks at the ends of the cells. Plicate junctions, defined as the gap junctions in a segment of the disk arranged in folds like a fan, are indicated by symbol b (in red). They connect cells A to B, C to D, and E to F end-to-end (longitudinally). As shown in the diagram, other gap junctions labeled interplicate (symbol a, in black) (between the fan shaped segments of the disk) connect cell A to C, C to E, B to D, D to F in the transverse direction. Although these junctions are located at the ends of the cells, they provide the major coupling in the transverse direction. There are only a few scattered gap junctions along the lateral segment of the sarcolemma that probably do not have a major role in transverse conduction (symbol labeled c, in blue). Therefore, both longitudinal (through plicate) and transverse (through interplicate) coupling occurs mostly at the ends of the muscle cell. Because of these gap junctions, the action potential can conduct in the transverse direction from one cell to the next cell alongside it, (A to C, C to E, B to D, D to F (black arrows)), as easily as it can in the longitudinal direction between one cell to another cell at its end, (A to B, C to D, and E to F (red arrows)). Nevertheless, over a distance of many cells, transverse propagation is significantly slower than longitudinal propagation.

Transverse conduction is slower than longitudinal conduction because in the transverse direction, an impulse encounters many more gap junctions than over an equivalent distance in the longitudinal direction. This is because cell diameter is much less than cell length and, therefore, the impulse must traverse more cells transversely per unit distance and conduct through an increased number of gap junctions (compare gap junctions traversed per distance unit indicated by the green lines in Figure 9-10). Because gap junctions are a resistance to current flow, there is a greater resistance to axial current flow (axial resistivity) transversely than longitudinally.

In summary, therefore, although the definition of uniform anisotropy is an advancing wavefront that is smooth in all directions relative to the long axis of the myocardial fiber bundles as shown in Figure 9-9, this definition is based on the characteristics of activation at a macroscopic level where the spatial resolution encompasses numerous myocardial cells and bundles. Because of the irregularities in cell geometry and irregular distribution of the gap junctions of normal ventricular cells, as diagrammed in Figure 9-10, activation at a microscopic level, where the spatial resolution is comparable to individual cells, is irregular. The slow conduction in the direction transverse to the longitudinal axis occurs despite action potentials with normal resting potentials and upstroke (phase 0) velocities. This is similar to slow conduction caused by gap junction uncoupling (Figure 9-8) and unlike slow conduction caused by inactivation of I_{Na} where phase 0 is decreased (Figure 9-4).

In uniform anisotropic tissue, the extracellular unipolar electrogram has a large amplitude, smooth biphasic, positive–negative morphology during propagation in the longitudinal direction reflecting the rapid conduction. In the transverse direction, this electrogram has a low-amplitude triphasic (negative-positive-negative) morphology reflecting the slow irregular conduction with delays between cell activation.

Nonuniform anisotropy. Anisotropic conduction properties are affected by other structural features in both normal and diseased heart muscle that influence the extent and location of gap junction coupling. In some regions of the normal atria (crista terminalis) and ventricles (papillary muscles), myocardial cells are grouped in bundles comprised of 2–30 cells and surrounded by a connective tissue sheath, which prevents extensive lateral connections. Parallel bundles are connected to each other in a lateral direction by branches of muscle through perforations in the connective tissue sheaths. Similarly, in myocardium, where there is increased connective tissue because of aging or pathology, transverse gap junctional connections between cells and bundles of cells are disrupted by the expanding connective tissue septae. Then, conduction in the transverse direction is impeded, giving rise to a conduction pattern called "nonuniform anisotropy."

Nonuniform anisotropy is defined as the maintenance of tight electrical coupling between cells in the longitudinal direction with a paucity of side-to-side (transverse) electrical coupling, leading to an irregular pattern of transverse conduction. Instead of a smooth transition from longitudinal to transverse conduction velocities as in Figure 9-9, there is an abrupt transition from the rapid longitudinal velocity to very slow transverse velocity. The anisotropic ratio of fast to slow conduction velocities is increased because of a decrease in transverse velocity.

Figure 9-11 compares uniform anisotropy in tissue with sparse connective tissue septa (Panel A), to nonuniform anisotropy in tissue in which muscle bundles are separated by increased connective tissue (Panel B). In Panel B, increased connective tissue (brown shading) either precludes or disrupts the lateral gap junction connections, and transverse connections are provided by bridges of myocardium that penetrate the large amounts of connective tissue. In both panels, longitudinal conduction is indicated by the red arrows and transverse conduction by the blue arrows. In Panel A (uniform anisotropy), there are abundant connections in the transverse direction. Because of the connective tissue barriers in Panel B, transverse conduction occurs only in regions that bridge the connective tissue barriers, in an irregular zig-zag pattern, while a relatively normal pattern of longitudinal conduction is maintained (nonuniform anisotropy).

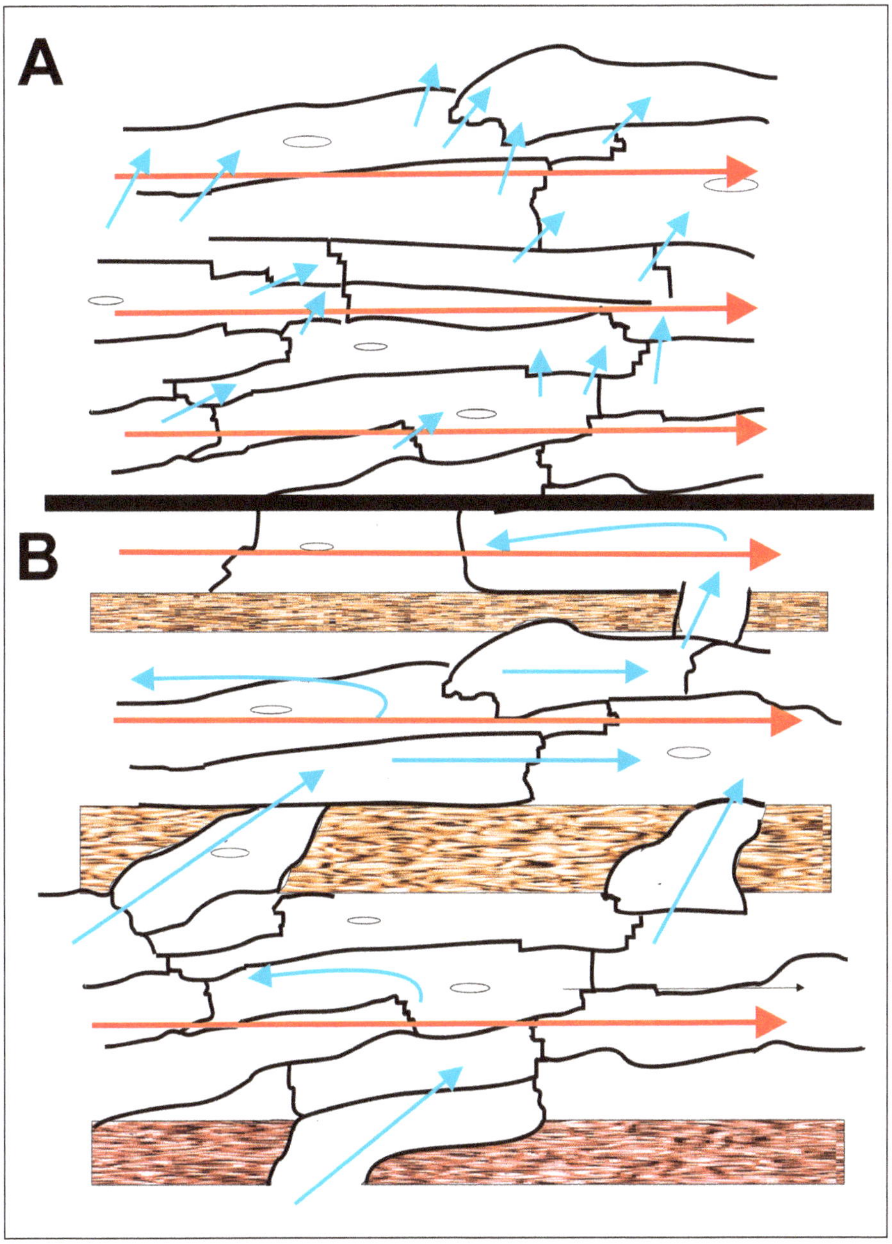

Figure 9-11 Comparison of uniform anisotropy (**Panel A**) and nonuniform anisotropy (**Panel B**).

Conduction in the transverse direction in regions with nonuniform anisotropic conduction can be slower than the slowest conduction associated with partial depolarization of the resting potential and inactivation of Na^+ channels. In fact, it can be as slow as the slow conduction caused by gap junction uncoupling shown in Figure 9-8. At a critical degree of gap junction uncoupling, conduction block can occur in the transverse direction while conduction is maintained in the longitudinal direction.

Characteristic electrograms. Bipolar electrograms recorded from nonuniform anisotropic myocardium have multiple components and long durations and are called "fractionated electrograms." This is a result of the fewer transverse connections between muscle bundles and the zig-zag nature of propagation when a region has a large, abnormal amount of connective tissue as described above. Slow transverse activation is dependent on the structural alterations rather than abnormalities in transmembrane potentials. The multiple components are caused by irregular and slow activation of muscle fibers within the recording field of the bipoles. Electrograms with this characteristic can be located in regions where reentrant circuits form and are a marker for circuit location (see Chapter 12) but may also be located anywhere that there is slow and nonuniform activation. A simplified explanation for the relationship of irregular, slow, activation in nonuniform anisotropic myocardium, to the occurrence of fractionated electrograms is shown in **Figure 9-12**, which shows a diagram of three myocardial bundles (yellow cylinders, a, b, and c) composed of many individual cells (which are not shown) separated by an expanded amount of connective tissue (dark brown regions between the bundles). Connections between the bundles are sparse because they have been disrupted by the connective tissue and are located in other areas outside the diagram. The location of a bipolar electrode is shown by the two red circles. This model assumes circuitous transverse conduction (the wavefront meanders back and forth through the three bundles rather than moving in a straight line across the bundles) in the vicinity of the bipolar electrode, from one bundle to the other as indicated by the curved black arrows. Conduction velocity in each of the three bundles might be normal because action potentials are normal but total activation of the region is slow because of the circuitous pathway of propagation made necessary by the lack of transverse connections. Individual deflections in the electrogram (EG) at the right (a, b, and c) are from activation of each of the bundles. Intervals between the larger deflections (with little activity) occur during the time the impulse is out of the recording field of the bipolar electrode. Activation of the small region around the electrode (several mm) is very slow, causing a long duration of the electrogram.

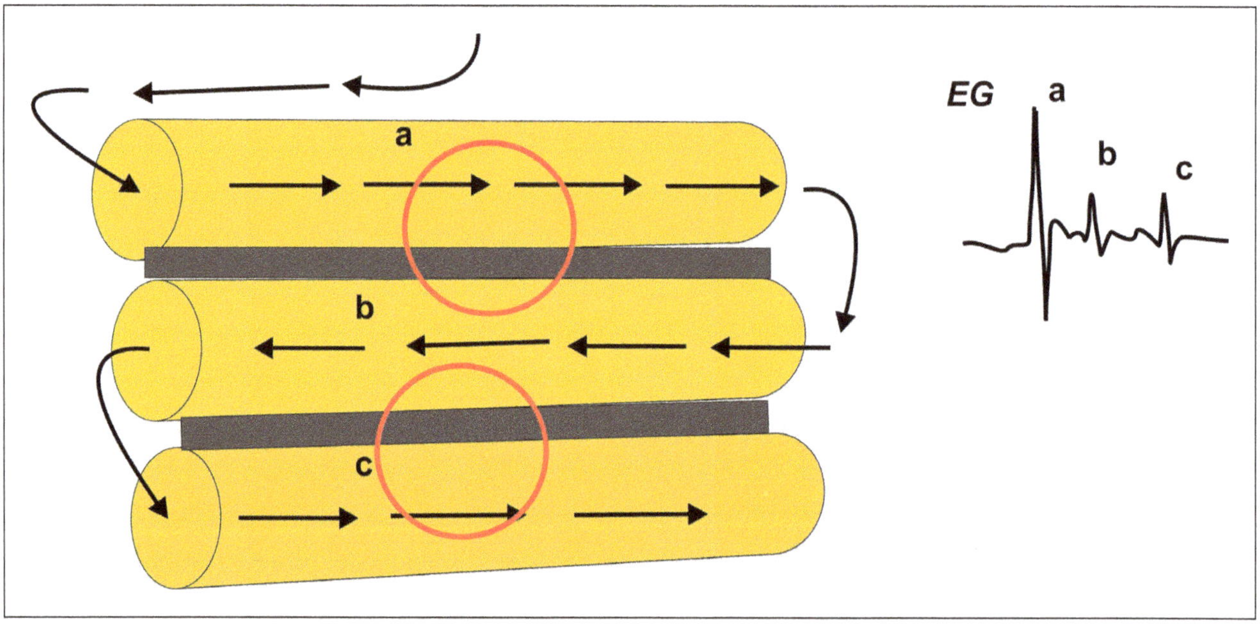

Figure 9-12 Mechanism for fractionated electrograms.

The characteristics of the electrogram change when the direction of activation changes. In the simple model shown in Figure 9-12, the electrogram recorded when propagation occurs longitudinally (from left to right) would not be as fractionated as during transverse activation, since activation of each bundle occurs nearly simultaneously in this direction. Electrogram characteristics also are influenced by the distance between the bipoles since, when they are farther apart, they sense electrical activity over a larger region. In actuality, there would be many more bundles of interconnected muscle than shown in Figure 9-12 leading to more deflections and a longer duration of the fractionated electrogram. The amplitude of the electrograms can also be low when there large amounts of connective tissue and the size of the muscle bundles are small as occurs in diseased myocardium. In this situation, recording electrodes are further from the muscle bundles and extracellular current flow in the vicinity of the electrodes is decreased. Unipolar electrodes can also detect fractionation but the multiple local deflections can also be masked by large extrinsic (far-field) deflections, particularly when fractionated electrogram amplitude is small.

Slow Conduction Caused by Wavefront Curvature

Figure 9-4, Panel D describes the slow conduction and block that occurs when the axial current that the source generates is reduced relative to the requirements to excite the sink. Slow conduction and/or conduction block can also result from source current to sink mismatch (impedance mismatch) resulting from an increase in the size of the current sink relative to the source. The shape of the wavefront is an important determinant of the source-sink relationship. **Figure 9-13** compares conduction of a flat (planar) wavefront (A) to a convexly curved wavefront (B) with the excitation front of current flow indicated by small arrows curving outward, and to a concavely curved wavefront (C) with the excitation front indicated by the small arrows, curving inward.

Figure 9-13, Panel A, is a diagram of a planar wavefront (indicated by the horizontal black line) that might be initiated by a broad source or multiple sources (red dots). When the wavefront is planar, depolarizing current (small arrows) flows only in the direction of propagation (long blue arrow) and is only required to depolarize cells in this direction. In Panel B, the convex-curved wavefront, current from the source is dispersed not only in the direction of propagation but also along the entire front of the curvature (small arrows). Examples of this wavefront pattern can result when the initiating stimulus is at a point such as a small pacemaker focus (red dot), or when a wavefront emerges from a narrow pathway into a wide area (from an A-V bypass tract, Figure 11-15, or from an isthmus in a reentrant circuit in a healed infarct, Figure 12-4). When the wavefront is convex, a larger area must be excited for propagation in the direction of the blue arrow. Conduction velocity is slowed compared to the planar wave because of the greater dispersion of current of the wavefront over this larger area that provides a larger sink. The larger sink offers greater impedance to current flow. The greater the curvature (smaller the radius of curvature), the more the current is dispersed leading to more slowing. At a critically small radius of curvature, conduction blocks because the source current is not sufficient to depolarize the large sink to threshold. When the excitation front is concave (Panel C), the excitatory currents converges in front of the propagating wave, producing a more rapid membrane depolarization and a faster conduction velocity than a planar wave.

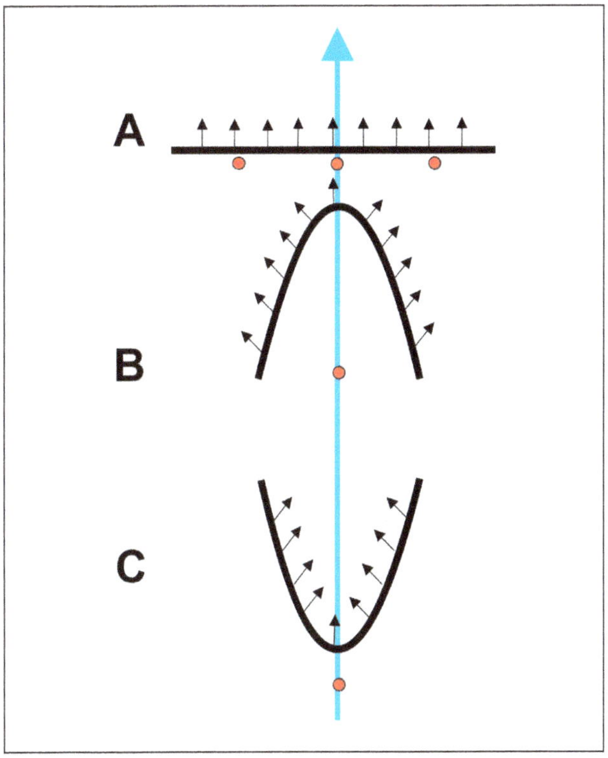

Figure 9-13 Effect of the shape of conducting wavefronts on conduction.

Curvature of wavefronts plays an important role in conduction slowing and block in reentrant circuits. The contribution of curvature to reentry in different models is described in detail later in this chapter (see Figure 9-18 and Figure 9-19).

Unidirectional Conduction Block

Unidirectional conduction block, defined as block of conduction in one direction through a conduction pathway but maintained conduction in the opposite direction, is necessary for the initiation of most forms of reentry. The model of circus movement in Figure 9-1 relies on unidirectional conduction block caused by transient block of the initiating impulse in snapshot A2, in the right-to-left direction (clockwise). The block prevents excitation of the left pathway in the ring and leaves this pathway as an excitable return pathway through which the impulse can conduct to reenter previously excited areas. There are a number of mechanisms that can cause unidirectional block. Unidirectional block can be transient during the initiating impulse as in Figure 9-1, or it can be persistent.

Unidirectional Block Caused by Regional Differences (Heterogeneities) in Recovery of Excitability

Regional differences in recovery of excitability, also referred to as heterogeneity or dispersion of refractory periods, can result in transient unidirectional conduction block that initiates reentry. **Figure 9-14** is a schematic model of how this occurs when there is heterogeneity in the time course for action potential repolarization. It shows initiation of reentry in an anatomically defined circuit. Important features are differences in the effective refractory period duration in different regions of the circuit; long action potential durations and refractory periods in the left pathway; and shorter action potential durations and refractory periods in the right pathway. In Figure 9-14, Panel A, conduction of an impulse at a relatively long cycle length (green action potential and green arrow above) is not affected by the heterogeneity in repolarization in the circuit because it enters after complete repolarization of even the longest duration action potentials (curved green arrows in the circuit and green action potential in the left pathway). This occurs when the cycle length is longer than the longest effective refractory period in the circuit. It is analogous to a sinus impulse arriving at a potential reentrant circuit without initiating reentry (green arrows).

Figure 9-14, Panel B, diagrams conduction of an impulse occurring at a shorter cycle length such as a premature impulse (green arrow and green action potential above) with a coupling interval less than the long effective refractory period in the left pathway. Conduction of this impulse is blocked in the left pathway at the horizontal gray bar (long curved green arrow and action potential followed by a subthreshold small depolarization in the repolarization phase indicated by small curved green arrow). However, this same premature impulse conducts in the right pathway with shorter refractory periods (long, curved, green arrow and green action potential in the right pathway). In order for block to occur, the premature impulse must also arise in a region with a short refractory period so that it occurs before the action potentials in the left pathway repolarize. Conduction of the premature impulse continues from the right pathway retrogradely into the left pathway indicated by the red arrow in Panel B, since the distal part of the left pathway is excitable owing to the block proximal to it.

Panel C is a continuation of the events in Panel B; the blocked left pathway is retrogradely invaded by the reentrant impulse conducting from the right pathway (red arrows beginning at the asterisk, and action potential). The proximal region where the premature impulse originates is then reexcited (red arrow and action potential above). For successful reexcitation of the region where the premature impulse originates, the myocardial cells in the circuit at the region of initial block and proximal to it (toward the site of origin) must have regained their excitability by the time the impulse that is conducting through the reentrant pathway, arrives there. Conduction velocity of premature impulses is also decreased because of activation during phase 3 of repolarization (Figure 9-6) shortening the wavelength and facilitating successful reexcitation of the region proximal to the unidirectional block. The unidirectional block of the premature impulse is transient, occurring only during the initiating premature impulse. After the wavefront is launched in the clockwise direction around the circuit, the region of initial unidirectional block recovers excitability and resumes its original property of bidirectional conduction, although during reentry the impulse conducts only in one direction (from right to left) through it. This reentrant impulse once again enters the right pathway and continues to circulate clockwise in the reentrant circuit causing another action potential in the right pathway (Panel C, blue arrow and third blue action potential of the right pathway). Continuation of reentry induced by a premature impulse is also facilitated because action potential and refractory period duration of the premature action potential may be shortened by the short cycle length (Figure 7-9). On the next excursion of the reentrant impulse around the circuit (blue arrows in Panel C), it conducts in a circuit with a shorter refractory period. If the initiating premature impulse arises too early (Panel D) (green action potential and green arrow above) it would block in both pathways of the circuit (curved green arrows), not initiating reentry. Therefore, there is a window of vulnerability characterized by a critical time period and range of membrane potentials in the circuit during which reentry can be initiated.

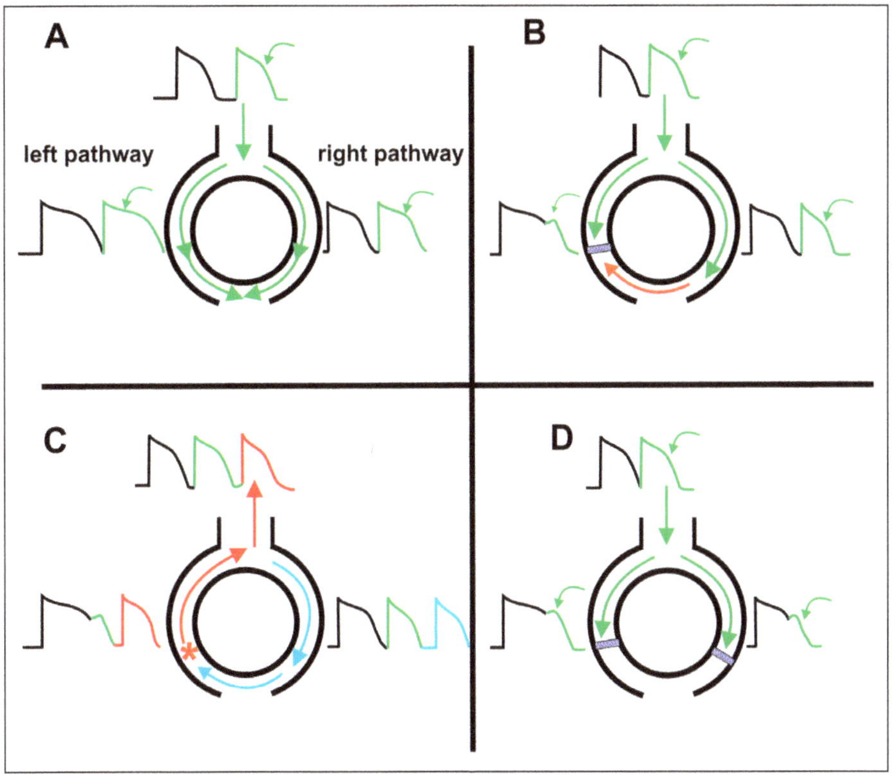

Figure 9-14 Model of unidirectional block and reentry caused by heterogeneous refractory periods.

Differences in repolarizing membrane currents: the "substrate" for heterogeneity. Heterogeneity of action potential duration and dispersions of refractory periods can result from qualitative and/or quantitative differences in repolarizing membrane currents. Natural differences occur in the A-V node leading to dual pathways of conduction (Figure 11-3). Heterogeneities also occur in the ventricle among epicardium, midmyocardium, and endocardium, between the base and apex, and between Purkinje cells and muscle cells. These differences can be exacerbated by genetic changes (e.g., long QT syndromes), or pathological changes such as changes in repolarization that accompany heart failure and myocardial infarction (Chapter 12). Natural differences in action potential duration in the atria occur between the crista terminalis and atrial free wall, or atrial trabeculae and between left and right atria. However, in closely adjacent regions in atria or ventricles, intrinsic repolarization differences may be minimized by the flow of electrotonic current through gap junctions where current flowing from cells with the longer action potential prolong the shorter action potentials and shorten the longer action potentials (Figure 1-3). Gap junctional uncoupling that reduces this current flow can enhance dispersions in repolarization sufficiently to cause unidirectional block. The likelihood of conduction block is greater if there is an abrupt change in adjacent regions rather than a gradual change.

Other causes of heterogeneity in excitability in addition to differences in the time for action potential repolarization, are different amounts of resting membrane potential depolarization causing differences in postrepolarization refractoriness (Figure 9-7) and different anisotropic properties (Figure 9-11). These properties have the same effects as heterogeneity in action potential duration in causing unidirectional block and reentry.

Premature depolarizations as the stimulus for reentry. For reentrant arrhythmias to arise because of regional differences in refractory periods, a premature depolarization that initiates reentry (often called a "trigger," but not to be confused with triggered activity caused by afterdepolarizations) is as necessary a requirement as the circuit with appropriate electrophysiological properties in which reentry occurs (the substrate). This is one reason why reentrant tachycardias often begin with a premature impulse with a different ECG morphology than the tachycardia.

The mechanism causing the premature depolarization may be quite different from the arrhythmia it initiates; it might arise spontaneously by automaticity or be a result of triggered activity. For example, as described in Chapter 7, a possible mechanism of torsades de pointes is initiation by an EAD-generated premature impulse, and perpetuation by reentry owing to a dispersion of refractoriness caused by differences in time course for repolarization in different regions of the ventricles. The premature impulse that initiates reentry might also be induced by an electrical stimulus during programmed stimulation protocols (see Figure 9-27).

Although the example of unidirectional block caused by heterogeneity in Figure 9-14 diagrams an anatomical reentrant circuit, similar heterogeneities can cause unidirectional block in functional circuits that do not have an anatomic barrier (a comparison of anatomical and functional circuits is presented below (in Figure 9-18 and Figure 9-19).

Unidirectional Block Caused by Asymmetrical Depression of Excitability

Persistent unidirectional block can be associated with a reduction of excitability. A common cause is depressed, less negative, resting potentials and reduced I_{Na} causing a slow action potential phase 0 in regions affected by disease (mechanism described in Figure 4-5 and Figure 9-7). Unidirectional block occurs when the depression of the resting potential and action potential, and thus excitability, is asymmetrical, that is, depression of both gradually becomes more severe in the direction from a normal region to a very depressed region. This might occur, for example, in regions with variable coronary perfusion in ischemic heart disease.

A model of persistent unidirectional block caused by asymmetrical depression of action potentials in a muscle bundle is shown in **Figure 9-15**. Below the muscle bundle, the action potentials show conduction block of an impulse arising outside the bundle (action potential a, below the bundle) propagating in the left-to-right direction, where the degree of depression gradually becomes more severe indicated by the progression of pink to black shading. Resting potentials and phase 0 of action potentials b–d in the bundle (below) become more depressed (lower and slower) and axial current gradually decreases indicated by the decreasing size of the arrows (decremental conduction).

The black-shaded area is a region of conduction block associated with a small electrotonic response (d, below). A normal region at the right outside the depicted bundle (e) is not excited by the weak electrotonic (axial) current from region (d) (small arrow). Conduction, therefore, blocks in the left-to-right direction even though the region (e) is normal and excitable.

However, in Figure 9-15, conduction in the opposite direction (action potentials above the bundle from right to left), still succeeds because the large axial current generated by stimulation of a normal action potential at site (e) can flow for a considerable distance through the depressed region (curved blue arrows above d) and depolarize to threshold muscle at some distance from the most severely depressed region (c). The normal action potential (e, above) is a more effective stimulus in the right-to-left direction since it encounters an abrupt region of depression, than the abnormal action potential c (below)) in the left-to-right direction of gradual depression. Propagation continues successfully from site c to sites b and a (at the top) as axial current increases (indicated by the size of the arrows above). In other words, in the series of action potentials below, the action potential (c) is too attenuated to conduct through the most depressed region (d). But in the series above, the normal action potential (e) generates enough axial current to circumvent the severely depressed excitability in (d).

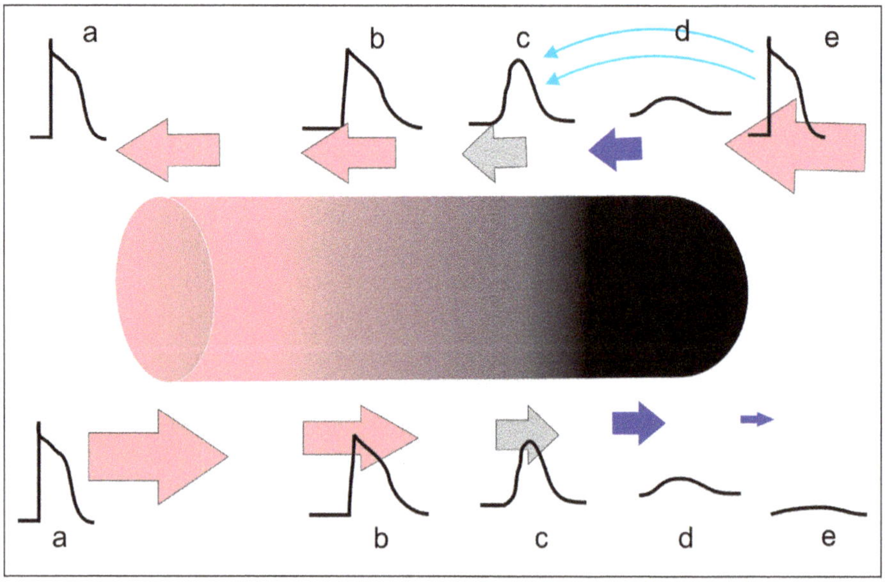

Figure 9-15 Unidirectional block in a muscle bundle with progressively more severe depression from **left to right** (**pinkish to black shading**).

Geometrical Factors Causing Unidirectional Block

Geometrical factors related to tissue architecture, particularly muscle bundle diameter and branching patterns, under certain conditions can lead to persistent unidirectional block. In bundles of atrial, ventricular, or Purkinje fibers, there is usually some asymmetry in conduction even under normal conditions; conduction in one direction may be slightly faster than in the other direction. An impulse conducting in one direction encounters a different sequence of changes in muscle bundle diameter, branching and frequency and distribution of gap junctions than it does when traveling in the opposite direction. These structural features influence conduction by affecting the axial current and the source sink relationship. **Figure 9-16** illustrates simple models to show how the geometrical organization can result in directional differences in conduction and unidirectional block. In real tissue the structure is much more complex than what is diagrammed. In Panel A, a muscle bundle with a small diameter (1) joins a larger diameter bundle (2) and in Panel B, a muscle bundle with a small diameter (1) branches into two bundles (2, 3). Panel C represents both situations as a cylinder with a small surface area (1, small diameter bundle) connecting with a cylinder with a large surface area representing either a large diameter bundle (such as [2] shown in Panel A above), or a branched region (such as [2, 3] in Panel B).

In Figure 9-16, going from left to right, the conduction velocity of an impulse (red arrows) passing from the small diameter bundle (the source, 1) to a larger one (the sink, 2) (Panel A), or to the branched region (the sink, 2, 3) (Panel B), transiently slows at the junction because the larger bundle or branched region has more total membrane for the axial current from the smaller bundle to depolarize to threshold. The current from the smaller bundle is dispersed over a larger area indicated by the red arrows (Panel C, top), weakening or slowing its effects to depolarize the larger area. In addition as indicated by the dashed purple line in Panel A, the wavefront changes from planar to highly convex at the junction where the bundle size expands also slowing conduction (see Figure 9-13 for description of effects of wavefront curvature on conduction).

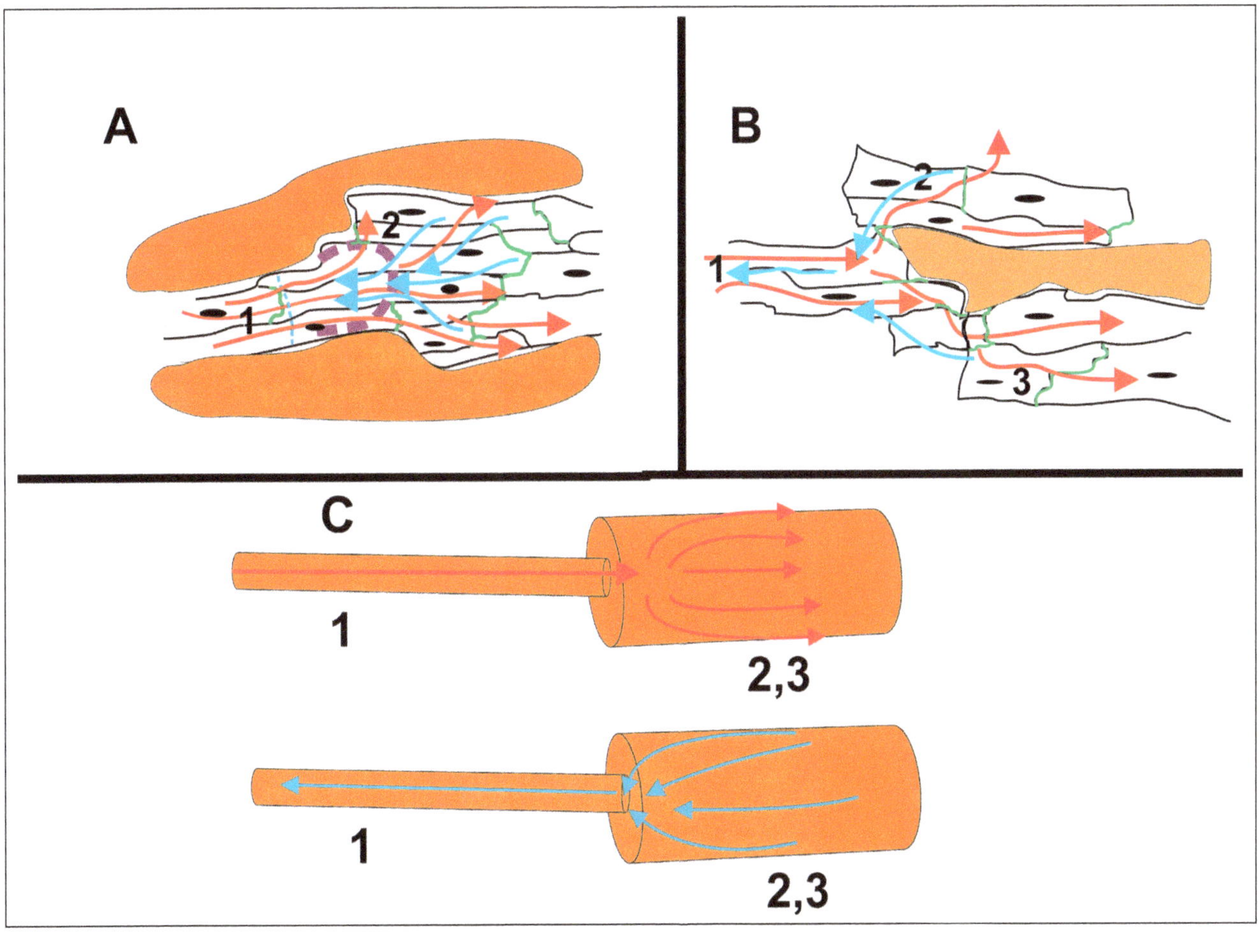

Figure 9-16 Diagrams of tissue structure that can cause unidirectional conduction block.

In the opposite direction, (Figure 9-16; going from right to left), going from the large-diameter bundle, to the small-diameter bundle (blue arrows in Panels A and C), or from the branched bundles to the single bundle (blue arrows in Panels B and C), conduction speeds up transiently because the smaller membrane area (the sink) is depolarized more rapidly to threshold by the large amount of current from the source with the larger membrane area.

Theoretically, an impulse conducting in the small bundle from left to right, could block at the junction with the larger bundle or branches if there is a large enough increase in the membrane area that must be depolarized (source-sink or impedance mismatch). In the opposite direction, however, excitation proceeds because the current from the larger membrane area is more than enough to depolarize the smaller membrane area. Thus, there is unidirectional block. An example of unidirectional block based on these geometrical factors in the normal heart occurs at the junctions between some small Purkinje bundles in the peripheral ventricular conducting system and the larger mass of ventricular muscle. At these junctions propagation from muscle with the large membrane area to Purkinje bundles (small membrane area) is possible while propagation from Purkinje bundles to muscle is not. However, abrupt changes as diagrammed in Figure 9-16 of the magnitude required to cause block of the normal action potential might not occur because the safety factor for conduction is large. Depression (decrease) of the resting potential and phase 0 of the action potentials in the small bundle (1) enhances the likelihood of unidirectional conduction block. At a critical degree of depression of phase 0, the reduced axial current becomes insufficient to depolarize the membrane to threshold where the current sink is increased (in the left-to-right direction in Panels A, B, C) because of the increased membrane area, but the axial current is still more than adequate during conduction in the opposite direction.

Unidirectional Conduction Block Caused by Anisotropy

The possibility of preferential conduction block caused by a critical degree of gap junction uncoupling in the transverse direction is described in Figure 9-8 but block caused by this mechanism is probably bidirectional. Anisotropy can also lead to directional differences in conduction block related to myocardial geometry, which may facilitate initiation of reentry. This different type of block can occur in nonuniform anisotropic myocardium—block in the longitudinal direction with maintained conduction in the transverse direction. This type of block can occur if the source current is reduced by premature stimulation owing to initiation of action potentials with reduced phase 0 when they occur prior to complete repolarization (Figure 9-6). In nonuniform anisotropic myocardium there is a low safety factor in the longitudinal direction associated with low axial resistivity because of long distances between gap junctional connections that allows current to flow relatively unimpeded. On the other hand, there is a high safety factor in the transverse direction caused by the poorer gap junction coupling that prevents current from flowing for long distances because of a high impedance in this direction, and is responsible for very slow propagation (Figures 9-8 and 9-11). Block in the longitudinal direction occurs with a critical degree of reduction of source current in the form of a premature action potential with reduced I_{Na}, while transverse conduction is maintained at low source currents. The transverse propagating wavefront can then propagate to regions distal to the region of longitudinal block and then conduct retrogradely back through this blocked region after it has recovered excitability (see description of anisotropic reentry in Figure 9-20).

CLASSIFICATION OF REENTRANT CIRCUITS

Reentrant circuits that cause arrhythmias have different electrophysiological characteristics, sizes, and shapes, accounting for the different clinical features of the arrhythmias that they cause. They may be formed by anatomical structures (anatomical circuits) resulting in a fixed pathway. They may also be functional, formed because of specific electrophysiological properties of myocardial cells.

Anatomical Reentry

An anatomical reentrant circuit is comprised of conducting pathways around an inexcitable obstacle formed by an anatomical structure. The central obstacle prevents the reentrant impulse from "short circuiting" the reentrant pathway and preexciting a more distal part of the circuit, which would terminate the reentry process. The reentrant pathways around the central obstacle may be formed by distinct macro-anatomical structures, such as bundles of Purkinje cells in the peripheral conducting system or bundles of muscle cells surviving in an infarct scar that are separated (protected) from surrounding myocardium by structural barriers except for discrete connections to the surrounding myocardium. These connections provide an exit pathway through which the reentrant impulse leaves the circuit to excite adjacent myocardium. The connections also allow impulses from outside the circuit to enter the circuit, for example stimulated impulses during an electrophysiological study using programmed stimulation (Figures 9-23, 9-25, and 9-30).

In other situations, the reentrant pathways around the obstacles may have electrophysiological connections with surrounding myocardium around most or all of the circuit circumference (not in separated or protected bundles) such as the typical flutter reentrant circuit (Figure 10-2). The reentrant impulse, in this case, can exit the circuit at multiple sites around its circumference, and stimulated impulses outside the circuit can enter the circuit from sites around much of its circumference.

In its simplest form, an anatomical circuit is the substrate for circus movement reentry, propagation of the reentrant impulse in a pattern resembling a circle around the obstacle as illustrated in Figure 9-1. The occurrence of transient or unidirectional block in one of the pathways of an anatomical circuit, caused by any of the mechanisms previously described in this chapter, with maintained conduction in the other pathway, is a prerequisite for initiation of anatomical reentry (see Figure 9-1).

Reentrant Circuit Size Influences Necessary Electrophysiological Properties

Some anatomical circuit path lengths are long, allowing reentry to occur without the necessity for major alterations in conduction velocity or refractory periods to shorten the wavelength (wavelength must be less than the path length for reentry, Figure 9-2). Examples are the large circuit encompassing much of the right atrium, causing typical atrial flutter, although there is a region of natural slow conduction (see Chapter 10), and the circus movement reentry involving the A-V conducting system and an A-V bypass tract, although a region of naturally occurring slow conduction is provided by the A-V node (see Chapter 11). Other arrhythmias are caused by reentry over short paths where there must be major changes in conduction velocity (slowing) and/or refractory periods (shortening) to decrease the wavelength such as reentrant circuits in healed myocardial infarcts (Chapter 12).

Excitable Gap and Revolution Time

Fully excitable gap. When time for propagation of the reentrant impulse around the circuit (revolution time) is significantly longer than the effective and relative refractory periods (wavelength shorter than path length), a fully excitable (spatial) gap is present (Figures 9-1 and Figure 9-3). In this situation, the reentrant impulse is propagating in fully excitable tissue. When this occurs, revolution time will change with changes in conduction velocity but is insensitive to changes in refractory period unless lengthening of the refractory period causes disappearance of the fully excitable gap. If this occurs, then, propagation in a partially recovered (relatively refractory) myocardium will prolong revolution time.

Partially excitable gap. There can also be only a partially excitable gap in an anatomical circuit when the wavelength is only slightly shorter than the path length and the head of the wavefront propagates in the relatively refractory tail. In this case, revolution time is sensitive to changes in refractory period; revolution time slows with an increase in the relative refractory period. In most circuits conduction velocity and/or refractory periods change from one segment to another when the circuit involves myocardial tissue with different properties (Figure 9-3). Thus, the wavelength is different in different regions. This may lead to oscillations in the revolution time. When the wavefront first encounters more refractory tissue, conduction slows because of a decrease in phase 0 of the action potential. The wavefront then retreats from the refractory tail but then speeds up again when it propagates in regions where there is more complete recovery of excitability. When oscillations become severe, reentry may terminate if the wavefront propagates into effectively refractory tissue and conduction is blocked.

"Figure-Eight" Anatomy

A more complex form of an anatomical circuit is the "figure-eight" configuration. A diagram of this pattern is shown in **Figure 9-17**. Two circuits, A and B, coalesce in a central pathway that is common to both circuits, referred to as the central common pathway or isthmus. An impulse propagates around each of the circuits simultaneously, represented by the red and blue arrows. For reentry to occur in each circuit, the wavelength must be less than the path length.

In order for the two reentrant impulses to arrive at the entrance to the isthmus at the same time (Figure 9-17, left panel), the transit time around each circuit must be the same. For this to occur, either the distance around each circuit and the conduction properties in each circuit must be exactly the same, or if the length of each circuit is different, conduction time around the circuits must still be the same via faster conduction velocity in the longer circuit. When this occurs, the impulse formed in the isthmus by the two reentrant impulses that coalesce here can exit through a connection between the isthmus and surrounding myocardium (green arrow). Usually one circuit dominates as shown in Figure 9-17, right panel. The impulse in circuit B (blue arrow) arrives at the isthmus before the impulse in circuit A (red arrow) and is the

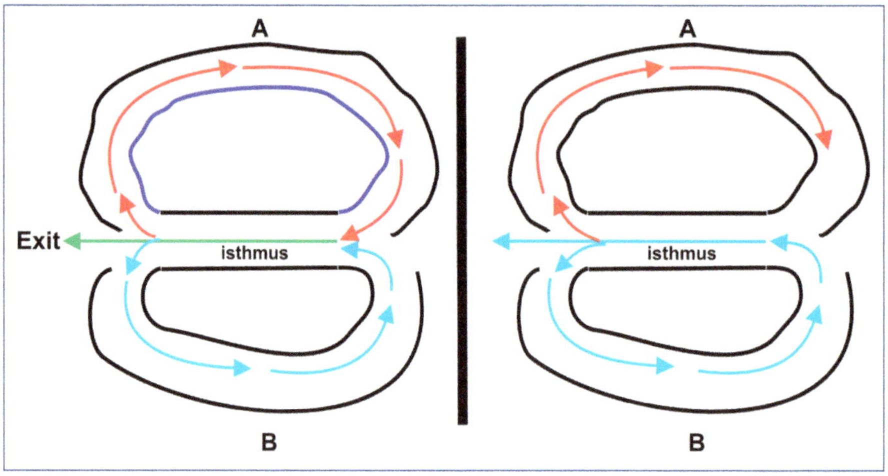

Figure 9-17 Diagram of an anatomical circuit with a figure-eight configuration.

cause of the tachycardia; circuit B is the dominant circuit, and circuit A is a "bystander." The blue arrow exiting from the isthmus in the diagram indicates the impulse from the dominant circuit B. However, if the reentrant impulse in circuit B is disrupted, the impulse in circuit A can become the dominant reentrant impulse since the electrophysiological requirements for reentry are present. Figure-eight reentrant circuits often occur in healed myocardial infarcts, the central isthmus is formed by an anatomical structure comprised of bundles of surviving myocardium. One or both of the circuits may also be formed by anatomical bundles embedded in the scar or by myocardium adjacent to the scar (see Chapter 12 for a more detailed description).

Functional Reentry

Functional reentrant circuits are dependent on the specific electrophysiological properties of the region of myocardium where they form and are not dependent on macro-anatomical structures or a central inexcitable anatomical obstacle. Micro-anatomical structures such as gap junction distribution or tissue anisotropy may still be a cause of the special electrophysiological properties that enable a functional reentrant circuit to form. While each kind of functional reentry described below (leading circle, rotor and anisotropic reentry) has some unique features, there is also significant overlap in the mechanisms. Because of the overlap, identification of the specific mechanism causing functional reentry in the clinical electrophysiology laboratory is not usually feasible.

Leading Circle Reentry

A type of functional reentry called "leading circle reentry," caused by heterogeneous refractory periods, is shown in **Figure 9-18**. Each panel shows a small region of atrial myocardium. In Panel A, a conducted impulse arising at a cycle length of 500 ms, such as might occur during sinus rhythm or electrical stimulation at a regular rate, originates in the center at the black dot. The stimulated wavefronts activate the region depicted in a relatively uniform pattern (indicated by the 5 ms isochrones and red arrows) in about 20 ms because the cycle length is longer than the local refractory periods. The effective refractory periods (ERP) are plotted in Panel D; the isochrones show that the longest refractory periods at the right are 60–70 ms.

In Figure 9-18, Panel A, there is no evidence of an anatomical obstacle or special anatomical reentrant pathways.

In Panel B, a premature impulse with a coupling interval of 56 ms initiated at the center black dot, blocks where there are long ERPs (60–70 ms), forming a line of block at the right (black arrowheads and yellow shading). This region becomes the region of unidirectional conduction block (see Figure 9-14). The premature impulse conducts around both ends of the block line indicated by the red arrows (isochrones 10–40 ms) where refractory periods are shorter (50–55 ms), returning to the distal side of the initial region of block at isochrone 50. Since excitability has recovered by this time, the circulating impulse conducts back through this region (Panel C) as a reentrant impulse (short red arrow beginning at the asterisk, isochrones 50 and 60). The size of the area of unidirectional block is important for successful initiation of reentry. Even in the presence of large differences in refractory period duration, reentry may not occur when the area with long refractory periods (the yellow barrier in B) is too small because the impulse traveling around the area of unidirectional block will not be delayed sufficiently to reexcite the region of origin at the end of its ERP.

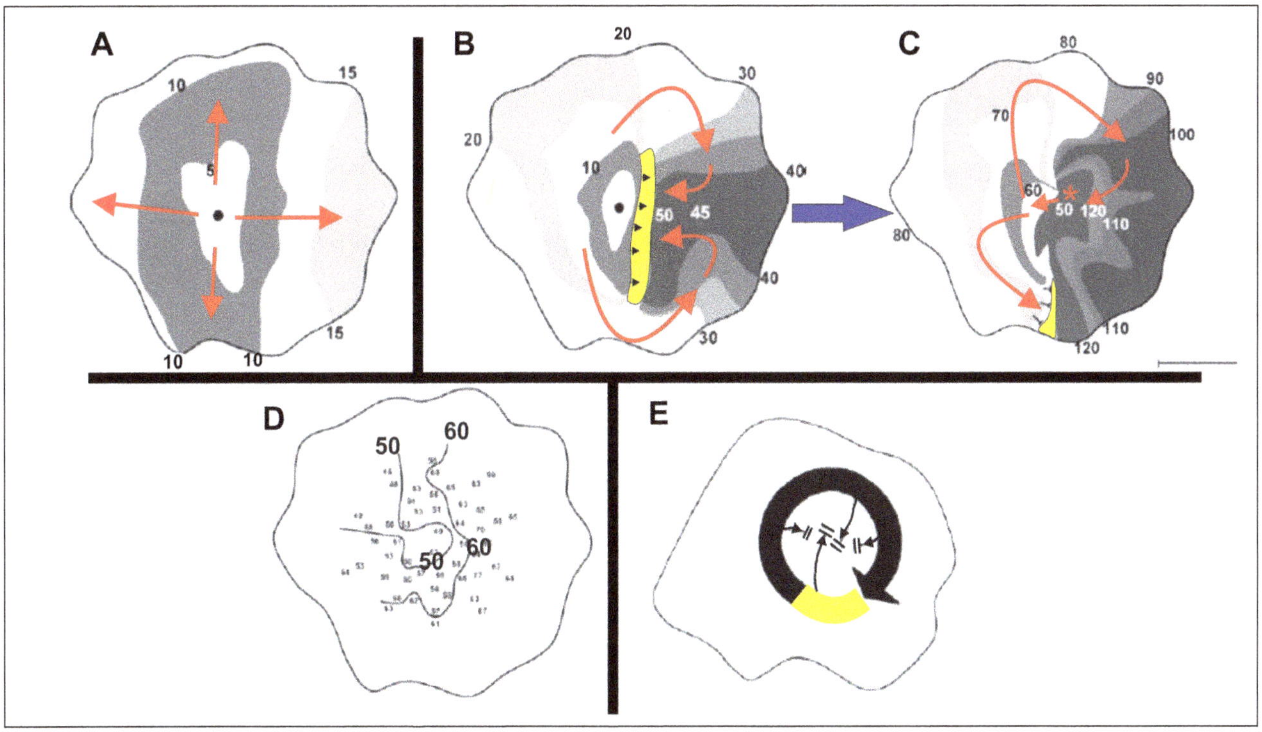

Figure 9-18 Functional leading circle reentry in right atrial myocardium. (Based on records published by Allessie MA, Bonke FIM. Circus movement in rabbit atrial muscle as a mechanism of tachycardia. II. The role of nonuniform recovery of excitability in the occurrence of unidirectional block as studied with multiple microelectrodes. *Circ Res.* 1976;39:168–177.)

In Figure 9-18, Panel C, two reentrant wavefronts then begin to circulate, one above and one below (long curved red arrows starting at isochrones 60). The one below blocks in the yellow-shaded region (at about isochrones 110 ms) leaving a single reentrant impulse that continues to circulate above and to the right (long curved red arrow). If the impulse conducting downward does not block, a figure-eight reentrant pattern similar to Figure 9-17 could be established. Panel E diagrams the reentrant impulse formed in Panels B and C. The thick curved black arrow represents the wavelength of the reentrant impulse from its head to the end of its inexcitable (ERP) tail. The yellow region is the partially excitable (relative refractory period) tail. The reentrant impulse is conducting around a central region that is kept refractory by constant bombardment with impulses propagating centripetally toward it from all sides of the circuit (Panel E, thin arrows and double bars). This central area provides a functional obstacle that plays the same role as the anatomical obstacle in an anatomical circuit; it prevents the reentrant impulse from short-circuiting (preexciting) the reentrant pathway. The circumferences of the smallest reentrant pathway, called "the leading circle," around the functional obstacle is dependent on the electrophysiological properties of the substrate and may be as little as 6–8 mm in the atria where the effective refractory period is very short. The leading circle represents a pathway in which the efficacy of stimulation of the circulating wavefront (arrowhead in Panel E) is just sufficient to excite the tissue immediately ahead of it that is still in its relative refractory phase (yellow-shaded region).

Slowed conduction and partially excitable gap in leading circle reentry. Conduction around the functional reentrant circuit in Figure 9-18 is slower than normal for several reasons: (1) the head of the wavefront (arrowhead in Panel E) propagates in the partially refractory tail (yellow region); (2) the reentrant wavefront is curved; and (3) if the circuit is in anisotropic myocardium, impulses conduct transversely to the long axis of the myocardial bundles in parts of the circuit. The size of the circuit and revolution time is determined mainly by the duration of the relative refractory period; e.g., shorter refractory periods result in smaller circuits with a faster revolution time. Wavefront curvature may also limit how small a circuit can be (see discussion in section on rotors). The circuit can shift from one region to another once it is established since its location is not dependent on an anatomical obstacle, as long as the new region has appropriate electrophysiological properties. Its size can also change, if the new region has different refractory periods. The circuit can be small enough to allow multiple circuits to exist simultaneously. Since the head of the wavefront is propagating in the relatively refractory tail, there is no fully excitable and only a partially excitable gap making it difficult for impulses originating outside the circuit such as stimulated impulses, to penetrate and affect the circuit. Leading circle reentry may be a cause of focal reentrant tachycardias or participate in atrial and ventricular fibrillation when the circuits are sufficiently small to allow multiple circuits to coexist as described further in Chapter 10.

Spiral Waves and Rotor Reentry

Another form of functional reentry was originally introduced into cardiac electrophysiology with the nomenclature of "spiral waves" based on its appearance in chemical excitable media. It is now usually referred to as "rotor reentry." The main (but not only) difference from leading circle reentry, is that slow activation in a reentrant circuit formed by a rotor is primarily caused by the wavefront curvature and not propagation in partially refractory tissue.

The properties of rotors are shown in **Figure 9-19**. In Panel A, the horizontal black line represents a narrow linear anatomical obstacle. The red arrow shows the path of a planar wavefront propagating along the upper side of the obstacle (5 ms isochrones) until it reaches the end of the obstacle. At this point (the pivoting point [pp]), the wavefront moving around the obstacle must assume a curved shape (see below), and conduction slows because of the curvature (described in Figure 9-13). The red asterisk in Panel A indicates the time point for the illustration of the wavefront (short blue arrows) in Panel B.

In Figure 9-19, Panel B, the curved thick black line shows the wavefront at the time of the red asterisk in Panel A, followed by refractory tissue it has excited represented in gray. The segment of the wavefront indicated by the black arrow (yellow dashes), blocks because of the critical radius of curvature (r_c) at the pivot point (pp). Curvature is less at point P, which enables propagation to continue (red arrow). The tip of the wavefront, P is detached from the original line of block and forms the head (wavefront) of the rotor, which conducts in a circular pattern around an unexcited central region (red arrow) and not around the original line of block. (Although unexcited, the central region is excitable as described further below). The yellow dashed line (t) shows the trajectory of the wave tip with the radius r_c. The tip (P) of the rotor is also called the "phase singularity" but in keeping with the terminology used in this chapter, it is the wavefront of the reentrant impulse. Wave breaks rotate around the phase singularity. The pivoting radius required for detachment from the pivot point (pp) is dependent on the tissue excitability. The radius is very small in normally excitable myocardium and might not initiate a rotor since the wavefront does not detach from the line of block. With some depression of excitability, for example caused by decreased I_{Na}, or gap junction uncoupling, the radius gets larger allowing the formation of the wave break and the wavelength to be less than the wavefront trajectory (path length).

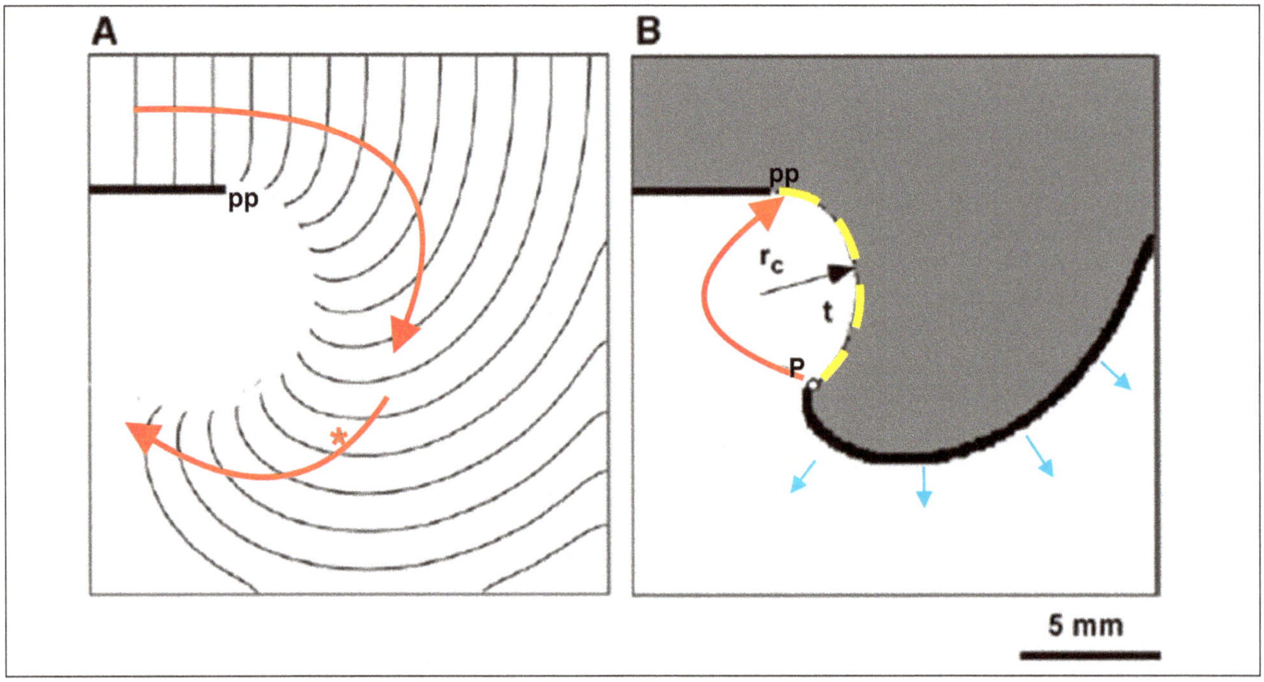

Figure 9-19 Formation of a rotor. **Panel A** shows an isochronal map of activation spread with an interval of 5 ms in a computer model. **Panel B** shows activation at the moment marked by the **red asterisk** in **Panel A**. (Reproduced from Kleber AG, Rudy Y. Basic mechanisms of cardiac impulse propagation and associated arrhythmias. *Physiol Rev.* 2004;84:431–488.)

Initiation of a rotor. Rotors can be initiated by several mechanisms, including the occurrence of a small inexcitable area (Figure 9-19), by interaction of several wavefronts in homogeneously refractory myocardium or by premature impulses propagating into regions with intrinsic differences in refractory periods as shown for the leading circle model. Rotors can also be initiated by electrical shocks that can render regions refractory by depolarizing them while exciting adjacent regions through a hyperpolarizing effect.

Additional properties of rotors. The central region around which the tip of a rotor rotates, is excitable unlike the leading circle model where the central region is refractory because of the propagation of impulses inward from the circuit. The high curvature of the rotor wavefront, where conduction is the slowest, prevents impulse propagation into the center. Rotors, therefore, revolve around an excitable core, which can have different shapes; circular, elongated, or complicated behavior, depending on the electrophysiological properties of the myocardium in which they occur.

Rotors are at the center of spiral waves. Excitatory wavefronts emanate from the rotor along the wavefront boundary (Figure 9-19, small blue arrows). In a uniform medium they form the appearance of a spiral with the rotor at the center, since the center with the greatest curvature conducts the slowest, while more peripheral wavefronts with less curvature conduct more rapidly. In three dimensions, a scroll-like shape is formed (scroll waves) that rotates around a three-dimensional filament. However, in the heart such uniform regions are rarely present so the peripheral spiral is distorted by the effects of heterogeneous refractoriness, anisotropic structure, anatomical obstacles and boundaries that dictate the pattern of excitation away from the rotor.

The spinning rate of the rotor determines the degree of turbulence (fractionation of wavefronts into multiple wavelets) around it. The higher the spinning rate, the greater the fractionation. This property is described in more detail in Chapter 10 on atrial fibrillation caused by rotors.

In addition to the wavefront curvature, anisotropy also can contribute to the slowing of conduction of a rotor where the direction of propagation is transverse to the long axis of the myocardium. Anisotropy causes rotors to assume an elliptical shape with the long axis of the ellipse in the direction of more rapid conduction along the long axis of the myocardial bundles.

Once a rotor is initiated, continuation of rotor reentry is dependent on the wavelength of the rotating impulse being less than the path length as in the other models of reentry. If the radius of the wavefront curvature is small, the circuit assumes a small size and the head of the wavefront may interact with the tail. This leads to the absence of a fully excitable gap and a small relatively excitable gap similar to leading circle reentry. Instability of the rotational cycle length can be caused by the head of the wavefront interacting with the tail. It also can result in a meandering wavefront trajectory (drift), as the rotor moves through the myocardium. Heterogeneity of excitability, repolarization and refractoriness also promotes rotor drift. Unstable rotors can break up into multiple reentrant wavelets.

If excitability is depressed, the radius of curvature (r_c) is larger because of slower conduction, leading to a larger rotor in which the head of the wavefront conducts in completely excitable tissue that has recovered from previous excitation, and a fully excitable gap. The rotor cycle length is more stable. The tip of a rotor (Figure 9-19, P) can also fix itself to an anatomical obstacle (not necessarily the obstacle responsible for its initiation) and the rotor revolves around the obstacle, thereby becoming stabilized similar to the role of an obstacle in an anatomical circuit. Rotors may also meander or drift over long distances if there is no anchoring point.

Anisotropic Functional Reentry

Nonuniform anisotropy can sometimes be the dominant cause of both the unidirectional conduction block as well as the conduction slowing in a functional circuit, giving rise to anisotropic reentry. (Anisotropy can also cause slow conduction in other kinds of functional reentry as well as in anatomical circuits as mentioned previously.)

Figure 9-20, Panel A diagrams the pattern of nonuniform anisotropic conduction in muscle bundles separated by connective tissue septae (brown shading) that is also described in Figure 9-11. The red arrows indicate longitudinal conduction and the blue arrows indicate slow transverse conduction caused by reduced transverse coupling. Figure 9-20, Panel B shows conduction of a premature impulse with a short coupling interval. Block occurs in the longitudinal direction (red arrows and vertical lines) because of the decreased stimulating efficacy and safety factor for conduction associated with the reduced phase 0 of the premature action potential (Figure 9-5). Slow transverse conduction still occurs at the short coupling interval (blue arrows) because of the higher safety factor of propagation in partially uncoupled nonuniformly anisotropic myocardium (Figure 9-8). If conduction delay of the transversely conducting impulse is sufficient, it can circulate through excitable myocardium to reexcite the region distal to the longitudinal block (Panel B, blue arrows) and then propagate retrogradely as a reentrant impulse (dashed green arrow). If the impulse continues to circulate, a major contribution to the slow conduction and reduced wavelength is provided by slow conduction in the transverse direction.

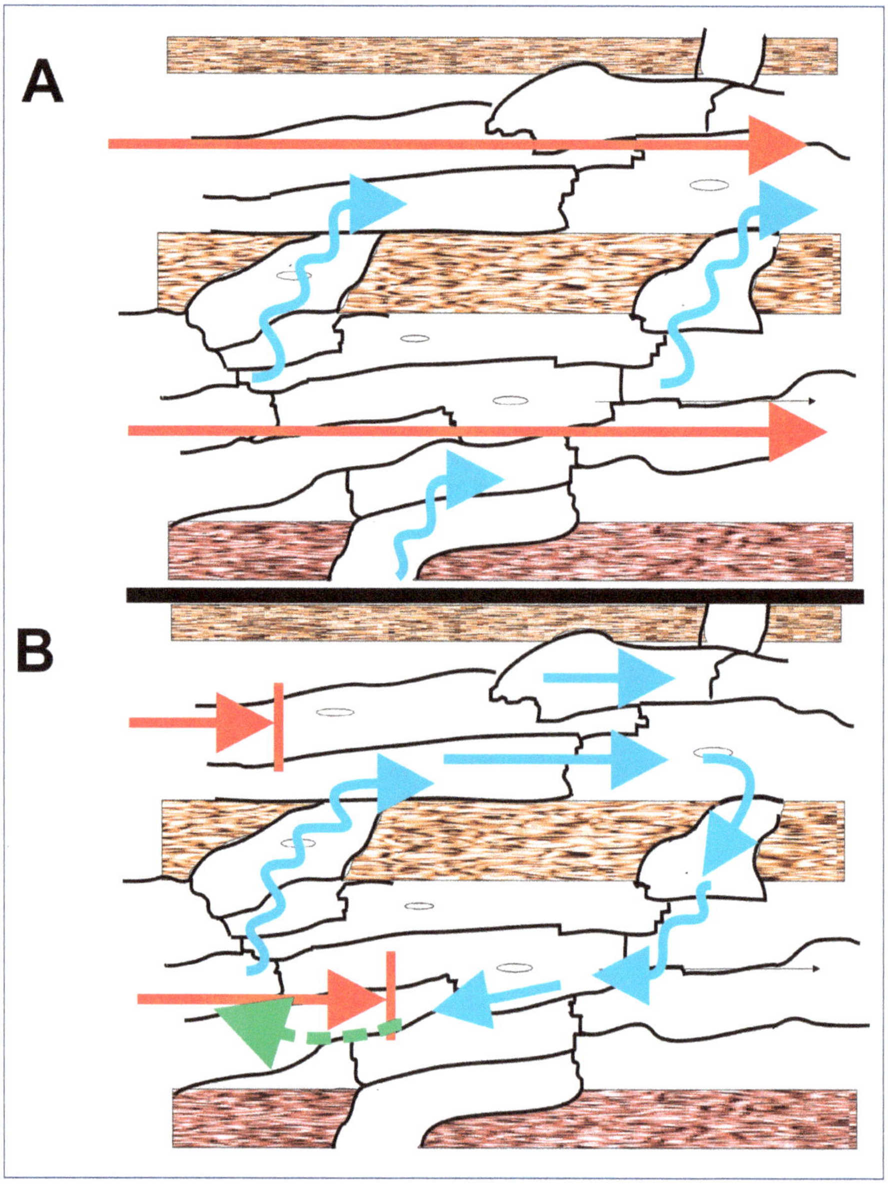

Figure 9-20 Anisotropic reentry. **Panel A** diagrams nonuniformly anisotropic conduction in bundles of muscle separated by connective tissue (**shaded regions**). **Panel B** diagrams conduction of an early premature impulse that initiates reentry.

Anisotropic reentrant circuits are oval in shape with the long axis in the direction of the long axis of the muscle bundles because of the more rapid conduction in this direction. Conduction velocity of the reentrant impulse changes as the direction of propagation changes, slowing in the transverse direction and speeding up in the longitudinal direction. Therefore, a spatial excitable gap can occur during transverse conduction when the wavelength decreases and disappears during longitudinal conduction when the wavelength lengthens. The properties at the center of the circuit around which the impulse circulates can resemble either leading circle reentry or rotor reentry, or can be a small anatomical obstacle. In Figure 9-20 Panel B, the circuit is a small anatomical barrier provided by a region of fibrosis.

Reentry Based on Reflection

Reflection describes a form of reentry in a linear bundle of myocardial cells with an area of depressed conduction. During reflection, excitation occurs in one direction along the bundle, which is then followed by continued propagation and excitation occurring in the opposite direction.

Figure 9-21, Panel A depicts a bundle of cells with an asymmetrically depressed region (reduced membrane potential and slow action potential upstrokes) in the shaded area (also see Figure 9-15). The degree of depression increasing from left to right is indicated by progression of the shading from yellow to brown. An impulse conducting from left to right in the bundle (red arrow) blocks in the more severely depressed region (small red arrows at vertical red lines) by the mechanism described in Figure 9-15. Conduction from left to right without block (green arrows) occurs adjacent to the depressed region. This impulse conducts transversely once it is past the region of severe depression. It then can conduct retrogradely through this severely depressed region which is a region of unidirectional block (see Figure 9-15). The blue arrows show the reflected impulse returning to reexcite the left end of the bundle. There is longitudinal dissociation of conduction. While this mechanism has been proposed to cause clinical arrhythmias, proof for its involvement is lacking since mapping this sequence of activation requires extremely high resolution. In laboratory experiments, continuous reflection of the kind that might cause tachycardias has not been described.

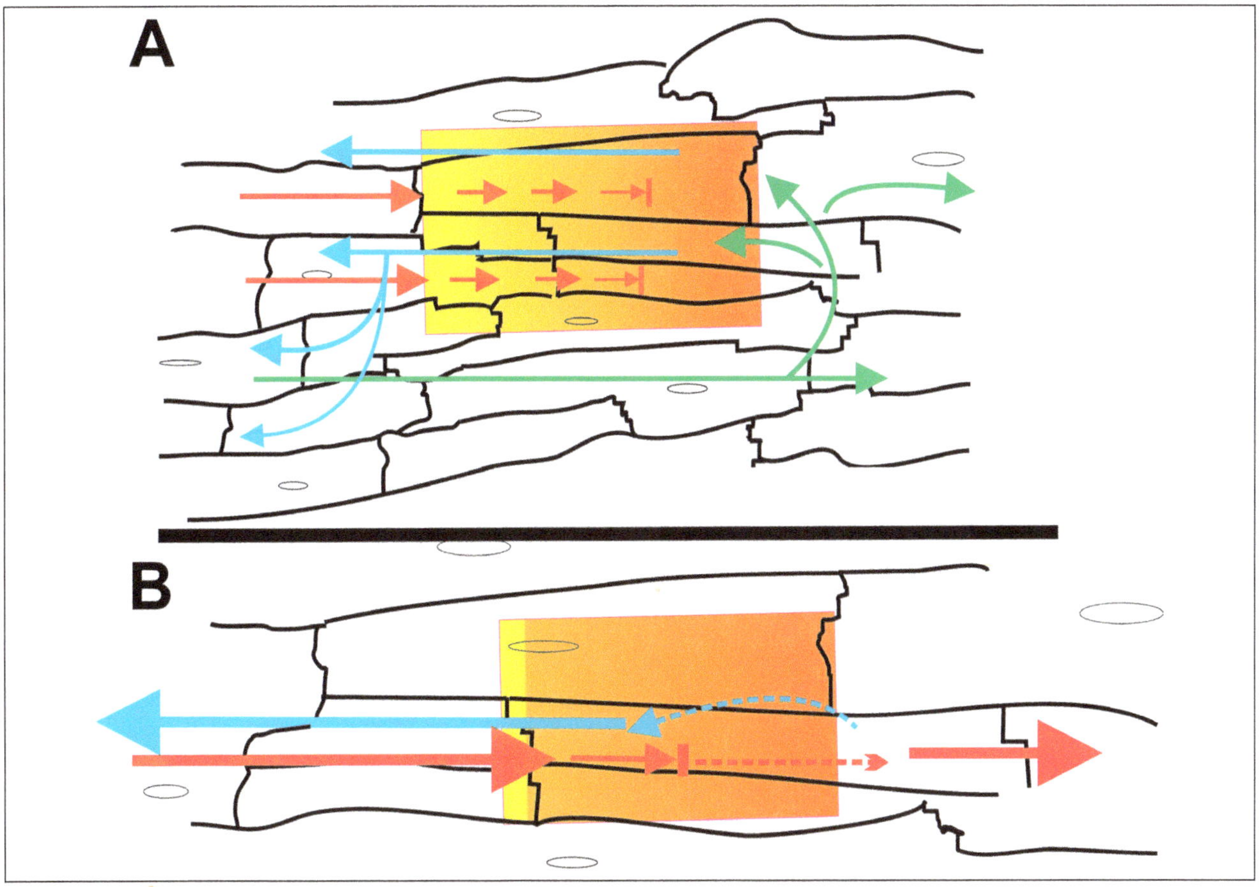

Figure 9-21 Reentry caused by reflection. **Panel A** shows longitudinal dissociation. **Panel B** shows electrotonic excitation.

A different model for reflection involves antegrade and retrograde conduction through the same muscle bundles. This mechanism is diagrammed in Figure 9-21, Panel B. An impulse initiated at the left, propagates into a depressed region (brown shading) and blocks (small red arrow and vertical red line). Electrotonic current flows through the inexcitable region distal to the block without generating an action potential (dashed red arrow) and then is able to excite cells distal to the inexcitable segment. The time delay before the occurrence of the distal action potential is dependent on the time-course and amplitude of the electrotonic current flow. The action potential initiated distal to the point of block conducts antegradely along the muscle (large red arrow at the right) but can also lead to retrograde conduction by generating electrotonic current to excite the proximal side of the region of block (dashed blue arrow) if the time delay is sufficient to allow the proximal side to recover excitability. The reflected or reentrant impulse is shown by the blue arrow. Impulse transmission in both directions occurs over the same pathway unlike the types of reentry discussed previously. As with the model of reflection shown in Panel A, no clinical data has verified the occurrence of this mechanism shown in laboratory models as a cause of clinical arrhythmias.

Combination Anatomical and Functional Circuits

Reentrant circuits can be part anatomical and part functional. The central region of block can have both an anatomical and a functional component. The conducting pathway around the central region of bock may or may not involve specific anatomical structures. For example, the circuit in the right atrium causing typical atrial flutter (Figure 10-2) has a central region of anatomical block formed by the inferior vena cava and coronary sinus orifice and a functional region of block in the crista terminalis. Other examples are described in in Chapters 10, 11, and 12.

IDENTIFYING REENTRANT EXCITATION AS A CAUSE OF CLINICAL ARRHYTHMIAS

ECG Characteristics of Reentrant Arrhythmias

The ECG characteristics of reentrant arrhythmias vary depending on the anatomic location of the reentrant circuits and the properties of the myocardium that form the circuits. Therefore, the ECG characteristics are described, along with the examples of reentrant arrhythmias occurring in different regions of the heart, in Chapters 10, 11, and 12.

Limited Use of Pharmacological Agents to Identify Reentry as a Mechanism of Arrhythmias

In general, most drugs that affect reentrant arrhythmias by changing their cycle length or terminating them also affect other mechanisms of arrhythmias, so they have limited use in identifying a reentrant mechanism in a clinical study. However, sometimes a drug effect can support the conclusion that an arrhythmia is reentrant when the occurrence of reentry is determined by programmed stimulation or mapping activation. Specific examples are described in Chapters 10, 11, and 12.

Electrical Stimulation to Determine That Arrhythmia Mechanism Is Reentry

Electrical stimulation is valuable for identifying mechanisms causing arrhythmias (see Chapters 1, 5, and 7). The responses to stimulation, either overdrive pacing or programmed premature stimulation, can distinguish automaticity from triggered activity. Electrical stimulation is also an important tool that can identify reentrant arrhythmias.

ELECTRICAL STIMULATION AND CHARACTERISTICS OF REENTRANT ARRHYTHMIAS

Initiation of Reentrant Arrhythmias

Overdrive pacing and programmed premature stimulation can initiate reentrant arrhythmias, which is a hallmark feature of this mechanism. However, failure to initiate an arrhythmia by stimulated impulses does not necessarily eliminate reentry, since there are several reasons for failure (see below). Delayed afterdepolarization (DAD)-triggered activity can also be initiated by electrical stimulation (Chapter 5), but automaticity cannot (Chapter 1). Therefore, additional characteristics of initiation of reentry described in this section are important in distinguishing between reentry and DAD-triggered arrhythmias.

Both overdrive pacing and programmed premature stimulation protocols can be implemented during sinus rhythm in a patient who has spontaneous episodes of tachycardia. The goal is to establish the conditions necessary for reentry that occur when the arrhythmia occurs spontaneously, specifically unidirectional conduction block and/or sufficiently slow conduction (see Figure 9-1). Of primary importance during these stimulation protocols is that the stimulated impulses reach the site where the potential circuit that causes the clinical arrhythmia is located. An important problem is refractoriness of myocardium between the stimulus site and the circuit location, which causes conduction block when the stimulus site is at a distance from the circuit. In the description that follows, the stimulus site is close to the circuit, so this problem is eliminated.

Overdrive Pacing

During overdrive pacing, either the cycle length or the duration of pacing can be varied (also see Chapters 1 and 5). **Figure 9-22** illustrates an overdrive protocol during sinus rhythm at three different cycle lengths, each for the same duration, as would be implemented in a heart that has periodic reentrant tachycardias. **Figure 9-23** shows possible effects of this stimulation protocol on impulse conduction in a model of an anatomical reentrant circuit with dispersion of refractoriness (similar to the model shown in Figure 9-1), for each of the stimulus cycle lengths (A, B, and C). The two figures are designed to be viewed in tandem.

In Figure 9-22, Panel A, sinus rhythm at the left (vertical black bars, 500-ms cycle length) is interrupted by overdrive pacing at a long cycle length of 375 ms (vertical blue bars) for 30 sec. This is followed by overdrive suppression of sinus node automaticity; the first cycle length after overdrive is prolonged to 620 ms (return cycle, horizontal black bar) without initiation of an arrhythmia.

Overdrive at this cycle length and duration activates the potential reentrant circuit without establishing the unidirectional block and slow conduction necessary to initiate reentry as diagrammed in Figure 9-23, Panels A1–A3.

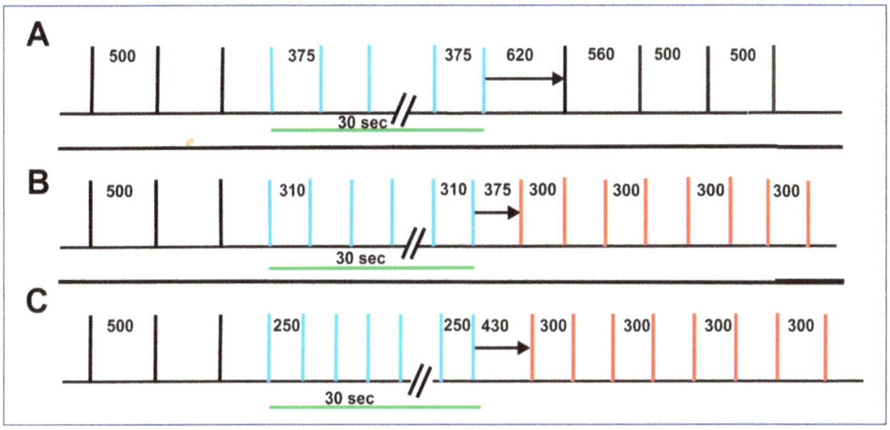

Figure 9-22 Diagrams of initiation of reentrant tachycardia by overdrive stimulation.

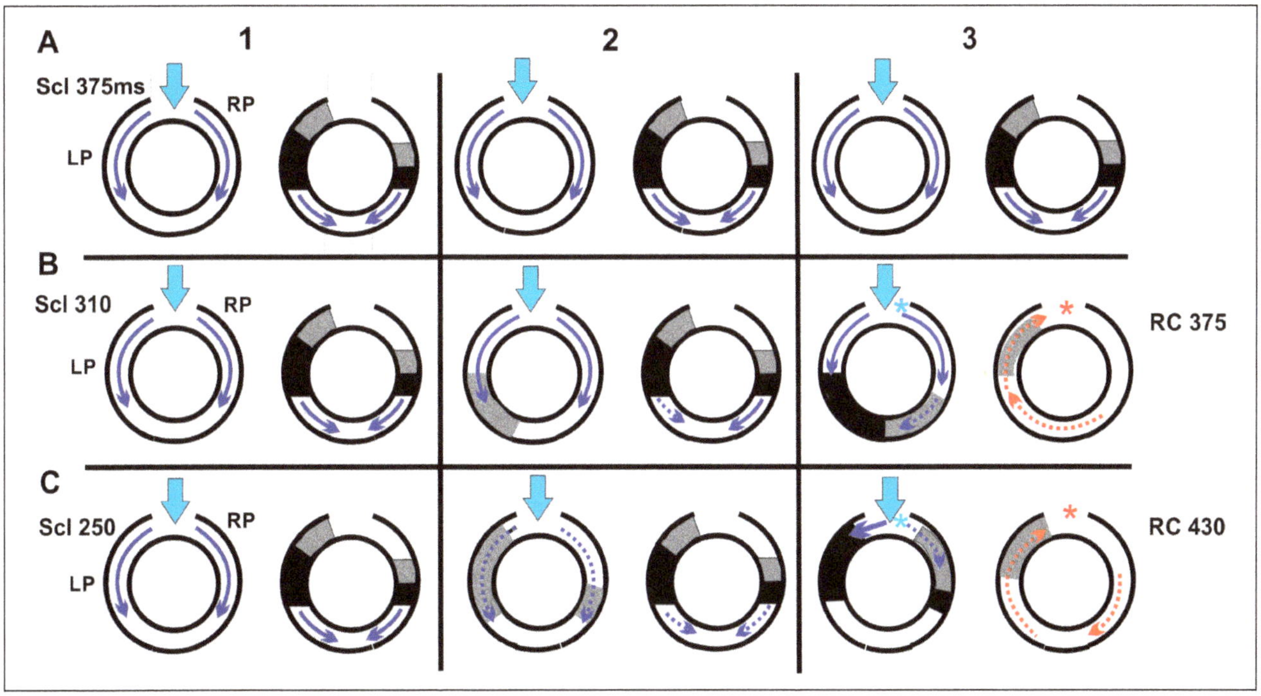

Figure 9-23 Mechanism for initiation of reentry by overdrive pacing in a model of an anatomical circuit with dispersion of refractoriness (longer in the left pathway [LP] than in the right pathway [RP]).

The model illustrated in Figure 9-23 has a central anatomic obstacle and a fixed circular pathway around that obstacle. Left pathway (LP) and right pathway (RP) in the circuit converge above and below. In this model, entrance into the circuit is above where the large blue arrow is located. Exit from the circuit for reentrant impulses propagating to the rest of the heart can also occur here. The model has dispersion of refractoriness, with refractory periods in the LP longer than refractory periods in the RP, similar to the model described in Figure 9-14. The concepts described in this model can be applied to some functional circuits as well.

Figure 9-23 Panel A (snapshot 1–3) shows the wavefront of excitation and refractory periods during the overdrive protocol illustrated in Figure 9-22, Panel A. Each snapshot in Figure 9-23, Panel A shows conduction of a stimulated impulse (large blue arrow) at the cycle length of 375 ms. Each snapshot (1, 2, or 3) has two paired diagrams of the circuit model. The one on the left shows the stimulated impulse as it enters the circuit, and the one on the right shows the pattern of conduction of the impulse when it has moved through the circuit as overdrive continues. A1 occurs near the beginning of the overdrive period, A2 near the middle, and A3 at the end. Because of the long cycle length of stimulation during overdrive (375 ms) each stimulated impulse (purple arrowheads indicate the wavefront) activates the potential reentrant circuit after it has completely recovered excitability from the previous stimulated impulse (left diagrams in snapshots A1, A2, and A3). The right diagrams of each pair illustrate continuation of conduction through these pathways in A1, A2, and A3. The dark black region following the stimulated impulse indicates completely refractory myocardium (the effective refractory period [ERP]) and the gray indicates partially refractory myocardium. Note the longer refractory periods in the LP than the RP. Reentry is not initiated because the left and right pathways of the potential circuit are activated in the same direction (from top to bottom) during each stimulated impulse.

In Figure 9-22, Panel B, a decreased overdrive cycle length of 310 ms (blue bars) initiates reentrant tachycardia (red bars), the return cycle from last stimulated impulse to the first tachycardia impulse is 375 ms (horizontal black arrow) and the tachycardia cycle length is 300 ms (red bars).

Figure 9-23, Panel B snapshots 1–3 shows the mechanism for initiation. The stimulated impulse near the beginning of the pacing (B1) conducts through the circuit without encountering refractory myocardium, similar to Figure 9-23, A1. In snapshot B2, the stimulated impulse near the middle of the pacing period at the shorter cycle length (310 ms) encounters relatively refractory myocardium in the LP (gray region, left diagram) where refractory periods are longer, but not in the RP with short refractory periods. In the right diagram in B2, conduction continues through both pathways. The stimulated impulse at the end of the pacing period (B3) blocks in the LP because of its long refractory period (impulse block indicated by purple arrowhead abutting effectively refractory myocardium indicated by black region in the left diagram) while conduction proceeds through the RP because of the shorter refractory periods, although the impulse is conducting more slowly in relatively refractory myocardium (dashed arrow and shaded region in Panel B3). The block region in the LP (B3) becomes a region of unidirectional block, allowing the impulse from the RP (dashed purple arrow in left diagram) to propagate through and complete an excursion through the circuit as a reentrant impulse (dashed red arrow in Panel B3, right diagram) 375 ms after it was initiated (time from blue asterisk in B3 left diagram to red asterisk, right diagram). This is the same as the return cycle shown in Figure 9-22, Panel B.

Conduction is slower around the circuit, resulting in the longer return cycle length (375 ms) than for the tachycardia impulse (cycle length 300 ms in Figure 9-22, Panel B) because the stimulated impulse conducts slowly (dashed arrow) in partially refractory tissue (shaded region) around the circuit, which is not the case once tachycardia is established. Reentry can then continue to cause subsequent impulses of the tachycardia. Instead of decreasing the stimulus cycle length to establish reentry, a similar effect can occur if the duration of overdrive at 375 ms is increased from 30 sec, which did not induce reentry (Figure 9-22, Panel A), to 60 sec (not shown).

The mechanism for reentry caused by overdrive stimulation is similar to that described in Figure 9-1. In overdrive initiation of reentry, the transient unidirectional block is established by a stimulated impulse at a short cycle length, entering the circuit during the ERP of one pathway.

There are several possible mechanisms for the gradual slowing and eventual block during overdrive pacing. At short overdrive cycle lengths, the normal shortening of APD (Figure 7-7) might not occur sufficiently to prevent block in regions with long APD, or in myocardium with postrepolarization refractoriness, refractory periods may lengthen at short cycle lengths (Figure 9-7). The resulting decrease in inward current during phase 0 (I_{Na} in atrial or ventricular myocardium, I_{CaL} in A-V node) can by itself slow conduction and lead to block or can interact with structural features such as nonuniform anisotropy or impedance mismatch (Figure 9-11 and Figure 9-16) to cause slow conduction and block. The predominant mechanism varies with the clinical substrate as described in the subsequent chapters on clinical arrhythmias.

In Figure 9-22, Panel C, the overdrive cycle length is decreased to 250 ms (vertical blue bars) for 30 sec, which initiates a reentrant tachycardia at a cycle length of 300 ms (vertical red bars). The cycle length from the last stimulated impulse to the first tachycardia impulse (the return cycle) is 430 ms (horizontal black arrow). The mechanism for tachycardia initiation is shown in Figure 9-23, Panel C, snapshots 1–3. Snapshot C1 shows a stimulated impulse at the beginning of the pacing period before slowing and block is established, similar to Panel A1 and B1. Panel C2 shows a stimulated impulse near the middle of the pacing period where the impulses in both the LP and RP propagate in relatively refractory myocardium (dashed purple arrows and shaded region in left diagram) with continuation of activation of the right and left pathway in the right diagram. In Panel C3, left diagram, block of the stimulated impulse occurs in the LP occurring later at the end of the overdrive (solid purple arrowhead encounters black region in the left diagram) while slow propagation in relatively refractory myocardium is maintained in the RP (dashed purple arrow in lightly shaded region in the left diagram). In Panel C3, the right diagram shows continued slow propagation of the impulse from the RP in partially refractory myocardium (dashed red arrow, shaded region) retrograde into the LP and around the circuit as the first reentrant impulse (dashed red arrow, red asterisk) at a return cycle of 430 ms. The increased return cycle is caused by still slower conduction of the stimulated impulse around the circuit at the shorter pacing cycle length (Panel C3, blue asterisk in left diagram to red asterisk in right diagram). Therefore, there is an inverse relationship between the overdrive cycle length and the return cycle. Clinical examples of the initiation of tachycardia by overdrive and this inverse relationship are shown in Chapters 10, 11, and 12.

Programmed Premature Stimulation

Programmed premature stimulation can also initiate reentry by causing unidirectional conduction block and slow conduction in potential reentrant circuits. The same clinical protocol in the investigation of reentry is used as described in Chapter 1 and Chapter 5, with a premature stimulus applied every 10 to 15 sinus impulses or during stimulation at a fixed basic cycle length, as illustrated in **Figure 9-24**. A diagram of conduction patterns of the stimulated impulses in the reentrant circuit model with heterogeneous refractory properties is shown in **Figure 9-25**.

In Figure 9-24, the basic cycle length of 800 ms (during sinus rhythm or basic stimulation) in each panel is indicated by the black vertical bars and the prematurely stimulated impulse is indicated by the blue vertical bar. In Panel A, after the premature stimulus with a 600 ms coupling interval (blue bar), the basic (sinus) rhythm is reset (return cycle length of 800 ms, horizontal arrow). At this long coupling interval, the premature impulse conducts without block and/or sufficiently slow conduction, and reentry does not occur.

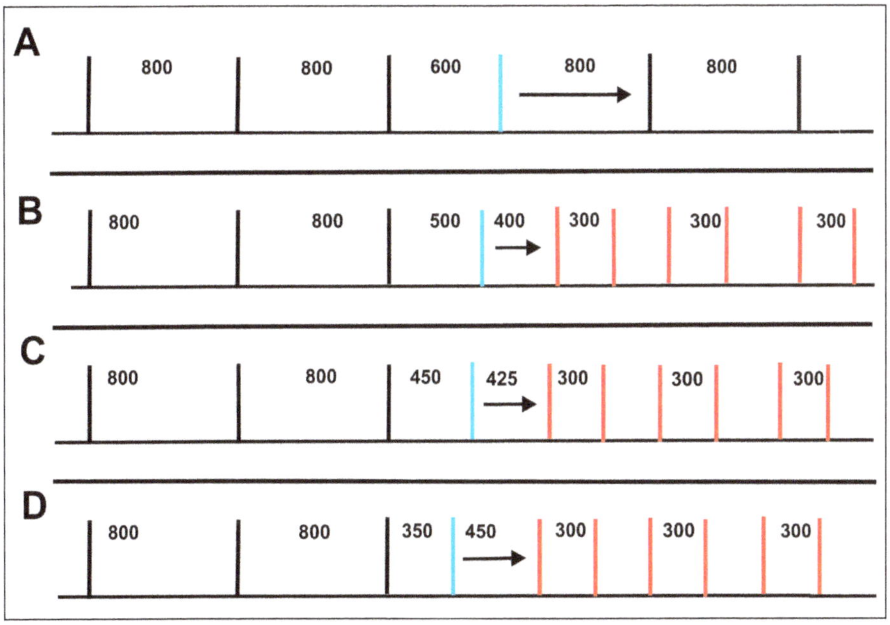

Figure 9-24 Diagrammatic representation of a reentrant tachycardia initiation by premature stimulation.

In Figure 9-25, Panel A, the large blue arrow shows entry into the circuit of the premature impulse in the left diagram, and continued conduction through the left (LP) and right pathway (RP) of the circuit in the right diagram (purple arrows; effective refractory myocardium is in black, relative refractory myocardium in gray) because there is sufficient time for recovery of excitability in the circuit from the previous sinus impulse. This pattern of activation is also the same as during the sinus impulse.

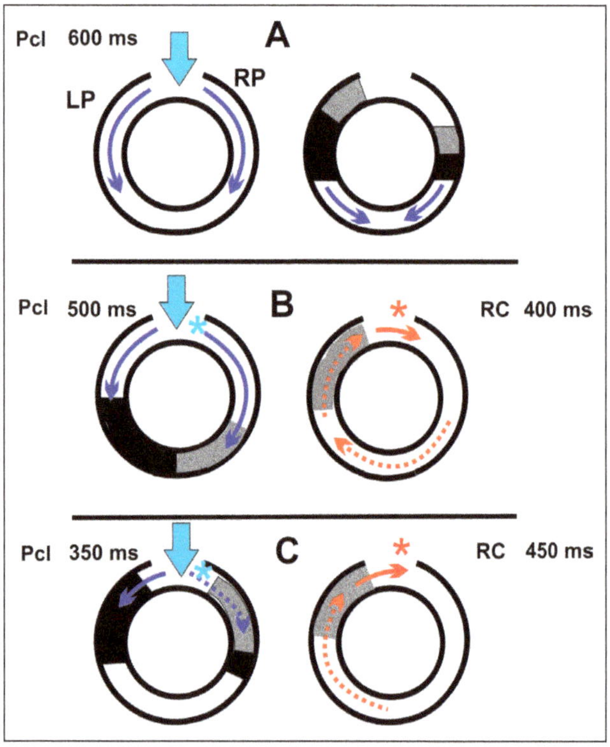

Figure 9-25 Initiation of reentry by a premature impulse in a model of an anatomical circuit with dispersion of refractoriness. Refractory periods in the left pathway (LP) are longer than the right pathway (RP). **Panels A, B,** and **C** show the patterns of propagation of three prematurely stimulated impulses (premature cycle lengths [Pcl] at **left**).

In Figure 9-24, Panel B, a reentrant tachycardia (vertical red bars) is initiated by the prematurely stimulated impulse (vertical blue bar) with a coupling interval of 500 ms and a return cycle of 400 ms (horizontal black arrow). In the model shown in Figure 9-25, Panel B, the premature impulse is sufficiently early to block in a region with long refractory periods (left diagram, purple arrow abutting black area in the LP) but still conducts slowly in partially refractory myocardium of the RP (gray region) with shorter refractory periods (dashed arrow in right diagram) to emerge as a reentrant impulse (dashed red arrow, right diagram). The return cycle (RC) from the premature impulse to the first tachycardia impulse of 400 ms is determined by the conduction time of the premature impulse from initiation (blue asterisk in left diagram) to completion of one revolution around the circuit (red asterisk in right diagram).

In Figure 9-24, Panels C and D, tachycardias (red bars) are initiated by premature stimuli (blue bars) with shorter coupling intervals (450 and 350 ms). The return cycle from the stimulated premature impulse to the first impulse of tachycardia increases to 425 and 450 ms (horizontal black arrows) showing an inverse relationship to the premature stimulus coupling interval. At these shorter coupling intervals, as shown in Figure 9-25, Panel C, block of the stimulated impulse occurs in the LP (left diagram, solid purple arrow abutting black-shaded region), and conduction of the premature impulse in the RP is slower (dashed purple arrow) than at longer coupling intervals because of conduction in relatively refractory myocardium (light gray-shaded area). Because of the slow conduction, the time from initiation (blue asterisk in left diagram) to completion of one revolution around the circuit (red asterisk in right diagram) is longer, thus accounting for the increased return cycle to the first tachycardia impulse. The cycle length and duration of the tachycardia itself are not influenced by the prematurity of the stimulated impulse, unlike DAD-triggered activity, where cycle length of tachycardia can be directly related to coupling interval. Although not shown in Figure 9-25, a shorter coupling interval will not initiate reentry if the premature impulse blocks in both the RP and LP of the potential circuit. Examples of initiation of clinical tachycardias by premature stimulation are shown in Chapters 10, 11, and 12.

Sometimes a single premature impulse may be unable to reach the circuit early enough to cause block and/or sufficiently slow conduction because of the refractoriness of myocardium between the stimulus site and the circuit. Adding a second prematurely stimulated impulse may then succeed, since the first one can shorten the refractory period of the intervening myocardium (refractory periods shorten at short cycle lengths), allowing the second one to conduct at a shorter coupling interval to the circuit.

Comparing Initiation of Reentrant and DAD-Triggered Tachycardia

The characteristics of initiation of reentry in an anatomical circuit by overdrive pacing and premature stimulation are summarized here and compared to initiation of DAD-triggered activity. Although there are detailed clinical studies on initiation characteristics of reentry, this is not the case for DAD-triggered activity. Therefore, much of the comparison is based on laboratory *in vitro* and *in vivo* studies on DADs.

Important differences between the two mechanisms are the following:

- Although arrhythmias caused by both mechanisms can be induced by overdrive and by premature stimulation at a critical coupling interval, it is usually easier to induce reentry by premature stimulation and easier to induce DAD-triggered activity by overdrive. Overdrive stimulation sometimes fails to initiate reentry when it cannot establish conduction block and/or sufficiently slowed conduction on account of refractory period shortening at decreased cycle lengths (Figure 7-7). On the other hand, overdrive loads triggerable cells with Ca^{2+} that causes DADs (Figure 5-4). Reentry is more easily induced by premature stimulation than triggered activity because unidirectional conduction block can be more readily established by a single premature impulse when there is dispersion of refractoriness Figure 9-14), whereas sufficient Ca^{2+} loading to initiate DAD-triggered activity may not occur after a single (premature) activation.
- The basic cycle length during a premature stimulation protocol can also have different influences on initiation of reentry and triggered activity. Repolarization and the duration of the effective refractory period decrease as basic cycle length shortens (Figure 7-7) as does dispersion of refractoriness. As a result, premature stimuli at short basic cycle lengths may be less effective for initiation of reentry, since establishing block is less likely. Therefore, clinical premature stimulation protocols are often carried out at the longest basic cycle length that reliably captures the rhythm of the heart. (Tachycardias can sometimes be induced at both long and short basic cycle lengths.) On the other hand, triggered activity is more likely to be initiated by premature stimulation during a short basic cycle length that increases Ca^{2+} loading.
- Initiation of reentry is related to establishment of a critical degree of slow conduction in the region where the arrhythmia originates. Detection of the slow conduction with electrogram recordings adds credence to the interpretation that the arrhythmia is caused by reentry. The induction of triggered activity caused by DADs is not dependent on slowed conduction and does not show this relationship.
- The coupling interval of the return cycle of reentrant tachycardia is inversely related to the overdrive or premature stimulus cycle length (Figure 9-22 and, Figure 9-24), whereas it is directly related for triggered activity (Figure 5-5). The return cycle for initiation of reentry is determined by conduction time of the stimulated impulse around the circuit, which is slower (takes a longer time) at shorter cycle lengths, whereas the return cycle of triggered activity is caused by the coupling interval of the DAD, which is shorter at short cycle lengths because of increased Ca^{2+} loading (Figure 5-4 and Figure 5-6).
- Gradual shortening of the cycle length (warm up) at the start and gradual slowing at termination as is characteristic of DAD-triggered activity, are not general features of reentrant tachycardia. However, if catecholamine-sensitive tissues such as the AV node are part of the reentrant circuit, gradual warm up and slowing may occur because changes in blood pressure affect sympathetic activity (see Chapter 11).
- The cycle length and duration of reentrant tachycardia is not usually related to the cycle length of the initiating stimuli as it sometimes is with DAD-triggered activity (Figure 5-4 and Figure 5-6).

Some of the above characteristics of anatomic reentry can apply to initiation of reentry in functional circuits. Leading circle reentry and rotors can be initiated by stimulation because of heterogeneities in electrophysiological properties. A more detailed description of characteristics of initiation in functional reentrant circuits is not available. However, since the size, shape, and location of functional circuits might change with different overdrive or premature cycle lengths, many of the features of initiation of functional reentry are likely to be different.

Premature Stimulation and Overdrive Pacing During Reentrant Arrhythmias

Programmed Premature Stimulation: Resetting and the Temporal Excitable Gap

Single stimulated premature impulses initiated close to a reentrant circuit can be used to evaluate resetting characteristics and properties of the excitable gap. As described in Figure 1-10, resetting occurs when the sum of the premature coupling interval and the first cycle of the returning basic rhythm (the tachycardia in this example) following the premature impulse (the return cycle) is less than two tachycardia cycles. The "temporal excitable gap" (the time interval between the head of activation of one reentrant impulse and tail of refractoriness of the prior impulse) (see Figure 9-1), is the interval between the longest coupled stimulated impulse that enters the circuit to reset it, and the coupling interval of the premature impulse that enters the circuit to terminate reentry. The temporal gap is comprised of relatively and completely excitable segments, the duration of which can be quantified based on conduction characteristics of the premature impulse in the circuit. Evaluation of the spatial excitable gap, which is the distance occupied by the excitable gap at any moment in time, requires high-density mapping of the circuit and local stimulation at multiple sites in the circuit—which, in general, is not feasible in clinical studies.

Figure 9-26 diagrams the protocol using single stimulated premature impulses (vertical blue bars) at different times in the basic cycle length of a tachycardia caused by reentry (vertical black bars, cycle length 320 ms), to evaluate resetting characteristics and properties of the temporal excitable gap.

Figure 9-27 diagrams the interaction of the prematurely stimulated impulse with the reentrant impulse in the anatomical model of reentry with the premature stimulation occurring at different times in the basic cycle length, as shown in Figure 9-26. The basic reentrant pattern causing the tachycardia with a 320-ms cycle length is shown in Figure 9-27, far left panel (with no letter indicator). In this snapshot, the reentrant wavefront is indicated by the black arrowhead. The completely refractory region following the wavefront is indicated by the black curved arrow tail, and the partially refractory region by the gray shading.

The unshaded area between the wavefront (arrowhead) and the end of the partially refractory tail (gray area) is the fully excitable gap, while the gray area is the partially excitable gap.

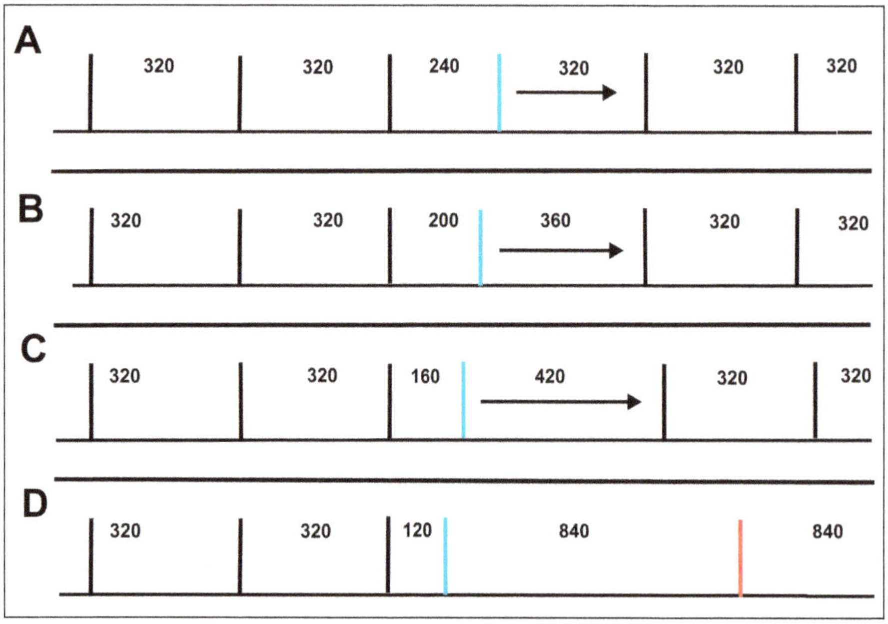

Figure 9-26 **Panels A–D** show effects of premature stimuli (**blue bars**) on reentrant tachycardia (**black bars**). Cycle lengths in ms are indicated.

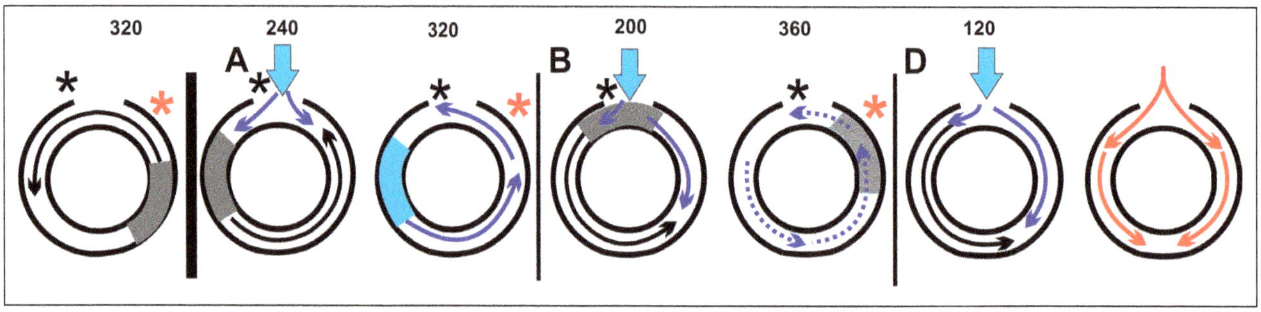

Figure 9-27 Diagram of effects of premature impulses on reentry in an anatomical circuit.

Compensatory return cycle. When the stimulated impulse is delivered late in the cycle length (not shown in Figure 9-26), it may be unable to enter the reentrant circuit, sometimes due to collision between the stimulated impulse and the reentrant impulse exiting from the circuit, and reentrant tachycardia is not affected. The next tachycardia impulse then comes precisely on time and is compensatory (the sum of the premature cycle and the return cycle equals two successive tachycardia cycles).

Activation pattern of the reentrant circuit in the resetting response. In Figure 9-26, Panel A, a prematurely stimulated impulse (vertical blue) with coupling interval of 240 ms resets the tachycardia. The return cycle of 320 ms (horizontal arrow) is less than compensatory; the sum of the premature cycle and the return cycle is less than two successive tachycardia cycles. The diagram in Figure 9-27, Panel A, shows the activation pattern of the circuit by the stimulated impulse (large blue arrow) at a coupling interval of 240 ms. In the left diagram in Panel A, the impulse initially excites the circuit (purple arrows) in a region completely recovered from prior excitation by the reentrant tachycardia impulse—the fully excitable gap. The reentrant tachycardia impulse is moving counterclockwise (black arrow). The stimulated impulse propagates in a clockwise direction (purple arrow to the right; "antidromic" is the term used to describe movement in the opposite direction to the tachycardia reentrant impulse) and collides with the oncoming reentrant impulse (black arrow). The stimulation also initiates an impulse that propagates in a counter clockwise direction (purple arrow to the left) ("orthodromic" is the term used to describe movement in the same direction as the tachycardia reentrant impulse). The orthodromic impulse conducts around the circuit (right diagram in Panel A, purple arrow) in the completely recovered myocardium of the fully excitable gap, at the same conduction velocity as the tachycardia reentrant impulse. It therefore completes one revolution around the circuit (to the black asterisk in Panel A) in 320 ms (the return cycle), which is the same as one revolution of the tachycardia reentrant impulse. In some circuits that have separate entrance and exit routes, the premature impulse can exit the circuit before making a complete revolution, and in those cases the return cycle can be less than the tachycardia cycle length. The red asterisk in Panel A at the right would be an example of the possible location of such a separate exit route.

The time for orthodromic conduction of premature impulses in the circuit remains constant over the range of premature coupling intervals at which the stimulated impulses conduct around the circuit in the fully excitable gap with the same activation pattern as in Figure 9-27, Panel A. In Figure 9-26, Panels B and C, prematurely stimulated impulses at shorter coupling intervals of 200 and 160 ms (blue bars) are followed by return cycles of 360 and 420 ms (horizontal arrows), which are longer than the tachycardia cycle but still less than compensatory; the tachycardia is still reset. The diagram in Figure 9-27, Panel B shows the earlier prematurely stimulated impulse at a 200 ms coupling interval, entering the circuit in a region still relatively refractory from prior activation (partially excitable gap) by the reentrant impulse (blue arrow, gray-shaded region in Panel B, left diagram). The stimulated impulse conducts antidromically (purple arrow to the right) to collide with the oncoming reentrant impulse (black arrow, left diagram). The stimulated impulse also conducts orthodromically (purple arrow to the left) around the circuit in relatively refractory myocardium (gray region) at a slower conduction velocity (indicated by dashed arrows in the right diagram) accounting for the longer transit time around the complete circuit (360 ms from black asterisk in left diagram to black asterisk in right diagram) than the basic tachycardia reentrant impulse (320 ms). Premature impulses with shorter coupling intervals conduct even more slowly orthodromically, causing a further increase in the return cycle (Figure 9-26, Panel C) because they conduct in more refractory myocardium. There is an inverse relationship between the premature cycle lengths and return cycle lengths.

Termination. In Figure 9-26, Panel D, an earlier premature impulse (120 ms, blue bar), is followed by sinus rhythm (red bar) because it stops reentry. The mechanism for termination is shown in Figure 9-27, Panel D. The prematurely stimulated impulse conducts antidromically (purple arrows to the right) and collides with the oncoming (orthodromic) reentrant impulse (black arrow). In the orthodromic direction, the premature impulse (purple arrow to the left) encounters completely refractory myocardium of the tail of the reentrant impulse and also blocks. The circuit is then activated by a sinus impulse without reentry (right diagram, red arrows).

Resetting curves. Resetting curves can be plotted from the results of premature stimulation studies shown in Figure 9-27 (described for automaticity in Figure 1-11). **Figure 9-28** shows an idealized situation where the site of stimulation and return cycle measurements are close to the circuit so that conduction properties between the site of stimulation and the circuit do not significantly influence the values. The sites of entrance and exit also remain constant over the range of premature coupling intervals.

The return cycles following long-coupled, premature impulses that do not affect the reentrant impulse fall along the slanted black line known as the "line of identity" (Figure 9-28), indicating a compensatory response. At shorter coupling intervals, at which premature impulses propagate in the fully excitable gap in the circuit, the return cycles are approximately equal to the tachycardia cycle lengths (horizontal blue line coincides with horizontal dashed black line which is the tachycardia cycle length of 320 ms), provided the premature impulse conducts completely around the circuit to the site where the return cycle is measured (see also Figure 9-27, Panel A).

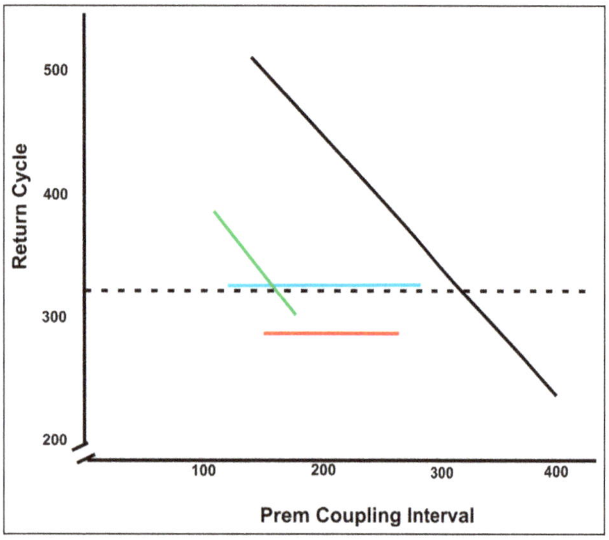

Figure 9-28 Resetting response of reentrant tachycardia. The premature cycle (Prem) coupling interval is on the abscissa, the return cycle is on the ordinate.

In a circuit with a separate entrance and exit pathway, the return cycles are dependent on the distance between entrance and exit and are less than the tachycardia cycle length, since the stimulated impulses do not conduct around the entire circuit before exiting the circuit (Figure 9-28, red line). The return cycles remain constant over the full range of coupling intervals when conduction is occurring in the fully excitable gap (horizontal blue and red lines), since conduction velocity is constant and independent of prematurity. When the premature impulses travel around the circuit in the partially excitable gap, conduction velocity slows (Figure 9-27, Panel B), and the return cycles increase and continue to increase with increased prematurity of the stimulated impulse (green line in Figure 9-28). The tachycardia is then terminated when the coupling interval is sufficiently premature (see Figure 9-26, Panel D and Figure 9-27, Panel D).

The interval between the longest and shortest coupling intervals that result in resetting is the resetting zone. The duration of the total (temporal) excitable gap that includes both the fully excitable and partially excitable components, is from the longest coupling interval that first resets tachycardia to the coupling interval that terminates it. When tachycardias have a well-defined flat segment (blue line) and ascending segment (green line) to the resetting curve, the durations of both fully and partially excitable gaps can be estimated.

For tachycardias with only a partially excitable gap, the entire response graph may show only the ascending green line, indicating an inverse relationship between premature cycle and return cycle before tachycardia termination at the shortest coupling interval. The range of coupling intervals between the longest that resets and the shortest that terminates is the duration of the partially excitable gap in this situation. Only if tachycardia is terminated by the shortest-coupled, premature impulse can it be concluded that the entire excitable gap has been determined.

Comparing the Resetting Responses for Reentry, Normal Automaticity, and DAD-Triggered Activity

The resetting responses described in Figure 9-28 has features that distinguish reentry in an anatomical circuit from normal automaticity and DAD-triggered activity. Data from clinical studies on DAD-triggered activity is limited, so the description combines characteristics obtained from laboratory animal studies with clinical studies.

1. A "flat segment" to the resetting curve (Figure 9-28, horizontal blue and red lines) occurs in both automaticity and reentry in circuits with a fully excitable gap. For reentry, the return cycle length is approximately equal to the tachycardia cycle length when the premature impulse conducts around the entire circuit before onset of the tachycardia ECG waveform (horizontal blue line). For reentrant circuits with a separate entrance and exit routes where the premature impulse conducts around only part of the circuit, the return cycle is less than the tachycardia cycle length (horizontal red line). For automatic arrhythmias, the return cycle is the same as the tachycardia cycle, since premature activation does not usually alter spontaneous diastolic depolarization (SDD). It is longer when there is conduction delay into and out of the automatic focus (Figure 2-14).
2. The "ascending segment" (increasing) of the reset curve of a reentrant circuit, where the return cycle is inversely related to the premature cycle (Figure 9-28, green line) indicating propagation in a partially recovered excitable gap, does not occur with automaticity or triggered activity.
3. A "descending" response is characteristic for triggered activity. The return cycle decreases with

decreased premature cycle length because of earlier occurrence of DADs at short cycle lengths. This does not occur with automaticity or reentry.

4. Reentry, and DAD-triggered activity can be "terminated" by early-coupled premature impulses. Termination of tachycardia in a stable reentrant circuit is often sudden whereas termination of DAD-triggered activity may occur several impulses after the premature impulse. Automaticity is not terminated by early premature impulses.
5. Resetting of reentrant circuits might occur when stimulating at some sites and not others (site specificity) since stimulation at certain sites may allow easier entry of the stimulated impulse into the circuit than others. Site specificity usually does not occur for automaticity and triggered activity since the stimulated impulse is likely to reach the focus no matter where it is located although exceptions can occur.

In conclusion, the above description provides a foundation for understanding the electrophysiology of the resetting response of reentrant circuits based on the model of an anatomically determined circuit with a large, fully excitable gap. There are, however, a number of exceptions and variations that are dependent on the properties of circuits in different regions of the heart. Resetting would not be measured if conduction time of the premature impulse in the circuit were sufficiently long. A long conduction time caused by slow conduction in a localized region of the circuit, might result in a long return cycle resembling a compensatory pause rather than a return cycle indicating resetting even though the premature impulse entered the circuit early. In the absence of a fully excitable gap and the presence of only a small, partially excitable gap—which can occur in an anatomical circuit but which is more characteristic of functional leading circle reentry—premature impulses may be unable to enter the reentrant circuit and reset or terminate a tachycardia. Therefore, only a compensatory pause occurs over the full range of premature coupling intervals. The effects of premature stimulation on rotors is not known. The expected effects of premature impulses on the cycle length of reentry might also be altered in a functional circuit if changes in the entry path into a circuit occurs with changes in prematurity of the stimulated impulse or if the premature impulse causes a change in the size or shape of the circuit or converts a single circuit into multiple circuits.

Overdrive Pacing and Entrainment

The description in this section covers basic features of the effects of overdrive pacing on reentry in an anatomical circuit with the specific properties of a large, fully excitable gap with uniform conduction velocity and wavelength (**Figure 9-29**). These basic effects of overdrive are modified in the reentrant circuits causing specific atrial (Chapter 10), AV junctional (Chapter 11), and ventricular (Chapter 12) reentrant tachycardias because of variations in circuit size, location, and electrophysiological properties. Examples of these variations include: circuits may be anatomical, functional, or partly anatomical and partly functional; circuits may have a region of slow conduction and/or long refractory periods causing changes in the wavelength; and circuits may have fixed or variable entry and exit routes, all of which affect some of the responses to overdrive pacing.

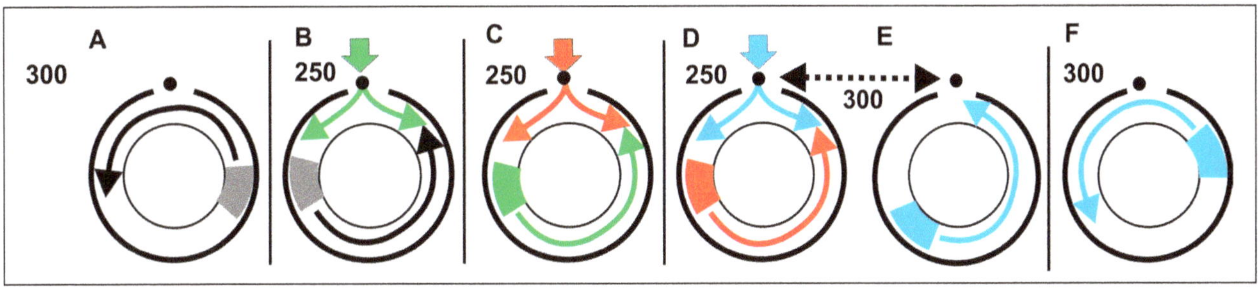

Figure 9-29 Entrainment of an anatomical reentrant circuit by overdrive pacing. **Panel A** shows the reentrant wavefront. **Panels B–D** show activation patterns of stimulated impulses during overdrive. **Panel E** shows propagation of the last stimulated impulse in the circuit. Panel F is the continuation of reentry after stimulation is stopped.

Entrainment; acceleration of the rate of activation of the circuit by overdrive pacing. Figure 9-29 diagrams a response pattern of a reentrant circuit (tachycardia) to overdrive pacing when the location of the pacing site and cycle length of pacing enables continuous interaction in the circuit between the paced impulses and the reentrant impulses. This response pattern where overdrive pacing accelerates the rate of activation of the reentrant circuit is called "entrainment."

In Figure 9-29, the pattern of impulse propagation in the circuit before overdrive pacing begins, shown in Panel A, is indicated by the curved black arrow with the wavefront (arrowhead) followed by the effective refractory tail (solid curved black line) and relative refractory tail (thick gray area). The unshaded area in the circuit is the fully excitable gap, the thick gray area is the partially excitable gap. The reentrant impulse propagates around a relatively large anatomical obstacle at the center. The 300-ms cycle length of tachycardia (above left) is determined by the conduction time of the reentrant impulse around the circuit that is longer than the wavelength, accounting for the large, fully excitable gap. Even though the circuit is diagrammed as having discrete well-defined boundaries, the boundaries may not always be fixed and protective. Connections between the circuit and surrounding myocardium can sometimes occur around its circumference.

Panel B shows the first stimulated impulse of overdrive pacing through electrodes located near the black dot, at a 250-ms cycle length (green arrow), that interacts with the circuit. (The first overdrive impulse is synchronized to the last tachycardia impulse during a clinical study to attain the first 250-ms cycle length.) The entry route into the circuit may not be fixed but may be dependent on the location of the stimulating electrodes. The region where the paced impulse first excites the circuit in the fully excitable gap (green arrows), is activated prematurely, before the arrival of the intrinsic reentrant impulse represented by the black arrow. The stimulated impulse (curved green arrow) collides with this reentrant impulse (curved black arrow) in the antidromic direction to the right, extinguishing that impulse while propagating through the circuit in the orthodromic direction (curved green arrow to the left in Panel B, and curved green arrow continued in Panel C) with the same conduction velocity as the reentrant impulse since it is propagating in fully excitable myocardium. The first overdrive impulse resets the reentrant wavefront in the circuit; the stimulated orthodromic impulse, which becomes the reentrant impulse (green arrow in Panel C), occurs 50 ms earlier than the expected arrival time of the intrinsic reentrant impulse. This is identical to the pattern of activation of reentrant circuits by single premature impulses that reset the reentrant circuit described in Figure 9-27.

The second stimulated impulse of overdrive in Figure 9-29 Panel C (red arrows, designated as the nth impulse, at the cycle length of 250 ms) collides in the antidromic direction (to the right) with the orthodromic impulse elicited by the previous stimulus (green arrow, designated as impulse n–1). Note that for descriptive purposes in these examples, the stimulated impulse is designated "n" and the previous impulse in the circuit (either previous overdrive or reentrant impulse) is designated "n–1". It also propagates in the circuit in the orthodromic direction (curved red arrow to the left in Panel C and curved red arrow continued in Panel D) with the same conduction velocity as the original reentrant impulse and the first stimulated impulse since it is also propagating in the fully excitable gap. It is again premature with respect to the orthodromic impulse propagating in the circuit caused by the preceding (n–1) stimulated impulse. Rather than resetting the original tachycardia circuit, this second stimulated impulse resets the circuit that has already been reset by the previous stimulated impulse, e.g., it is resetting the reset circuit. This pattern of activation continues with each stimulated impulse, antidromic collision with the previously stimulated orthodromic reentrant impulse with initiation of a new premature orthodromic impulse by the stimulated impulse (the same patterns as shown in Panels C and D). Each stimulated impulse conducts orthodromically in the circuit with the same conduction velocity, resetting activation of the already reset circuit. Overdrive pacing therefore is accelerating the rate of activation of the circuit in Figure 9-29, to the pacing cycle length of 250 ms, which is entrainment of the reentrant circuit When applied to clinical arrhythmias, entrainment affects the rate of activation of the entire chamber where the circuit is located in addition to the reentrant circuit. The recognition of entrainment of clinical arrhythmias is described in the next chapters.

The last stimulated impulse in a period of overdrive of variable duration, that causes entrainment, is represented by the blue arrows in Figure 9-29, Panel D. It again collides with the orthodromic wavefront from the next to last stimulated impulse (red arrow) and propagates around the circuit in the orthodromic direction in the pattern of the previous stimulated impulses (curved blue arrow to the left in Panel D) but is not met by another stimulated impulse (curved blue arrow in Panel E) since overdrive is stopped (there is no overdrive impulse originating at the black dot in Panel E). The last stimulated impulse (from Panel D) continues to propagate around the circuit, and reentry continues at the same cycle length (300 ms) as prior to overdrive (Panels E and F). The conduction time of the last stimulated impulse from its site of initiation (Panel D, black dot) back to that site (Panel E, black dot) is a measurement of the conduction properties and excitable gap of the reset circuit. In Figure 9-29, conduction time is the same as during reentry prior to overdrive, e.g., the last stimulated impulse takes 300 ms to conduct around the circuit (horizontal dashed arrow). Resumption of the original pattern and properties of reentry when the overdrive is abruptly terminated as in Figure 9-29, is part of the definition of entrainment, i.e., resumption of the original rate of tachycardia when pacing is stopped. The same phenomenon of tachycardia continuation occurs when overdrive rate is slowed below the entrainment cycle length; below the rate that "captures" the circuit.

The reset (entrained) circuit can sometimes have different properties than the original circuit since the more rapid activation during entrainment can change conduction velocity or refractory periods, the wavelength and the size of the excitable gap. The first cycle after overdrive ends can sometimes be longer than after a comparable premature impulse even though the reentrant circuit during tachycardia has a completely excitable gap. This occurs when the paced impulses propagate in partially excitable myocardium that is more likely to occur when the fully excitable gap is small. In spite of this possibility, overdrive suppression as described for normal automaticity (Figure 1-7), or overdrive acceleration described for DAD-triggered activity (Figure 5-7), does not usually occur, distinguishing reentry from these mechanisms. An exception to this is the reentrant circuit that is partially determined by functional properties that can be changed (pathway shortened) by overdrive to cause apparent overdrive acceleration.

Termination. At a critically short overdrive cycle length, the reentrant excitation pattern is disrupted as diagrammed in **Figure 9-30**, and the arrhythmia terminates.

Figure 9-30, Panel A shows the pattern of activation at the 250-ms pacing cycle length (PCL) (described in Figure 9-29); antidromic collision of the stimulated impulse (n) (green arrow to the right) with the orthodromic impulse in the circuit (black arrow, n–1) and orthodromic propagation (green arrow to the left). At a shorter PCL (230 ms) in Panel B, the stimulated impulse (n) (green arrow) in the orthodromic direction to the left runs into the relatively refractory tail of the reentrant impulse in the circuit (gray-shaded region) because it enters the circuit earlier in the cycle but propagation continues. The stimulated impulse (green arrow in Panel B) also penetrates further into the circuit in the antidromic direction (to the right) before colliding with the orthodromic impulse of the previously stimulated impulse (black arrow, n–1) because of its increased prematurity. In Panel C, because of its earlier entry into the circuit at a still shorter PCL (200 ms), the stimulated impulse in the orthodromic direction (green arrow to the left) collides with the refractory tail of the reentrant impulse in the circuit (black arrow), blocking in this direction while also colliding with the reentrant wavefront in the antidromic direction (green arrow to the right). Because block occurs in both the orthodromic and antidromic directions, the reentrant pattern of excitation is disrupted and reentry does not continue when stimulation is stopped. It may require several or more paced impulses at this cycle length during overdrive before block occurs, as shown in Panel C. After block occurs, there is no n–1 impulse in the circuit (no green arrow in Panel D). The following stimulated impulse (Panel D, black arrows), activates all regions of the circuit itself, in the same direction without encountering an n–1 impulse. When stimulation is stopped, sinus rhythm occurs. Termination of the reentrant pattern and the tachycardia that it causes at a critically short PCL is another criterion identifying entrainment. Its recognition during a clinical study is described in the following chapters.

Termination of reentry by overdrive also distinguishes it from automaticity. Termination is usually abrupt, occurring immediately after block in the circuit, which can differentiate a reentrant mechanism from termination of DAD-triggered activity that often occurs several or more impulses after overdrive is stopped (see Figure 5-7). Other features of overdrive and entrainment also distinguish reentry from these other mechanisms as described in the next section.

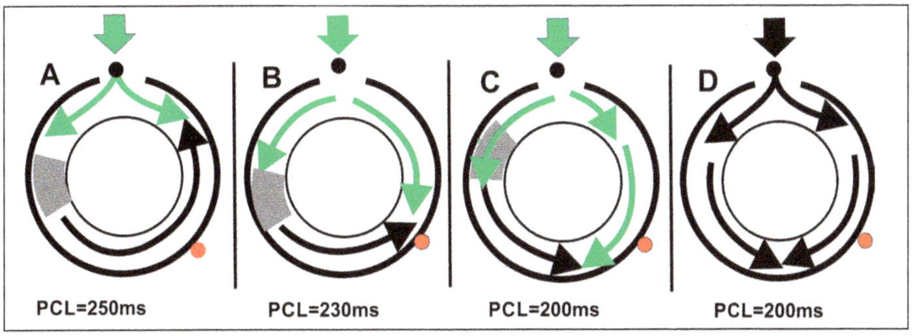

Figure 9-30 Overdrive termination of reentry. **Panel A** shows activation of the circuit during entrainment at a 250 ms pacing cycle length (PCL). **Panels B** and **C** show the activation patterns at shorter stimulus cycle lengths that terminate reentry. **Panel D** shows the activation pattern of a stimulated impulse after reentry is terminated. PCL = pacing cycle length.

Fusion activation during entrainment of reentrant circuits. An important feature of entrainment is the simultaneous activation of the reentrant circuit by two successive impulses in the overdrive train, the current paced impulse (n), and the previous paced impulse conducting orthodromically (n–1) (Figure 9-29). This pattern called "fusion activation" is also diagrammed in **Figure 9-31**. Sometimes fusion within the circuit itself might be manifested on the ECG. When fusion can be recognized on the ECG, entrainment is documented and reentry diagnosed during a clinical study, even when the pattern of activity in the circuit is not mapped. If the circuit is too small, fusion activation of surrounding myocardium may still be manifest on the ECG. In order to recognize fusion activation, the ECG patterns for the antidromic and orthodromic wavefronts must be sufficiently different.

Figure 9-31 diagrams patterns of fusion activation of a reentrant circuit that is large enough so that the impulses in the circuit can be detected on the surface ECG; for example, a circus movement tachycardia using both a left- and right-sided A-V bypass tract (see Chapter 11). In each panel, the orthodromic impulse and the region of the circuit activated by it are shown by the black arrows and isochrones. The antidromic impulse and the region of the circuit it activates is shown by the green arrows and isochrones. Panels A1–D1 represent progressively shorter pacing cycle lengths (PCLs) of stimulation at a site outside the circuit (black dot). At the longest PCL at which entrainment occurs in Panel A1, most of the circuit is activated by the orthodromic impulse (black arrow and isochrones) and the ECG morphology would closely resemble the morphology during the reentrant tachycardia. Fusion activation during all stimulated impulses at this cycle length is constant, called "fixed fusion." At shorter PCLs in Panels B1, C1, and D1, the stimulated impulse (n) enters the circuit earlier allowing the antidromic wavefront to penetrate further, activating more of the circuit (green arrows and isochrones), while the orthodromic wavefront (n–1; black arrows and isochrones) activates less of the circuit. Fusion is still fixed during a period of overdrive at each cycle length but the degree of fusion is changed with the antidromic wavefront contributing more to the fused ECG waveform. This is known as "progressive fusion." In Panel D1, most of the circuit is activated by the antidromic wavefront so the ECG would have a morphology characteristic of the pacing site. Clinical examples of fixed and progressive ECG fusion are shown in Chapters 10, 11, and 12.

Electrograms can also be recorded within the circuit (at a site indicated by the red dots in Figure 9-31), and fusion in the circuit can also be detected in these electrograms. In Figure 9-31, Panel A1, a local electrogram recorded at the site indicated by the red dot would have a morphology characteristic of the orthodormic direction of activation (black arrow). In Panel B1, at a shorter overdrive cycle, this site is activated both by the orthodromic (black arrow) and antidromic (green arrow) impulse, and would show an altered morphology representing fusion activation by both wavefronts. At a still shorter overdrive cycle length (Panel C1), this electrode is activated entirely by the antidromic impulse (green arrow). Not only would the electrogram morphology change to that characteristic of antidromic activation (fusion is no longer evident), but the time interval from stimulus to electrogram onset would markedly shorten. The electrogram is no longer activated by the orthodromic impulse conducting through a long pathway around the circuit, as shown in Panel A1, but is activated through a less circuitous antidromic pathway. Sometimes, when fusion cannot be detected on the surface ECG, it is detected in local electrogram recordings from the circuit enabling entrainment to be recognized.

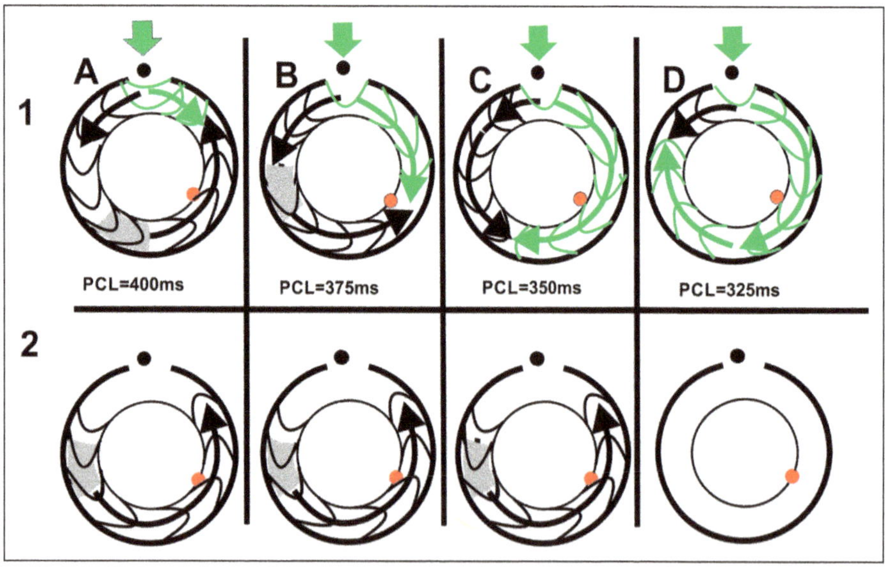

Figure 9-31 Fusion activation of a reentrant circuit. Each vertical panel (**A–D**) has two diagrams (**1** and **2**) that illustrate activation of the reentrant circuit during overdrive pacing at progressively shorter PCLs (**1**) and after pacing is stopped (**2**).

Another characteristic of entrainment related to fusion is also shown in Panels A–C in Figure 9-31. If the stimulated impulse that is diagrammed in Panels A1–C1 is the last one of the period of overdrive that does not terminate reentry, this stimulated impulse would travel around the circuit in the orthodromic direction (black arrows in Panels A2–C2) and cause an ECG morphology which is not fused since there is no subsequent stimulated impulse. The last stimulated impulse occurs at the overdrive cycle length but is not fused. In Panel D1, the reentrant pattern is terminated by the last stimulated impulses (see Figure 9-30) so no activity continues (Panel D2).

Propagation of different antidromic and orthodromic impulses in small circuits might not be detected on the ECG. However, fusion during entrainment of antidromic and orthodromic wavefronts outside the circuit might still be apparent on the ECG.

Figure 9-32 shows fusion activation outside a reentrant circuit that is depicted as being small and protected; it has barriers around most of its circumference but is attached to the myocardium by an entry (ENT) and exit pathway, which are widely separated. This model represents the features of some circuits causing ventricular tachycardia in infarcted hearts (see Chapter 12). The orthodromically conducting reentrant impulse is represented by the black arrows in each panel. Activation of the circuit during overdrive occurs with the same pattern shown in Figure 9-29: antidromic collision of the paced wavefront (n) with the previously paced orthodromic impulse (n–1). In Panel A1, an overdrive impulse (n, originating at the asterisk) entering the circuit during stable entrainment is indicated by the blue arrows. Shortly before it enters, an orthodromic wavefront from the preceding stimulated impulse (n–1) exits from the circuit (black arrow). The pacing stimulus occurs after the onset of the ECG waveform, since the reentrant impulse has already exited the circuit at the time of stimulation and has already activated a variable amount of myocardium. The amount of myocardium activated by the exiting wavefront is dependent on the time relationship between the exiting wavefront and the stimulated wavefront (n). A region outside the circuit shows fusion activation, partly activated by the stimulated wavefront (n) (blue isochrones) and partly by the orthodromic wavefront (n–1) exiting from the circuit (black isochrones). Recognition of fusion is dependent on sufficient separation of the entry and exit pathways so that separate regions of myocardium are activated by each wavefront. A diagram of the fused ECG waveform is shown in Figure 9-32 in the box above. The segment of the waveform generated by the stimulated impulse is shown in blue, and that generated by the impulse emerging from the circuit, in black. During entrainment, the fusion pattern is constant during each paced impulse (fixed fusion) as long as conduction of the orthodromic impulse is stable. If the paced impulse in Panel A1 is the last one, it continues around the circuit and is not met by another stimulated impulse, as diagrammed in Panel A2. The emerging wavefront (Panel A2) is the sole activator of the region outside the circuit (blue isochrones) and the ECG waveform (in the box) represents the morphology of the emerging orthodromic wavefront (blue curve in ECG inset box has a similar orientation as the black negative curve in Panel A1). This waveform is not fused.

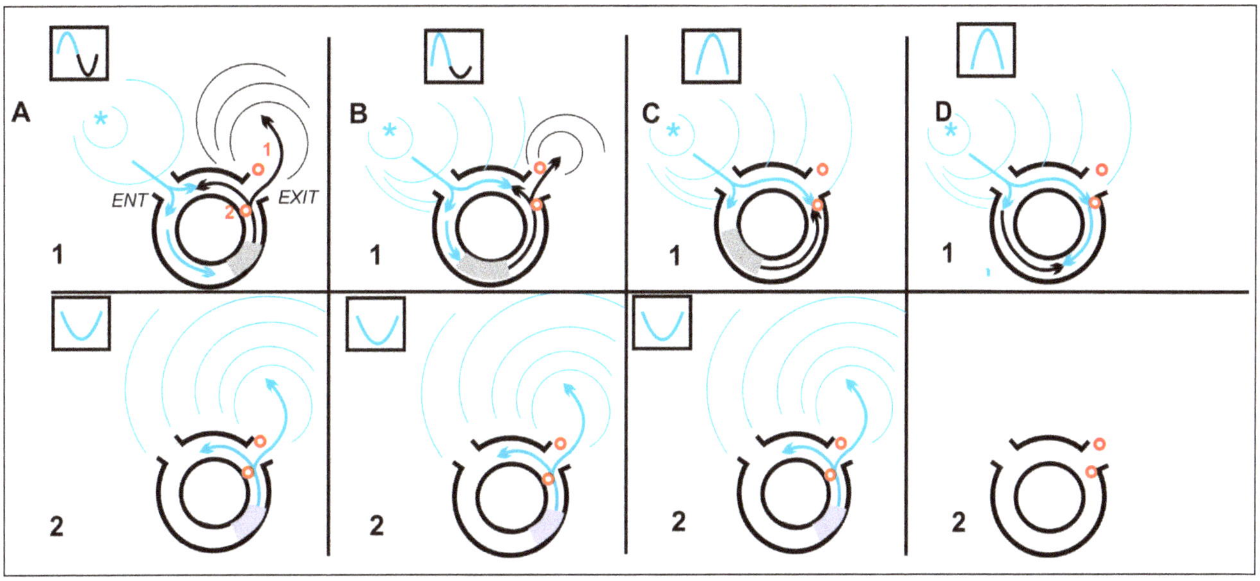

Figure 9-32 Mechanism for fusion during entrainment of a small anatomical circuit. **Panel A1–D1** at the top shows entrainment of the tachycardia at decreasing pacing cycle lengths. Bottom diagrams (**A2–D2**) shows activation by the last stimulated impulse.

The degree of fusion that occurs outside the circuit depends on the time the paced wavefront arrives at the circuit relative to the time the impulse emerges from the circuit and is, therefore, dependent on the stimulus cycle length. Figure 9-32, Panel B1, shows activation when the PCL is decreased. The general pattern remains the same; the stimulated excitation wave (n; blue arrow) enters the circuit and collides antidromically with the orthodromic impulse from the previous stimulus (n–1; black arrow) while propagating in the orthodromic direction (blue arrows). This time however, the stimulated impulse arrives at the circuit earlier at the shorter cycle with relation to emergence of the previous impulse from the circuit. It therefore activates more of the surrounding myocardium (blue isochrones) while the region activated by the emerging impulse is decreased (black isochrones). The ECG morphology (box above) still shows fusion but the paced segment (blue) is greater and the circuit segment (black) is decreased. The fusion pattern is constant (fixed) during each paced impulse as long as conduction of the orthodromic impulse is stable, but fusion is progressive. If this were the last paced impulse, it would emerge from the circuit (Panel B2) in the same way as described for Panel A2, with an ECG morphology that is not fused (shown in the box).

Figure 9-32, Panel C1, shows activation at a still shorter pacing cycle length. The stimulated impulse arrives at the circuit prior to the exit of the previous orthodromic impulse from the circuit, penetrating the circuit for a greater distance in the antidromic direction (blue arrows). The region outside the circuit is activated entirely by the paced wavefront (blue isochrones) and the ECG waveform is not fused but entirely representative of the paced wavefront (box above, blue waveform). It is still possible for the last stimulated orthodromic impulse to conduct through the circuit and emerge from the circuit (Panel C2) with an ECG waveform characteristic of the circuit (box above in Panel C2). This is a type of "concealed entrainment." Fusion is occurring in the circuit but is not detected (concealed) on the ECG.

In Panel D1, at a still shorter pacing cycle length, fusion also does not occur on the ECG. The antidromic stimulated impulse (n) (blue arrows), collides with the orthodromic wavefront from the previous stimulus (n–1) (black arrow) before it reaches the exit pathway, while the orthodromic stimulated wavefront (n) (blue arrow) blocks in the completely refractory tail of the orthodromic impulse (n–1) that is in the circuit (black arrow). Therefore, no propagating orthodromic wavefront is in the circuit when stimulation is stopped and reentry is terminated (Panel D2).

When the surface ECG does not show fusion, local electrogram recordings can be used to document entrainment in a small protected circuit similar to the description in Figure 9-30. In Figure 9-32, hypothetical sites of local electrogram recordings are indicated by the small red circles (1) outside the circuit and (2) inside the circuit. In Panels A and B, both are activated by the orthodromic wavefront, first in the circuit (2) and then emerging from the circuit (1). Activation of electrode 2 occurs before onset of the ECG waveform, while activation of electrode 1 coincides with the onset of the ECG waveform.

In Panel C1, at a stimulus cycle at which no ECG fusion occurs, electrode 1 is activated in the antidromic direction by the stimulated wavefront (n) and electrode 2 shows fusion activation from the antidromic (n; blue arrow) and orthodromic (n–1) impulses (black arrow) within the circuit. The antidromic impulse now causes the initial segment of the fused electrogram to occur earlier because the antidromic impulse reaches it directly and sooner than when it is only activated orthodromically. Compare Panel C1 to Panel B1, where the initial activating impulse has to conduct orthodromically around the circuit.

In addition to the example of concealed entrainment described in Figure 9-32, C1 above, entrainment without fusion on the ECG can occur when the stimulus site is within a protected circuit, since the ECG morphologies of the reentrant and paced impulses are identical (**Figure 9-33**).

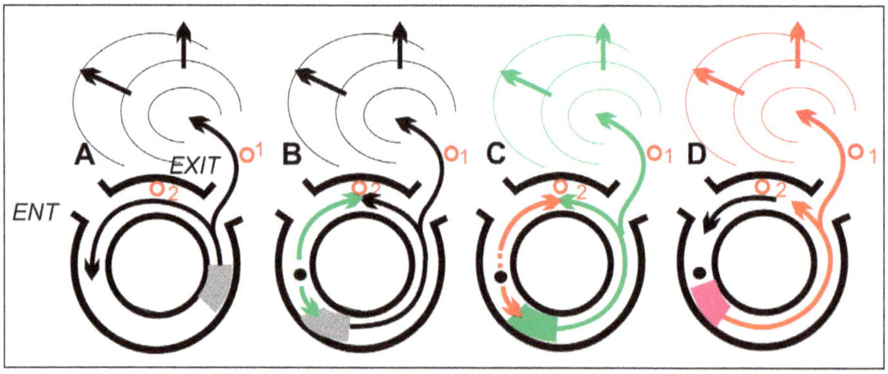

Figure 9-33 Entrainment without fusion on the ECG. **Panel A** shows the reentrant impulse. **Panels B** and **C** show activation during entrainment by stimulation in the circuit at the site indicated by the **black dot**. **Panel D** shows activation after the last stimulated impulse.

An example of entrainment without fusion (concealed or exact entrainment) on the ECG resulting in identical ECG waveforms during stimulation and tachycardia, in a small protected circuit with a separate entrance and exit route is diagrammed in Figure 9-33. Panel A shows the reentrant impulse (black arrows), exit route and isochrones of the exiting wavefront, as in Figure 9-32. Panel B shows the first stimulated impulse of overdrive from a site within the circuit (black dot and green arrows). Antidromic activation (long green arrow) collides with the orthodromic reentrant impulse in the circuit (black arrow), while the orthodromically stimulated impulse propagates around the circuit (short green arrow in Panel B and green arrow in Panel C). The orthodromically stimulated impulse emerges from the circuit through the exit pathway to activate the surrounding myocardium with the same pattern and therefore, the same ECG morphology, as the tachycardia impulses (Panel C, green arrow). All subsequent stimulated impulses follow the same pattern (red arrows in Panels C and D). Activation of surrounding myocardium comes entirely from the stimulated orthodromic impulse emerging from the circuit region. Fusion is restricted to an area without electrocardiographic representation (in the circuit).

During stimulation in the reentrant circuit, changes in electrogram morphology recorded from within the circuit itself can help identify concealed entrainment. In Figure 9-33 electrogram recording site 2 in the circuit is activated orthodromically during reentry in Panel A. During entrainment (Panels B and C), it shows fusion activation between the antidromically stimulated impulse (green and red arrows) and the orthodromically propagating impulse from the previous (n–1) stimulus (black and green arrow). An electrogram recorded at site 1 in the exit pathway is still activated orthodromically.

When stimulating within the circuit, as shown in Figure 9-33, the next activation of the site at which the stimulus is applied after stimulation is stopped (return cycle) will be the same as the cycle length of the tachycardia, since the stimulated impulse conducts around the complete circuit, if conduction velocity is the same as the tachycardia reentrant impulse.

Characteristics of Reentrant Circuits That Cannot Be Entrained

Overdrive stimulation is unable to entrain some reentrant circuits. Tachycardias caused by reentry in anatomical circuits either without a fully excitable gap or with a very small one might not be entrained, since stimulated impulses are unable to enter the circuits. If the tachycardia is rapid, reentry may be terminated at the longest cycle length at which a stimulated impulse does penetrate the circuit, because the pattern of activation shown in Figure 9-30, Panel D occurs. Even when the stimulated impulses succeed in entering the circuit, if the substrate forming the circuit is unable to conduct impulses at a cycle length less than the tachycardia, entrainment cannot occur because conduction of the stimulated impulses block.

Whether or not functional circuits can be entrained is uncertain due to lack of experimental and clinical data. Leading circle reentry has only a partially excitable gap, since the head of the wavefront propagates in the partially refractory tail (Figure 9-18). Although stimulated impulses might enter the circuit, it is predicted to be difficult and require rapid overdrive rates. A rapid rate of overdrive might also disrupt the circuit, or change its size and shape since the pathway is not fixed. It is uncertain whether reentry caused by a rotor mechanism can be entrained (Figure 9-19).

Entrainment of Clinical Tachycardias

The above description of the mechanism of effects of overdrive pacing on reentrant circuits can be translated into the following characteristics of entrainment of a clinical arrhythmia:

- Transient entrainment of a tachycardia was originally defined as an increase in the rate of a tachycardia to a faster overdrive pacing rate, with resumption of the tachycardia at its original rate either upon abrupt cessation of pacing or slowing of the pacing rate below the intrinsic rate of the tachycardia. In actuality, it is acceleration of activation in the reentrant circuit and the chamber in which the circuit is located, to the pacing rate. During entrainment the circuit is continuously reset by the pacing impulses. The ECG morphology can resemble the tachycardia morphology rather than having the morphology of the pacing site, because the pattern of activation of the circuit is the same as during tachycardia.
- During entrainment at cycle lengths that do not interrupt the reentrant circuit, there is constant (fixed) fusion on the ECG representing the paced wavefront (n) and the orthodromic reentrant wavefront (n–1). As the rate of overdrive increases, fusion is progressive but still constant (fixed) at any given rate, with more of the ECG representing activation characteristic of the site of pacing.
- During entrainment that does not interrupt the circuit, the last paced impulse occurs at the pacing

cycle length but is not fused and has the ECG morphology of the tachycardia, since there is no antidromic impulse to meet it.

- Concealed entrainment occurs when there is minimal activation by the antidromic impulse and the myocardium giving rise to the ECG waveform is instead activated by the orthodromically conducting impulse in/from the reentrant circuit. In this situation, fusion can still often be recognized in local electrogram recordings from within the reentrant circuit.
- At a sufficiently rapid pacing rate, the reentrant pattern of activation is disrupted and the ECG morphology reverts to the one characteristic of the pacing site. When pacing is stopped, tachycardia does not resume.

SUMMARY

Altered impulse conduction underlies reentrant excitation. During reentry the propagating impulse persists to reexcite (i.e., reenter) regions it has already excited by conducting in a circuitous pathway—the reentrant circuit. For reentry to occur, unidirectional conduction block usually exists in the reentrant pathway, at least transiently, to force the impulse to conduct in one direction around it. Mechanisms that cause unidirectional block include: (1) heterogeneities in refractory periods, (2) asymmetrical depression of excitability, (3) impedance mismatch caused by geometrical factors related to tissue architecture, and (4) nonuniform anisotropy. The impulse that is conducting around the circuit must also find excitable tissue in the direction in which it is propagating. In order for this requirement to be fulfilled, the conduction time around the pathway must be longer than the effective refractory period of the myocardium that comprises it; that is, the wavelength of the conducting impulse (conduction velocity × refractory period) must be less than the path length. The excitable region of the circuit in front of the propagating impulse forms the spatial excitable gap.

A slow conduction velocity can be a consequence of a reduction of the resting membrane potential, which reduces inward I_{Na}, or it can be a consequence of a decrease in the flow of axial current between cardiac cells through gap junctional channels. Other contributors to slowing of conduction velocity are anisotropy of cardiac muscle and wavefront curvature.

An anatomical reentrant circuit is comprised of conducting pathways around an inexcitable obstacle formed by an anatomical structure. Functional reentrant circuits are dependent on the specific electrophysiological properties of the region of myocardium where they form. Mechanisms for functional reentry include: (1) leading circle reentry caused by heterogeneous refractory periods, (2) spiral waves and rotors in which slow activation is primarily caused by the wavefront curvature, (3) anisotropic reentry in which nonuniform anisotropy is the predominant cause of both unidirectional block and slow conduction, and (4) reflection, which is a form of reentry in a linear bundle of myocardial cells characterized by excitation occurring in one direction along the bundle followed by continued propagation and excitation occurring in the opposite direction.

The responses of arrhythmias to programmed stimulation can distinguish a reentrant mechanism from automaticity and triggered activity. Programmed stimulation can initiate reentrant arrhythmias when it establishes unidirectional conduction block and/or sufficiently slow conduction. Additional characteristics of initiation are important in distinguishing between reentrant and DAD-triggered tachycardias. The return cycle length for initiation of reentry is longer at shorter cycle lengths resulting in an inverse relationship between the cycle length of the initiating impulse(s) and the first cycle length of tachycardia. In comparison, the return cycle length of triggered activity is caused by the coupling interval of the DAD, which is shorter at short cycle lengths resulting in a direct relationship between the cycle length of the initiating impulse(s) and the first cycle length of triggered tachycardia

Resetting, termination, and entrainment responses to overdrive pacing and premature stimulation of reentry also enables this mechanism to be distinguished from automaticity and DAD-triggered activity. Prematurely stimulated impulses can interact with the reentrant impulse in a circuit with an excitable gap to cause resetting and termination. The basic mechanism is collision of the stimulated impulse in the antidromic direction with the reentrant impulse and, at the same time, conduction of the stimulated impulse in the orthodromic direction around the circuit. A flat segment to the resetting curve indicates conduction of the stimulated impulse around the circuit in a fully excitable gap while an ascending segment indicates conduction in a partially excitable gap.

Continuous resetting of a circuit by each overdrive-stimulated impulse results in entrainment of the circuit, a process that can be identified on the ECG. The last stimulated impulse continues to propagate around the circuit, and reentry continues at the same cycle length as prior to overdrive. An important feature of entrainment is fusion complexes on the ECG, resulting from the simultaneous activation of the reentrant circuit by two successive impulses in the overdrive train, the current paced impulse, and the previous paced impulse conducting orthodromically in the circuit. Fusion is progressive; that is, as the overdrive cycle length is decreased, the stimulated ECG complexes resemble more the site of overdrive stimulation and less the reentrant tachycardia. The last stimulated impulse is entrained but not fused. At a critically short cycle length of overdrive the ECG reverts entirely to the complex morphology of the pacing site indicating entrainment is ended. Reentry is terminated and tachycardia does not continue when overdrive is stopped. During overdrive stimulation from within the circuit, ECG fusion is not evident although fusion still occurs within the circuit, called concealed fusion. Whether or not functional circuits can be entrained is uncertain due to lack of experimental and clinical data. However, their very small or absent fully excitable gap would seem to make it difficult.

SOURCES

Carmeliet E, Vereecke J. *Cardiac Cellular Electrophysiology.* Boston, MA: Kluwer Academic Publishers; 2002.

Fleischhauer J, Lehmann L, Kleber AG. Electrical resistances of interstitial and microvascular space as determinants of the extracellular electrical field and velocity of propagation in ventricular myocardium. *Circulation.* 1995;92:587–594.

Heath B, Gingrich K, Kass RS. Ion channels in the heart. Cellular and molecular properties of cardiac Na, Ca, and K channels. *Handbook of Physiology. Section 2. The Cardiovascular System Volume I. The Heart.* Rockville, MD: American Physiological Society/Oxford University Press, 2002: 548–567.

King JH, Huang CLH, Fraser JA. Determinants of myocardial conduction velocity: Implications for arrhythmogenesis. *Front Physiol.* 2013;4:1–14.

Kleber AG, Janse MJJ, Fast VG. Normal and abnormal conduction in the heart. In Page E, Fozzard HA, Solaro RJ. *Handbook of Physiology. Section 2. The Cardiovascular System Volume I. The Heart.* Rockville, MD: American Physiological Society/Oxford University Press, 2002: 455–530.

Hoyt RH, Cohen ML, Saffitz JE. Distribution and three-dimensional structure of intercellular junctions in canine myocardium. *Circ Res.* 1989;64:563–574.

Josephson ME. *Josephson's Clinical Cardiac Electrophysiology: Techniques and Interpretations* (5th ed.). Philadelphia, PA: Wolters Kluwer; 2016.

Makielski JC, Fozzard H A. Ion channels and cardiac arrhythmia in heart disease. *Handbook of Physiology. Section 2. The Cardiovascular System Volume I. The Heart.* Rockville, MD: American Physiological Society/Oxford University Press, 2002: 709–740.

Rudy Y. The cardiac ventricular action potential: *Handbook of Physiology. Section 2. The Cardiovascular System Volume I. The Heart.* Rockville, MD: American Physiological Society/Oxford University Press, 2002: 531–547.

Spach MS, Josephson ME. Initiating reentry: The role of nonuniform anisotropy in small circuits. *J Cardiovasc Electrophysiol.* 1994;5:182–209.

Spach MS, Miller WT, Dolber PC, et al. The functional role of structural complexities in the propagation of depolarization in the atrium of the dog. Cardiac conduction disturbances due to discontinuities of effective axial resistivity. *Circ Res.* 1982; 50:175–191.

Spach MS, Miller WT, Geselowitz DB, et al. The discontinuous nature of propagation in normal canine cardiac muscle. Evidence for recurrent discontinuities of intracellular resistance that affect the membrane currents. *Circ Res.* 1981;48:39–54.

Spach MS, Miller WT, Miller-Jones E, et al. Extracellular potentials related to intracellular action potentials during impulse conduction in anisotropic canine cardiac muscle. *Circ Res.* 1979;45: 188–204.

Spach MS, Heidlage F, Dolber PC, Barr RC. Electrophysiological effects of remodeling cardiac gap junctions and cell size. Experimental and model studies of normal cardiac growth. *Circ Res.* 2000;86:302–311.

Toure A, Cabo C. Effect of cell geometry on conduction velocity in a subcellular model of myocardium. *IEEE Trans Biomed Eng.* 2010;57:2107–2114.

CHAPTER 10

Atrial Reentrant Arrhythmias

Reentry in the atria is a cause of atrial tachycardias. Atrial tachycardias are regular atrial rhythms at a rate equal or greater than 100 beats per minute (bpm), originating outside the sinus node region. They can also be caused by automaticity (Chapters 3 and 4), and triggered activity (Chapter 6). Although traditionally diagnosed and classified on the basis of their rate and ECG characteristics, a recent classification used in this chapter takes into account electrophysiological mechanisms in the classification. It subdivides atrial tachycardias into macroreentrant tachycardia that includes atrial flutter (Section 10A) and focal tachycardia (Section 10B). Although the tachycardias caused by automaticity and triggered activity are focal, some focal tachycardias are caused by reentry in small (micro) circuits. Atrial fibrillation is described separately in Section 10C, owing to uncertainties concerning its mechanism(s).

SECTION 10A Atrial Tachycardias Caused by Reentry in Macroreentrant Circuits

Macroreentrant atrial tachycardias are arrhythmia caused by reentry in circuits around a large central obstacle that is generally several centimeters in diameter in at least one of its dimensions. The obstacles provided by the normal atrial structure can be functional and/or anatomical. Anatomical obstacles may also result from disease or surgery (lesion reentry), a separate situation described below.

MACROREENTRANT CIRCUITS AROUND OBSTACLES PROVIDED BY NORMAL ATRIAL STRUCTURE

ECG Characteristics

Figures 10-1 shows two examples of typical atrial flutter (Panels A and B), which is a form of macroreentrant atrial tachycardia that has a regular atrial rate of approximately 250–350 bpm (cycle length 190–250 ms). Typical flutter is sustained by a macroreentrant circuit in the right atrium. Conduction delays within the circuit can prolong cycle length to as long as 300 ms, making it overlap with focal atrial tachycardia (Section 10B). The classic "sawtooth" pattern of atrial activity on the ECG, called flutter waves, is a hallmark of typical flutter; atrial complexes have a constant morphology, polarity, and cycle length and usually lack an isoelectric baseline between deflections in leads II, III, aVF, and V_1. Neither the rate nor lack of an isoelectric baseline is specific for any atrial tachycardia mechanism, since under certain conditions focal atrial tachycardia may show these ECG features (see Section 10B).

Electrophysiological Foundations of Cardiac Arrhythmias: A Bridge Between Basic Mechanisms and Clinical Electrophysiology, Second Edition.
 Cardiotext Publishing, ISBN: 978-1-942909-42-2.

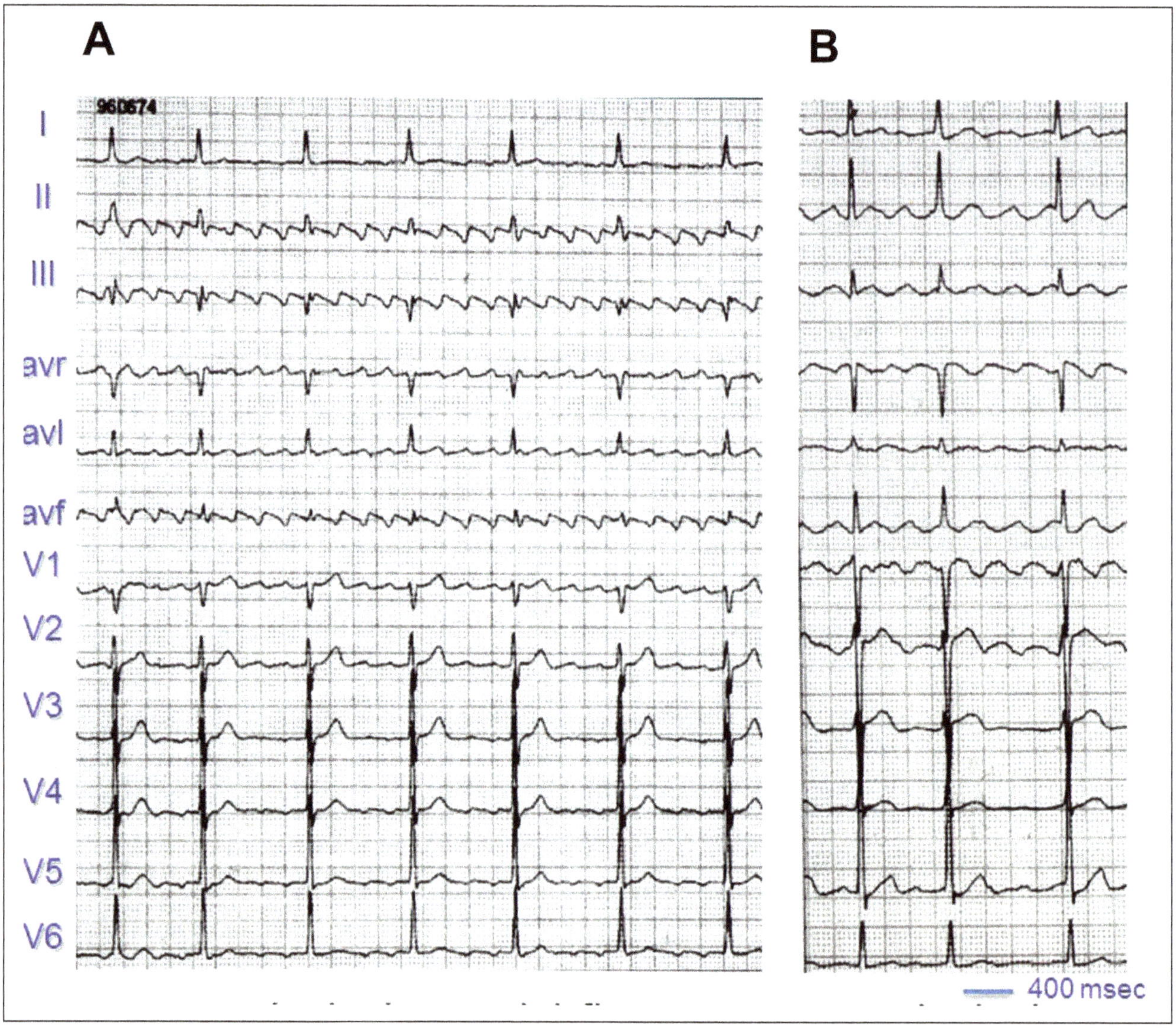

Figure 10-1 A 12-lead ECGs recorded from two different patients (**Panels A** and **B**) with typical atrial flutter (Wellens' ECG collection).

Counterclockwise and Clockwise Flutter

"Typical flutter" is a term used to describe the most common form of flutter (90% of flutter), as compared to atypical flutter (described later). Typical flutter is further subdivided into counterclockwise flutter and clockwise flutter. Counterclockwise flutter (the more common variety) is caused by rotation of the reentrant impulse around the tricuspid annulus in the right atrium in the counterclockwise direction when viewed in the left anterior oblique projection (Figure 10-1, Panel A). Clockwise flutter (also called "reverse typical flutter") is caused by rotation of the reentrant impulse around the tricuspid annulus in the clockwise direction (Figure 10-1, Panel B). Typical flutter is also called "isthmus-dependent flutter," based on the characteristics of the reentrant circuit that causes it (see location and description of circuits below and Figure 10-2).

Counterclockwise can be distinguished from clockwise flutter by the morphology of the flutter waves on the ECG, which is dependent on the direction of rotation of the reentrant impulse (Figure 10-1, Panel A). In counterclockwise flutter atrial activation is in the cranial–caudal direction in the right atrial anterior and lateral free walls and caudal–cranial in the posterior wall and atrial septum (see Figure 10-2). This is characterized in the inferior leads II, III, and aVF by negative deflections—either an initial negative followed by positive deflections that are of approximately equal size or small negative deflections followed by positive deflections of higher amplitude. These varieties coexist with tall, positive P waves, smaller positive P waves, or biphasic P waves in V_1. This flutter pattern also indicates inferior activation of the left atrium, which is not part of the circuit but an important contributor to flutter-wave morphology, by inferior breakthrough of the right atrial reentrant impulse, through the atrial septum. The degree to which positivity in the inferior leads is present appears to be related to the coexistence of heart disease and an enlarged left atrium.

Clockwise flutter in which activation of the right atrial anterior and lateral free wall is in the caudal–cranial direction and activation of the posterior wall and septum is in the cranial–caudal direction, generally has positive deflections in leads II, III, and aVF and negative deflections in lead V_1 (Figure 10-1, Panel B) indicating activation of the left atrium by superior breakthrough from the reentrant circuit into the left atrium through the atrial septum.

Other Features

The regularity and rate of the ventricular rhythm during typical atrial flutter depend on the characteristics of atrial impulse transmission through the A-V node. Regular patterns of 2:1 or 4:1 are common. Group beating resulting from A-V nodal Wenckebach can occur. Sometimes, A-V conduction is irregular with no fixed pattern.

Location of Reentrant Circuits Causing Typical Atrial Flutter

Counterclockwise Reentry

Typical counterclockwise atrial flutter is caused by reentry in a large (macro) reentrant circuit in the right atrium. The circuit is formed by specific structural features of this chamber.

Figure 10-2 shows the reentrant circuit (large black arrows) in relation to the right atrial anatomy in a right anterior oblique view of the endocardial surface. The reentrant impulse travels counterclockwise in the cranial–caudal direction in the pectinated anterolateral free wall, anterior to the crista terminalis (large black arrow 1). The crista acts as one of the regions of block around which the reentrant impulse rotates; it does not usually cross the crista from the trabeculated region (at the left) towards the septal side (at the right). The electrophysiological mechanism causing block is described below. The reentrant impulse then turns in the inferior region of the triangle of Koch (see Figure 3-12) and enters a narrow isthmus (large black arrow 2). This isthmus (arrow 2) is bounded posteriorly by the inferior vena caval orifice (IVC), the Eustachian valve and ridge (the Eustachian valve is the embryonic remnant of the sinus venosus valve), the coronary sinus ostium, and anteriorly by the tricuspid valve annulus (dashed green arrows). This region is referred to as the inferior, cavotricuspid, or "flutter isthmus." It is the target for ablation of typical flutter since a lesion that spans the narrow isthmus stops reentry. The reentrant impulse then emerges from the isthmus into the smooth region of the interatrial septum and the septal side of the tricuspid annulus (large black arrow 3). Propagation continues in the circular muscle along the tricuspid annulus superiorly (black arrows 3 and 4). The upper turnaround point completing the flutter circuit is near the superior vena cava (SVC) between the crista terminalis that lies just anterior to it and the tricuspid annulus (black arrow 4). The reentrant circuit is completed by connections superiorly either anterior or posterior to the SVC. The smooth septum above the Eustachian ridge and posterior to the fossa ovalis is usually not part of the reentrant circuit; transverse conduction blocks in this region (blue arrows 6).

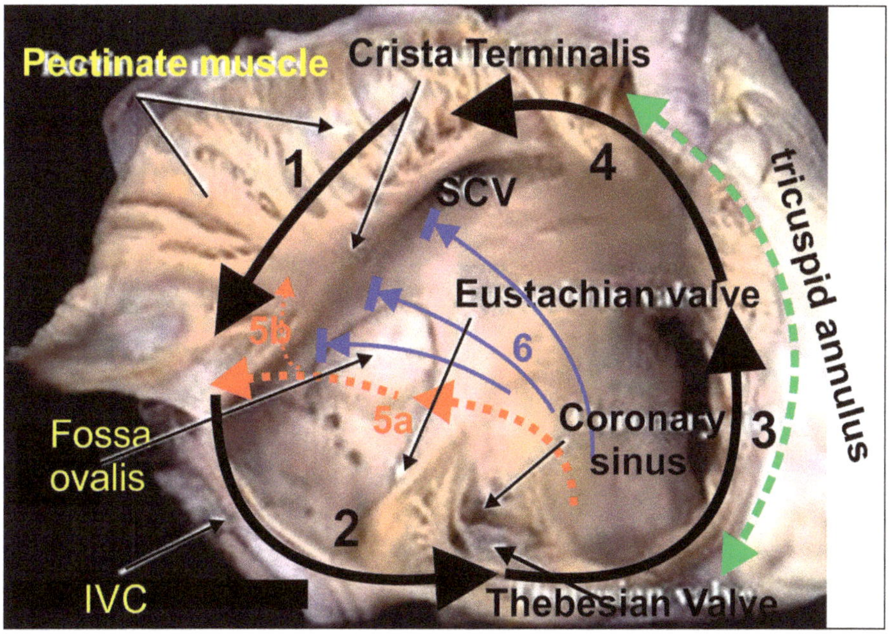

Figure 10-2 Right anterior oblique view of endocardial surface of the right atrium. Large **black arrows** show the pattern of impulse propagation of typical counterclockwise flutter. **Arrows** in this and subsequent figures indicate the pattern of impulse propagation only. The length of the arrows does not indicate the wavelength as in some previous figures unless it is specifically indicated as such.

The pathway of the reentrant circuit is around several obstacles formed by anatomical structures. The crista terminalis and the Eustachian ridge form lines of block (Figure 10-2) that force the reentrant impulse to go superiorly in myocardium around the tricuspid annulus (large black arrows 2 and 3), preventing the impulse from short circuiting the long pathway of the reentrant circuit (blue arrows 6). The obstacle formed by the crista terminalis (and possibly the Eustachian ridge) is functional, although the location of the functional block is dictated by this anatomic structure. Impulses can conduct across the crista (from left to right in Figure 10-2) during sinus or slow-paced rhythms but not during reentry causing flutter. A detailed description of possible mechanisms for the functional block is described in Figure 10-6.

Additional obstacles around which the reentrant impulse rotates, shown in Figure 10-2, are anatomic and fixed. These are formed by the orifices of the vena cavae (IVC and SVC), coronary sinus os, and tricuspid A-V orifice. The important role of the tricuspid A-V orifice as an obstacle is shown in **Figure 10-3** in a view of the inferior right atrial chamber from above, which shows the reentrant circuit from a different perspective. The reentrant impulse (black arrow numbers in Figure 10-3 are comparable to numbers in Figure 10-2) rotates in circular bundles of atrial muscle around the tricuspid annulus, which is parallel to the crista terminalis. The reentrant impulse indicated by black arrow 1 propagates in the lateral free wall segment of the circuit, through the flutter isthmus (black arrow 2) and then through the septal side of the annulus (black arrows 2 and 3) to complete the circuit.

Clockwise Reentry

During typical clockwise flutter, the reentrant impulse travels in the same circuit but in the opposite direction with caudocranial spread along the anterolateral wall adjacent to the crista and craniocaudal activation down the septal side of the tricuspid annulus and across the flutter isthmus from CS os toward the orifice of the inferior vena cava.

The left atrium is not part of the reentrant circuit causing typical flutter and is activated mostly by impulses conducting from the right atrium through coronary sinus musculature inferiorly in counterclockwise flutter and across the upper atrial septal wall in clockwise flutter.

Lower Loop Reentry

A variant of the counterclockwise macroreentry is "lower loop" reentry. As diagrammed in Figure 10-2, during "lower loop reentry," the impulse that emerges from the flutter isthmus, turns around the Eustachian valve and ridge in the smooth surface of the atrium (red dashed arrow 5a), travels back toward and through a gap in the line of block normally formed by the crista terminalis, and then continues in a circuit indicated by black arrow 2 and red arrow 5a, around the orifice of the IVC. This wavefront may split, also forming an ascending wavefront (dashed red arrow 5b) that collides with the counterclockwise activation in the superior right atrium. Activation of the left atrium is the same as in typical flutter.

Electrograms in Typical Flutter

Figure 10-4 shows electrograms recorded around an entire typical flutter reentrant circuit. The sequence of activation is from electrogram 1 to 10 (upward black arrow a).

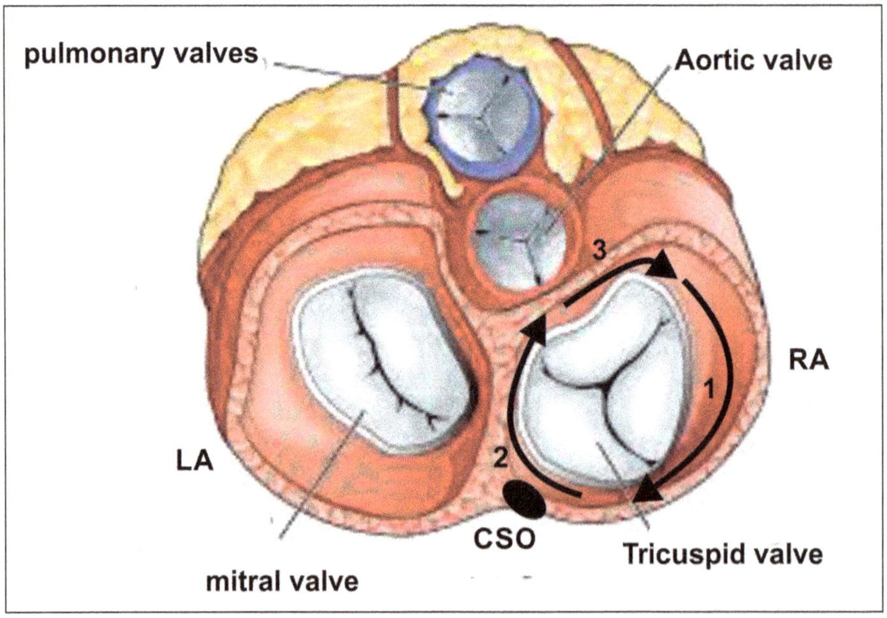

Figure 10-3 View of the inferior right atrial chamber from above, which shows the same circuit (**black arrows**) as in Figure 10-2. LA, left atrium; RA, right atrium; CSO, coronary sinus ostium.

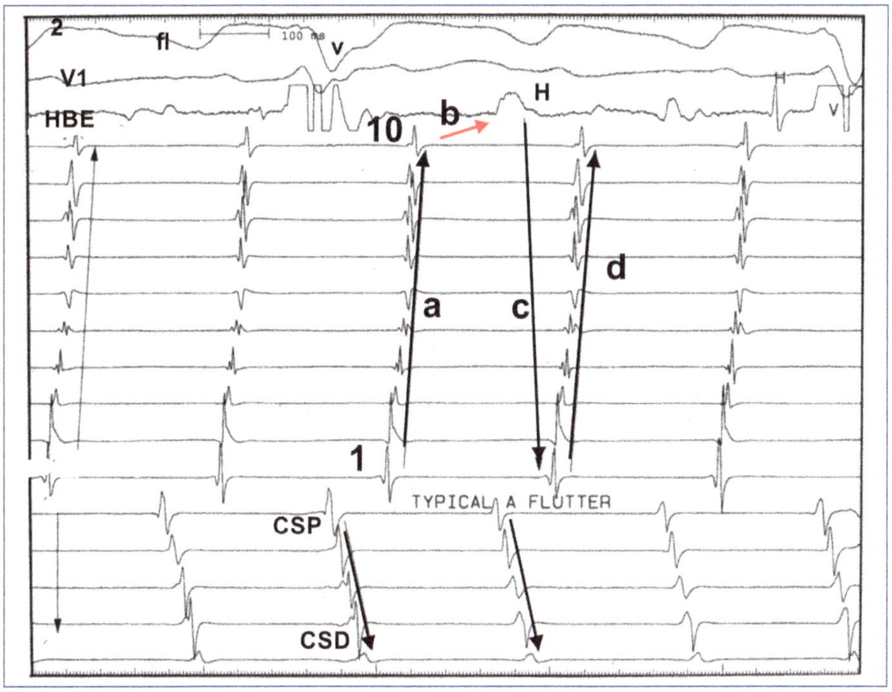

Figure 10-4 ECG leads 2 and V_1, flutter wave (fl), ventricular QRS (v),His bundle electrogram (HBE), and 10 electrograms recorded around the circumference of a typical flutter reentrant circuit. **Arrows** show sequence of activation. Lower five electrograms recorded from coronary sinus musculature (CSP is proximal in right atrium, CSD is distal in left atrium). (Reproduced from Josephson ME. *Josephson's Clinical Cardiac Electrophysiology. Techniques and Interpretations* (5th ed). Philadelphia, PA: Wolters Kluwer; 2016.)

In Figure 10-4, the impulse at recording site 10, which is just anterior to the coronary sinus os, propagates through the A-V node to activate the His bundle (H) (red arrow b) (the His bundle is not part of the circuit). Soon after activation of site 10, electrode 1 is again activated (downward arrow c) and the impulse begins another excursion around the circuit (upward arrow d). During propagation in a reentrant circuit, electrical activity (electrograms) span the entire systolic and diastolic intervals, unlike during focal impulse initiation, where much of diastole can be quiescent. The recordings show activation occurring during isoelectric intervals on the ECG. The concept of early activation indicating the site of origin of focal activity—defined as the earliest electrical activity prior to systole (see Figure 2-3 and Figure 3-6)—does not apply during reentry, since any electrogram during diastole can be interpreted as being either late in relation to the previous systolic activity or early in relation to the following systolic activity.

The bottom five electrograms in Figure 10-4 show activation in coronary sinus musculature that connects right and left atrium, progressing from the proximal coronary sinus os (CSP), toward the distal coronary sinus (CSD); this sequence of activity shows propagation of an impulse from the right atrial circuit to the inferior left atrium.

Electrophysiological Properties of Reentrant Circuits

Conduction Block and Spontaneous Initiation of Flutter

The spontaneous initiation of typical counterclockwise atrial flutter is described in **Figure 10-5**, which shows simplified diagrams of the right atrial flutter circuit based on Figure 10-2. During sinus rhythm (Panel A), the right atrium is activated predominantly in a superior (cranial) to inferior (caudal) direction. A rapidly conducting pathway from the sinus to the A-V node is provided by the crista terminalis (CT, solid red arrow). The crista terminalis is a nonuniformly anisotropic structure (see Figure 9-11) formed by distinct parallel-oriented muscle bundles that are well connected in the longitudinal direction but separated by intervening connective tissue septae with sparse lateral connections between bundles in the transverse direction. The pectinate muscles (PM), atrial septum, and the muscle bundles adjacent to the tricuspid annulus are also activated in a similar direction although more slowly (dashed red and black arrows). The activation pattern does not permit reentry in the potential flutter circuit, since there is no return pathway in the region that forms the circuit. The occurrence of typical flutter necessitates the occurrence of unidirectional block in a segment of the potential circuit in order to establish conduction in one direction (see Figure 9-1). It also requires the establishment of the long line of block along the crista terminalis (Figure 10-2). These necessary components of the flutter circuit during spontaneous onset of flutter appear to be caused by a transitional period of a very rapid rhythm, usually atrial fibrillation (AF), which often precedes the onset of flutter. Occasionally, the line of block along the crista may be present already at slow heart rates and the period of antecedent fibrillation may not be necessary.

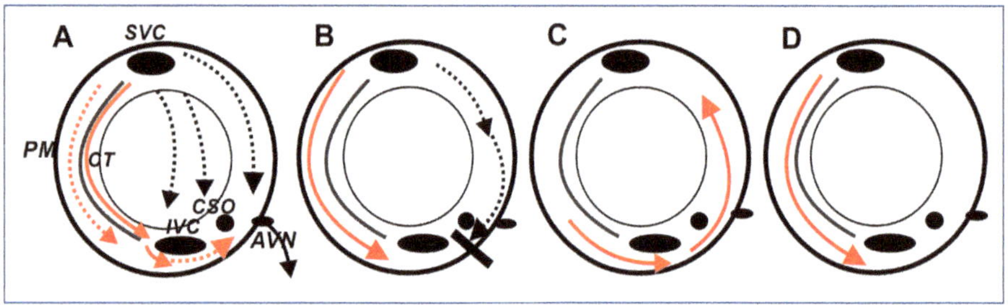

Figure 10-5 Diagrams of initiation of typical atrial flutter. AVN, A-V node; CSO, coronary sinus ostium; CT, crista terminalis; IVC, inferior vena cava; PM, pectinate muscles; SVC, superior vena cava. **Panel A** is activation during sinus rhythm, **Panel B** is block of rapidly occurring impulses, and **Panels C** and **D** are counterclockwise reentry.

Transient unidirectional block that initiates conduction in one direction through the reentrant circuit is most likely to occur in the confined region of the narrow isthmus where the thick myocardial bundles of the crista terminalis end in smaller bundles that are irregularly arranged. This structure is analogous to the diagram in Figure 9-16 that shows the impedance mismatch that occurs when large myocardial bundles with a large membrane area connect with smaller bundles with a smaller membrane area. Although conduction in both directions can occur during slow (sinus) rhythms since there is adequate axial current, a reduction of current can occur during rapid rhythms such as AF. Decreased phase 0 occurs when successive depolarizations occur at less negative membrane potentials before complete repolarization of the previous action potential. This results in insufficient axial current generated in the small bundles (in the isthmus) to excite the large bundles (forming the crista), causing block. The block is unidirectional, since axial current is still sufficient in the opposite direction to allow conduction from large bundles of the crista to its small terminal bundles in the isthmus.

Unidirectional block of an initiating impulse at rapid rates is diagrammed in Figure 10-5, Panel B. The wavefront indicated by the dashed black arrows toward the septal side, blocks in the flutter isthmus (black bar). When block occurs, it permits a properly timed impulse from the anterior wall side (Figure 10-5, Panel B, red arrow) to propagate through the isthmus and then in a caudocranial direction up the septal side of the flutter circuit (Panel C, red arrows) to initiate counterclockwise flutter (Panel D, red arrow). The clinical predominance of counterclockwise flutter may be a result of the anatomical structure at the termination of the crista that favors block in the direction from the CS os toward the orifice of the SVC (direction of small to larger muscle bundles). However, block can also occur in the other direction, resulting in clockwise flutter. The initiation of flutter by programmed electrical stimulation is dependent on unidirectional block in the same region (see below).

Mechanisms for Functional Conduction Block Along the Crista Terminalis During Flutter

As shown in Figure 10-2, the crista terminalis provides an important region of conduction block in the typical flutter reentrant circuit. The reentrant impulse conducting in the anterior free wall during counterclockwise flutter cannot conduct transversely across the crista, forcing the impulse to conduct through the flutter isthmus. Since transverse conduction does occur across the crista during sinus rhythm or atrial pacing at rates comparable to sinus rates, the transverse block during atrial flutter must be functional, caused by rapid activation. **Figure 10-6** diagrams several theoretical mechanisms for the functional block based on the electrophysiological properties of the crista.

In Figure 10-6, Panel A, during sinus rhythm, activation occurs both longitudinally (green arrows) and transversely (red arrows) through the crista. Longitudinal conduction is more rapid than transverse conduction that is slow because of sparse gap junction connections in the transverse direction (nonuniform anisotropy). When rate increases such as during the period of AF that initiates flutter, both longitudinal and transverse conduction may slow. However, in patients with a history of atrial flutter, slowing of transverse conduction is more severe as indicated by the squiggly red arrows in Panel B. Rate-related exaggeration of slowing of transverse conduction may be related to a higher degree of nonuniform anisotropy resulting from the poorer transverse connections. Increased intracellular Ca^{2+} that can occur at rapid rates decreases gap junction conductance likely contributing to conduction slowing. In Panel B, the very slowly propagating transverse impulses would reach the septal side of the crista after the reentrant impulse (green arrows on the septal side) had already reached it—and therefore, would not prevent reentry. Slowly propagating transverse "wavelets" from the reentrant impulse traveling in the opposite directions on the septal side of the crista (squiggly blue arrows) can also collide with the transverse conducting impulses from the free wall side, causing a functional line of block.

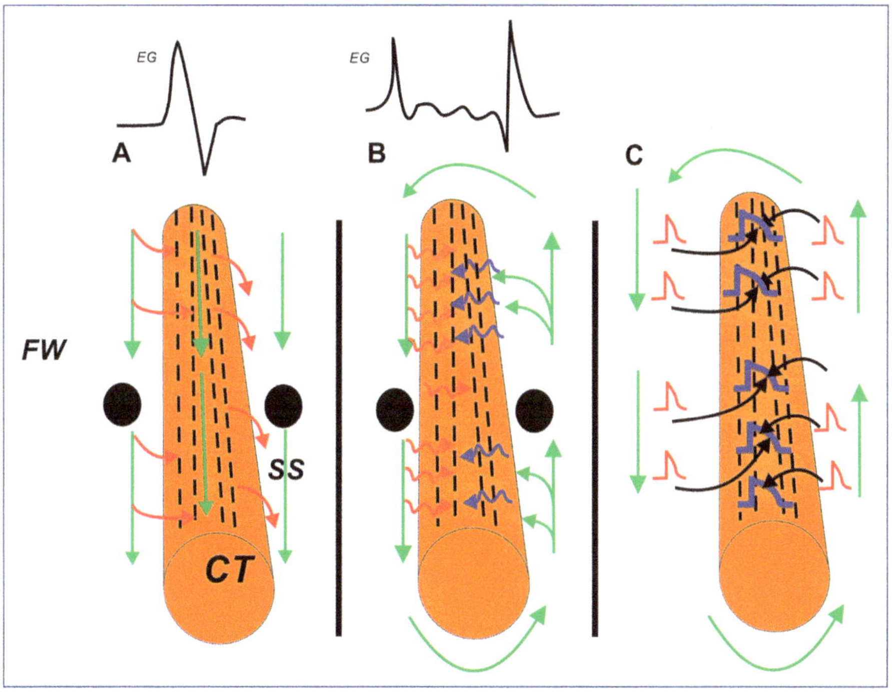

Figure 10-6 Possible mechanisms for conduction block in the crista terminalis (CT) during typical flutter. FW is free wall. SS is smooth septal side. **Dashed lines** in the CT indicate the long axis of the muscle bundles. **Large black circles** show location of a bipolar electrode and EG is electrogram. **Panel A** diagrams sinus rhythm. **Panels B** and **C** are during reentry.

Figure 10-6, Panel C diagrams another possible mechanism for functional conduction block in the crista terminalis. The transverse block in the crista may also be related to the longer action potential duration and refractory periods in this region, resulting from a distinct plateau phase of repolarization (blue action potentials), compared to pectinate and septal muscle (red action potentials), which have a shorter refractory period because they lack a plateau. At short cycle lengths, the reentrant impulse (green arrows) cannot conduct transversely across the crista because it blocks in myocardium that has not completely repolarized (Panel C, solid black arrows). A combination of the different mechanisms shown in Figure 10-6 might also occur.

Crista terminalis electrograms. Electrograms recorded from the region of the crista terminalis during flutter have special features that are indicative of block in a reentrant circuit. Whereas during sinus rhythm, they have a single deflection (Figure 10-6, electrogram (EG) above Panel A), during flutter they are characterized by double or split potentials (Figure 10-6, EG above Panel B). In the two-component electrogram above Panel B, the first component is caused by the reentrant impulse conducting in one direction and the second component caused by the reentrant impulse conducting in the opposite direction. The duration of the segment between the two components is a function of the time it takes for the impulse to conduct around the line of block. If the recording poles of a bipolar electrode straddle the crista as diagrammed by the large black circles in Figure 10-6, low amplitude deflections may be recorded between the two large deflections, from the slow transversely conducting impulse. Similar electrograms can be recorded from the Eustachian ridge, which also may be a region of functional block in the circuit.

Mechanisms for Slow Conduction in the Flutter Circuit

The wavelength of the reentrant impulse (conduction velocity × refractory period) that causes typical flutter is significantly shorter than the path length resulting in a large fully excitable temporal gap that is 15%–30% of the cycle length (see next section). The wavelength in the flutter circuit changes from one region to another. Since muscle bundle orientation in the reentrant pathway can range from longitudinal to oblique to transverse, changes in conduction velocity caused by anisotropy contribute to some of the changes in the wavelength.

Pectinate muscles on the anterior wall are arranged nearly perpendicularly to the crista with interlacing small trabeculations interconnecting the major musculature bundles, leading to slow transverse conduction. On the venous side, inter caval musculature also changes direction at the juncture with the crista and potentially is a substrate for slow conduction. On the other hand, conduction in muscular bundles around the tricuspid annulus is in the longitudinal direction and more rapid. The flutter isthmus may also be a region of conduction slowing and delay because of the irregular arrangement of interconnecting small muscle bundles in this region and resultant nonuniform anisotropy. In the region where the narrow isthmus expands into a wide segment of the pathway, slowing may occur because of impedance mismatch (see Figure 9-16). As the reentrant impulse emerges from the narrow isthmus into a broader expanse of myocardium, significant wavefront curvature is also likely to occur and cause slowing of conduction (see Figure 9-13). Spontaneous termination of isthmus-dependent flutter often occurs in the isthmus in either counterclockwise or clockwise flutter, likely because of these factors which slow conduction. Wavefront curvature in other segments of the circuit, for example in the region of the superior vena cava, can also cause slowing of conduction. In some patients with flutter, disease alterations may also contribute to slowing of conduction velocity.

Different refractory periods reflecting the different action potential durations in different regions of the circuit also contribute to the changing wavelength. Remodeling of ion channels may also accelerate repolarization and shorten refractory periods that promote reentry by shortening the wavelength.

Effects of Electrical Stimulation

Initiation of Reentry

Initiation of tachycardia by electrical stimulation is a general characteristic of reentrant arrhythmias, which can distinguish them from other mechanisms (see Chapter 9). Isthmus-dependent typical atrial flutter can be initiated by programmed premature stimulation with 1 to 2 premature stimuli and by rapid pacing from the right atrium in a majority of patients with a history of this arrhythmia. It is more difficult to initiate flutter from the left atrium because of the distance a left atrial stimulation site is from the circuit. Flutter induction in a patient without a history of flutter is rare, suggesting that the right atrium in these patients lacks the necessary electrophysiological properties to develop unidirectional block in the isthmus region or block in the crista terminalis.

Figure 10-7 shows the initiation of typical counterclockwise flutter by a premature atrial impulse (S2) with a coupling interval of 170 ms during atrial pacing from the smooth septal right atrium, at a cycle length of 600 ms (S1–S1 interval). **Figure 10-8**, Panels A–C diagram the patterns of impulse propagation for typical counterclockwise atrial flutter that might occur as a result of this stimulation.

As diagrammed in Figure 10-8, Panel A, impulses initiated by the basic stimuli at the blue circle and arrow, on the atrial septum (SS) activate the potential circuit mainly from right to left (S1 black arrows). The premature impulse initiated at the blue circle (blue arrow) blocks in the isthmus (Panel B, black arrow, black bar), enabling reentry of the premature impulse to occur (Panel B, red arrows 1 and 2), (Panel C, red arrows 3 and 4).

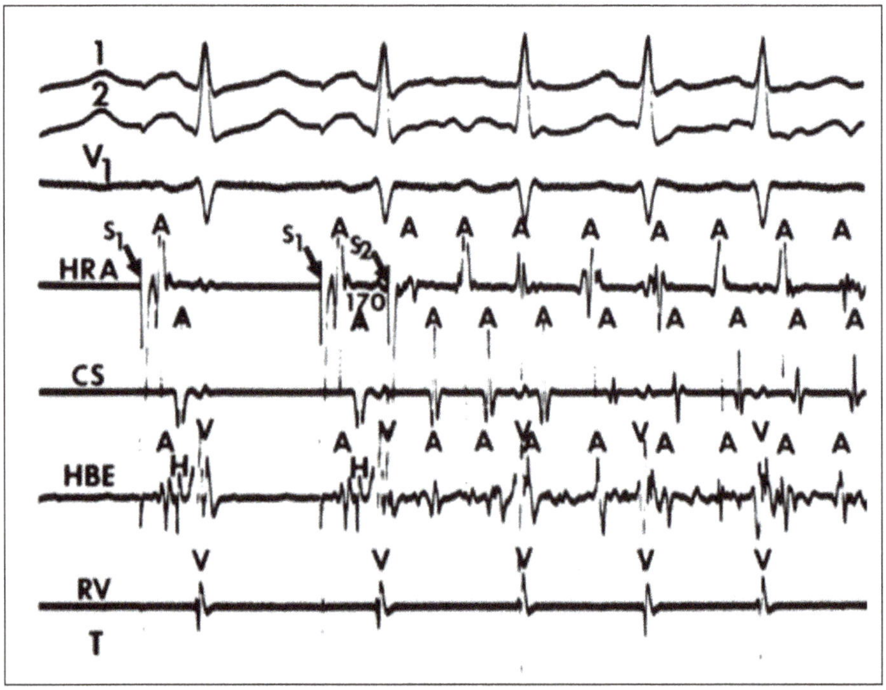

Figure 10-7 Initiation of atrial flutter with a premature atrial stimulus (S2) during basic stimulation (S1). ECG leads 1, 2, and V_1, and electrograms from the high right atrium (HRA), coronary sinus (CS), His bundle (HBE), and right ventricle (RV). A, atrial; H, His bundle; V, ventricular electrograms. (Reproduced from Josephson ME. *Josephson's Clinical Cardiac Electrophysiology. Techniques and Interpretations* (5th ed). Philadelphia, PA: Wolters Kluwer; 2016.)

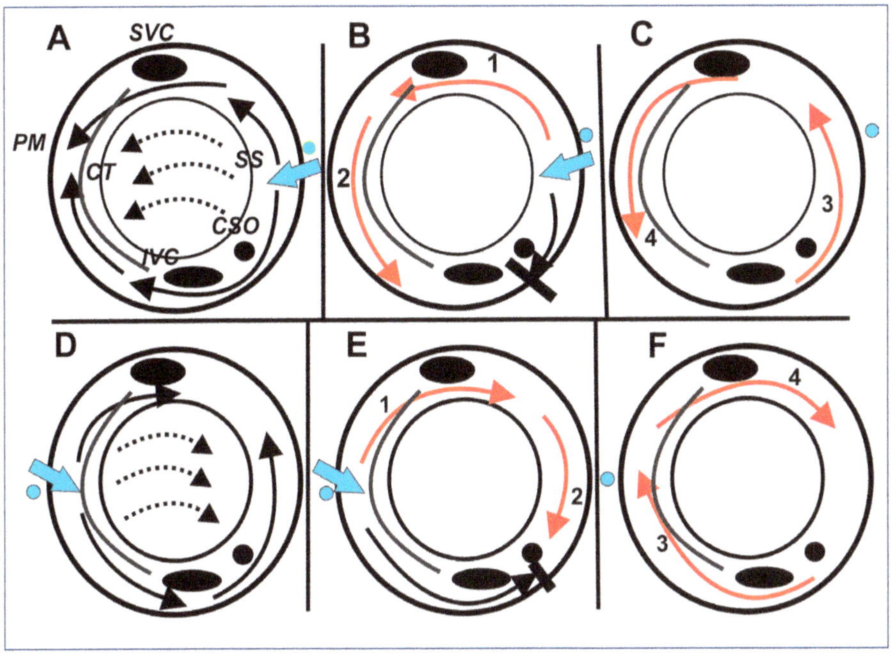

Figure 10-8 Initiation of flutter by electrical stimulation. A typical flutter circuit is pictured. CSO, coronary sinus ostium; CT, crista terminalis; IVC, inferior vena cava; PM, pectinate muscles; SS, smooth septal wall; SVC, superior vena cava.

The activation pattern is the same as during spontaneous onset of flutter following a period of AF. Similarly, rapid pacing can lead to block in the isthmus and reentry. In fact, the stimulation protocol may occasionally initiate a short period of unstable rhythm resembling AF prior to flutter onset.

Clockwise, isthmus-dependent flutter is also inducible by electrical stimulation in patients who have this arrhythmia. While the isthmus is the site of block regardless of whether clockwise or counterclockwise flutter is induced, the direction of rotation may be dependent on the site of stimulation. Figure 10-8, Panels D–F, diagram the initiation of clockwise flutter during stimulation from the trabeculated free wall (blue circle and arrow). Panel D shows activation in the left to right direction by the basic stimulus (black arrows). Block of premature or rapid paced impulses occur in the isthmus (Panel E, black arrow and black bar), allowing the stimulated impulse conducting in the caudal–cranial direction (Panel E, red arrow 1) to conduct around the circuit initiating reentry (Panel E, red arrow 2 and Panel F, red arrows 3 and 4).

Resetting, Entrainment, and Termination

The reentrant circuit that causes typical atrial flutter has a large temporal excitable gap. This property enables stimulated impulses to enter the circuit to reset, entrain, and terminate flutter.

Resetting. When the site of stimulation is in the right atrium, near to or within the circuit, resetting can occur at long premature stimulus cycle lengths because of easy access of the stimulated impulse to the circuit. This property is illustrated in **Figure 10-9**. In Panel A, an atrial premature stimulus (S) during flutter at a cycle length 285 ms, is delivered to the high right lateral atrium (HLRA), at a coupling interval of 265 ms. It is followed by a return cycle (RC) of 285 ms, the same as the flutter cycle length. The sum of the premature cycle and return cycle is less than two times the basic cycle, indicating resetting (Chapter 9).

In Figure 10-9 the pattern of propagation of the stimulated premature impulse is shown in the diagrams of the reentrant circuit at the right. The stimulation site is at the large red arrow in Panel C. The black arrow represents the reentrant impulse in the circuit. The premature impulse enters the circuit (red arrows), collides with the reentrant impulse (black arrow) to the right (antidromically), and conducts in the counterclockwise direction (red arrow 1 to the left) (orthodromically). Panel D shows continuation of conduction of the premature impulse (red arrows 2, 3, and 4) around the circuit. Conduction time from stimulation (red arrow 1 in Panel C), to return of the stimulated impulse to the site of stimulation (red arrow 4 in Panel D) is the same as the conduction time of the flutter reentrant impulse since the stimulated impulse is conducting in completely excitable myocardium (the fully excitable gap). The return cycle length is, therefore, the same as the flutter cycle length.

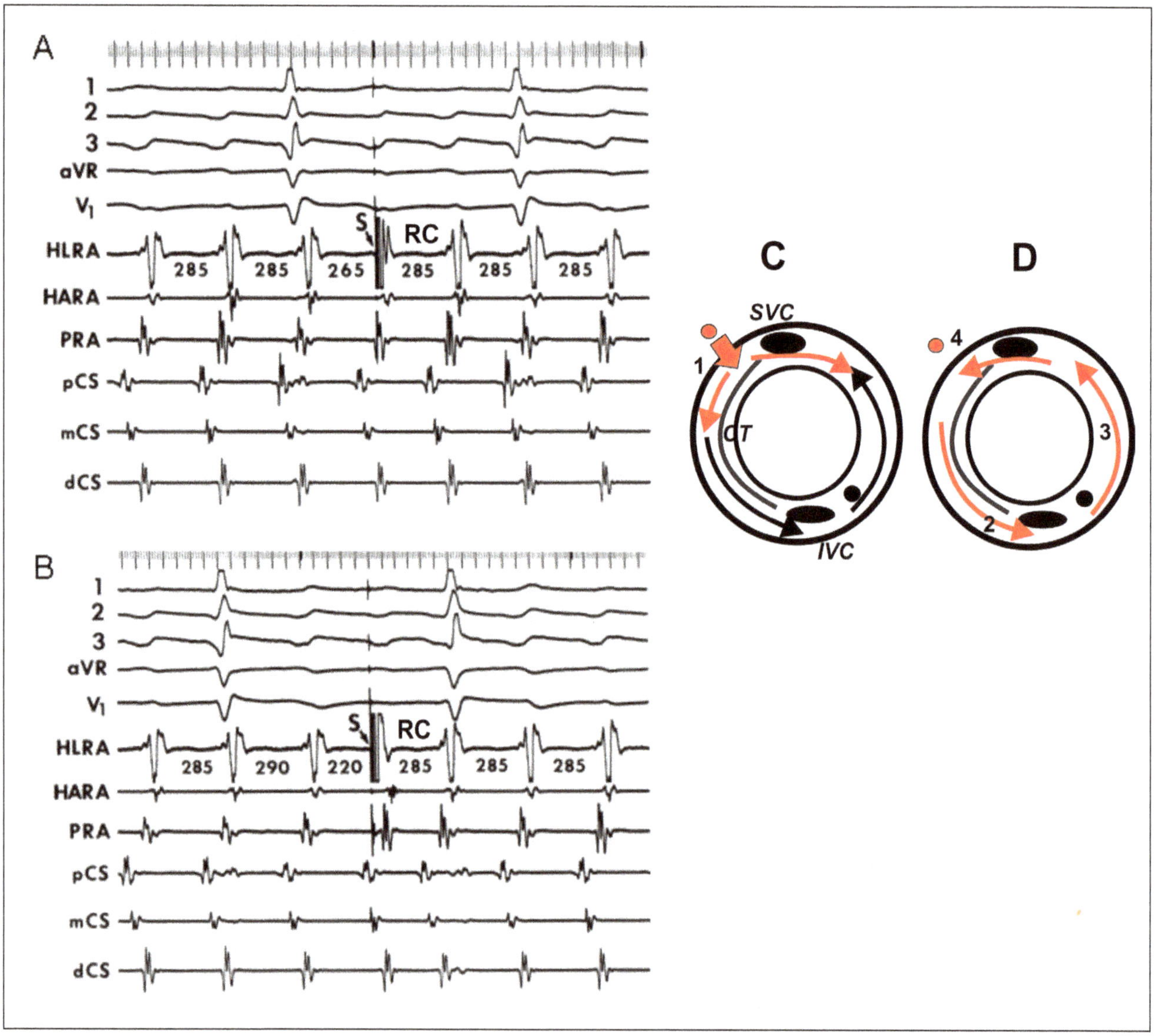

Figure 10-9 Resetting response of typical flutter circuit. **Panels A** and **B**; ECG leads 1, 2, 3, aVR, and V_1, and electrograms from high lateral right atrium (HLRA), high anterior right atrium (HARA), posterior right atrium (PRA), proximal, mid, and distal coronary sinus (pCS, mCS, dCS). S, premature stimulus; RC, return cycle. At the right are diagrams of the pattern of propagation of the premature impulses.

The stimulated impulse (S) in Panel B has a shorter coupling interval of 220 ms. The return, reset cycle (RC) is still 285 ms. This earlier premature impulse still propagates around the circuit in the fully excitable gap, with the same conduction velocity as the flutter impulses, resulting in the return cycle measured at the stimulus site, being the same as the flutter cycle. The pattern of propagation of the premature impulses is the same as described in Panels C and D. The return cycle remains at this constant value over a range of coupling intervals, as long as the premature impulses propagate in the completely excitable gap. Thus, the completely excitable gap of the flutter circuit in Figure 10-9 is at least 45 ms long, from a coupling interval of 265 to 220 ms. This flat response pattern is characteristic of reentrant circuits with large excitable gaps (see Figure 9-28). The flat response occurs at all stimulus sites within or adjacent to the flutter circuit. Very early premature impulses propagate in the partially refractory gap at a slower velocity than the flutter impulse, leading to a prolonged return cycle and an increasing response, but nevertheless are reset (Figure 9-28).

Resetting by premature impulses initiated at sites distant from the circuit such as in the left atrium, requires shorter premature coupling intervals or even double premature impulses. The return cycle, if measured at the stimulus site, is longer than the flutter cycle even when the premature impulses propagate in the fully excitable gap of the circuit because of additional conduction time from stimulus site to the circuit and from the circuit back to the stimulus site.

Termination. Although in general, short-coupled premature impulses can terminate reentrant arrhythmias by blocking in reentrant circuits (Chapter 9), premature impulses cannot usually terminate atrial flutter, perhaps because of the very long excitable gap that precludes block in the orthodromic direction.

Entrainment. Overdrive pacing can reset and entrain reentrant circuits that cause atrial flutter. The basic concepts of entrainment are described in Figure 9-29 to Figure 9-31.

Figure 10-10, shows entrainment of typical counterclockwise flutter in a patient who developed the arrhythmia during open-heart surgery. Panel A shows atrial flutter with a cycle length of 264 ms and 2:1 A-V conduction (ECG lead II). The thick red bar underlines the flutter wave that has a predominantly negative morphology. In Panel B, during overdrive pacing at a cycle length of 254 ms (horizontal black bar, S), the interval between flutter waves shortens to the pacing cycle length, and the R-R interval decreases as 2:1 A-V conduction is maintained. The pattern of activation of the flutter circuit during pacing is shown in diagram (a) at the right. The current paced impulse (n) (red arrows), collides with the previous paced impulse (n-1) (green arrow) in the antidromic direction (to the right) and propagates around the circuit in the orthodromic direction (to the left, red arrow 1). During pacing, although the circuit is activated by both the current paced antidromic impulse (in red, n) and the previous (n-1) orthodromic impulse (green) (fusion activation) the flutter waves (red bar) are almost the same as the spontaneous flutter waves because orthodromic propagation of the paced impulses in the circuit predominates in causing the ECG waveform.

Spontaneous flutter continues after pacing is abruptly stopped (end of horizontal black line in Panel B) due to continued propagation of the orthodromic wavefront from the last paced impulse around the circuit. This pattern is diagrammed by red arrows 2 and 3 in (b) at the right.

In Figure 10-10, Panels C and D, at pacing cycle lengths of 242 and 232 ms, the atrial cycle length again decreases to the pacing cycle length, and the R-R interval further decreases as 2:1 A-V conduction is maintained. Despite pacing from a site near the sinus node which should produce positive P waves in lead II, the morphology of the flutter waves in the ECG during pacing (horizontal red bar) is still negative, similar to the spontaneous flutter waves. Flutter continues after pacing is terminated (end of horizontal black bar) because of continued propagation of the last paced orthodromic impulse around the circuit. The patterns of impulse propagation during entrainment and after termination of stimulation are the same as described for Panels A and B and diagrammed in (a) and (b).

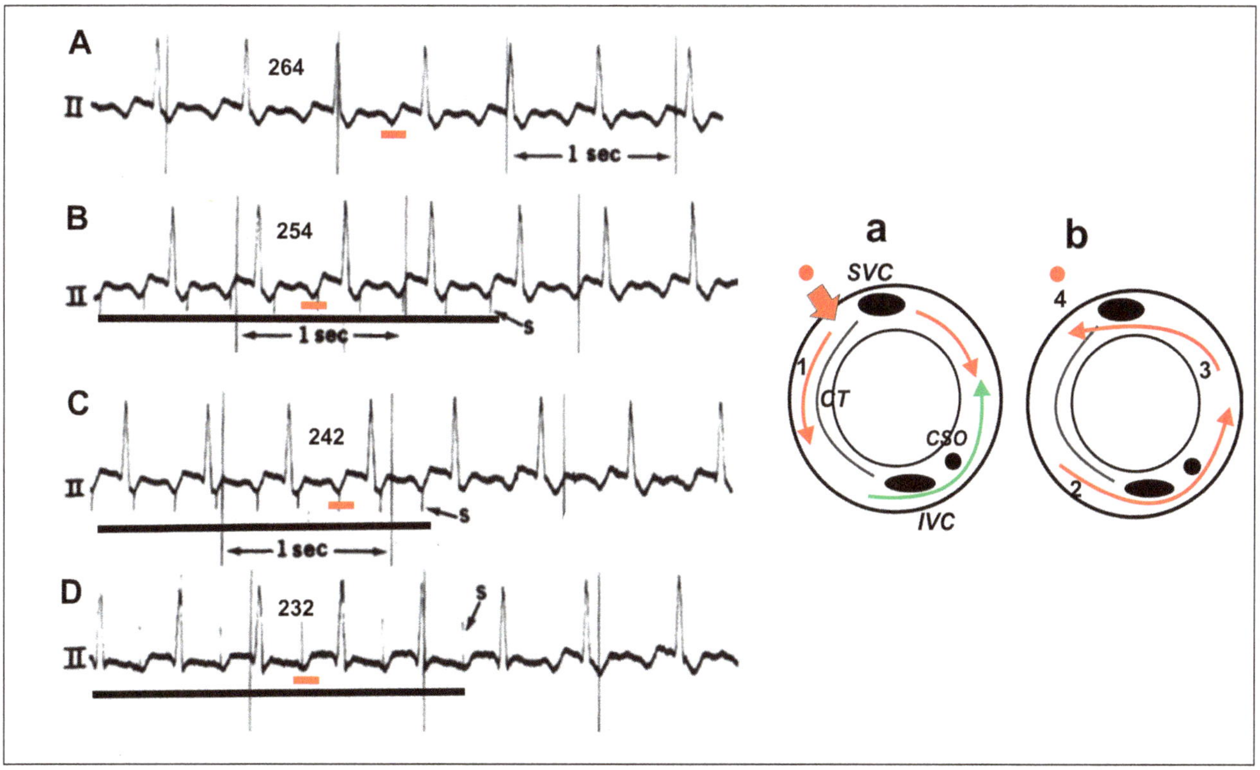

Figure 10-10 ECG lead II showing atrial flutter (**Panel A**) and entrainment (**Panels B, C, D**). Diagrams (**a**) and (**b**) at the right show impulse propagation in the circuit. (Panels A–D are reproduced from Waldo AL. From bedside to bench: Entrainment and other stories. *Heart Rhythm.* 2004;1:94–106.)

Fusion. A comparison of Panels D and C in Figure 10-10 shows changes in the paced flutter-wave morphology that is characteristic of fixed fusion at each cycle length that is progressive as cycle length is decreased, another property of entrainment described in Figure 9-31. The fusion is between the current stimulated wavefront (n) from the high right atrium moving in the cranial–caudal direction (red arrows in (a)) and the orthodromic impulse from the previous stimulus (n–1) both in the circuit (green arrows in (a)) and left atrium where activation is in the caudal–cranial direction. The stimulus artifact (S) occurs after the onset of the flutter wave because the orthodromic wavefront initiated by the previous stimulus (n–1) is contributing to the onset of the atrial ECG waveform before the current (n) stimulus occurs.

As described in Figure 9-31, a characteristic of entrainment is that the last paced impulse is entrained but not fused. In Figure 10-10 the last paced impulse, indicated by the (s) and arrow gives rise to the next flutter wave that is entrained since it still occurs at the stimulus cycle length (in Panel D, it is hidden in the QRS). It is also not fused since there is no longer activation by another paced impulse.

Stimulation at any site along the circumference of the circuit results in a post-pacing interval measured at that site, that is equal to the flutter cycle length since the stimulated impulse travels around the entire circuit before returning to that site. For example, in Figure 10-10, stimulation of a site near the CSO by the last paced impulse (red arrow 2 in (b)) requires the impulse to travel around the entire circuit before that site is activated again (the flutter cycle length). Stimulation at sites outside the circuit have a post-pacing cycle length greater than the flutter cycle length because the stimulated impulse travels around the circuit plus outside the circuit to reach the stimulation site.

Fusion is more apparent when comparing the atrial complexes during entrainment with the atrial complexes that are characteristic of the high right atrial pacing site shown in **Figure 10-11**. In this figure, Panel A shows the ECG from the same patient as in Figure 10-10 during high right atrial pacing at a shorter cycle length of 224 ms, which initially entrains the flutter. At the arrow in Panel A, the atrial complexes suddenly become positive, the expected morphology of the high right atrial pacing site. The change in morphology indicates that the reentrant pattern of activation has stopped. This is caused by collision of the antidromic paced wavefront (red arrow to the right in (a)) with the orthodromic wavefront from the previous stimulated impulse (green arrow) in the circuit and block of the orthodromic wavefront in the refractory tail of the impulse in the circuit (red arrow to the left in (a)). Activation of the entire circuit by the paced impulses then occurs in the cranial–caudal direction (red arrows in diagram (b)) causing the positive P-wave morphology. In Panel B, the same positive morphology continues until pacing is stopped (last paced impulse indicated by red arrow). Resumption of sinus rhythm occurs (asterisk) because reentry has been terminated by overdrive.

Concealed entrainment. Entrainment from a stimulation site in the protected isthmus of the flutter circuit results in concealed entrainment where the paced atrial wave form on the surface ECG is identical to the spontaneous flutter-wave morphology (see Figure 9-33). **Figure 10-12** shows surface ECG recordings during concealed entrainment resulting from pacing in the isthmus.

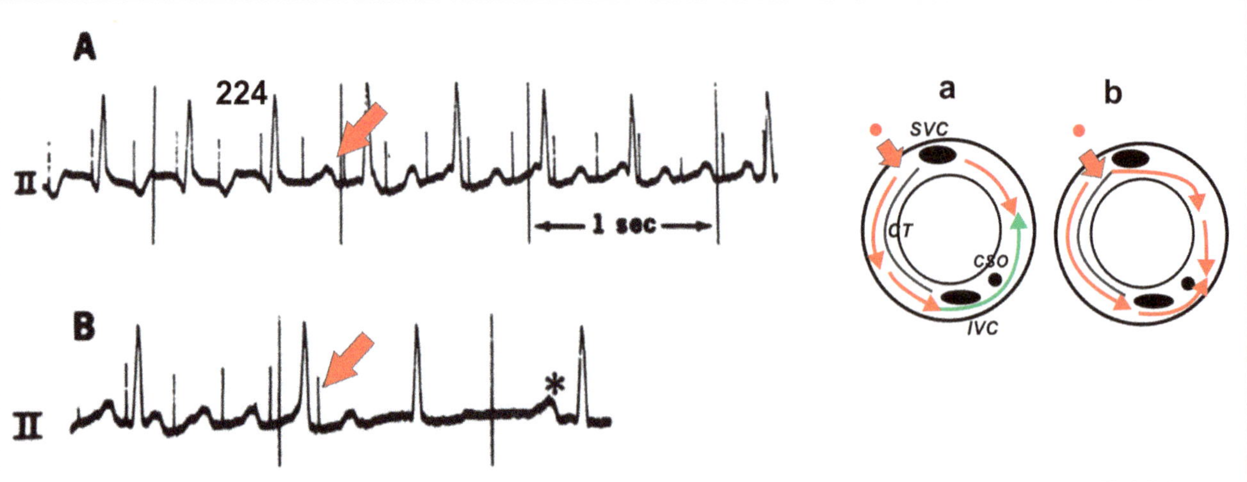

Figure 10-11 **Panel A:** ECG lead II at a pacing cycle length of 224 ms. **Panel B** show continuation of pacing. Diagrams at the **right** (**a** and **b**) show the propagation pattern when reentry terminates. (ECGs in Panels A and B are reproduced from Waldo AL et al. *Circulation.* 1977;56:737–745.)

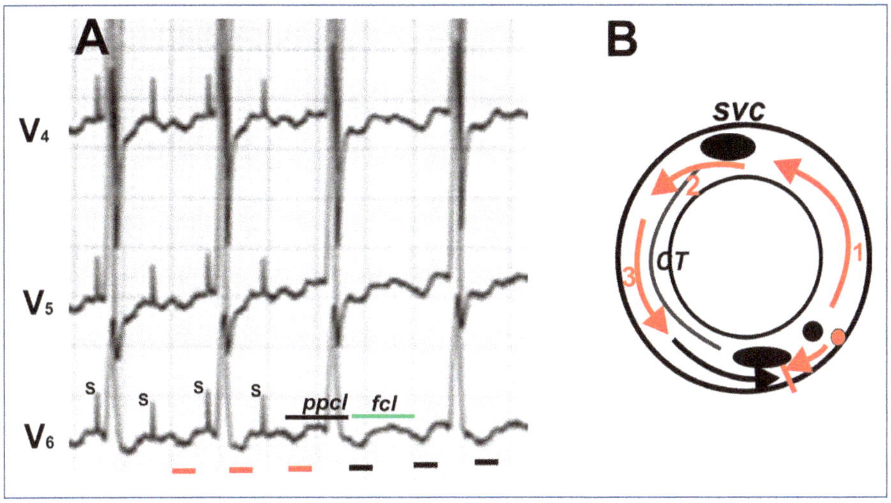

Figure 10-12 **Panel A:** ECG leads V_4, V_5, and V_6 during concealed entrainment of typical atrial flutter. **Panel B:** Diagram of flutter reentrant circuit and pattern of impulse propagation (**arrows**) during entrainment.

In Figure 10-12, the paced (s is stimulus artefact) flutter waves (horizontal red bars in lead V_6) are identical to the spontaneous flutter waves (horizontal black bars in lead V_6) occurring after pacing is terminated. Also, the post-pacing cycle length (ppcl) is the same as the flutter cycle length (fcl) since the last paced impulse propagates around the flutter circuit. The diagram at the right shows the pattern of impulse propagation during concealed entrainment. Stimulation in the isthmus (at the red dot), results in an antidromic impulse (red arrow to the left) that either collides with the reentrant impulse in the circuit (black arrow) or blocks in the isthmus because this is a region prone to block (see above). The orthodromic impulse propagates around the circuit (red arrows 1, 2, 3 to the right) in the same pathway as the spontaneous flutter reentrant impulse. The barriers to conduction that bound the isthmus prevent other patterns of impulse propagation.

Effects of the Autonomic Nervous System and Pharmacological Agents

This section only describes effects that help diagnose the mechanism of atrial tachycardia that has ECG characteristics of typical atrial flutter. Although mapping and entrainment clearly document a reentrant mechanism, the ECG features of typical flutter alone do not prove reentry. Automatic or delayed afterdepolarization (DAD)-triggered tachycardias at flutter rates sometimes mimic the typical flutter ECG.

Vagal and Sympathetic Stimulation

The effects of vagal stimulation differentiate between focal impulse initiation by automaticity or DAD-triggered activity and reentry in the typical flutter circuit. Vagal stimulation transiently suppresses automaticity (see Figure 3-10) and stops DAD-triggered activity (see Figure 6-12). On the other hand, it has little effect on reentry in the typical flutter circuit. **Figure 10-13** shows the ECG during typical flutter. Carotid sinus massage (CSM) was applied during the horizontal bar above. A-V block is increased as expected from the depressant effect of the vagus on A-V nodal conduction but the flutter rate is not changed (best seen in leads II and III). Shortening of the atrial refractory period that is a predominant effect of vagal stimulation, does not affect the reentrant cycle length because the circuit has a large excitable gap and the reentrant impulse is propagating in fully excitable myocardium. Although acetylcholine (ACh) can also increase the negativity of the membrane potential (by increasing outward K^+ current, I_{KACh}) and speed conduction, this effect is minimal in normal atrial myocardium. Vagal stimulation can sometimes convert atrial flutter to AF. Rather than being an effect on the flutter circuit, it results from a generalized shortening of the refractory period of atrial myocardium, enhancing fibrillatory conduction (see Figure 10-20). Similarly, sympathetic stimulation has little effect on reentry in the typical flutter circuit while significantly accelerating the rate of impulse initiation by automaticity and DAD-triggered activity.

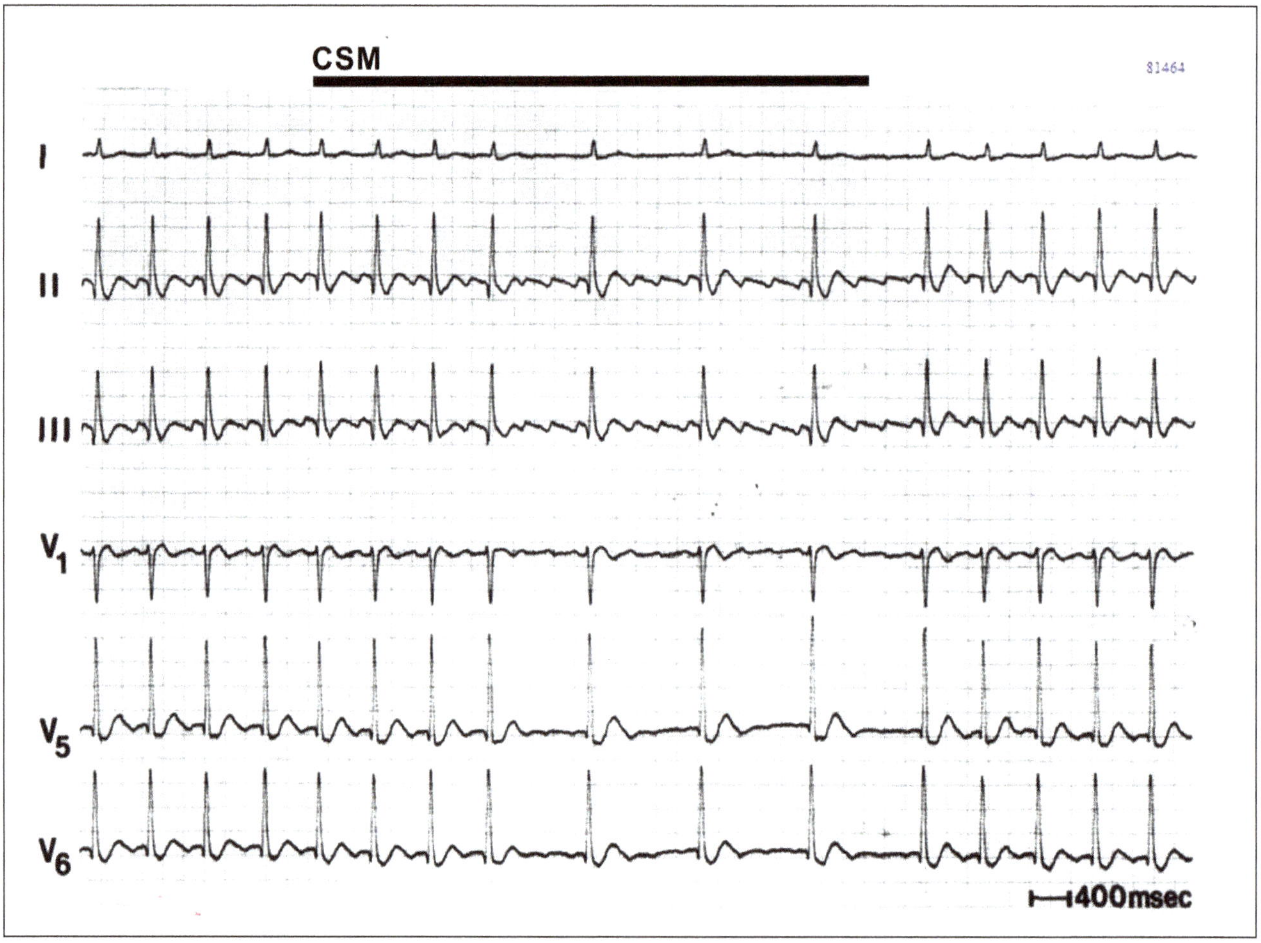

Figure 10-13 ECG leads I, II, III, V_1, V_5, and V_6 during typical flutter at the **left** and during carotid sinus massage (CSM) (**horizontal black bar**) (Wellens' ECG collection).

Pharmacological Agents

Pharmacological agents that might help in distinguishing among automaticity, triggered activity, and reentry include adenosine and verapamil. As described in Figure 3-11 and Figure 6-13, adenosine transiently suppresses normal automaticity and stops DAD-triggered activity. In comparison, during typical flutter caused by reentry, it decreases the ventricular rate because of the increase in refractoriness of the A-V node, but usually does not affect the atrial rate for the same reasons that vagal stimulation does not affect it. Shortening of atrial refractory periods does not affect impulse propagation during reentry when there is a large fully excitable gap.

The Ca^{2+} channel-blocking drug, verapamil, suppresses DADs and stops DAD-triggered tachycardia because of the important role of Ca^{2+} in the genesis of DADs (see Figure 5-2 and Figure 6-22). It also has little effect on normal automaticity. It does not affect typical flutter, which is not dependent on Ca^{2+}.

The Na^+ channel-blocking antiarrhythmic drugs have variable effects on the typical flutter circuit, dependent on alterations of conduction and/or refractory periods. However, these effects do not help in identifying a reentrant mechanism since these drugs also affect automaticity and DAD-triggered activity.

MACROREENTRANT CIRCUITS AROUND OBSTACLES CAUSED BY SCARS AND/OR SURGICAL LESIONS

Macroreentrant circuits causing atrial tachycardia can occur around large anatomical obstacles created by scarring of multiple etiologies. This includes lesions and scars from surgical interventions (lesion-related reentry) such as right atriotomy during repair of congenital heart disease, left atriotomy for mitral valve surgery, surgical or post catheter ablation of AF, or atrial flutter. It also includes right or left atrial scarring resulting from coronary artery disease, myocarditis, tachycardia-mediated cardiomyopathy, or idiopathic arrhythmogenic cardiomyopathy. The reentrant circuits that form in either the right or left atria sometimes also incorporate natural obstacles such as A-V valves or caval or pulmonary vein orifices.

ECG Characteristics

The morphology of the atrial complex on the ECG of lesion or scar related macroreentrant atrial tachycardia can range from typical atrial flutter to a more "classic" form of atrial tachycardia with a slower rate (150–250 bpm) described below (**Figure 10-14**). Atypical atrial flutter is a macroreentrant tachycardia fulfilling the classic ECG definition of a continuously undulating (sawtooth) pattern of atrial activity at a rate of approximately 250–350 bpm but not fitting the typical flutter ECG patterns described in Figure 10-1. In general, atypical flutter has positive flutter waves across the precordium. It is called "atypical" because it is caused by reentrant circuits other than the typical ones described in Figure 10-2.

Macroreentrant atrial tachycardia is differentiated from atypical flutter by a slower rate (150–250 bpm) and isoelectric intervals between discrete P waves on the ECG, even though it can be caused by similar reentrant circuits. An ECG of macroreentrant atrial tachycardia with characteristics different from atypical flutter is shown in Figure 10-14. The arrhythmia, with 2:1 A-V conduction, was caused by reentry around a right atrial scar resulting from the repair of an atrial septal defect. The slower rate of atrial tachycardia compared to atypical flutter is related to larger circuits/ slower conduction in the circuit or a combination of the two.

Location of Reentrant Circuits Causing Scar-Related Atypical Flutter and Macroreentrant Tachycardia

Figure 10-15 diagrams several of the many possible reentrant pathways that can cause either atypical flutter or macroreentrant atrial tachycardia.

In Figure 10-15, Panel A shows a reentrant circuit (red arrows, 1) around a suture line caused by an atriotomy in the right atrial free wall (dashed black line). The size of the obstacle provided by the lesion can be expanded by scarring around the suture line (light gray shading) caused by damage to muscle, mechanical stresses or decreased coronary flow as a result of the surgery. Reentrant circuits may also occur in damaged regions at a distance from the surgical incision, for example a circuit in the right atrial free wall instead of the septum after repair of an atrial septal defect. Such damage might be related to stretching or ischemia. A narrow conducting pathway called a channel or isthmus sometimes forms between areas of scarring (asterisks).

Also shown in Panel A is a circuit (black arrows, 2) around prosthetic material (dashed blue line) used to repair an atrial septal defect. In some cases, a figure-eight circuit (see Figure 9-17) may occur with another reentrant pathway around the tricuspid annulus (blue arrows, 3).

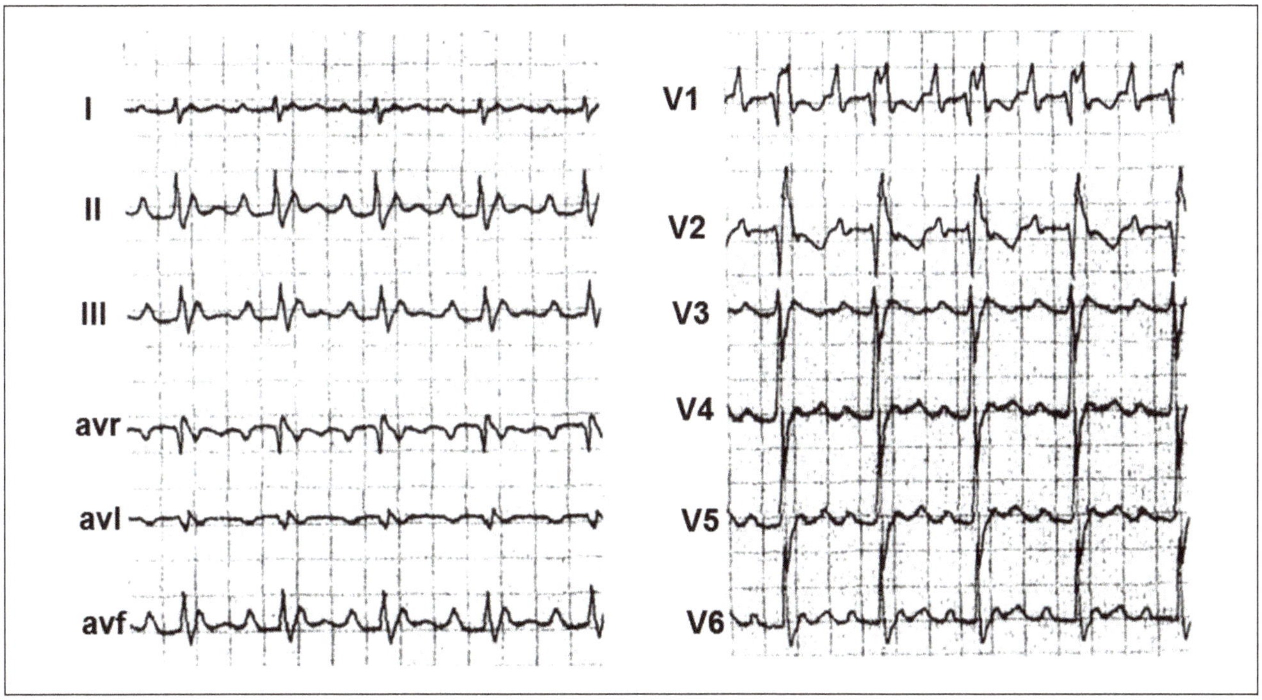

Figure 10-14 A 12-lead ECG recorded during scar-related macroreentrant atrial tachycardia with 2:1 A-V block.

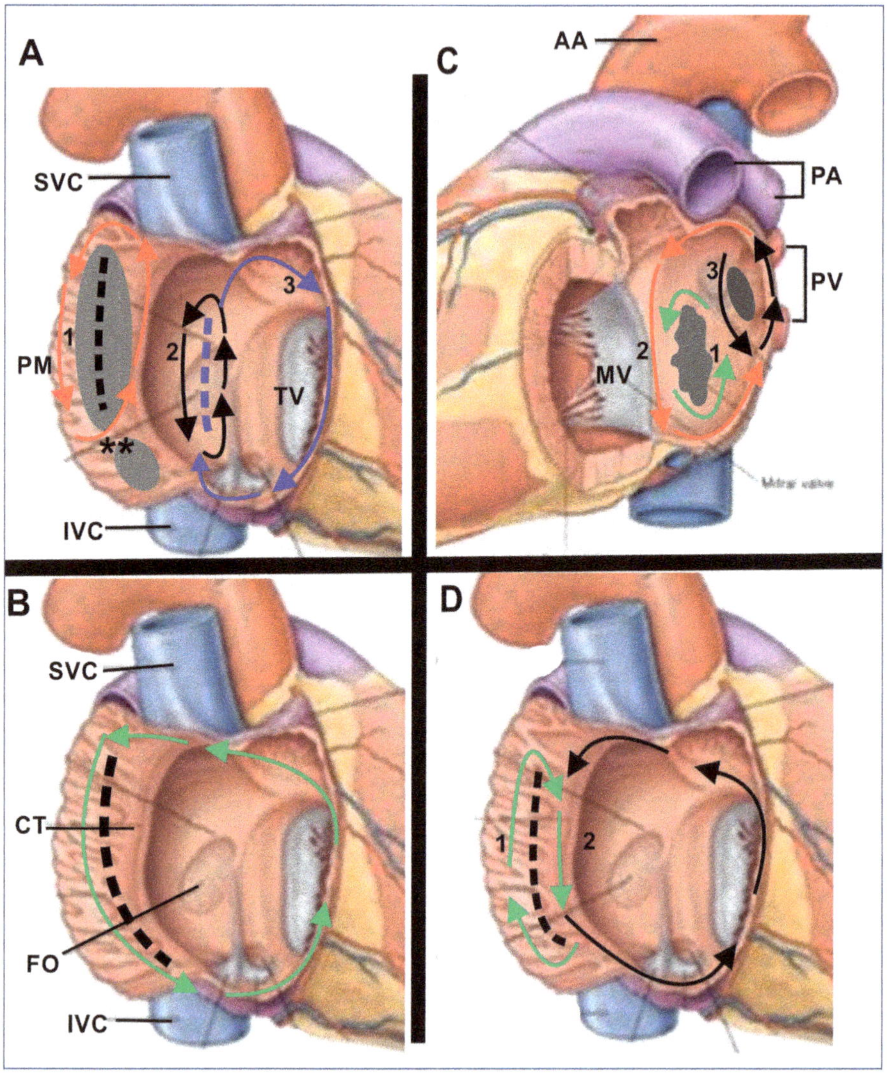

Figure 10-15 Macroreentrant circuits. **Panels A, B,** and **D** show a view of the endocardial surface of the right atrium. CT, crista terminalis; FO, fossa ovalis; IVC, inferior vena cava; PM, pectinate muscles; SVC, superior vena cava; TV, tricuspid valve. Thick **dashed black lines** indicate lesions, curved arrows show impulse conduction patterns. **Panel C** shows a view of left atrial endocardial surface. AA, aortic arch; MV, mitral valve; PA, pulmonary arteries; PV, pulmonary veins. **Gray regions** indicate scar and **curved arrows** are patterns of impulse propagation.

If a large incision is made in the right atrial free wall so that it provides a sufficiently long line of block between the vena cavae, diagrammed in Panel B (dashed black line), atrial flutter of the classic type can develop (green arrows) since the long region of conduction block caused by the incision, forces the impulse to conduct through the cavo tricuspid flutter isthmus, much like the crista does for typical flutter (see Figure 10-2). Figure-eight reentry can also occur after a right atrial atriotomy diagrammed in Panel D with one reentrant pathway through the cavo tricuspid isthmus, up the atrial septum and then down the right atrial free wall anterior to the atriotomy (counterclockwise flutter, black arrows, 2) whereas the other circuit rotates around the atriotomy in a clockwise direction (green arrows, 1) with both circuits sharing the pathway anterior to the atriotomy.

Figure 10-15, Panel C, diagrams reentrant circuits in the left atrium. These can occur after mitral valve surgery or in the presence of significant structural heart disease. In the case of heart disease, anatomical circuits form around regions of fibrosis that form a central anatomical obstacle (Panel C indicated by green arrows, 1). A reentrant circuit around the mitral annulus associated with atrial enlargement caused by heart failure causes perimitral flutter (Panel C indicated by red arrows, 2). Left atrial flutter or tachycardia can also involve circuits around the pulmonary veins or around pulmonary veins and areas of scar caused by pulmonary vein ablation (Panel C indicated by black arrows, 3).

Reentrant circuits can also form in the right atrium associated with atrial scarring not related to surgery. **Figure 10-16** shows an activation map of a macroreentrant circuit causing atrial tachycardia with a cycle length of 355 ms (ECG above the map) in a patient with idiopathic dilated scarred right atrium caused by arrhythmogenic atrial myopathy, a condition associated with extensive atrial scarring of unknown origin.

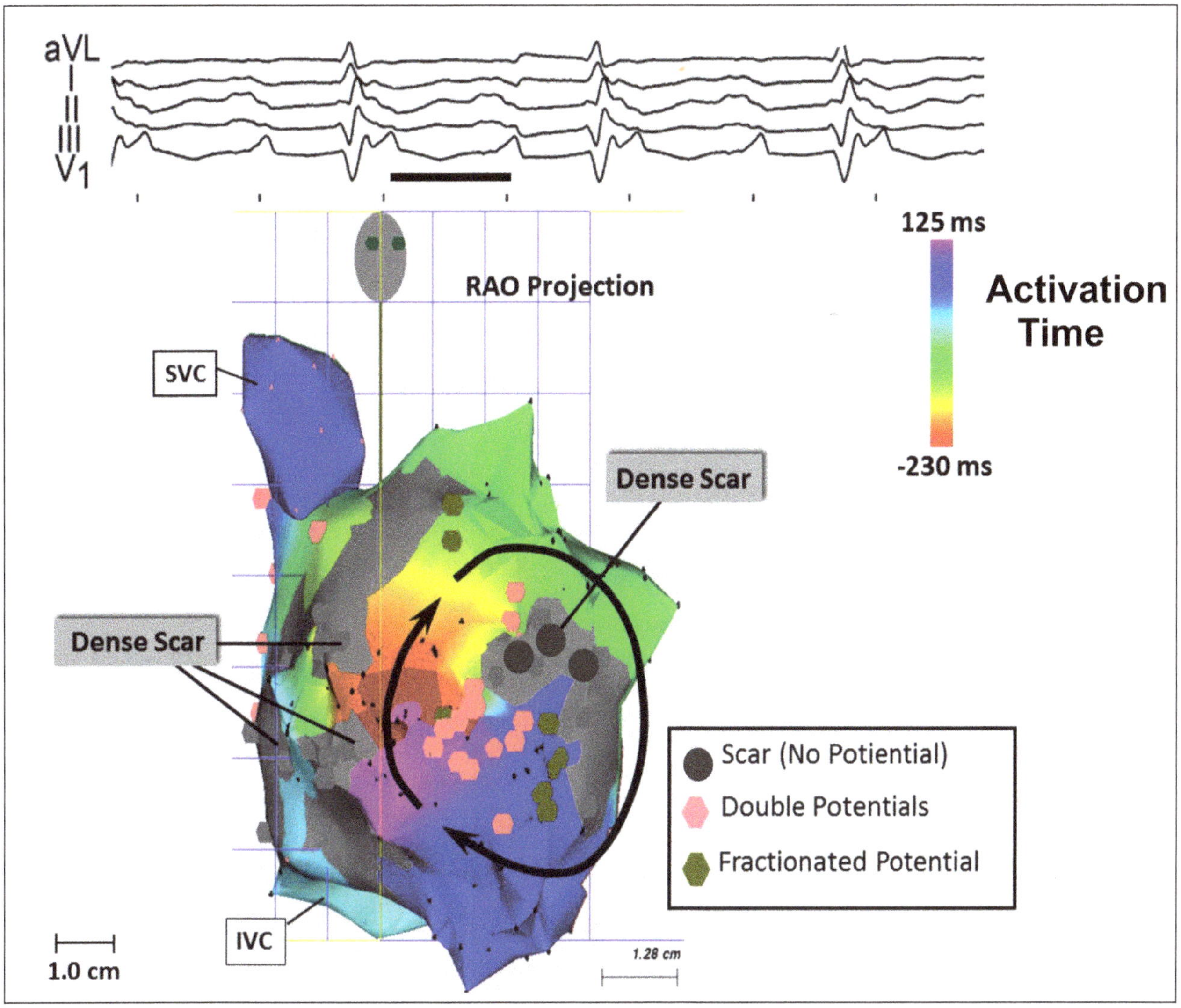

Figure 10-16 ECG Leads aVL, I, II, III, and V_1 during macroreentrant atrial tachycardia (**top**) and atrial activation map (right anterior oblique atrial projection (RAO) **below**). Isochrone scale and colors at right. IVC, inferior vena cava; SVC, superior vena cava. Box at lower right provides color code for location of electrograms with different characteristics.

In Figure 10-16, the extensive scarring is indicated by the gray areas (dense scar). The reentrant pathway is shown by the black arrows and the sequence of red, orange, yellow, green, blue, and purple isochrones. Earliest activation is red (–230 ms). As is characteristic of activation maps of reentry, the latest area activated (purple) is adjacent to the earliest (red). The region of scarring to the right is part of a large central anatomical obstacle around which is the reentrant pathway. The region of scarring to the left forms a boundary that confines the circuit to a narrow isthmus between the scarred areas.

Electrophysiological Properties of Reentrant Circuits

Electrogram Characteristics of Scar

Areas of dense scarring often have no detectable electrical signals owing to an absence of viable muscle bundles, and therefore provide an obstacle to conduction. (Very low voltages of < 0.05 mV in bipolar electrograms are considered to indicate no local activity, recorded at sites indicated by gray circles in Figure 10-16). However, sometimes, bundles of viable myocardium can penetrate the scar and are identified by electrical signals with higher amplitudes in recordings obtained with closely spaced bipoles (~0.1–0.5 mV). Conduction through these bundles may sometimes form part of the reentrant pathway. Adjacent to scars and extending into damaged regions, electrograms also have a very low voltage (0.05–0.1 mV) indicating regions of depressed action potentials (slow phase 0 depolarization and low amplitudes) and slow conduction. Low-voltage electrograms can also be generated by muscle bundles with normal action potentials, trapped deep in scarred areas.

Electrograms adjacent to scars are often fractionated (olive green hexagons in Figure 10-16), indicating slow nonuniform anisotropic conduction (Figure 9-12). Double potentials (pinkish hexagons in Figure 10-16) are a general characteristic of the center of reentrant circuits, caused by wavefronts moving in opposite directions on each side of the recording site as shown in Figure 10-6.

Similarities to Typical Flutter Circuits

Other factors slowing conduction are similar to those in typical flutter circuits including the natural directional differences in atrial muscle bundle orientation and the resultant effects of anisotropy and wavefront curvature. The influence of these factors resulting in changes in conduction velocity and wavelength is evident in the varying width of the isochrones in Figures 10-16. Propagation through a narrow isthmus such as between the two scars in Figure 10-15, Panel A, also leads to slow conduction through the mechanism of impedance mismatch (Figure 9-16). As a result of the slow conduction, the wavelength is significantly less than the path length resulting in a large fully excitable gap.

The onset of macroreentrant tachycardia requires the occurrence of unidirectional block in a segment of the reentrant circuit. This might be achieved by spontaneously occurring premature impulses or repetitive impulses at short cycle lengths similar to the initiation of typical atrial flutter (see Figure 10-5). The site of block is likely to vary according to the location and properties of the circuit, and is not necessarily in a readily predictable region like typical flutter circuits.

Effects of Electrical Stimulation, Autonomic Nervous System, and Pharmacological Agents

The effects of stimulation to initiate, entrain, and terminate macroreentrant circuits causing typical atrial flutter are described in Figures 10-7 to Figure 10-12. This description also applies to macroreentrant tachycardia related to lesions and scarring.

In general, the lack of effect of vagal stimulation and adenosine that is characteristic of the circuits that cause typical flutter, might also be expected for macroreentrant circuits caused by scarring because of the large excitable gap (Figure 10-13). However, these agents can increase the negativity of the resting membrane potential in atrial cells that have depressed (less negative) membrane potentials caused by damage or disease. Atrial myocardium with this property is expected in these macroreentrant circuits. When this occurs, conduction velocity increases because of an increase in phase 0 depolarization and tachycardia cycle length shortens. Nevertheless, the effects are different from those on automaticity that is transiently depressed (Chapter 2) and DAD-triggered activity that is terminated (Chapter 3).

Sympathetic stimulation can also increase the resting potential, and conduction velocity in diseased myocardial cells, shortening the cycle length of reentrant scar related tachycardias similar to its effects on automatic and DAD-triggered tachycardias.

SECTION

10B Atrial Tachycardia Caused by Reentry in Small (Micro) Reentrant Circuits; Focal Reentrant Tachycardia

FOCAL REENTRANT ATRIAL TACHYCARDIA

ECG Characteristics

The ECG characteristics of focal reentrant atrial tachycardia (Figure 10-17, right) are similar to those described in Chapter 3 for automatic atrial tachycardia, which also arises in a focus; discrete P waves at rates between 130–160/min with morphologies dependent on the site of origin (Figures 3-6, 3-7, and 3-8). ECG characteristics are not specific enough to distinguish reentry in small circuits or foci from reentry in large circuits or from automatic or DAD-triggered atrial tachycardia. Additional electrophysiological characteristics are necessary to distinguish focal atrial reentry from these other mechanisms.

Location and Mapping

Although ECG characteristics can approximate the location of tachycardia origin, the mapping of atrial activation confirms that tachycardia originates in a focus, arbitrarily defined as a region of less than approximately 2 cm^2.

Sinus Node and Perinodal Reentry

Supraventricular tachycardias that are focal can be caused by reentry in small circuits involving the sinus node-perinodal region (Figure 2-5). Slow conduction in the perinodal region provides a substrate in which reentry can occur to cause single reentrant (echo) impulses in response to atrial premature impulses or, more rarely, sinus node reentrant tachycardia. The P waves and atrial activation sequence during sinus node reentry are similar to sinus rhythm.

Atrial Reentry

Small reentrant circuits in a focus of atrial myocardium can exist most anywhere in the atria when certain electrophysiological properties are present. Fibrosis is a normal aging process that can enhance the nonuniformities in anisotropy that naturally exist. Unidirectional block and slowed conduction are promoted by impedance mismatch in regions of confluence of muscle bundles of different diameters (Figure 9-16), and dispersions of refractoriness caused by different regional characteristics of action potentials (Figure 9-14). Superimposed on these features can be alterations caused by disease such as additional fibrosis, changes in action potentials caused by ion channel remodeling, and decreased gap junction coupling caused by gap junctional remodeling.

Pattern of Atrial Activation of Focal Tachycardia

Figure 10-17 shows an activation map of a focal atrial tachycardia originating at the base of the right atrial appendage. Since this region does not have normal automaticity and probably no DAD-triggered activity, a mechanism of focal reentry is likely. Spread of activation is radial away from a small site of origin indicated by the white arrow and red isochrones. There is nonuniform conduction away from this site as indicated by the different isochrone widths. The nonuniformity is a result of the influence of a complicated atrial structure and different orientation of muscle bundles.

In Figure 10-17, earliest activity occurs well before onset of the P wave (red isochrones occurring at –105 ms). Activation of the entire atria is usually complete within about 25% of the tachycardia cycle with a significant portion of the cycle length electrically silent, as shown in the activation map, where activation for one impulse is 95 ms. (The ECG at the right of the map shows a tachycardia cycle length of 400 ms.) This pattern is different than that of macroreentrant atrial tachycardia, where electrical activity over a large part of the atrium occurs throughout the cycle length as shown in the activation map in Figure 10-16. The last region activated during focal tachycardia (blue and purple isochrones in Figure 10-17) is at a distance from the origin, whereas in macroreentrant tachycardia, the last region activated is adjacent to the first region activated (Figure 10-16) because of the circular pattern of activity. Within the focus, however, the activation pattern of the reentrant circuit should occupy the entire cycle length.

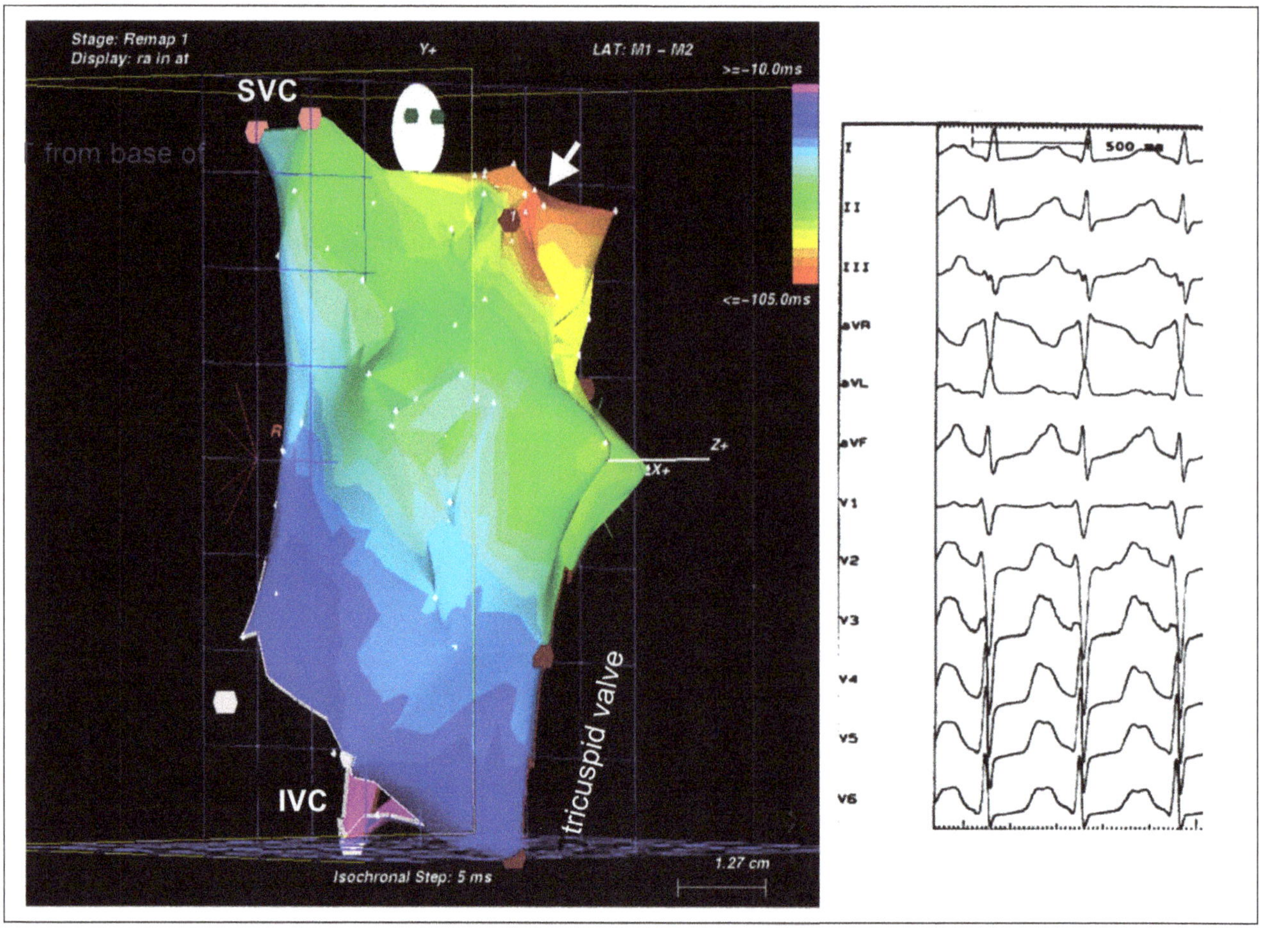

Figure 10-17 Electroanatomic activation map (**left**) of the anterolateral right atrium during focal tachycardia. Color code at the **upper right** indicates the sequence of atrial activation from earliest (**red**) to latest (**purple**) in 8-ms intervals. At the **right** is the ECG.

Electrophysiological Properties

Conduction Abnormalities

Regions in which focal reentry occurs often have low-amplitude electrograms and fractionated electrograms, features indicative of slow, nonuniform, anisotropic conduction (Figure 9-12). However, conduction abnormalities are not a requirement for automatic or triggered focal tachycardias.

When reentry is occurring within the focal site of origin, it can be caused by either leading circle (Figure 9-18), rotors (Figure 9-19), or anisotropic reentry (Figure 9-20). Each of these models has different mechanisms causing the slow conduction and short wavelength necessary for reentry in small circuits. Within the small circuits, no matter the mechanism, electrical activity is occurring throughout the tachycardia cycle that is detectable with electrodes placed in the vicinity of the circuit. This concept of continuous electrical activity as a marker for reentry is described in more detail in Chapter 12 on ventricular tachycardia.

Electrical Stimulation

Premature Stimulation

Focal atrial tachycardia caused by reentry is usually spontaneously initiated by an atrial premature depolarization, a characteristic consistent with a reentrant mechanism. Initiation is not related to conduction delay in the A-V node, as is the case in supraventricular tachycardia caused by A-V nodal reentry (described in Chapter 11). Reentrant focal atrial tachycardia can also be initiated by programmed atrial electrical stimulation (**Figure 10-18**). Sites of stimulation must be close enough to the region of origin to ensure that the stimulated impulse reaches it. Initiation usually occurs when the premature impulse occurs during the relative refractory period, causing slow conduction at the site of reentry.

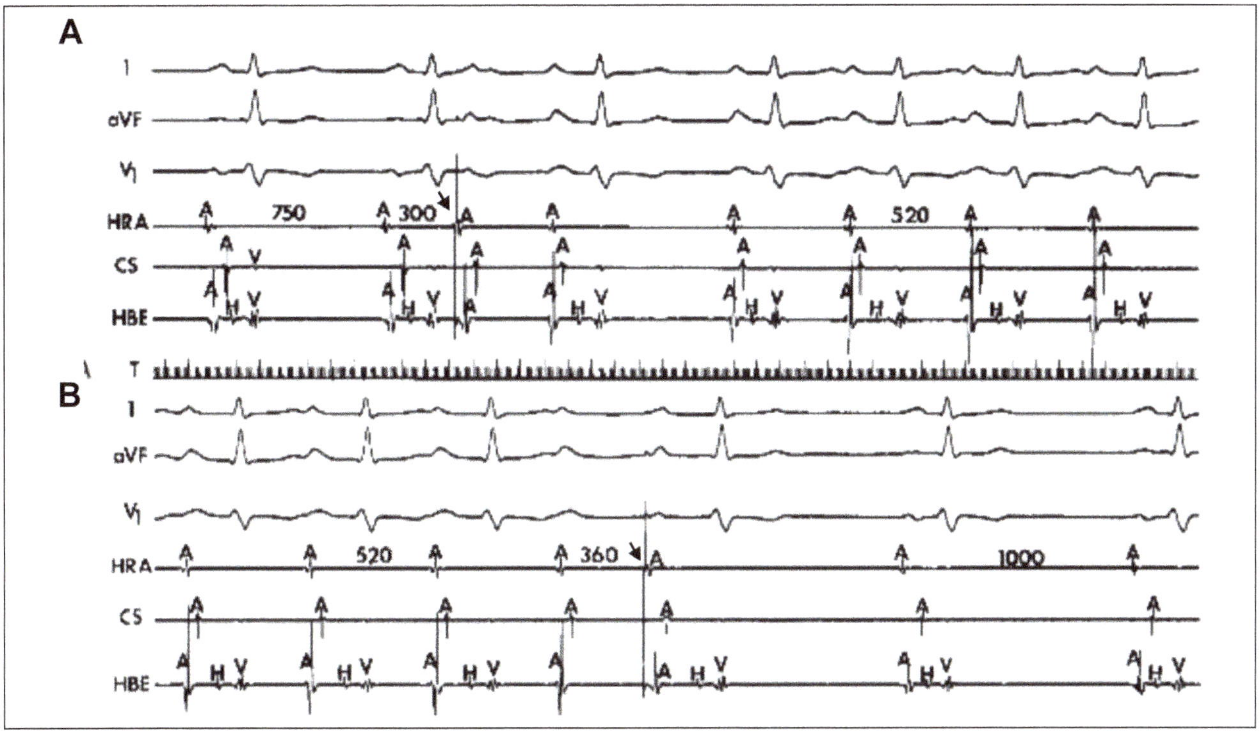

Figure 10-18 ECG leads I, aVF, and V_1, and electrograms from high right atrium (HRA), coronary sinus (CS), and His bundle region (HBE). A, atrium; H, His bundle; V, ventricle. (Reproduced from Josephson ME. *Josephson's Clinical Cardiac Electrophysiology. Techniques and Interpretations* (5th ed). Philadelphia, PA: Wolters Kluwer; 2016.)

Figure 10-18, Panel A, shows the initiation of focal tachycardia by a stimulated premature atrial impulse (arrow) delivered to the high right atrium at a coupling interval of 300 ms, during a basic paced cycle length of 750 ms. The tachycardia has a cycle length of 520 ms. The atrial activation sequence during tachycardia shows simultaneous activation of the high right atrium (HRA), and the inferior right atrium (note the A deflection in the HBE electrogram), which is distinctly different from sinus rhythm where the A deflection in the HBE occurs later than HRA. Also shown is that initiation of tachycardia occurs despite A-V block of the premature impulse (there is no QRS following the premature atrial impulse), suggesting that the A-V junction is not the site of reentry (see Chapter 11). Tachycardia is terminated by another premature atrial stimulus in Panel B (coupling interval 360 ms, arrow). Reentrant focal tachycardia is characterized by an inverse relationship between the cycle length initiating tachycardia and the cycle length between the last stimulated impulse and first impulse of tachycardia (Figure 9-24) that is not a characteristic of triggered activity, even though atrial tachycardia caused by DAD-triggered activity can also be initiated by stimulation (Figure 6-5). Focal reentrant tachycardias can also be initiated and terminated by overdrive pacing.

Resetting, Entrainment, and Termination

The occurrence of resetting, entrainment, and termination of reentrant focal atrial tachycardia by stimulation suggests that focal reentrant circuits have an excitable gap. This leads to a conundrum in assigning a reentrant mechanism. Leading circle reentry should be difficult to reset or entrain because of its small partially excitable gap, although stimulated impulses might still enter a circuit during the partially excitable gap. Rotor reentry and anisotropic reentry have fully excitable gaps that might enable stimulated impulses to enter the circuits although there are no experimental data to support this conjecture. The response to stimulation and the reentrant mechanism may also differ in different clinical cases depending on the reentrant mechanism.

Autonomic Stimulation and Pharmacological Agents

The response of reentrant focal atrial tachycardia to autonomic stimulation or selective pharmacological agents can sometimes be helpful in distinguishing focal reentry from focal automaticity and DAD-triggered activity. However, it provides limited insights into the possible mechanisms for reentry, i.e., leading circle, rotor, or anisotropic. Some tachycardias are not affected by vagal stimulation (carotid sinus pressure) or by adenosine. This property suggests a reentry mechanism and distinguishes these tachycardias from automatic and DAD-triggered tachycardia; transient suppression of the former and termination of the latter.

Adenosine and vagal stimulation accelerate repolarization of atrial cells and shorten the refractory period. This effect shortens the wavelength of the reentrant impulse. A lack of an effect on tachycardia cycle length suggests a fully excitable gap in those circuits. Leading circle reentry has only a partially excitable gap that should lead to a shortening of the tachycardia cycle length with shortening of the refractory period by adenosine or vagal stimulation. Rotor reentry appears to have a small fully excitable gap as does anisotropic reentry, possibly rendering these circuits insensitive to shortening of the wavelength. In general, adenosine and vagal stimulation have no effect on atrial macroreentrant circuits with large fully excitable gaps.

On the other hand, some focal reentrant atrial tachycardias are terminated by vagal activation and by adenosine, similar to the effects of these agents on DAD-triggered activity. In this situation, gradual prolongation of the atrial cycle length occurs before termination. Even though A-V block can occur, it is not related to tachycardia termination. These focal tachycardias are generally localized to the right atrium and are distinguished from those that cannot be interrupted by longer cycle lengths (~430 ms). Adenosine and vagal activation might be able to terminate small reentrant circuits in the tricuspid annulus where atrial action potentials have low membrane potentials and slow rates of depolarization (phase 0) that is dependent on I_{CaL} similar to the A-V node. Both adenosine and vagal activation decreases this current leading to conduction block. This agrees with the observation that some of these tachycardias are also terminated by verapamil, which diminishes I_{CaL}.

SECTION

10C Atrial Fibrillation

ECG OF ATRIAL FIBRILLATION

Figure 10-19 shows an ECG recorded from a patient with AF.

Well-defined P waves are absent. Only fine undulations during diastole are evident in most leads. The QRS complexes occur at irregular intervals. The absence of P waves is a result of the absence of a uniform wavefront activating the atria during fibrillation. Different regions are activated in a discordant manner at rapid rates by multiple wavefronts. The irregular small deflections represent uncoordinated atrial activation. These fibrillatory small deflections can be either fine (amplitude < 0.5 mm) or coarse (amplitude > 0.5 mm) depending on the number of wavefronts; the more individual wavefronts, the smaller the amplitude. Multiple wavefronts bombard the A-V node at a higher frequency than can be conducted to the ventricles. Concealed conduction and block in the A-V node lead to the irregular ventricular rate with a normal QRS in the absence of ventricular conduction system disease. Ventricular rate is usually < 120 bpm under resting conditions but can be faster during sympathetic activation that shortens the A-V nodal refractory period or slower during parasympathetic activation that lengthens the A-V nodal refractory period.

Clinical Significance

Atrial fibrillation is the most frequent arrhythmia for which patients are hospitalized. It is associated with an increase in sudden cardiac death, congestive heart failure, stroke risk, impaired quality of life, and overall mortality.

AF can occur in the absence of overt structural disease. It is also associated with a variety of conditions that cause fibrosis such as aging and diseases such as ischemic heart disease, hypertension, valvular heart disease, heart failure, cardiomyopathy, and congenital heart disease. All of these can cause changes in atrial electrophysiology and structure, called remodeling that are related to the mechanisms causing AF.

Although there are well-defined clinical risk factors for AF, a significant heritable component also exists. Heritable substrates are most likely important in early onset familial AF. As yet, the majority of heritable factors for AF is unknown. At least 30 genes have been identified to be associated with AF. Some of these genes encode ion channel proteins and others general transcription factors.

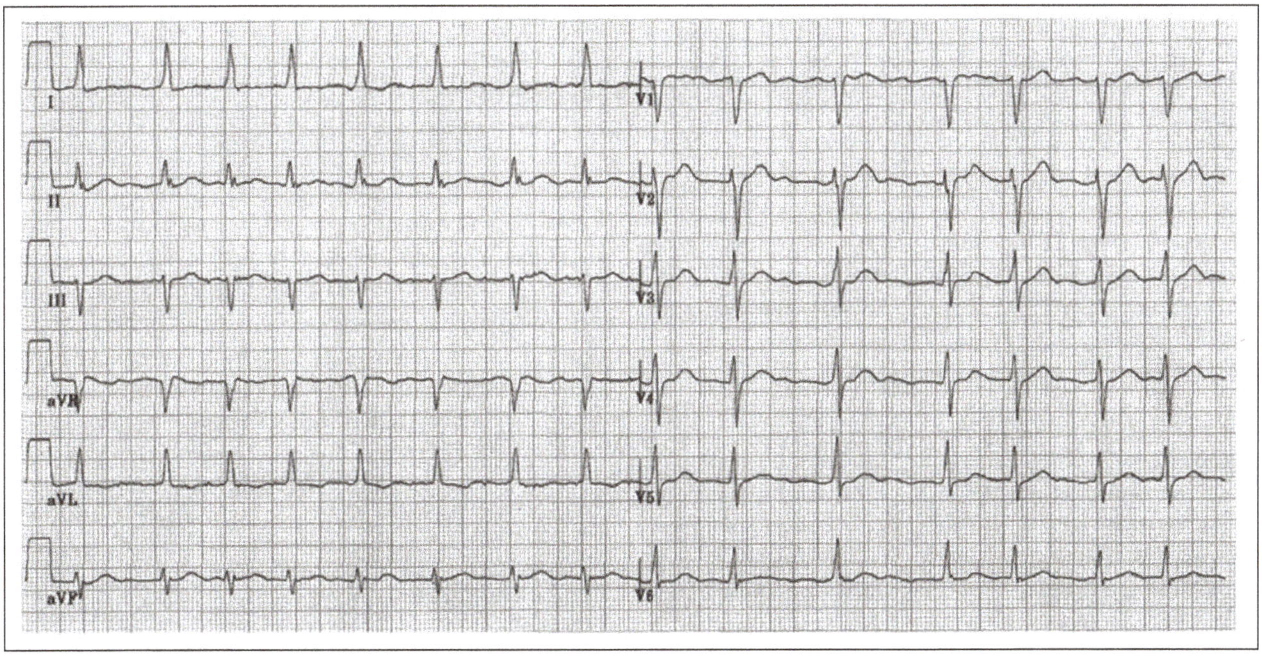

Figure 10-19 A 12-lead ECG recorded from a patient with AF.

Classifications of Atrial Fibrillation

AF can be divided into paroxysmal (self-terminating within 7 days), persistent (lasting greater than one week or requiring electrical or pharmacological cardioversion), and permanent (duration longer than one year, failed cardioversion, or cardioversion not attempted). The occurrence of numerous episodes of paroxysmal AF may eventually lead to persistent AF because of changes in morphological and electrophysiological properties (electrophysiological remodeling) of the atria related to the fast rate of activation during the paroxysmal episodes, as described later in this section. Likewise, persistent AF may eventually become permanent because of continuation of these changes. However, there is a large variability in progression from paroxysmal to persistent to permanent. Some patients have paroxysmal AF that never becomes permanent and some patients initially present with persistent AF. The electrophysiological mechanisms causing AF can change with time because of remodeling of the atria caused by both disease progression and the periods of rapid rate.

ELECTROPHYSIOLOGICAL MECHANISM(S) OF ATRIAL FIBRILLATION

The electrophysiological mechanisms causing AF probably differ depending on the history (paroxysmal, persistent, permanent) and the disease (heart failure, hypertension, etc.). Several different models for initiation and perpetuation of AF are described below, each of which has supporting experimental and clinical evidence. There is currently considerable controversy concerning the mechanism of AF. The controversy is fueled by the likelihood that different mechanisms may be operative in different clinical conditions. All models involve a "substrate" that is basically the mass of the right and left muscular tissue conducting fibrillatory impulses. Some models also involve a focus or "driver" that initiates impulses at a rapid rate. Most models include the involvement of reentry. Models that involve both a substrate and focus are described first.

Focal Initiation and Perpetuation: A Driver and Fibrillatory Conduction

Figure 10-20 shows a model for AF that involves two major components: a focus, also called a "driver" indicated by the red asterisk/red circle, and a substrate indicated by the gray rectangle. In some instances, the location of the focus may be anatomically distinct from the substrate and in some instances it may occupy a small region of the substrate.

The Focus

The focus is a small, circumscribed region that initiates impulses at a rapid rate that acts as a "driver" of AF. If the impulses activated the atria with a uniform wavefront as diagrammed in Panel A, the typical ECG features of AF would not occur. However, the rapidly occurring impulses emanating from the focus conduct in an irregular pattern throughout the atria that is called fibrillatory conduction (Figure 10-20, Panels B and C). (The mechanism for the irregular pattern is described below.) This pattern is responsible for the characteristic appearance of AF on the ECG. Continued activity of the focus is one mechanism that maintains this irregular conduction pattern. The focus has the highest frequency of electrical activity and the impulses arise in the focus at a regular cycle length, called the "dominant frequency." Regions at a distance from the rapid driver have a slower and irregular rate of activity because of the various degrees of conduction block between driver and distant sites, characteristic of fibrillatory conduction. Without the focal driver in this model, AF does not occur even when the substrate has the necessary electrophysiological properties for fibrillatory conduction (see below).

In clinical studies, AF can sometimes be terminated by locating and ablating the dominant frequency focus, located by recording electrograms throughout the atria. When a focus of rapid activity is the cause of AF, repetitive atrial premature impulses or atrial tachycardia often occur before AF onset, representing activity in the focus before fibrillatory conduction occurs in the substrate. (See Section 10B describing focal atrial tachycardia.) There are several prevalent sites where a rapidly active focus can occur to initiate and perpetuate AF.

Focal pulmonary vein activity. An important location of the focus is in the posterior left atrium around any of the four pulmonary vein–atrial junctions, or in the atrial muscle that extends into and lines the pulmonary veins. Focal pulmonary vein activity is most prevalent in paroxysmal AF but also can occur in persistent and permanent AF. The region with the highest frequency (the dominant frequency), is at the junction of the pulmonary vein and left atrium where the focus is located. The frequency decreases going from this site to the left atrium and then to the right atrium, caused by conduction block of impulses conducting away from the focus.

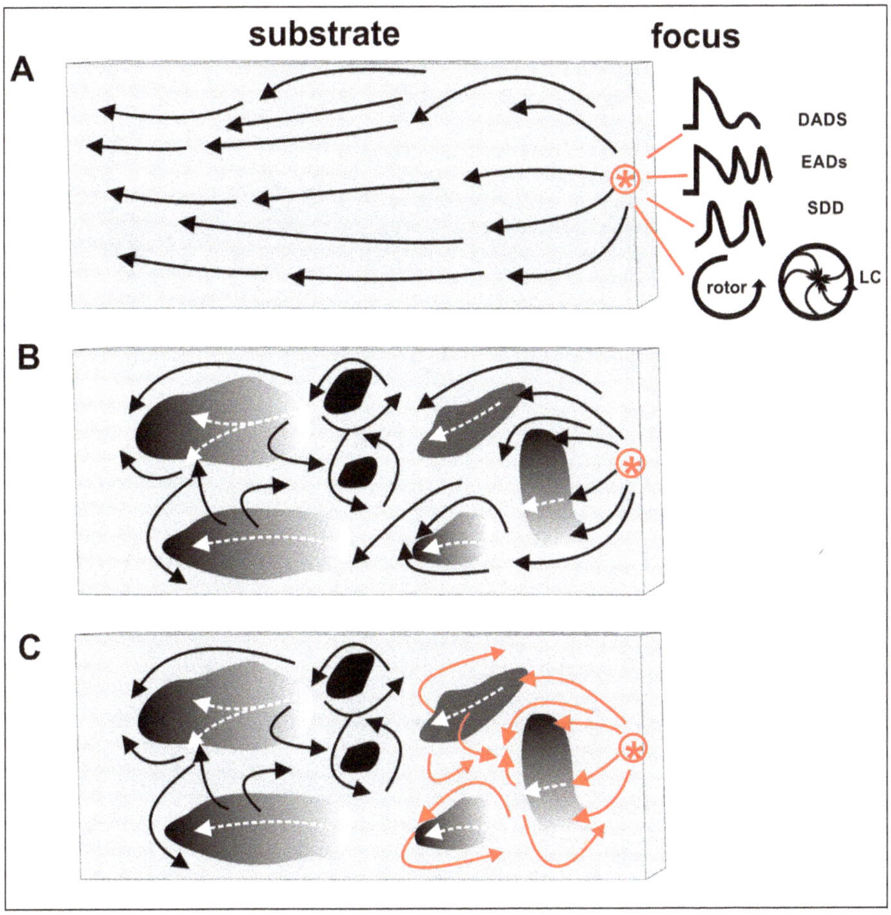

Figure 10-20 Mechanism of AF involving a focus of rapid impulse initiation (**red asterisk and circle**) and a substrate (**shaded rectangular region**, which represents atrial myocardium).

Figure 10-21 shows two examples of the onset of AF caused by rapid activity in foci in pulmonary veins. In Panel A, the electrogram recorded in the right inferior pulmonary vein (RIPV) during a sinus impulse (first ECG complex at the left) has two components, the first caused by atrial activity around and outside the vein (red arrow) and the second by atrial muscle in the vein (black arrow) which is delayed because of conduction time of the sinus impulse from outside to the inside of the vein. The asterisks indicate the onset of rapid firing of pulmonary vein musculature at a cycle length of 170 ms (the pulmonary vein component of the electrograms (asterisk, black arrow) now occurs before the atrial deflection (red arrow) since the impulses are conducting from inside the vein to the atria). The rapid pulmonary vein activity precedes the onset of coarse AF on the ECG. Continuous fractionated electrical activity then occurs in the pulmonary vein that indicates rapid irregular activity in the vein musculature.

In Panel B on the left, the electrogram recorded from the left superior pulmonary vein (LSPV) shows an initial slow depolarization caused by activity in surrounding atrial myocardium (red arrow) and a sharp deflection from electrical activity within the vein (black arrow) during a sinus impulse. It is followed by an isolated atrial ectopic impulse at a coupling interval of 240 ms (without AF) that does not conduct to the ventricles. The sharp deflection caused by pulmonary vein muscle (black arrow) precedes the lower-amplitude atrial activity (red arrow), and indicates an origin within the vein. In Panel C, after an initial sinus impulse, a series of rapidly occurring impulses originating in the pulmonary vein at a cycle length of 160 ms initiates AF; large pulmonary vein electrograms (asterisks and black arrow) precede smaller atrial electrograms (red arrow) during rapid activity. Rapid regularly occurring pulmonary vein electrograms (asterisks) continue to occur during AF that are likely involved in perpetuating AF.

Other sites of focal drivers (nonpulmonary vein). Focal drivers can also occur in atrial myocardium at sites in the left or right atria not related to the pulmonary veins. Focal activity in the right atria can originate in atrial muscle extending into the vena cavae or coronary sinus os, although less commonly than the pulmonary veins. The dominant frequency is then located in the right instead of the left atrium. A single atrial focus can cause paroxysmal AF. The number of foci can increase during remodeling and mediate the transition from paroxysmal to persistent AF.

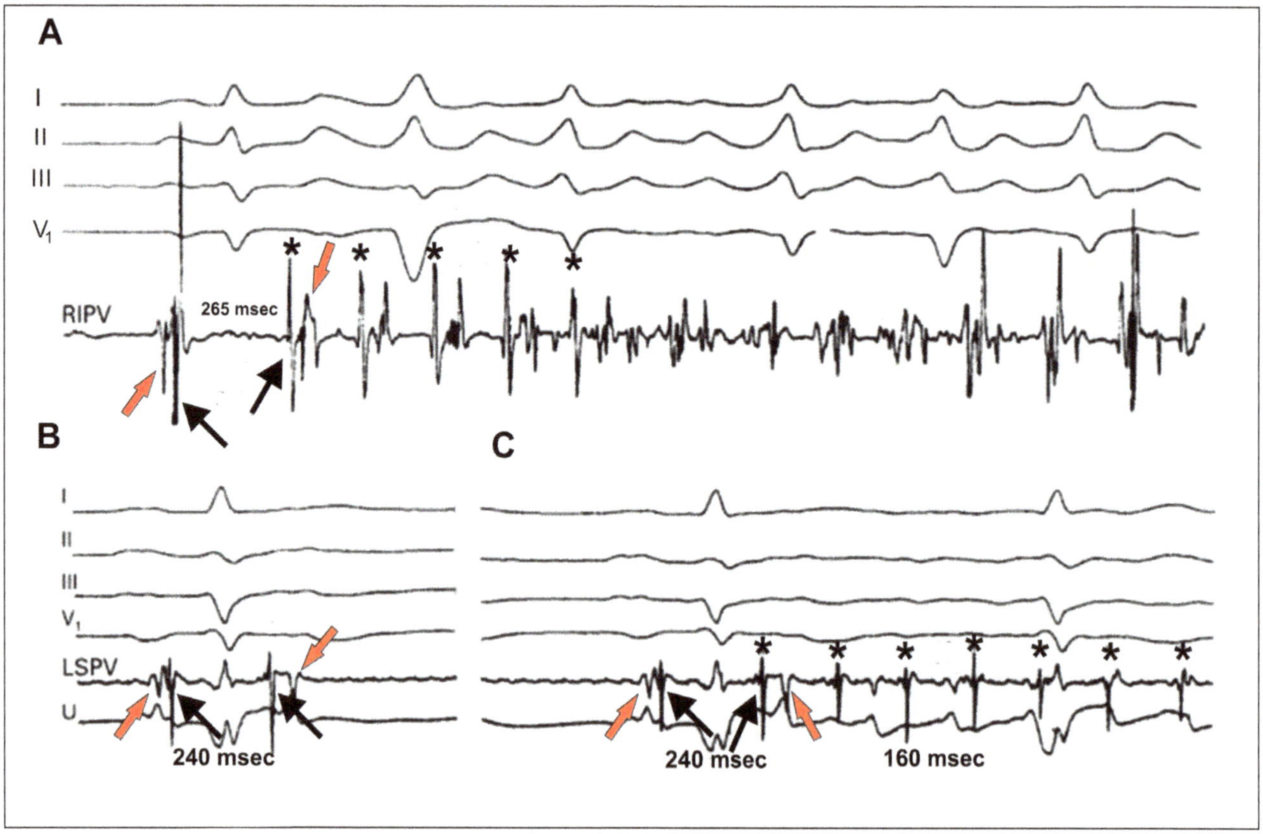

Figure 10-21 Pulmonary vein initiation of AF. (Reproduced with permission from Haissaguerre M, Jais P, et al. Spontaneous initiation of atrial fibrillation by ectopic beats originating in the pulmonary veins. Reproduced from *N Engl J Med.* 1998;339:659–666.)

Mechanisms for rapid focal driver activity. There are several proposed mechanisms for rapid focal driver activity. It may be caused by normal or abnormal automaticity (Chapters 3 and 4), early afterdepolarization- (EAD-) or DAD-triggered activity (Chapters 6 and 8), or reentry in small circuits (Chapter 9) (Figure 10-20, Panel A).

Reentry in or around the pulmonary veins or at other atrial sites can act as a driver. The muscle in the pulmonary veins is in the form of small bundles coursing in different directions with sparse gap junction connections between bundles forming a nonuniform anisotropic structure in which transverse conduction is very slow. Anisotropy may be enhanced by structural remodeling caused by increased connective tissue separating muscle bundles and/or decreased gap junction coupling. This property can lead to formation of very small anisotropic circuits described in Figure 9-20, that can be less than several mm in diameter. Similar small circuits might also form in remodeled atrial myocardium not related to the pulmonary veins.

Rotor reentry (Figure 9-19) may also form a focus in pulmonary vein musculature or atrial muscle outside the veins. A rotor forming a focus of rapid activity that is a driver of AF can be stationary or can change location. A stationary rotor is anchored to a specific region by discontinuities such as those caused by local variations in wall thickness, fibrosis, or heterogeneous refractory periods (Chapter 9). Rotors can move when not anchored, which also may occur during AF. The rate of the impulses generated by a rotor depends on its circumference; smaller rotors generate impulses at a more rapid rate conducting into the atria. The faster the rate, the more fragmented are the wavefronts conducting in the atria (fibrillatory conduction). Fragmented wavefronts may be detected as fractionated electrograms (Figure 9-12) near the site of the rotor but are not specific for rotor location. Rotors can be initiated by a premature impulse, perhaps arising in a pulmonary vein. In some cases, there may be more than one rotor initiating and sustaining AF.

Leading circle reentry (Figure 9-18) may also cause rapid activity in an atrial focus. Like rotors, the smaller the circuit, the faster the revolution rate and the more fragmented are the emanating wavefronts. More than one leading circle circuit might exist simultaneously and be drivers of AF.

The occurrence of small reentrant circuits caused by either rotors or leading circle reentry is favored by a decreased effective refractory period of atrial muscle in patients with AF, which contributes to the shorter wavelength necessary for formation of small circuits. Shortening of refractory periods may be related to acceleration of repolarization caused by remodeling of the repolarizing ion channels (see Figure 10-22). Shortening of the refractory period also occurs in atrial muscle in the pulmonary veins, where it becomes less than the left atrial muscle refractory period (normally it is longer). This difference in refractory periods between veins and atrial muscle enhances the likelihood of slow conduction and block of rapidly occurring impulses emanating from the veins into relatively refractory atrial myocardium that serves to break up the wavefront into small wavelets. This fibrillatory conduction is described in Figure 10-20. A decrease in refractory periods caused by vagal activation may also promote the occurrence of small reentrant circuits that act as drivers.

The Substrate

In the model of the mechanism for AF in Figure 10-20, the substrate is the mass of atrial myocardium represented by the rectangular area. The electrical activity of the substrate gives rise to the ECG characteristics of AF when the impulses arising in the focus at a rapid rate activate the substrate in an uncoordinated or heterogeneous pattern, called fibrillatory conduction.

Figure 10-20, Panel B shows the activation pattern of impulses arising from the focus conducting in a heterogeneous substrate (arrows) with marked regional differences in refractory periods and conduction properties indicated by the different shades of gray; lighter to darker shading indicates shorter to longer refractory periods and faster to slower conduction. The heterogeneities result from electrophysiological and structural remodeling described below. Slow conduction and block occur in regions where there are longer refractory periods (dashed white arrows), while more rapid conduction occurs in regions with shorter refractory periods (black arrows), leading to a chaotic pattern of activation by multiple wavelets. In some regions circular activation occurs resembling rotors or leading circle reentry but the regions showing this pattern are constantly shifting and are not drivers of fibrillation. In this model, when the focus generates impulses by a rotor, it is sometimes referred to as the "mother wave rotor" with "daughter waves" caused by the fibrillatory conduction.

In Panel C, at more rapid rates of the focus, the chaotic activation pattern is increased when a second impulse enters the substrate (red arrows,) while the previous impulse is still activating it (black arrows) and before all regions have recovered from the previous activation. In addition, the cycle length of activation differs in different regions of the substrate because of conduction block in some regions, further increasing the heterogeneities because of the relationship of recovery of excitability to cycle length. When there is more than one focus, there is fragmentation of wavefronts emanating from each one, contributing to the chaotic behavior.

Electrophysiology of the atrial substrate. Natural heterogeneities in both refractory periods and conduction velocities exist in the normal atria because of their complicated electrophysiology and anisotropic structure. Both cellular electrophysiology and structure undergo changes (remodeling) in patients with AF that promote fibrillatory conduction.

Normally action potentials in different regions of the atria have different time courses for repolarization that cause differences in refractory periods. Some of these differences are illustrated in **Figure 10-22**.

For example, the crista terminalis has a well-defined plateau phase (2) caused by a prominent inward I_{CaL} that contributes to a relatively long action potential duration (~250 ms) (Figure 10-22, Panel A, bottom action potential, I_{CaL} (red arrow)). Repolarization occurs when this current diminishes and outward K^+ currents (I_K (orange arrow), I_{K1} and I_{KACh} (blue arrow) dominate. In comparison, cells in the free walls and septum lack a plateau (Figure 10-22, Panel A, top trace) because of a smaller I_{CaL} (red arrow) and have short action potential durations (~150 ms) caused by the prominent repolarizing K^+ currents (orange and blue arrows). Similar disparities occur in other regions. The natural differences in repolarization and refractoriness can lead to slow conduction of impulses occurring at short cycle lengths (such as a premature impulse) propagating from regions of short action potential durations and refractory periods, into regions with longer action potential durations and refractory periods (Figure 10-22, Panel A indicated by a green dashed arrow from septum to crista).

Natural disparities in conduction also exist because of the structural complexities of atrial myocardium. Local variations in wall thickness caused by pectinate muscles result in regions where these thick bundles make contact with thinner bundles, providing natural sites of impedance mismatch (Figure 9-16) that can slow conduction. Conduction in some regions is parallel to the long axis of the muscle bundles (along the crista terminalis), while in other regions it is transverse or intermediate (in the septum), leading to a spectrum of conduction velocities caused by anisotropic properties.

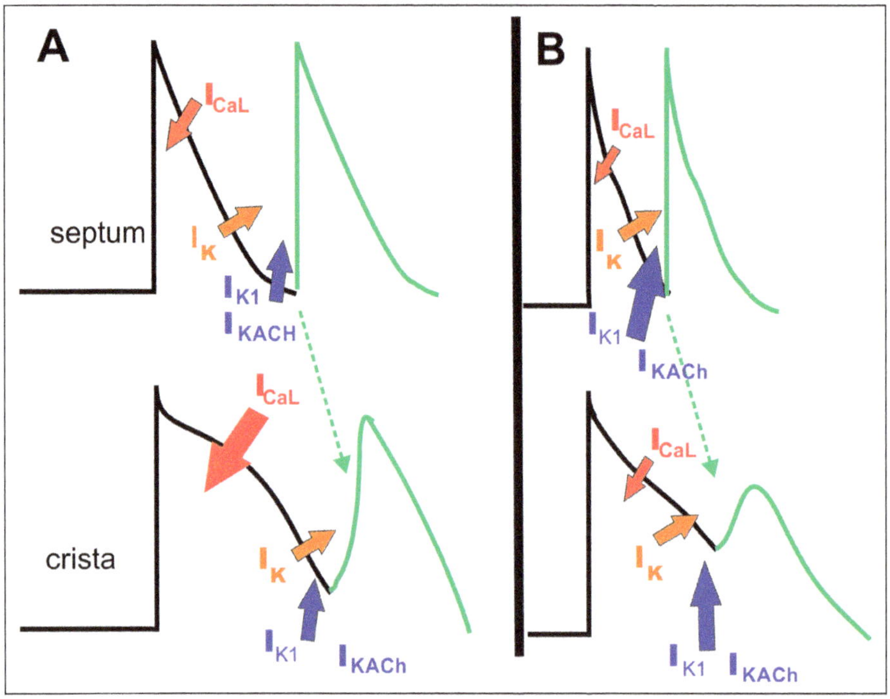

Figure 10-22 Action potentials and ionic currents from normal atrial cells (**Panel A**) and after remodeling (**Panel B**).

These natural heterogeneities of refractoriness and conduction are not sufficient to sustain long periods of AF, although short periods lasting several seconds can be initiated in normal atria by rapid electrical stimulation. The short periods of AF may be prolonged by additional changes due to vagal activation. In addition to shortening the wavelength, vagal activation can increase the heterogeneities of refractoriness in normal atria by acceleration of repolarization, more in some regions than others because of regional differences in the number of nerve endings, leading to more sustained AF.

Remodeling. The substrate for AF undergoes remodeling changes in both structure and electrophysiology caused by aging, progression of disease and periods of rapid atrial activity that create a more favorable environment for initiation and perpetuation of AF.

Remodeling due to paroxysmal AF: The periods of rapid activity that occur during paroxysmal AF can initiate the remodeling process by the concept of AF begets AF. This means that short periods of paroxysmal AF cause the remodeling that leads to longer periods of persistent AF and eventually to permanent AF. This electrophysiological remodeling process is attributed to the increased entry of Ca^{2+} via I_{CaL} into cells because of the increased frequency of action potentials during the initial short periods of AF. The increased cellular Ca^{2+} alters a number of processes involved in ion channel formation and function. Increased Ca^{2+} also triggers fibrosis and hypertrophy.

Ion channel remodeling and membrane currents: The remodeling of ion channels result in changes in magnitude and time course of membrane currents that control repolarization (see Figure 7-2). The currents that are most significantly remodeled are I_{CaL}, I_{K1}, and I_{KACh}. Figure 10-22, Panel B, shows a decrease in I_{CaL} after remodeling (indicated by smaller red arrows) because of decreased formation of one of the components of the channel that leads to acceleration of repolarization by decreasing the duration of the plateau phase 2. The acceleration of repolarization is greater in cells with a more prominent plateau such as the crista cells (Figure 10-22, compare crista action potential in Panel B after remodeling with crista action potential in Panel A before remodeling). This change also decreases atrial contractility. The decrease in I_{CaL} does not negate the effect of increased action potential frequency to increase intracellular Ca^{2+}. Remodeling is also characterized by an increase in I_{K1} related to an increase in protein sub-units that make up this channel. This makes the membrane potential more negative, while also accelerating the terminal phase of repolarization (Panel B, increased size of blue arrow). Another current that influences the time for repolarization is I_{KACh} (ACh-activated channel), which has a constitutively active component that contributes outward current during the terminal phase of repolarization and the resting potential even in the absence of ACh and a component that is activated to increase outward current by ACh. The constitutively active component is increased during remodeling because of abnormal channel phosphorylation (increased size of blue arrow) accelerating repolarization while the ACh-activated component is not, and may even be reduced. Increases in other currents involved in repolarization, such as I_K are inconsistent. Mutations in genes controlling K^+ currents are sometimes implicated. The amount of acceleration caused by these changes in membrane currents vary in different regions contributing to an increase in heterogeneity of refractory periods. Acceleration of repolarization enables atrial rate to increase. Changes in the function of channels involved in repolarization may also lead to decreased shortening of action potential duration with decreased cycle lengths (rate adaptation) (Figure 7-7). The increased heterogeneity leads to slower conduction and block of impulses conducting from regions of short to longer refractory periods (Figure 10-22, Panel B, dashed green arrow) facilitating fibrillatory conduction or formation of reentrant circuits. A reduction of I_{Na} may also be part of the remodeling process to cause slow conduction that promotes reentry.

Structural changes in remodeling: In addition to the remodeling of ion channel function, remodeling of the substrate structure contributes importantly to the development of persistent and permanent AF. One important change is an increase in connective tissue, and another change is caused by gap junction remodeling.

Increased cell Ca^{2+} caused by rapid rates can activate enzymes causing breakdown of proteins and stimulate fibrosis, leading to structural remodeling. During normal aging, there is an increase in connective tissue between bundles of atrial myocardium disrupting lateral gap junction connections and increasing nonuniform anisotropy. Increased fibrosis is also a common feature of the various diseases that are associated with the occurrence of AF, further disrupting connections among atrial cells and bundles.

Another feature of structural remodeling is changes in the number of gap junctions and distribution of gap junction connections in addition to their disruption by fibrosis. Atrial myocardium has two principal connexins forming gap junctions, Cx40 and Cx43, unlike ventricles, which have mainly Cx43. These gap junction connections disappear in some regions while being maintained in others. Although the total quantity of gap junctions does not always decrease, the increased heterogeneity in their location leads to more disparities in conduction in different regions of the atria. The increased fibrosis and gap junction remodeling become more prominent during persistent and prominent AF.

Perpetuation of AF by Substrate Mechanisms Without Focal Drivers

Figure 10-23, Panels A and B show two models for AF perpetuated in the substrate without drivers. These models also rely on the substrate remodeling of ion channels and structure described above.

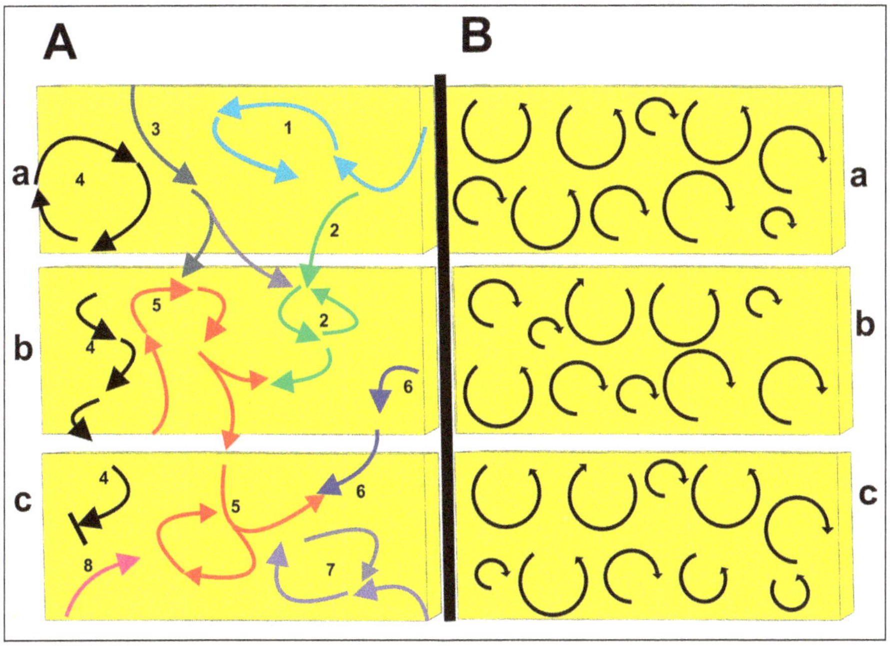

Figure 10-23 Two models of AF perpetuation in the atrial substrate without a "driver." **Panel A** shows the multiple wavelet model. **Panel B** shows multiple reentrant circuits.

Multiple Reentrant Circuits Model

One model of a proposed mechanism causing AF is multiple reentrant circuits, either rotors or leading circle reentry (Figure 10-23, Panel B). In this model small functional reentrant circuits are dispersed throughout the atria (curved arrows). The number of circuits is so numerous that conduction of the reentrant impulse in each circuit is directly responsible for activation of only a small segment of the atria surrounding it rather than fibrillatory conduction of impulses emanating from a limited number of circuits. The number of reentrant circuits that can simultaneously exist in the atria is dependent on the conduction velocities and refractory periods of the atrial myocardium, which determines the wavelength and therefore, the size of the circuits. In normal-sized atria, only a few circuits can exist because of a relatively long wavelength that determines circuit size. The limited number of circuits cannot cause the rate and activation patterns characteristic of sustained AF. Factors that decrease the wavelength—such as shortening of the refractory period and slowing of conduction that occur in the substrate during remodeling—decrease the size of the circuits, allowing many more circuits to coexist causing AF. Although the occurrence of multiple reentrant circuits have not been directly proven by mapping, it has been postulated that this mechanism might appear as multiple foci that have been mapped in some kinds of AF (focal reentry). Origin of impulses in the foci are indicated by a QS form on local electrograms which is a marker of early activity. It is possible that the multiple circuits shown in Panel B might have a stable size and location appearing as stable foci (as in the top diagram, (a)). Another possibility is that the circuits are not stable and the location of the foci are constantly changing. A comparison of Figure 10-23 Panel B, a, b, and c shows a change in circuit size and location at different times. The circuits are not stable but move from one location to another with some dying out and new ones forming. An increase in the area of atrial myocardium accompanying atrial dilation, that is available for circuit formation, also increases the number of simultaneous circuits that can exist at any one time. The initiation of AF in this model may be an early premature impulse or a short period of rapid impulse initiation in a focus, but as indicated above, this focal activity is not involved in perpetuation.

Multiple Wavelet Model

A second mechanism for perpetuation of AF shown in a computer model, that is dependent on the properties of the substrate is the multiple wavelet model diagrammed in Figure 10-23, Panel A. In this model, AF is dependent on breakup of atrial excitation into multiple small wavelets as occurs with fibrillatory conduction of very early premature impulses or impulses with short cycle lengths, arising from a focus. The difference is that after initiation, the focus disappears. The multiple wavelets then propagate perpetually in random patterns at different velocities through the atria around continually changing functional lines of block determined by the heterogeneous electrical and structural properties caused by remodeling. The process is self-sustaining as diagrammed in Figure 10-23. In Panel A, at the top (a), 4 separate wavelets indicated by the different colored arrows (1-4), randomly propagate through a region of atrial myocardium. Some of these wavelets (1 and 4) have circuitous patterns of conduction that might resemble rotors or leading circle reentry. Later in time (b) these circuits disappear and new circuitous patterns of conduction form (2). Some wavelets disappear (3) when they collide with others and new ones appear from other regions (wavelets 5 and 6). Still later in time (c), wavelet 5 forms a functional reentrant circuit, wavelet 4 blocks (black arrow with horizontal line) and disappears. Wavelets 7 and 8 appear from other regions, while wavelet 7 forms a new functional circuit. The diagram shows that the number of wavelets present at any one time is constantly changing and the meandering wavelets may transiently form reentrant circuits but there are no fixed reentrant pathways. Circuits that develop in widely scattered areas, shift position, frequency, and direction, disappear, and are replaced by others without repetition of patterns. A minimal number of wavelets are required to prevent AF from stopping. The arrhythmia is assumed to sustain itself when the number of wavelets is so great that chance of coalescence is improbable. In persistent and permanent AF, the number of wavelets is greater than in electrically induced AF in normal atrium. This is because of the increased electrophysiological and structural remodeling in persistent and permanent AF that leads to a decreased wavelength (slowing of conduction and shortening of refractory periods) and increased area of myocardium that allow an increased number of wavelets. Structural separation of epicardium and endocardium by fibrosis, but with connecting bundles of myocardium between the two, allow more wavelets to simultaneously exist. Wavelets can propagate from endocardium to epicardium and epicardium to endocardium through transmural connections. When this occurs, the appearance of the wavelet on the surface seems to arise from a focal source even though it does not.

ELECTRICAL STIMULATION

The effects of electrical stimulation do not identify the electrophysiological mechanism of AF. In some patients with normal atria and without a history of spontaneously occurring AF, rapid pacing can initiate short periods of AF of only several seconds. More sustained periods of AF can be induced by rapid pacing or premature stimulation in patients with a history of paroxysmal or permanent AF, likely because some substrate remodeling has occurred. An example of induction of AF with a single premature stimulus from the high right atrium (HRA), is shown in **Figure 10-24** (at the arrow). Induction can occur from stimulation at one site but not another. For example, initiation of AF by stimulation from the high right atrium or pulmonary veins is often easier than from the coronary sinus region. The shorter refractory period in these regions as compared to the coronary sinus or body of the left atrium allows for earlier premature impulses to propagate into more refractory surrounding regions resulting in multiple wavelets or atrial reentrant circuits (Figure 10-23). On the other hand, stimulation might also initiate rapid activity in a driver caused by DAD-triggered activity or reentry, such as in pulmonary veins that persists after the stimulated impulse and causes AF by the mechanism in Figure 10-20.

Overdrive or premature stimulation from random atrial sites do not terminate AF. Although stimulation can terminate DAD-triggered activity or reentry in circuits with excitable gaps, it may not be able to access the mechanism of AF because of the complicated activation of the atria. The effects of stimulation at a site of dominant frequency are not known.

Paroxysmal and persistent AF can be terminated by defibrillation, which is a procedure that stimulates the entire atria simultaneously. The shocks terminate reentry, either in focal reentrant drivers (rotors or leading circle, Figure 10-20) or multiple reentrant circuits in the substrate (Figure 10-23, Panel B). Defibrillation is also expected to block fibrillatory conduction of multiple wavelets (Figure 10-23, Panel A) enabling a coordinated wavefront to activate the atria until conditions develop to initiate AF again. Defibrillation is not expected to stop focal drivers that have automaticity but might terminate DAD-triggered activity.

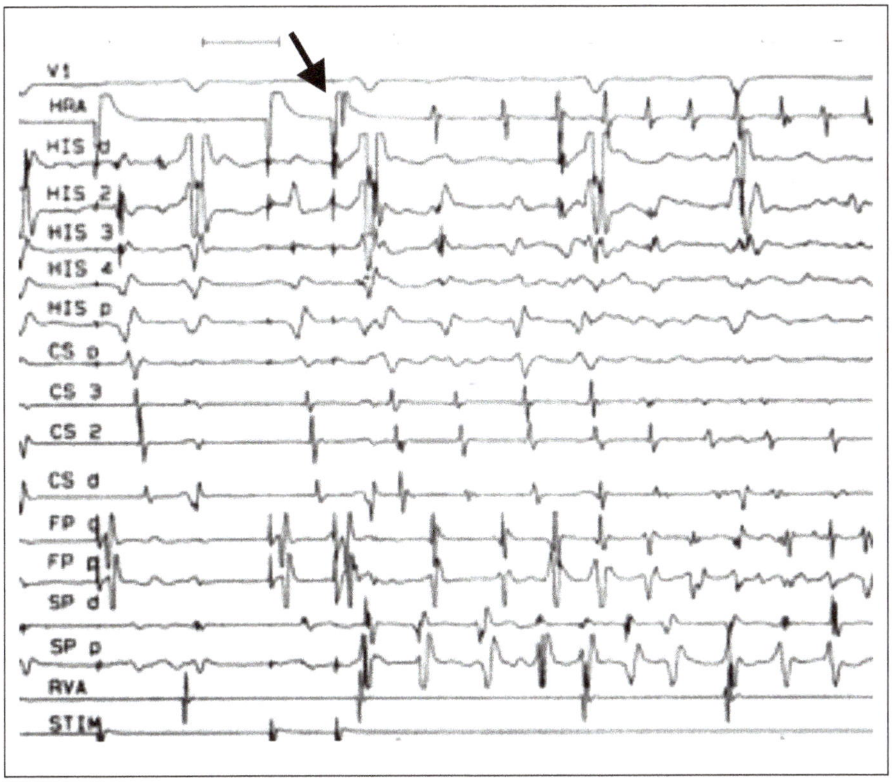

Figure 10-24 Induction of AF by a premature stimulus (**arrow**) at the high right atrium (HRA) in a patient with persistent AF. ECG lead V_1 and electrograms from various sites are shown. CS electrograms from coronary sinus region show atrial activity; RVA electrograms from right ventricular apex show ventricular activity.

PHARMACOLOGY

The use of drugs to establish mechanisms of AF is complicated by the different kinds of AF and the different diseases with which AF is associated. In Chapters 3 and 6 it is described how adenosine is helpful in establishing an automatic or triggered mechanism by transiently suppressing spontaneous diastolic depolarization or inhibiting DADs. Adenosine has been shown to accelerate the fibrillatory rate rather than suppress it. This would seem to eliminate automatic or DAD-triggered drivers in those cases. Adenosine favors reentrant drivers or multiple circuits/wavelets because adenosine shortens the refractory period and the wavelength. However, limited data is available so the occurrence of automaticity or triggered activity is still a possibility in some cases.

It is also described in Chapter 4 how Ca^{2+}-channel blockers such as verapamil can identify abnormal automaticity and in Chapters 5 and 6 how they are useful in identifying DAD-triggered activity. Verapamil does not usually terminate AF, seemingly eliminating triggered activity in those cases in which it was administered. However, data is limited.

Vagal stimulation and cholinergic agonists can accelerate or perpetuate AF. The effects of these agents indicate that perpetuation of AF is unlikely to result from focal mechanisms of automaticity or triggered activity, which should be suppressed. On the other hand, acceleration of repolarization and shortening of refractoriness decrease the wavelength and allow the presence of faster or more rotors, leading circle circuits or fragmented wavelets.

Certain antiarrhythmic drugs are important in the clinical management of AF either by stopping AF or by reducing the ventricular rate by their effect on A-V nodal conduction. They, however, in general do not establish the electrophysiological mechanisms of AF.

SUMMARY

Reentry in the atria is subdivided into macroreentrant circuits that cause macroreentrant atrial tachycardias, which include atrial flutter, and small reentrant circuits that cause reentrant focal tachycardia. Such small circuits also may play a role in the genesis of AF.

Atrial flutter is subdivided into typical and atypical flutter. Typical atrial flutter results from reentry in large anatomical circuits around natural obstacles formed by the crista terminalis and the orifices of the vena cavae, coronary sinus os, and tricuspid A-V orifice. The reentrant impulse can travel either in the counterclockwise or clockwise direction in this circuit causing counterclockwise or clockwise typical flutter. Reentry is initiated by transient conduction block in the narrow isthmus region between the coronary sinus os and tricuspid orifice, often caused by an initial period of AF. Similar unidirectional block enables typical flutter to be initiated by overdrive or premature stimulation. The typical flutter reentrant circuit has a large completely excitable gap enabling reentry to be reset and entrained. The lack of response of flutter circuits to autonomic agonists and adenosine distinguish this reentrant mechanism from automaticity and DAD-triggered activity.

Macroreentrant circuits around obstacles formed by scars caused by disease and/or surgical lesions (lesion-related reentry) also cause atrial tachycardias including atypical flutter. Reentry can be initiated and terminated by programmed electrical stimulation. These circuits also have large fully excitable gaps that enable resetting and entrainment.

Focal atrial tachycardia can be caused by reentry in small circuits most anywhere in the atria. The electrophysiological mechanisms that might cause reentrant focal tachycardia are anisotropic reentry, rotor reentry, or leading circle reentry. Focal reentrant tachycardias can be initiated by programmed electrical stimulation and can sometimes be entrained, depending on the mechanism for reentry and the properties of the excitable gap in the circuit. Some tachycardias are not affected by vagal stimulation or by adenosine, distinguishing them from automatic (transient suppression) and DAD-triggered focal tachycardia (termination). The lack of an effect suggests a fully excitable gap in those reentrant circuits. On the other hand, some focal atrial tachycardias are terminated by vagal activation and by adenosine, similar to the effects of these agents on DAD-triggered activity.

Atrial fibrillation can be divided into paroxysmal, persistent, and permanent. Different electrophysiological mechanisms for initiation and perpetuation of AF may be operative in different clinical conditions. One mechanism is characterized by a focal region that initiates rapid impulses (the driver) and a substrate formed by the mass of atrial muscle, in which there is fragmented, heterogeneous (fibrillatory) conduction of those impulses that are responsible for the fibrillatory waves on the ECG. The location of the focus may be anatomically distinct from the substrate, such as in the atrial muscle that extends into the pulmonary veins or it may occupy a small region of the substrate. The mechanism for impulse initiation in the driver might be automaticity, triggered activity, or reentry in small circuits (anisotropic, rotor, or leading circle reentry). For long lasting fibrillatory conduction to occur, the substrate must undergo electrophysiological and structural remodeling that fosters an increase in heterogeneous refractory periods and conduction.

The cause of AF may also involve substrate mechanisms without focal drivers, relying on the remodeling of electrophysiology and structure that causes enhanced heterogeneities of refractory periods and conduction. One possible mechanism causing AF is multiple reentrant circuits, either rotors or leading circle reentry that might be stable but are more likely constantly changing in size and location. A second possible mechanism based on a computer model is the multiple wavelets hypothesis dependent on breakup of atrial excitation into multiple small wavelets that propagate perpetually in random patterns at different velocities through the atria. Sustained periods of AF can be induced by rapid pacing or premature stimulation in patients with a history of paroxysmal or permanent AF which can be caused by either a reentrant or DAD-triggered mechanism. In general, the response of AF to the selected pharmacological agents that have been utilized to determine mechanisms of other arrhythmias have not been helpful in defining the mechanisms of AF.

SOURCES

Allessie MA, de Groot N, Houben RPM, et al. Electrophysiology of long-standing persistent atrial fibrillation in patients with structural heart disease: Ongitudinal dissociation. *Circ Arrhthm Electrophysiol.* 2010;3:606–615.

Allessie MA, de Groot N. Rotors have not been demonstrated to be the drivers of atrial fibrillation. *J Physiol.* 2014;592.15:3167–3170.

Cabrera JA, Sanchez-Quintanna D, Farre J, et al. The inferior right atrial isthmus: Further architectural insights for current and coming ablation technologies. *J Cardiovasc Electrophysiol.* 2005;16:402–408.

Friedman PA, Luria D, Fenton AM, et al. Global right atrial mapping of human atrial flutter: The presence of posteromedial (sinus venosa region) functional block and double potentials. A study in biplane fluoroscopy and intracardiac echocardiography. *Circulation.* 2000;101:1568–1577.

Jalife J, Berenfeld O, Mansour M. Mother rotors and fibrillatory conduction: A mechanism of atrial fibrillation. *Cardiovasc Res.* 2002;54:204–216.

Kindre C, Kall J, Kopp D, et al. Conduction properties of the inferior vena cava-tricuspid annular isthmus in patients with typical atrial flutter. *J Cardiovasc Electrophysiol.* 1997;8:727–737.

Lee G, Sanders P, Kalman JM. Catheter ablation of atrial arrhythmias: state of the art. *Lancet.* 2012;380:1509–1519.

Liu T-Y, Tai C-T, Huang B-H, et al. Functional characterization of the crista terminalis in patients with atrial flutter: Implications for radiofrequency ablation. *J Am Coll Cardiol.* 2004;43:1639–1645.

Moe GK, Rheinboldt WC, Abildskov JA. A computer model of atrial fibrillation. *Am Heart J.* 1964;67:200–220.

Narayan SM, Jalife J. Rotors have been demonstrated to drive human atrial fibrillation. *J Physiol.* 2014;592(Pt 15):3163–3166.

Nattel S, Maguy A, Le Bouter S, Yeh Y. Arrhythmogenic ion-channel remodeling in the heart: Heart failure, myocardial infarction and atrial fibrillation. *Physiol Rev.* 2007;87:425–456.

Schotten U, Verheule S, Kirchhoff P, Goette A. Physiological mechanisms of atrial fibrillation; A translational appraisal. *Physiol Rev.* 2011;91:265–325.

Shadevan LS, Khrestian CM, Durand DM, Waldo AL. High density mapping of atrial fibrillation during vagal nerve stimulation in the canine heart; restudying the Moe hypothesis. *J Cardiovasc Electrophysiol.* 2013;24:328–335.

Shah D, Jaïs P, Takahashi A, et al. Dual-loop intra-atrial reentry in humans. *Circulation.* 2000;101:631–639.

Waks JW, Josephson ME. Mechanisms of atrial fibrillation. Reentry, rotors, and reality. *Arrhythm Electrophysiol Rev.* 2014;3:90–100.

CHAPTER

11

Atrioventricular (A-V) Junctional Reentrant Arrhythmias

Supraventricular tachycardias (SVT) can be caused by reentry in circuits that utilize anatomical connections between the atria (A) and ventricles (V). These A-V junctional circuits can involve only the grossly anatomically normal A-V conducting pathway, which are a cause of A-V nodal reentrant tachycardia (AVNRT). They can also comprise the normal conducting pathway and an accessory pathway or bypass tract that forms an additional anatomical and electrophysiological pathway between atria and ventricles, causing circus movement reentrant tachycardia.

AVNRT is the most common form of SVT, accounting for approximately 50% of cases. Automaticity in the A-V junction (Chapter 3, Section 3B), triggered activity in the A-V junction (Chapter 6, Section 6B), and reentry utilizing a bypass tract constitute the other 50% of SVTs.

Reentrant Excitation in the Normal A-V Junction

AV NODAL REENTRANT TACHYCARDIA (AVNRT)

ECG Characteristics

The ECG in **Figure 11-1** shows the onset of typical A-V nodal reentrant tachycardia (AVNRT) (see Figure 11-2 below for comparison of "typical" and "atypical" AVNRT and a description of the reentrant circuits).

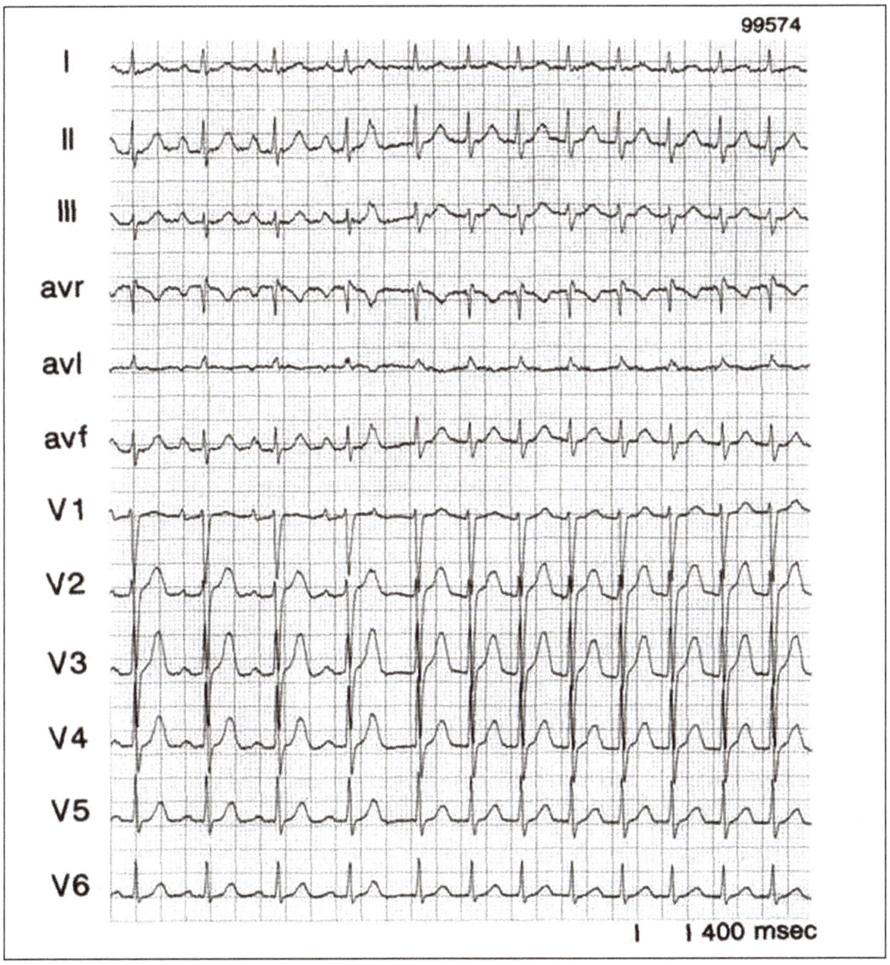

Figure 11-1 A 12-lead ECG recorded during onset of typical A-V nodal reentrant tachycardia (Wellens' ECG collection).

Electrophysiological Foundations of Cardiac Arrhythmias: A Bridge Between Basic Mechanisms and Clinical Electrophysiology, Second Edition.
 Cardiotext Publishing, ISBN: 978-1-942909-42-2.

The first four complexes have a sinus origin. A premature atrial impulse follows the fourth sinus impulse, indicated by a P wave superimposed on the T wave. The P-R interval of the premature impulse is prolonged and followed by a tachycardia with a supraventricular QRS morphology and inverted P waves in the inferior ECG leads. Typical AVNRT has a long P-R and a short R-P interval (also see Figure 11-2, left panel) because the reentrant circuit has a slowly conducting antegrade pathway through which the ventricles are activated and a much more rapidly conducting retrograde pathway through which the atria are activated (described in detail below). It is therefore also referred to as "slow/fast AVNRT."

Supraventricular tachycardia (SVT) caused by AVNRT has rates that range from 100–280 bpm with a mean of approximately 170 bpm. Rates are usually slower in patients over the age of 50. Holter monitoring in such patients demonstrates atrial premature depolarizations (APDs) and isolated atrial echo beats between episodes. The SVT in Figure 11-1 begins after an APD that is characteristic of this arrhythmia.

P Waves in AVNRT

The P waves during typical (slow/fast) AVNRT are inverted in the inferior leads, indicating earliest atrial activation in the inferior atrial septum where the atrial exit route from the junctional reentrant circuit begins to depolarize atrial myocardium (**Figure 11-2**, left panel).

Nearly simultaneous activation of both atria usually leads to a narrow (40–50 ms) P wave. In most patients with typical AVNRT, the onset of atrial activation occurs after onset or in the middle of the QRS. Occasionally, the P wave begins early enough to give the appearance of a Q wave in the inferior leads. This is most likely to occur when there is delay between the time the impulse exits the reentrant circuit and the time it begins to activate the ventricles. When this occurs, it is usually because there is delay between activation of the His bundle and ventricles (H-V prolongation) due to conduction system disease. More frequently, however, atrial activation begins within the QRS. In these patients, either no discrete P waves are noted on the surface ECG, or the terminal part of the QRS is slightly distorted, appearing as a "pseudo-S wave" in the inferior leads, and a "pseudo-R" in V_1. Rarely, the P waves occur just after the end of the QRS. A 1:1 relation usually exists between atrial and ventricular events in slow/fast AVNRT, but occasionally 2:1 block occurs with block either in the A-V node or in the His-Purkinje system.

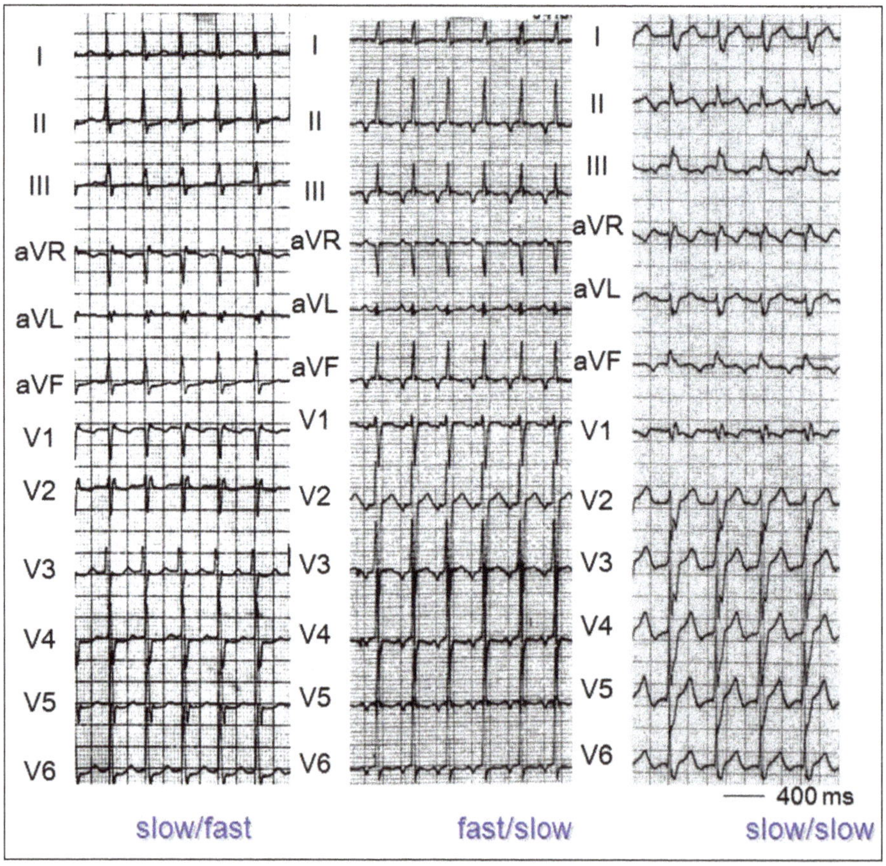

Figure 11-2 P-wave location in different types of A-V nodal reentrant tachycardia (Wellens' ECG collection).

ECG in Atypical AVNRT

As explained below, the fast conduction pathway in the reentrant circuit may sometimes conduct antegradely and the slow pathway retrogradely. This tachycardia is referred to as atypical, uncommon, or "fast/slow AVNRT." As shown in Figure 11-2, middle panel, the ECG in patients with this type of tachycardia exhibits a long R-P interval (retrograde conduction) and a short P-R interval (antegrade conduction) with negative retrograde P waves in leads II, III, and aVF.

Rarely, both antegrade and retrograde conducting pathways in the circuit are slowly conducting leading to "slow/slow AVNRT" (Figure 11-2, right panel). Inverted P waves in the inferior leads occur well after the QRS, usually in the middle of two QRS complexes.

Location, Anatomy, and Electrophysiological Properties of Reentrant Circuits

The anatomy and cellular electrophysiology of the normal A-V conducting system is described in Chapter 3, Section 3B and depicted in Figure 3-12 and Figure 3-13. The precise location of reentrant circuits causing AVNRT within this conducting system is uncertain. Although referred to as A-V nodal reentry, only part of the circuit may involve the actual node or compact node (CN in Figure 3-12) and the remaining segments may reside elsewhere within the triangle of Koch or even partly outside the triangle. In addition, whether the circuits have discrete anatomical pathways (anatomical circuit) or are formed by the functional properties (functional circuit) caused by different conduction and refractory properties of A-V junctional myocardium is also a subject of debate. However, the basic electrophysiological characteristics and requirements of the reentrant circuit causing AVNRT can still be described independently of its exact location and the exact nature of the circuit using a dual-pathway model.

A Model of Reentry Using Dual Pathways in the A-V Node

In its simplest form, a model for A-V nodal reentry consists of two conducting pathways within the A-V junction, between the connection of the circuit to the atria above and ventricles below (**Figure 11-3**). This model is referred to as dual A-V nodal conducting pathways even though the two pathways may not be in the anatomical A-V node. In Figure 11-3, the pathways are pictured as discrete entities, which might be determined either by anatomical structures, functional electrophysiological properties alone, or a combination of both (see below). One pathway, referred to as the slow pathway, has slow conduction and shorter refractory periods. The other pathway, referred to as the fast pathway, has faster conduction and longer refractory periods. (Note the similarity to the model described in Figure 9-1). The two pathways connect with each other at the atrial and ventricular ends to form the reentrant circuit, although the exact location of the connections is arguable. In this and all subsequent figures in this chapter, arrows are used only to show the pathway of impulse propagation. The length of the arrow tails are not meant to show the duration of the wavelength as depicted in some of the figures in Chapter 9.

During sinus rhythm, the atrial impulse conducts through both pathways (Figure 11-3, Panel A) but reaches the ventricles first through the fast pathway (green arrow) to produce the QRS. The impulse conducting simultaneously, but more slowly, down the slow pathway (dashed red arrow) reaches the lower part of the A-V node or His bundle after it has been depolarized and rendered refractory by the fast pathway impulse, and therefore does not contribute to ventricular activation. The P-R interval on the ECG (above in Panel A) is determined by conduction time in the fast pathway.

Figure 11-3, Panel B shows conduction through the A-V junction of a premature atrial impulse occurring at a short coupling interval to the previous sinus impulse. The premature impulse blocks in the fast pathway due to its longer refractory period (green arrow and horizontal bar) and proceeds slowly down the slow pathway (dashed red arrows). The ventricles are now activated through the slow pathway that leads to a sudden prolongation in the P-R interval (ECG above Panel B). This shift from fast to slow pathway caused the prolonged P-R interval of the premature impulse in Figure 11-1. Figure 11-3, Panel B also shows the impulse from the slow pathway entering the fast pathway in the retrograde direction but blocking (dashed red arrow and horizontal bar).

Figure 11-3, Panel C, diagrams conduction of an earlier premature atrial impulse (green arrow). The impulse blocks in the fast pathway (small green arrow and horizontal bar). Conduction through the slow pathway is slower (dashed red arrow) because it has had less time to recover full excitability from the previous sinus impulse. The additional slowing allows the previously refractory fast pathway time to recover (wavelength is shorter than path length), and an atrial reentrant impulse (an "atrial echo," indicated by red QRS complex above) results from retrograde propagation of the impulse in the fast pathway to the atria (solid red arrow). If the slow pathway does not recover excitability in time to permit subsequent antegrade conduction, only the single atrial echo occurs (block in the slow pathway indicated by red arrow and horizontal bar). However, if conduction around the circuit is sufficiently slow, which happens at a critically short premature cycle length, the impulse returning to cause the atrial echo can again enter

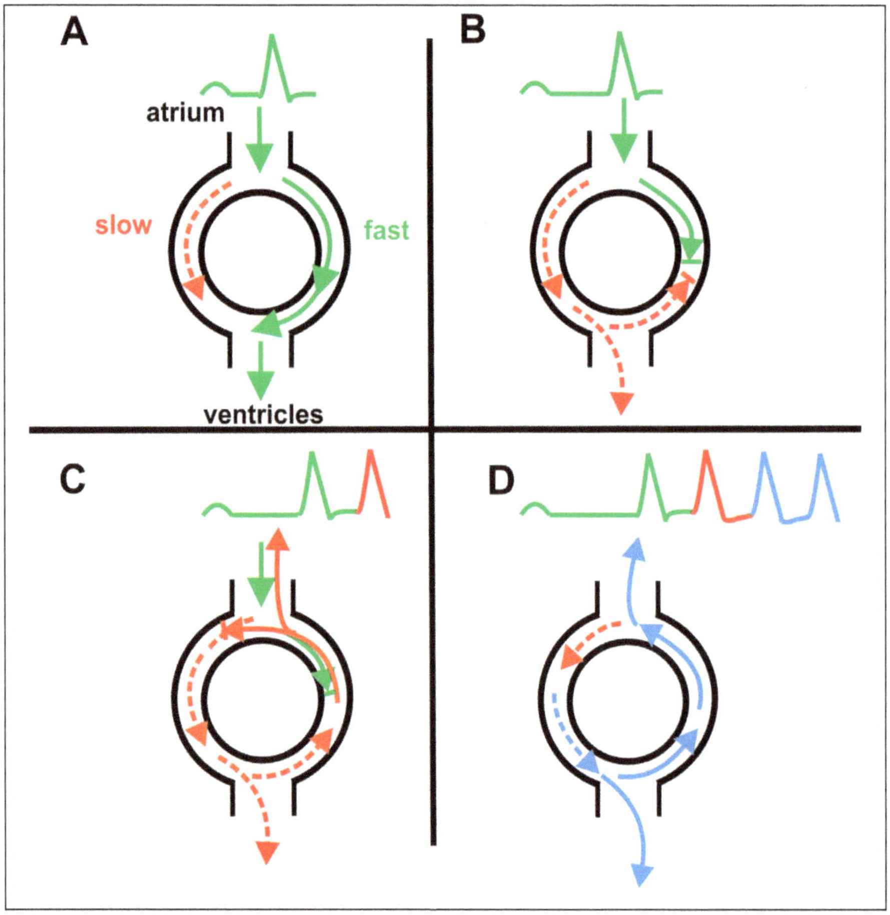

Figure 11-3 Model of a reentrant circuit in the A-V junction causing typical AVNRT. **Panel A** represents a sinus impulse, **Panel B** a premature atrial impulse, **Panel C** an earlier premature impulse, and **Panel D** depicts initiation of continuous reentry.

the slow pathway (Figure 11-3, Panel D, dashed red arrow) and travel through the reentrant circuit repetitively (blue arrows), causing AVNRT (blue QRS complexes above). Once reentry is initiated, the slow pathway must be able to conduct repetitively at short cycle lengths (less than about 350 ms) for sustained tachycardia to occur. Spontaneous termination of typical AVNRT occurs because of block of the reentrant impulse—either retrogradely in the fast pathway or antegradely in the slow pathway.

The two (dual) pathways of the reentrant circuit in patients with typical AVNRT can be revealed by a sudden increase ("jump") in the A-H interval in the His bundle recording that precedes the onset of AVNRT as shown in **Figure 11-4**.

The first two sinus beats (sinus cycle 970 ms) have an A-H interval of 70 ms that represents conduction through the fast pathway (red arrow) (see Figure 11-3, Panel A). An atrial premature depolarization (APD) with a coupling interval of 420 ms (black arrow above lead III) conducts to the ventricles with a sudden increase of the A-H interval to 240 ms (red arrow) that indicates block in the fast pathway and a shift in conduction to the slow pathway (diagrammed in Figure 11-3, Panels B and C). This leads to the onset of AVNRT (horizontal bar above lead I) when the impulse returns to the atria via the fast pathway (short blue arrow). During tachycardia conduction in the slow pathway of the circuit is indicated by the red arrows and conduction in the fast pathway by the blue arrows in Figure 11-4.

The ECG in Figure 11-4 also shows that the interval from the R wave to the atrial electrogram (R-P interval) is short because retrograde conduction in the circuit is through the fast pathway (from His bundle (H) to atrium (Ae) indicated by the blue arrow). Conduction from the atrial (Ae) to His bundle electrogram (H) and R wave (P-R interval, red arrow) is long because of antegrade conduction through the slow pathway. As a result, the P wave occurs at the end of the QRS (see lead I).

Atypical AVNRT. Occasionally, the fast pathway may have a shorter refractory period than the slow pathway. As a result, block of premature atrial impulses occur in the slow pathway, resulting in atypical AVNRT.

In atypical AVNRT, the P-R interval is only modestly prolonged because of modest slowing in the fast pathway while block in the slow pathway is concealed. There is no sudden, large jump in conduction time from atrium to ventricles to reveal the presence of dual pathways, as explained in **Figure 11-5**.

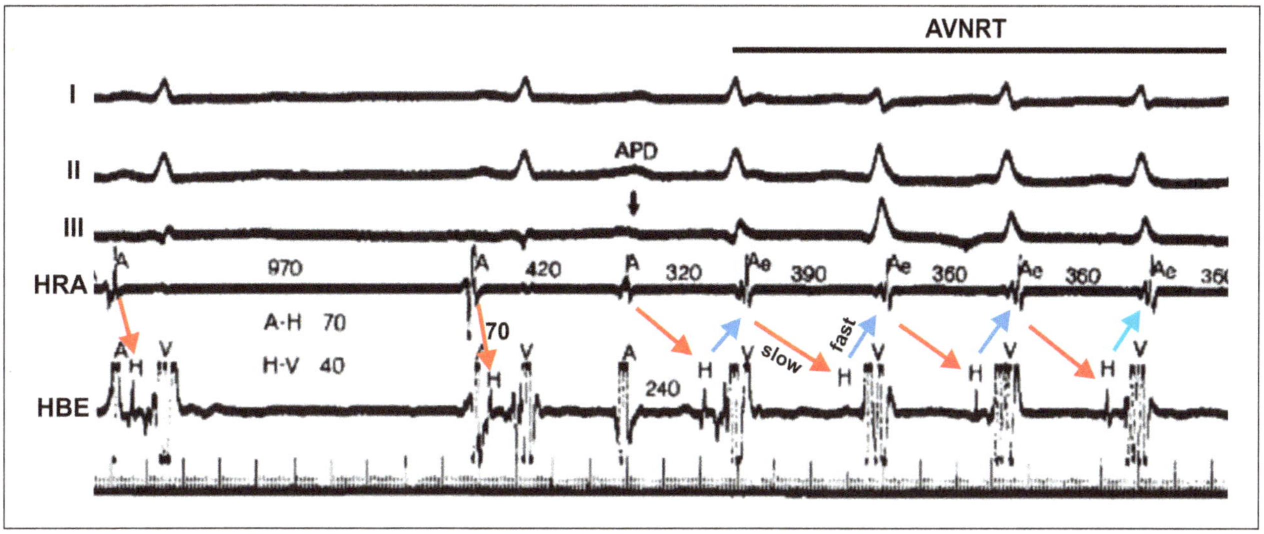

Figure 11-4 Onset of typical AVNRT. ECG leads I, II, and III are shown with electrograms from the high right atrium (HRA; A is atrial electrogram of sinus and atrial premature depolarization [APD]; Ae is atrial electrogram during AVNRT) and His bundle (HBE; A is atrial, H is His bundle, V is ventricular electrogram). (Reproduced from Josephson ME. *Josephson's Clinical Cardiac Electrophysiology: Techniques and Interpretations* (5th ed.). Philadelphia, PA: Wolters Kluwer; 2016.)

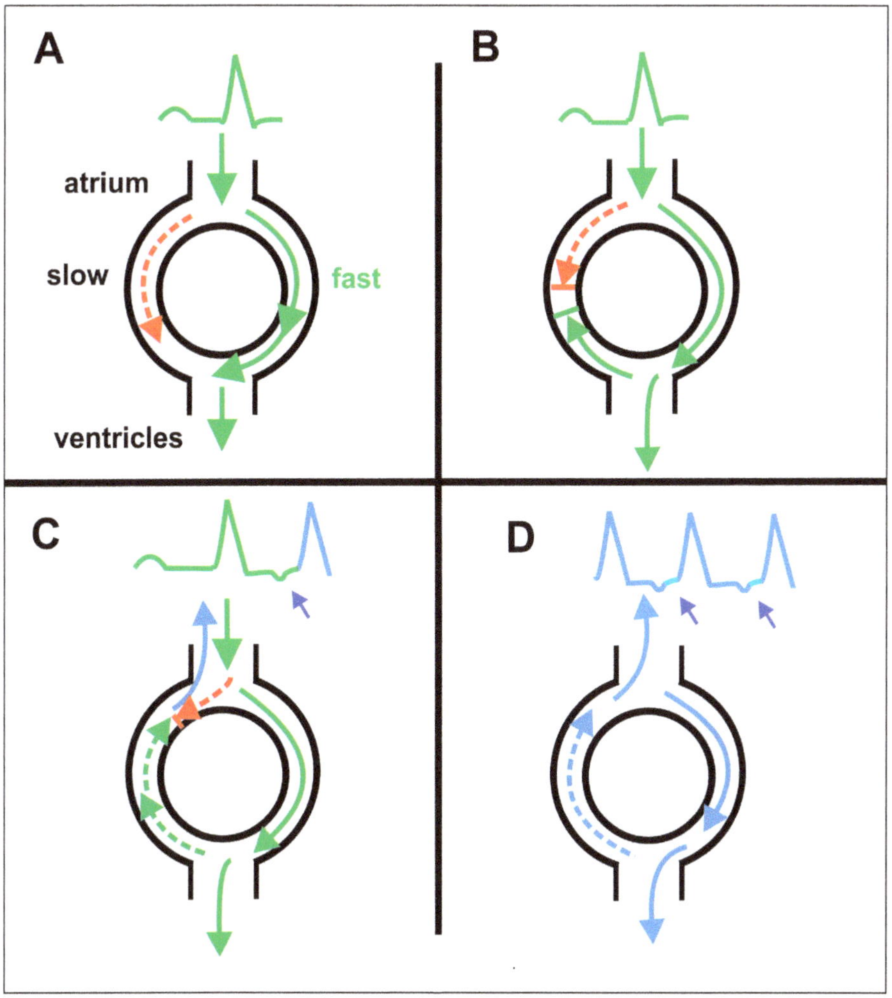

Figure 11-5 A model of reentrant circuit causing atypical AVNRT. **Panel A** shows sinus impulse. **Panels B** and **C** show premature atrial impulses. **Panel D** illustrates the initiation of AVNRT.

The initiation of atypical AVNRT is diagrammed in Figure 11-5. Panel A shows conduction of a sinus impulse through the A-V junction with the impulse conducting through the fast pathway (green arrow) activating the His bundle and ventricles as previously described in Figure 11-3. During sinus rhythm the shorter refractory period of the fast pathway is not evident. In Panel B, conduction of an early premature impulse blocks in the slow pathway (dashed red arrows and horizontal red bar) while still conducting through the fast pathway (green arrows) because of its shorter refractory period. Retrograde conduction of this impulse blocks if it arrives at the distal end of the slow pathway too early (Figure 11-5, Panel B, green arrow and horizontal bar). At a sufficiently short cycle length (Panel C) block of the premature impulse occurs in the slow pathway (dashed red arrow), and successful conduction antegrade occurs through the fast pathway (green arrow) and retrograde through the slow pathway (Panel C, dashed green arrow). This leads to a reentrant atrial echo (Panel C, blue arrow and ECG above). The occurrence of a reentrant impulse without a large jump in the P-R interval is the only evidence that block must have occurred in the slow pathway. The reentrant impulse can then continue to conduct again into the fast pathway (Panel D, blue arrow) and around the circuit (dashed blue arrow) to cause atypical AVNRT. For this atypical AVNRT to occur, the slow pathway must be able to conduct retrogradely at short cycle lengths (less than about 400 ms). During atypical AVNRT, the P-R is short because of fast antegrade conduction, resulting in P waves before the QRS (arrows on ECG above in Panel D) and a long R-P interval because of slow retrograde conduction.

Electrophysiological Mechanisms for Reentry and Location of Reentrant Circuits Causing AVNRT

Figures 11-3 and 11-5 show simplified descriptions of the characteristics and properties of reentrant circuits causing AVNRT. However, it is uncertain if the dual pathway properties reside in different well-defined anatomical pathways (anatomical circuits) or if these properties are caused by the electrophysiological properties of the different types of myocardial cells that occur in the triangle of Koch (functional circuits). Also, the exact location of the different components of the circuit is controversial.

Are Reentrant Circuits Causing AVNRT Functional? Functional reentrant circuits described in Chapter 9 (Figures 9-18, 9-19, and 9-20) result from electrophysiological properties of the myocardial cells rather than anatomically defined pathways. As described in Figure 3-13, variations in resting potentials, and phase 0 depolarization of transitional (AN cells in Figure 3-13) and compact nodal cells (N cells in Figure 3-13) contribute to regional differences in conduction velocities within the A-V junction. There are also large variations in refractory periods in different regions of the A-V junction due to the different characteristics of the action potentials. These variations in conduction properties and refractory periods can provide a substrate, without the presence of anatomically discrete pathways, where cells with more rapid conduction and longer refractory periods form the fast pathway and cells with slower conduction and shorter refractory periods form the slow pathway.

Reentry in a substrate characterized by heterogeneities in conduction and refractory periods can occur by mechanisms similar to the "leading circle" (Figure 9-18). A premature impulse entering the junctional region blocks in the region with long refractory periods that represents the fast pathway. Slowed conduction continues through regions with shorter refractory periods representing the slow pathway. Slow conduction in the circuit is attributed to propagation of the reentrant wavefront in partially refractory transitional and nodal cells. Functional reentry caused by this mechanism might occur either in more than one region within the A-V junction or at a specific anatomical site. A region of slow conduction coincides with the right (posterior) extension (Figure 3-12) that has been proposed to be the location of the slow pathway, and a region of faster conduction forming a fast pathway may coincide with the AN cells connecting the anterior atrial septum to the CN.

Another possible functional mechanism for reentry in the A-V junction is anisotropic reentry caused by nonuniform anisotropy (see Figure 9-11 and Figure 9-20). In the A-V junction and A-V node, it is caused by the irregular distribution of gap junctions, the mix of different connexins with different conductances that form the gap junctions, and the presence of fibrous septae that separate myocytes into bundles. Conduction properties in a nonuniformly anisotropic substrate can mimic the properties of dual A-V nodal pathways. Fast conduction in the (longitudinal) direction that is better coupled forms the fast pathway. Slow propagation in the more poorly coupled (transverse) direction forms the slow pathway. The properties of nonuniform anisotropic myocardium also explain the longer refractory periods associated with the direction of faster conduction and shorter refractory periods associated with the direction of slower conduction. As explained in Figure 9-20, conduction block of premature impulses in the fast direction occurs at longer cycle lengths because of the excessive electrical load than conduction block in the transverse direction. In the transverse direction, slow transverse conduction is associated with shorter refractory periods because in this direction conduction is more resistant to decreases in the membrane depolarizing currents of premature action potentials. These properties coincide with the properties of the dual A-V nodal pathways described in Figure 11-3. The AN and the right (posterior) extension of the node have nonuniform anisotropic structure and conduction properties suggesting they might form part of the substrate for anisotropic reentrant circuits.

Some data from clinical electrophysiology studies support a functional model. AVNRT induced by programmed premature stimulation (see Figure 11-6) can have different cycle lengths depending on the atrial site of stimulation, indicating changes in a functional reentrant circuit and not a fixed anatomical circuit. Also, earliest atrial activation during AVNRT may occur at multiple or changing sites or over a wide region. Activation spreads superiorly without a fixed pattern that could be interpreted to indicate the absence of a specific anatomical atrial pathway between the retrograde and antegrade pathways.

There is also controversy concerning the location of the connection between slow and fast pathways at the atrial end of the circuit. This connection might be through AN transitional cells within the triangle of Koch. Alternatively, atrial myocardium outside the triangle could be involved. Lack of atrial myocardial participation in some reentrant circuits is suggested by the occurrence of A-V nodal echoes and AVNRT in the absence of atrial depolarization.

The connection between slow and fast pathways at the lower part of the circuit toward the ventricles might occur proximal to the CN, in the CN or in the NH region. The connection is proximal to the His bundle and bundle branches since bundle branch block can occur during AVNRT without affecting the tachycardia cycle length and AVNRT can occur with various degrees of A-V block proximal to the His bundle.

Are Reentrant Circuits Causing AVNRT Anatomical? An alternative model is AVNRT caused by an anatomical reentrant circuit formed by discrete anatomical structures. A possible anatomical circuit causing slow/fast AVNRT utilizes antegrade conduction in the right (posterior nodal) extension as the slow pathway, turn around from the antegrade to retrograde limb in the lower nodal (NH) region where AN transitional cells that form the fast pathway insert into the lower CN and retrograde conduction through a fast pathway beginning in these transitional AN cells, which gradually turn into atrial cells. Retrograde conduction through the fast pathway activates the left atrial septum, propagating inferiorly to activate atrial myocardium in the coronary sinus that acts as a bridge to the right side through the coronary sinus ostium through which the impulse enters the right (posterior) extension slow pathway to complete the circuit. In this model, atrial myocardium forms an important part of the reentrant circuit.

Evidence leading to the formulation of this model is sometimes contrary to evidence for the functional models described above and the differences remain to be resolved. Evidence for the anatomical model includes: (1) the fast pathway can be ablated at the apex, and the slow pathway at the base of the triangle of Koch remote from the compact AVN, (2) retrograde activation of the atria during slow/fast and fast/slow AVNRT occurs at discrete regions consistent with the anatomical connections of the fast and slow pathways in the model.

Effects of Electrical Stimulation

A property that is characteristic of reentrant arrhythmias is initiation by electrical stimulation, either premature stimulation or overdrive pacing.

Initiation of Typical AVNRT by Premature and Overdrive Stimulation

Figure 11-6 illustrates initiation of typical AVNRT in a patient with a history of this arrhythmia, by premature stimulation from the right atrium during sinus rhythm.

In Panel A, a stimulated premature impulse with a coupling interval of 390 ms (black arrow) has an A-H interval of 105 ms (see HBE recording), compared to the A-H of 35 ms of the previous sinus impulse. Conduction of the premature impulse from atrium (A) to His bundle (H) is through the fast pathway (see Figure 11-3, Panel A). The A-H interval of the premature impulse increases modestly to 145 ms in Figure 11-6, Panel B at a premature coupling interval of 380 ms (black arrow) with conduction still through the fast pathway. In Panel C, a further small decrease in coupling to 365 ms (black arrow) results in a large increase of the A-H interval to 500 ms (first slanted red arrow), representing block in the fast pathway and maintained conduction through the slow pathway as diagrammed in Figure 11-3, Panels B–D. This jump is followed by a reentrant impulse returning to the atrium (short blue arrow) and typical slow/fast AVNRT during which antegrade conduction is through the slow pathway (red arrows from A to H) and retrograde conduction through the fast pathway (blue arrows from H to A). The slowly conducting impulse in the slow pathway allows sufficient time for recovery of the fast pathway for retrograde propagation as diagrammed in Figure 11-3. The jump in A-H interval indicates a switch from the fast to slow pathway. In this case the increase in A-H interval is unusually large although sudden increases in the A-H interval from 70 to 300 ms can occur.

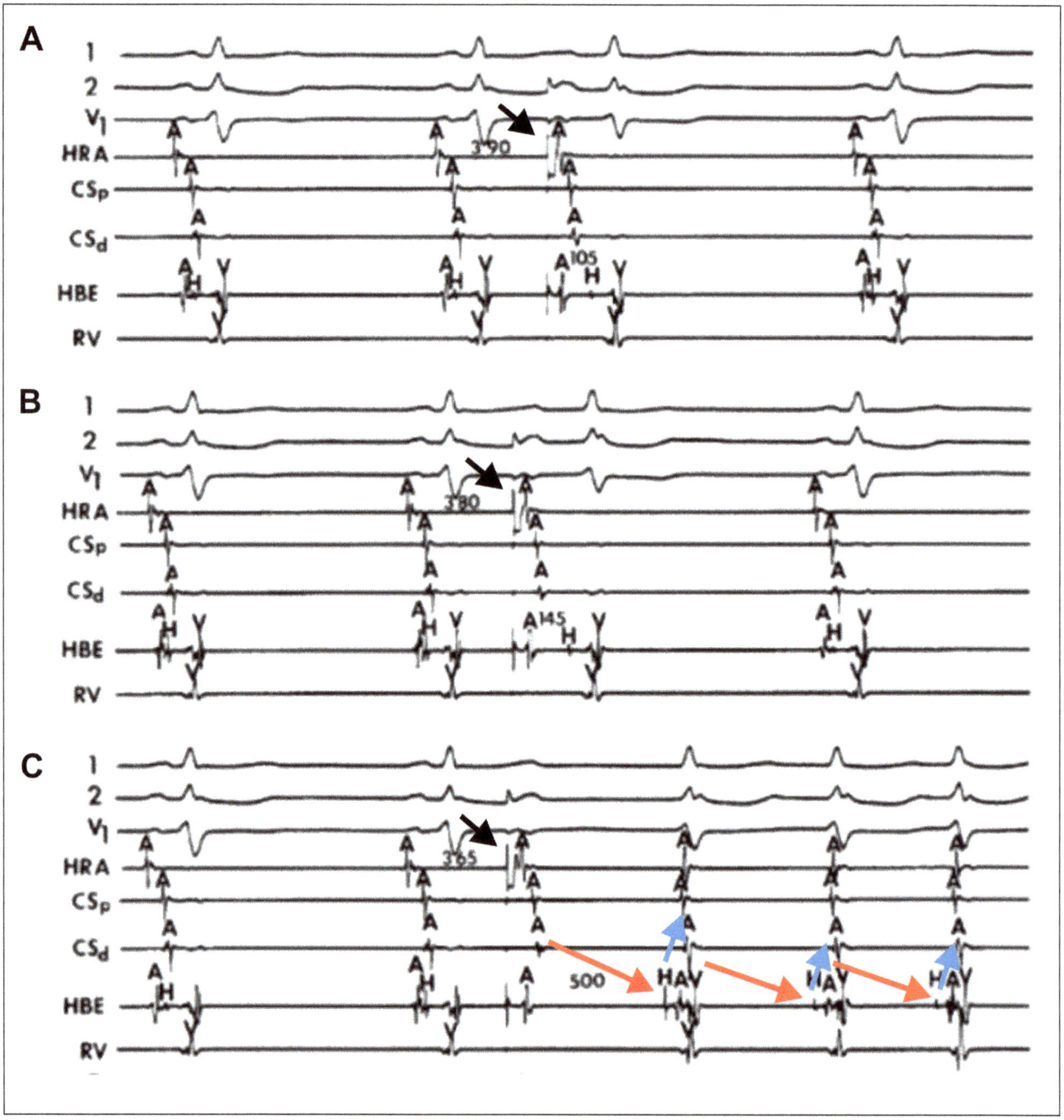

Figure 11-6 Initiation of typical AVNRT by premature stimulation. ECG leads I, II, and V_1, and electrograms from high right atrium (HRA), proximal and distal coronary sinus (CSp and CSd), His bundle (HBE), and right ventricle (RV) are displayed. A, atrial electrogram; H, His bundle electrogram; V, ventricular electrograms. (Reproduced from Josephson ME. *Josephson's Clinical Cardiac Electrophysiology: Techniques and Interpretations* (5th ed.). Philadelphia, PA: Wolters Kluwer; 2016.)

Typical (slow/fast) AVNRT can also be initiated by overdrive pacing. A large increase in the A-H interval representing the switch from fast to slow pathway conduction also precedes onset of AVNRT.

The "jump" in A-H interval as an indicator of dual pathways. A graph showing the relationship of A-V nodal conduction of the premature impulse (A_2-H_2 interval) to the premature coupling interval (A_1-A_2) for another patient with AVNRT is shown in **Figure 11-7**.

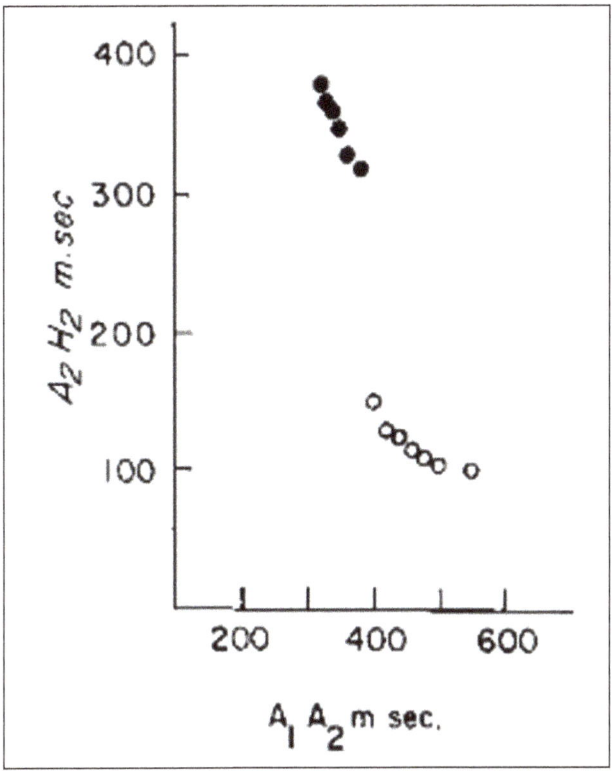

Figure 11-7 Relationship between atrial premature coupling interval (A_1-A_2) on the abscissa vs. A-V junctional conduction time of the premature impulse to the His bundle on the ordinate (A_2-H_2). (Reproduced from Josephson ME. *Josephson's Clinical Cardiac Electrophysiology: Techniques and Interpretations* (5th ed.). Philadelphia, PA: Wolters Kluwer; 2016.)

There is a modest increase in A_2-H_2 conduction time as A_1-A_2 coupling interval decreases from 575 to 370 ms representing an increase in conduction time over the fast pathway that occurs as the premature impulse encounters increasing relatively refractory tissue. At an A_1-A_2 of 370 ms, a marked increase (a "jump") occurs in A_2-H_2 as the atrial impulse blocks in the fast pathway and conduction proceeds through the slow pathway. AVNRT is associated with this sudden increase in A_2-H_2 interval (filled circles). This sudden jump in the A_2-H_2 interval indicates dual A-V nodal conducting pathways. An increase of at least 50 ms in the A-H interval with a small (i.e., 10 ms) decrease in the coupling interval of the atrial premature impulse is considered to be the criterion for dual pathways, although arbitrary. A further decrease in the A_1-A_2 interval from 370–230 ms in Figure 11-7 causes further prolongation of the A_2-H_2 interval representing slowing of conduction of the premature impulse in the relative refractory period of the slow pathway. All coupling intervals in this range are associated with initiation of AVNRT (filled circles). Because of this increase in conduction time through the slow pathway, there is an inverse relationship between the premature coupling interval (A_1-A_2) and the coupling interval to the first impulse of tachycardia (A_2-A_3), a hallmark of initiation of reentry as explained Figure 9-25.

Initiation of Atypical (Fast/Slow) AVNRT

Initiation of atypical AVNRT (Figure 11-5) either by premature or overdrive atrial stimulation is not associated with the sudden increase in the A-H interval. In atypical AVNRT antegrade conduction remains through the fast pathway during onset of tachycardia and does not switch to the slow pathway that is responsible for the sudden increase ov A-V nodal conduction time in typical AVNRT. This characteristic is illustrated in **Figure 11-8** during initiation of atypical AVNRT by atrial overdrive pacing at a cycle length of 400 ms (horizontal black bar). There is only a modest increase in A-H that proceeds the onset of tachycardia (compare diagonal red arrow at left which is A-V conduction during pacing with second red arrow to the right which is A-V conduction time at initiation of AVNRT). Onset of tachycardia occurs when there is retrograde conduction through the slow pathway indicated by the longer diagonal blue arrow.

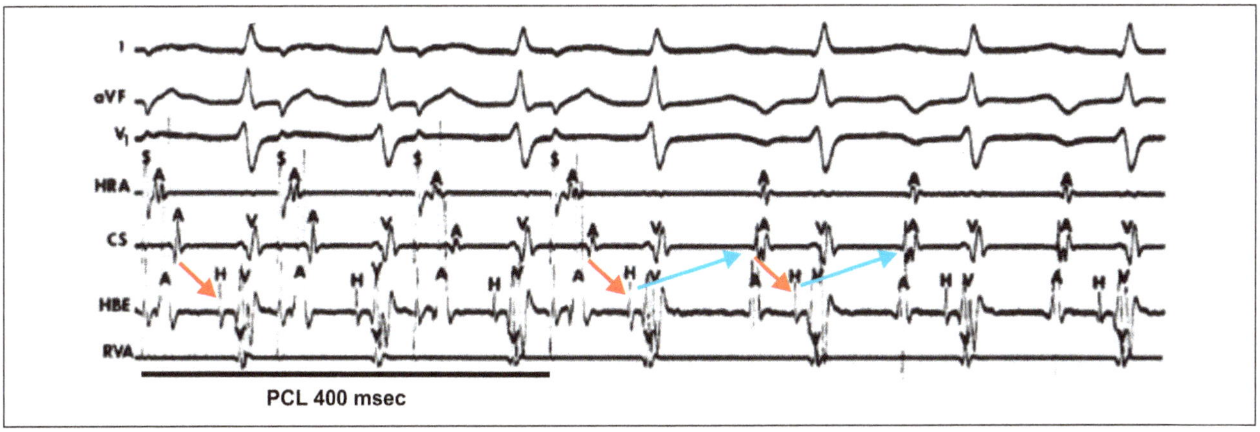

Figure 11-8 Initiation of atypical AVNRT by overdrive pacing. ECG leads I, aVF, and V_1, and electrograms from the high right atrium (HRA; S, stimulus artifact; A, atrial electrogram), coronary sinus (Cs; A, atrial; V, ventricular), and His bundle (HBE; A, atrial; H, His bundle; V, ventricular). (Reproduced from Josephson ME. *Josephson's Clinical Cardiac Electrophysiology: Techniques and Interpretations* (5th ed.). Philadelphia, PA: Wolters Kluwer; 2016.)

Initiation by Ventricular Stimulation

AVNRT can also be initiated by ventricular stimulation during ventricular pacing. During ventricular stimulation, initiation of typical AVNRT occurs less frequently than that of atypical AVNRT. Diagrams of impulse conduction for both typical and atypical AVNRT during ventricular stimulation are shown in **Figure 11-9**.

In Figure 11-9, Panels A–C diagram conduction for initiation of typical AVNRT. Impulses initiated by ventricular stimulation conduct more rapidly to activate the atria through the fast pathway (solid green arrow, Panel A). (Conduction in the slow pathway is represented by the dashed green arrow). Induction of typical AVNRT by rapid pacing or by a premature stimulated impulse depends on retrograde conduction block in the slow pathway (dashed green arrow with horizontal bar in Panel B). Therefore, the refractory period of the slow pathway must exceed the fast pathway in this retrograde direction from ventricle to atrium. This usually occurs in patients with spontaneously occurring atypical AVNRT since the slow pathway has a longer effective refractory period than the fast pathway in these patients. However, a longer retrograde effective refractory period in the slow pathway than the fast pathway occasionally occurs in patients in whom the fast pathway has a longer refractory period in the antegrade direction. Directional differences in refractory periods may be related to variations in axial current flow in different directions, as explained in Figure 9-15 and Figure 9-16. In Panel C, reentry then results from antegrade conduction through the slow pathway (dashed blue arrow) and retrograde conduction through the fast pathway (Panel C, blue arrow).

Ventricular premature impulses or ventricular pacing induce typical AVNRT in the absence of a sudden increase in A-V junctional conduction time that usually is the indicator of dual pathways (see simulated ECG above Panels A and B where the R-P interval does not significantly change). Retrograde conduction proceeds up the fast pathway both during the basic rhythm (Panel A) and after retrograde block in the slow pathway (Panel B). Block in the slow pathway is concealed and only inferred by initiation of tachycardia. Retrograde block in the slow pathway is easier to achieve with ventricular pacing than premature ventricular impulses. If the slow pathway is comprised mostly of typical A-V nodal cells, a decrease in basic pacing cycle length would readily cause rate-dependent conduction delay and block.

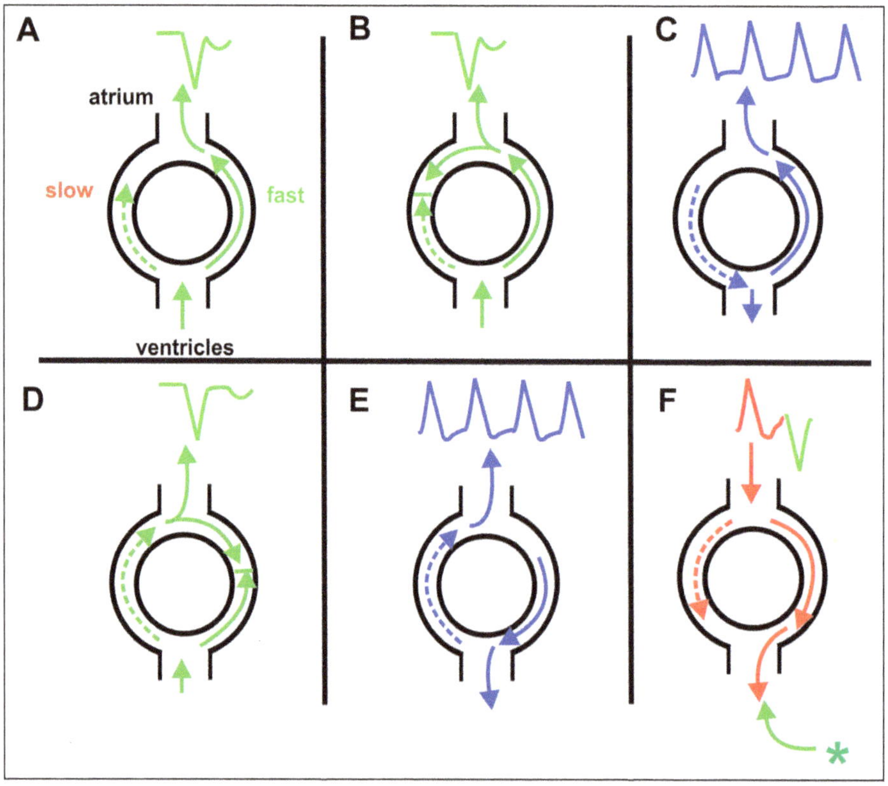

Figure 11-9 **Panels A–C:** Pattern of propagation of ventricular impulses to cause typical AVNRT. **Panels D** and **E:** Pattern of propagation of ventricular impulses to cause atypical AVNRT. **Panel F:** Failure of ventricular stimulated impulses to propagate into the circuit when it is activated by sinus impulses.

In contrast to typical AVNRT, atypical AVNRT can be induced almost as frequently from the ventricle as from the atrium. Figure 11-9, Panels D and E, diagrams the pattern of impulse propagation during initiation when the fast pathway has a longer refractory period. Retrograde block in the fast pathway during rapid pacing or premature stimulation is indicated in Panel D by the green arrow and horizontal bar. Retrograde conduction through the slow pathway is indicated by the dashed green arrow. Subsequent antegrade conduction of the impulse from the slow pathway that propagates into the fast pathway (Panel E, blue arrow), results in reentry and atypical AVNRT.

Figure 11-9, Panel F, shows why AVNRT is usually not initiated by ventricular stimulation (or spontaneously occurring ventricular premature impulses) when the A-V junction is being activated in the antegrade direction from atria to ventricles such as during sinus rhythm or atrial pacing. Ventricular stimulated impulses (green asterisk and arrow) collide with atrial impulses (red arrows), emerging from the A-V node, in the His bundle or bundle branches. The stimulated impulses cannot reach the A-V nodal pathways to initiate reentry as shown in Panels B and D.

Resetting, Entrainment, and Termination

Premature atrial impulses can reset the reentrant circuit causing both typical and atypical AVNRT because the circuit has a spatial and temporal excitable gap. The wavelength of A-V junctional reentrant impulses causing AVNRT changes as they propagate around the circuit. The spatial excitable gap is largest during slow pathway conduction when the wavelength is shortest and smallest during fast pathway conduction when the wavelength is longest (see Figure 9-3 for explanation).

A model of resetting and termination of typical AVNRT by a premature atrial impulse is described in **Figure 11-10.** Panel A diagrams a long coupled atrial premature impulse that does not penetrate the circuit. The blue arrow depicts the reentrant impulse with the inexcitable segment of the wavelength indicated by the solid blue tail, partially excitable segment by the dashed blue line and fully excitable gap by the clear region. The green arrow indicates the stimulated atrial impulse arriving at the circuit while the entrance is refractory and therefore, not resetting the circuit. In this case, the next reentrant impulse comes precisely on time, that is, the cycle length to the next impulse is compensatory.

Figure 11-10, Panel B, shows that earlier (shorter coupled) premature impulses penetrate the circuit to reset it. The stimulated impulse (green arrow) collides with the reentrant impulse in the fast pathway (blue arrow) and conducts antegradely in the slow pathway (B_1) to traverse the entire circuit (B_2) and emerge in the atrium as the reset impulse (green arrow in B_2). An inverse relationship is expected between the premature cycle length (coupling interval between the premature impulse and the previous tachycardia impulse, A_1-A_2) and the return cycle length (coupling interval between the premature impulse and the next tachycardia impulse, A_2-A_3) such that the return cycle length increases as the premature impulse occurs earlier (see Figure 9-28) even though there is a fully excitable gap. The earlier the premature impulse, the more slowly it conducts in the slow pathway because of its A-V nodal characteristics of time dependent refractoriness. Conduction of very early premature impulses may be so slow that there may be no evidence of resetting on the ECG even though the premature impulse successfully penetrated the circuit. If the atrial premature impulse (green arrow) penetrates the circuit early enough (Figure 11-10, Panel C), it will block antegradely in the slow pathway (green arrow and horizontal bar) and collide with the reentrant wavefront (blue arrow) in the fast pathway to terminate reentry and the arrhythmia.

Termination of AVNRT by a premature atrial impulse (A_1) in a clinical study is illustrated in **Figure 11-11** (premature stimulus indicated by the arrow).

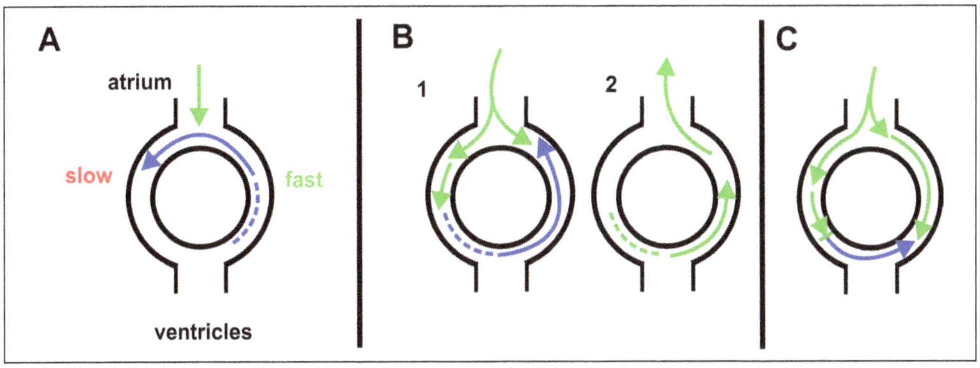

Figure 11-10 Resetting of typical AVNRT. **Panel A** shows a late coupled premature impulse. **Panel B (1 and 2)** shows an earlier premature impulse. **Panel C** shows termination of reentry.

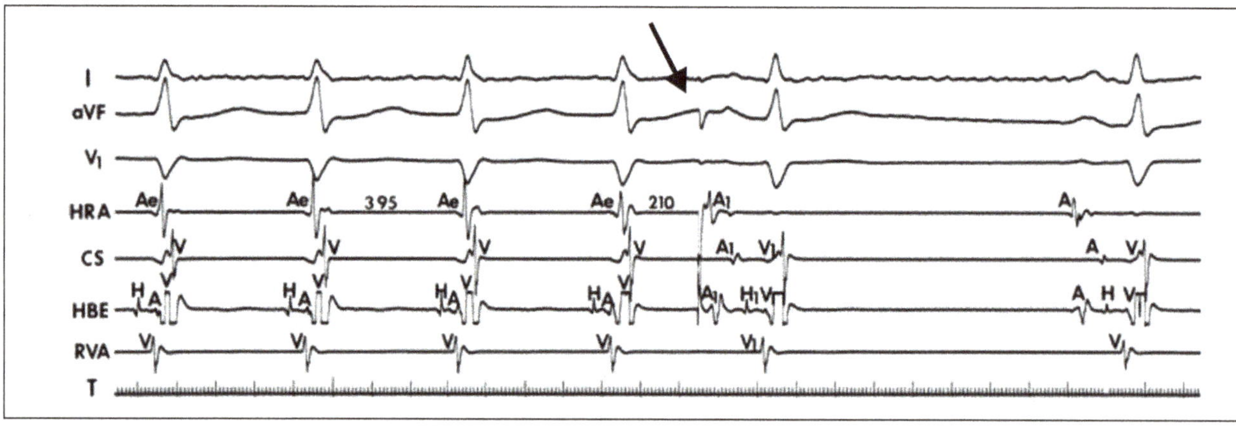

Figure 11-11 ECG leads I, aVF, and V_1, and electrograms from the high right atrium (HRA, Ae), coronary sinus (A, atrial; V, ventricular), His bundle (HBE), and right ventricular apex (RVA). Stimulus that terminates typical AVNRT shown by arrow. (Reproduced from Josephson ME. *Josephson's Clinical Cardiac Electrophysiology: Techniques and Interpretations* (5th ed.). Philadelphia, PA: Wolters Kluwer; 2016.)

Ventricular stimulation. Stimulated ventricular impulses may not be able to enter the reentrant circuit to reset and terminate AVNRT because they collide with antegradely conducting impulses from the NH part of the reentrant circuit similar to the pattern shown in Figure 11-9, Panel F.

Entrainment. A specific characteristic of reentrant arrhythmias is transient entrainment by overdrive pacing. In Chapter 9, the basic electrophysiological concepts are described. To briefly reiterate, entrainment is continuous resetting of a circuit during overdrive pacing with each stimulated impulse resetting the circuit that was reset by the previous stimulated impulse. Reentrant circuits causing both typical and atypical AVNRT can be entrained. The pattern of impulse propagation during entrainment of typical AVNRT from the atria are the same as described in Figure 11-10, Panels B_1 and B_2 during resetting. Each stimulated impulse during entrainment enters the circuit (green arrow in B_1), collides in the antidromic direction with the reentrant impulse (blue arrow) (which is from the previous stimulated impulse) in the fast pathway (B_1), and propagates in the orthodromic direction through the slow pathway (B_2). When pacing is stopped, the last stimulated impulse emerges from the circuit as shown in Panel B_2 at the pacing cycle length and tachycardia continues. At a short pacing cycle length, the reentrant tachycardia is terminated by the mechanism shown in Figure 11-10, Panel C. There is collision of the paced impulse (green arrow) in the antidromic direction with the previous paced impulse (blue arrow) in the circuit and block of the stimulated impulse in the orthodromic direction, in the slow pathway (green arrow and horizontal bar). Entrainment may be difficult to demonstrate since even at a modest overdrive pacing cycle length, rate-dependent conduction slowing and block may occur quickly to terminate the tachycardia.

Autonomic Nervous System and Pharmacology to Help Distinguish A-V Nodal Reentry from Other Mechanisms Causing Supraventricular Tachycardia (SVT)

Sympathetic Stimulation

Sympathetic stimulation shortens the cycle length of AVNRT. It speeds conduction through the A-V node by increasing the L-type Ca^{2+} current (I_{CaL}) that is primarily responsible for phase 0 of A-V nodal (N cell) action potentials. However, this feature does not identify a reentrant mechanism since sympathetic stimulation also accelerates A-V junctional automaticity by enhancing spontaneous phase 4 depolarization and DAD-triggered activity by increasing DAD amplitude. Unlike A-V nodal reentry, the acceleration of automaticity and triggered activity are not directly correlated with more rapid conduction in the A-V node.

Sympathetic stimulation can also decrease the range of cycle lengths that initiate AVNRT by shortening A-V nodal refractoriness related to the effects of norepinephrine to decrease the time for recovery of I_{CaL}. This decrease prevents block of long coupled premature impulses that is necessary to initiate reentry. Short coupled premature impulses are needed to cause block and reentry. Contrary to AVNRT, DAD-triggered SVT is predicted to occur at longer initiating cycle lengths because sympathetic stimulation increases DAD amplitude thereby increasing the range of cycle lengths that initiate tachycardia. This characteristic distinguishes triggered activity from A-V nodal reentry.

Parasympathetic Stimulation

Parasympathetic stimulation has effects on the A-V node that may sometimes assist in distinguishing A-V nodal reentry from the other mechanisms causing SVT. ACh released from parasympathetic nerve endings slows conduction and prolongs refractoriness by decreasing L-type Ca^{2+} current (I_{CaL}) in nodal cells and enhancing outward ACh-sensitive K^{+} current (I_{KACh}). By slowing conduction, the cycle length of AVNRT is lengthened. Parasympathetic stimulation can increase the range of stimulation cycle lengths that initiate AVNRT. Because of its effect to lengthen the refractory period, even longer coupled premature impulses can block and conduct slowly enough in the circuit to cause reentry whereas they would not do so in the absence of parasympathetic stimulation. Parasympathetic stimulation is also expected to increase the cycle length of DAD-triggered SVT. Since it suppresses DAD amplitude, long cycle lengths will not be able to increase DAD amplitude sufficiently to cause triggered activity. Shorter stimulation cycle lengths are needed, thereby decreasing the range of cycle lengths that initiate triggered activity in contrast to initiation of AVNRT. By prolonging A-V nodal refractoriness parasympathetic stimulation can prevent initiation of AVNRT by blocking conduction of premature impulses. It can also prevent initiation of DAD-dependent triggered activity by suppressing DADs.

Parasympathetic stimulation can terminate AVNRT by slowing conduction in the A-V node and causing conduction block. In contrast, parasympathetic stimulation transiently slows A-V nodal automaticity by decreasing the slope of phase 4 depolarization but does not terminate it. Parasympathetic stimulation can terminate triggered SVT by decreasing the amplitude of delayed after depolarizations. Therefore, this response to parasympathetic stimulation does not distinguish triggered activity from reentry. The effects on automaticity and triggered activity are not correlated with changes in conduction in the A-V node in contrast with the effects on AVNRT.

Pharmacological Effects

Information on the pharmacology of A-V nodal reentry and drug therapy of AVNRT is extensive and is not described here. The description below only points out a few differences between the responses of A-V nodal reentry, automaticity, and DAD-triggered activity that are sometimes helpful in identifying the different mechanisms.

Drugs that antagonize the effects of the sympathetics (such as β-receptor blockers) and antagonize the effects of the parasympathetics (such as muscarinic blockers) have the opposite effects compared to ANS stimulation described above.

Drugs that are useful in elucidating automatic and DAD-triggered mechanisms described in Chapters 3 and 6, such as adenosine and verapamil, also affect AVNRT by their actions on the A-V node. Both drugs slow A-V nodal conduction increasing the cycle length of AVNRT and can cause A-V nodal block, thus terminating the arrhythmia. They can also prevent initiation of reentry. Adenosine slows automaticity transiently but does not terminate it, distinguishing automaticity from A-V nodal triggered activity and A-V nodal reentry. Adenosine does terminate triggered activity, similar to its effect on A-V nodal reentry. The effects of adenosine on automaticity and triggered activity are not correlated with changes in A-V nodal conduction as they are for AVNRT.

Reentrant Excitation Utilizing an Accessory A-V Conducting Pathway

PREEXCITATION AND SUPRAVENTRICULAR TACHYCARDIA (SVT) USING AN ACCESSORY A-V PATHWAY

ECG Characteristics

The ECG in **Figure 11-12** shows the onset of SVT, in a patient with a preexcitation syndrome, also called the Wolff-Parkinson-White syndrome. Preexcitation occurs when the atrial impulse conducts to the ventricles in the normal conducting pathway and an additional pathway called an A-V accessory pathway or bypass tract (the terms are used interchangeably). The atrial impulse conducting through the accessory pathway can reach the ventricles prior to the impulse conducting through the normal A-V conducting system. A region of the ventricles is then activated early (preexcited) by the bypass tract impulse before the impulse conducting through the normal conducting system reaches the ventricles. The anatomy and electrophysiology of bypass tracts and their involvement in reentrant arrhythmias are described in detail below.

The first four complexes in Figure 11-12 have a sinus origin. The presence of a bypass tract is indicated by the slurred upstroke of the QRS complex called a delta wave particularly prominent in lead I (small black arrow), caused by the ventricular muscle that is depolarized early by the impulse from the bypass tract. The early depolarization results in a wide QRS complex (~0.12 sec). Early ventricular activation using the bypass tract is also responsible for a short P-R interval.

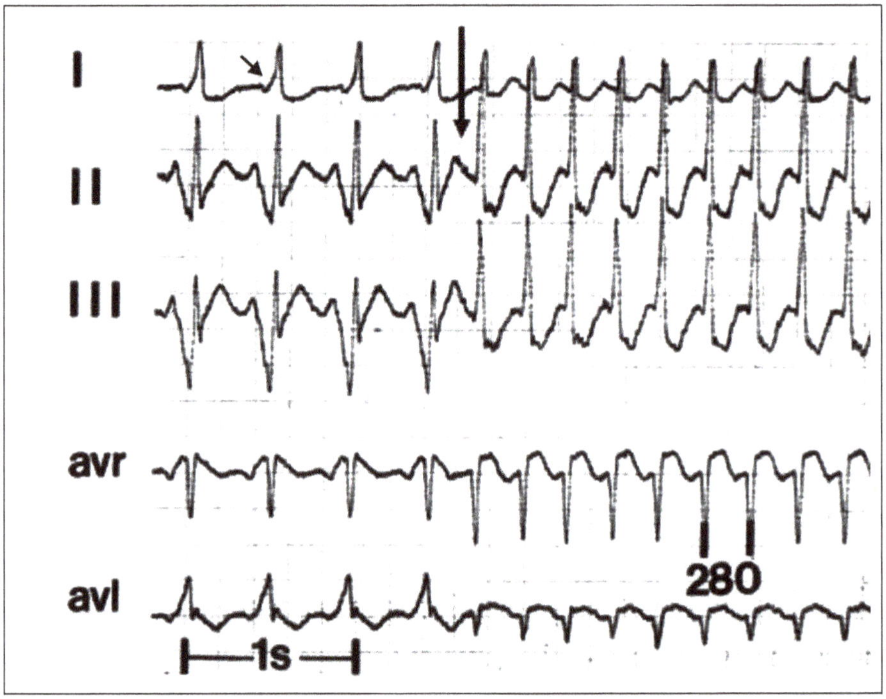

Figure 11-12 Initiation of SVT by a premature atrial impulse (**large arrow**) in a patient with a bypass tract (Wellens' ECG collection).

A premature atrial impulse follows the fourth sinus impulse, indicated by a P wave superimposed on the T wave (large black arrow) with a short coupling interval to the previous atrial impulse. The premature atrial impulse conducts through the normal A-V conducting system resulting in a normal QRS (no delta wave) that occurs after an increased P-R interval because of conduction delay in the A-V node. SVT then follows. The inverted P wave morphology during tachycardia (superimposed on the S wave) indicates retrograde atrial activation (see below). The ECG shows the characteristics of an "orthodromic tachycardia" caused by reentry (280-ms cycle length) in a circuit comprised of antegrade conduction from atria to ventricles over the normal A-V conducting system causing a long P-R interval, normal ventricular activation (normal QRS), and retrograde conduction from ventricles to atria over the bypass tract causing a short R-P interval since there is rapid conduction through this pathway. The reentrant circuit is completed by propagation through part of the atria back to the A-V node (Figure 11-17 shows diagrams of the circuit which is described in detail later). Conduction in the reentrant circuit is called "circus movement," describing a circular reentrant pathway, and hence the tachycardia is often referred to as "circus movement tachycardia."

Bypass tracts are not associated with heart disease but may have a genetic component, since there is a familial occurrence. Of patients with A-V bypass tracts, 40% to 80% manifest tachyarrhythmias, the most common being orthodromic circus movement tachycardia. Antidromic tachycardia is less frequent.

Antidromic Preexcited Tachycardia

In some patients with preexcitation, an "antidromic" or "preexcited tachycardia" occurs (**Figure 11-13**), in which the ventricles are activated by antegrade conduction from the atria to ventricles through the bypass tract and retrograde conduction occurs from the ventricles to atria over the normal conducting pathway (described in detail in Figure 11-17).

As shown in Figure 11-13, Panel A, the QRS complex during antidromic tachycardia typically shows preexcitation with a delta wave and a wide QRS. The P-R interval is short reflecting the rapid antegrade conduction from atria to ventricles over the bypass tract and the R-P interval is long reflecting the slower retrograde conduction from ventricles to atria in the normal A-V conducting system. Figure 11-13, Panel B, also shows an orthodromic tachycardia in the same patient. Note the narrow QRS because antegrade A-V conduction is now through the A-V node. The short R-P interval indicates ventricular to atrial conduction over the bypass tract. Like orthodromic tachycardia, antidromic tachycardia can also be initiated by a premature atrial impulse (not shown).

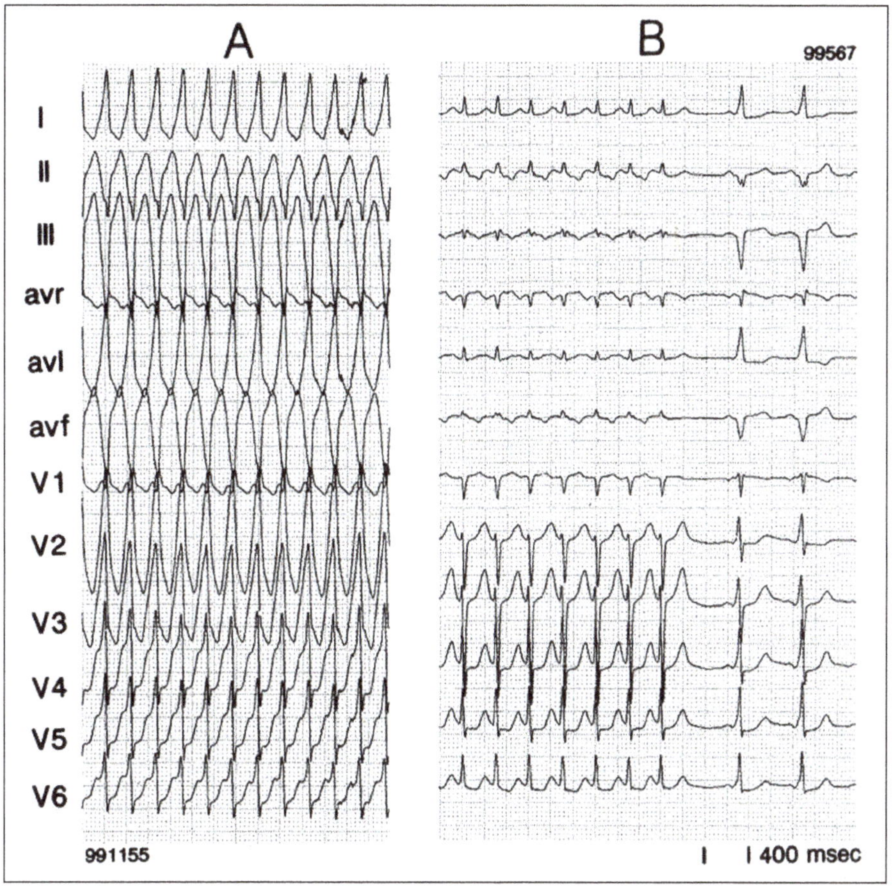

Figure 11-13 12-lead ECG showing antidromic (**Panel A**) and orthodromic (**Panel B**) tachycardia in the same patient with a left posteroseptal accessory pathway. Tachycardia in **Panel B** terminates followed by sinus rhythm showing ventricular preexcitation (Wellens' ECG collection).

Location and Conduction Properties of Bypass Tracts and Reentrant Circuits

Origin of Bypass Tracts

During early embryological development, the atrial and ventricular chambers in the tubular heart have muscular connections around their entire circumference. Later, normal development of the fibrous ring separates the atria from the ventricles, leaving only the A-V connection through the A-V node and His bundle. However, occasionally other pathways remain as well that form the bypass tracts.

Location of Bypass Tracts

Bypass tracts can occur in different regions, resulting in different preexcitation patterns, distinguished one from another by their characteristic ECGs and arrhythmias. The different tracts are shown schematically in **Figure 11-14.**

In Figure 11-14, an A-V accessory pathway (AV Acc. Pathway in red) connects the left lateral atrial wall and left posterolateral ventricular free wall (about 50% of preexcitation cases). Although not shown in the figure, A-V accessory pathways also can connect the right lateral atrial and ventricular free walls (~15% of cases) and the atrium anteriorly (~5%) or posteriorly (~30%) with the ventricular septum. A-V accessory pathways are usually formed by ventricular myocardial cells, not A-V junctional (nodal) cells. They are characterized by the normal conduction velocity in this cell type (~0.5 m/sec) that is more rapid than that of the A-V node (~0.05 m/sec). Conduction time from atria to ventricles in A-V accessory pathways varies in different hearts because of different pathway lengths but, nevertheless, is shorter than through the normal A-V conducting system. Most A-V accessory pathways conduct both antegradely and retrogradely but some conduct only antegradely or retrogradely (see below). The effective refractory period may be shorter or longer than the A-V node and decreases when the heart rate increases because of cycle length-dependent action potential shortening (sometimes dependent on sympathetics) characteristic of ventricular muscle (see Figure 7-7).

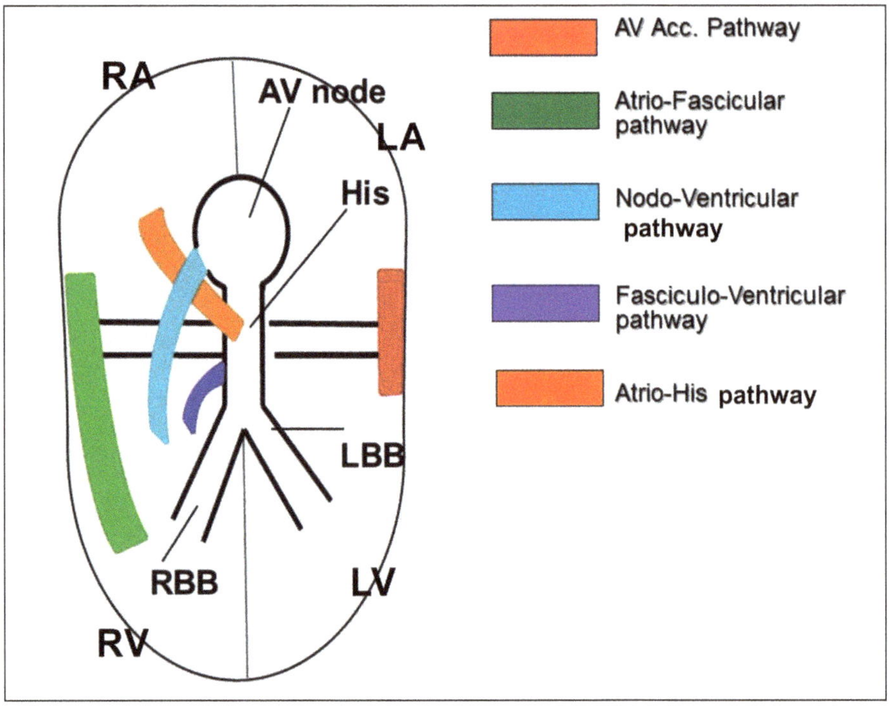

Figure 11-14 Diagram showing location of different bypass tracts. His, His bundle; LA, left atrium; LBB, left bundle branch; LV, left ventricle; RA, right atrium; RBB, right bundle branch; RV, right ventricle.

Atrial impulses occurring at short cycle lengths either conduct to the ventricles without delay in the accessory pathway because of a short relative refractory period (no change in P-to-delta wave as atrial cycle length decreases) or block suddenly at a critically short cycle length without prior slowing. This characteristic contrasts with the A-V node where conduction slows with decreases in atrial cycle length (because of an increase in the relative refractory period) before a cycle length is reached at which block occurs. The A-V nodal relative and effective refractory periods increase with decreased cycle length reflecting the dependence of recovery of excitability on time (time-dependent) rather than action potential duration (voltage-dependent).

Concealed A-V Bypass Tracts

A-V bypass tracts can also be concealed, not conducting antegradely from atria to ventricles but having the ability to conduct retrogradely from ventricles to atria. Concealed bypass tracts are functionally silent during sinus rhythm, with no apparent delta wave. The P-R interval is normal during sinus rhythm since conduction from atria to ventricles occurs only through the normal A-V conducting system. Concealed bypass tracts can be diagnosed during ventricular stimulation or orthodromic tachycardia (see below). They usually have rapid conduction retrograde (analogous to the antegradely conducting A-V bypass tracts described above) and participate in reentrant circuits causing orthodromic tachycardia where they form the rapid retrograde conducting pathway (short R-P interval) of the circuit (see Figure 11-17). Slowly conducting, concealed bypass tracts (with slow A-V nodal like conduction properties) are much less common and cause tachycardia with a long R-P interval. The electrophysiological mechanism for unidirectional conduction in concealed bypass tracts may relate to the pattern of branching of the muscle bundles that form the bypass tracts, resulting in impedance mismatch in the antegrade but not the retrograde direction, analogous to the mechanism for unidirectional block described in Figure 9-16.

Other Accessory Pathways

Other accessory pathways are diagrammed in Figure 11-14. They include: atrio-fascicular pathways between atrial myocardium and a segment of the right bundle branch (in green); atrial-His connections (in brown) that bypass the A-V node; nodofasicular or nodoventricular tracts (in light blue) that originate in the compact node and insert into the proximal right bundle branch or ventricular muscle; fasciculo-ventricular pathways from the His bundle; or a fascicle to ventricular myocardium bypassing part of the conducting system (in purple). Some of these accessory pathways can be part of complex reentrant circuits resulting in tachycardia involving more than one pathway.

The description of electrophysiological properties of reentrant circuits and effects of stimulation in the remainder of this chapter focuses only on lateral A-V bypass tracts (red AV accessory pathway in Figure 11-16).

Fusion of Ventricular Activation; Origin and Prominence of the Delta Wave

The relative time of arrival in the ventricles of impulses conducting through the normal A-V conducting system and bypass tract determines how much of the ventricles are activated by each pathway. **Figure 11-15** illustrates activation in a heart with a left lateral bypass tract (BT) during sinus rhythm (red arrows). The QRS in the ECG at the top is a fusion complex of wavefronts arriving through the normal A-V conducting system (AVN, H) and the bypass tract (BT). Conduction times between the various locations are indicated. Panels A and B diagram the effect of changes in relationship between activation times through the two pathways.

In Figure 11-15 Panel A, total conduction time from sinus node (red dot) to ventricular muscle through the normal A-V conducting system (red arrows) is 160 ms—the sum of conduction times from the sinus node to the atrial end of the A-V node (AVN) (35 ms), conduction time through the A-V node (80 ms because of slow conduction), and conduction time through the His-Purkinje system (H) (45 ms). Conduction time through the left lateral accessory pathway (BT) to ventricular myocardium (red arrow) is only 95 ms because of more rapid conduction (dependent on conduction time from the sinus node to the atrial end of the bypass tract (65 ms) and conduction time through the bypass tract (30 ms)). The rapid conduction through the bypass tract results in earlier activation of the lateral left ventricular wall by this route (dark blue shading) than through the normal conducting system (light blue shading). Fusion activation is evident on the ECG above, which shows a prominent delta wave (small arrow) generated by the preexcited region of the ventricle, also resulting in a short P-R interval. In this example, the His bundle electrogram (H) occurs after the onset of the QRS because of delayed activation through the A-V node (His bundle is activated 115 ms after HRA compared to the earlier onset of the preexcited QRS at 95 ms after activation of HRA).

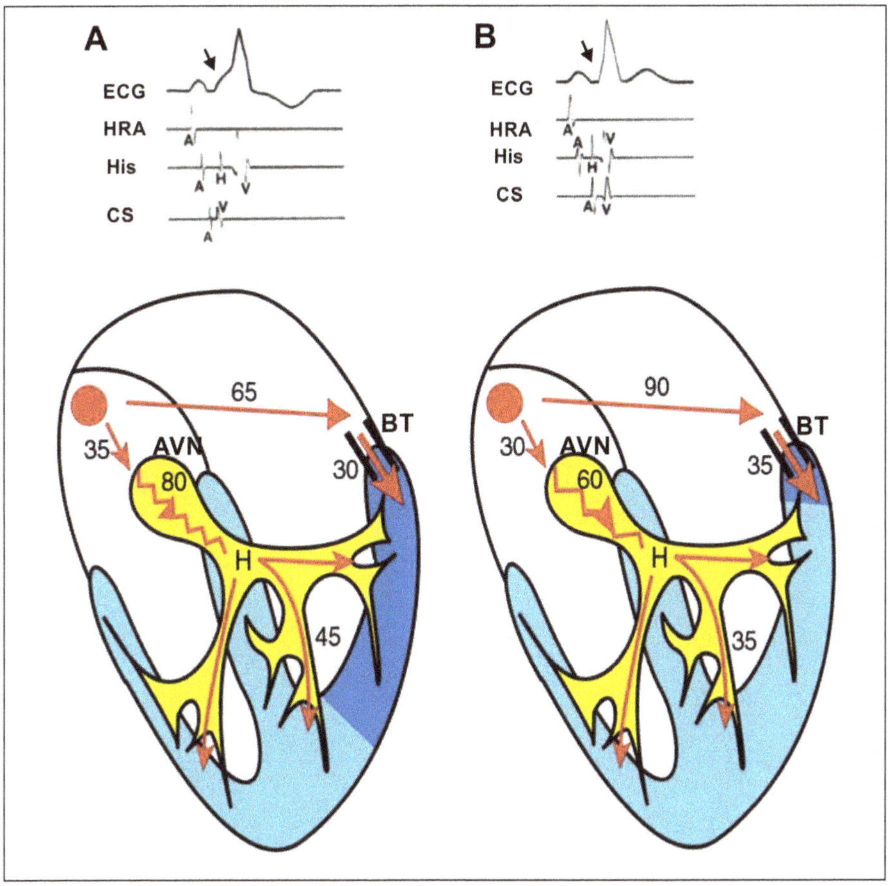

Figure 11-15 Comparison of ventricular activation in a heart with a left lateral bypass tract (BT) and different activation times.

Panel B diagrams an example where most of the ventricle is activated through the normal A-V nodal pathway. In Panel B conduction time through the normal A-V conducting system is shortened to 125 ms (atrium = 30 ms + AVN = 60 ms +H = 35 ms) and conduction time through the accessory pathway is lengthened to 125 ms (atrium = 90 ms + BT = 35 ms). In this situation, less of the ventricles are activated by the bypass tract impulse (dark-blue shaded area) and more by the normal A-V impulse (light-blue shaded area). The QRS has lost most of the delta wave (arrow on ECG above). The His bundle electrogram (H) occurs before the onset of ventricular activation indicating earlier activation through the normal conducting system.

A change in relationship between activation times through the two pathways can be caused by any factors that change conduction differentially in the two pathways. Slowing of conduction in the normal conducting system increases preexcitation, faster conduction decreases preexcitation. Slowing conduction in the bypass tract decreases preexcitation, while faster conduction enhances it. Differential changes can occur because of the different electrophysiological properties of the two pathways. Increased A-V nodal conduction delay without increasing bypass tract delay can result from atrial premature impulses, increased atrial rates, vagal activation, L-type Ca^{2+}-channel blockers, and digitalis, any of which results in more ventricular activation by the impulse from the bypass tract. During an electrophysiological study, atrial stimulation near the atrial end of the bypass tract will also increase ventricular activation through the bypass tract. On the other hand, some antiarrhythmic drugs that block Na^+ channels can slow bypass tract conduction while not affecting conduction through the normal A-V conducting system, which can decrease or eliminate preexcitation.

Figure 11-16 illustrates the effects of decreasing atrial cycle length, which preferentially slows conduction in the A-V node, on preexcitation of the ventricles in a patient with a left lateral bypass tract.

In Figure 11-16, Panel A, during atrial pacing at a cycle length of 500 ms, a delta wave is not evident since the ventricles are activated entirely through the normal A-V conducting system. The A-H interval is normal and the His bundle (H) electrogram occurs before ventricular activation. In Panel B, at a pacing cycle length of 400 ms, conduction through the A-V node is slowed prolonging the A-H interval. There is a small delta wave because slowing of A-V nodal conduction results in some early activation through the bypass tract since conduction here is not slowed. At shorter stimulus cycle lengths (300 ms in Panel C and 240 ms in Panel D), the QRS shows a larger delta wave because of very slow conduction through the A-V node without slowing of conduction through the bypass tract. The H electrogram is no longer visible because His bundle activation occurs after the start of ventricular activation. The impulse conducting through the bypass tract reaches the ventricles earlier than the impulse from the normal A-V conducting system.

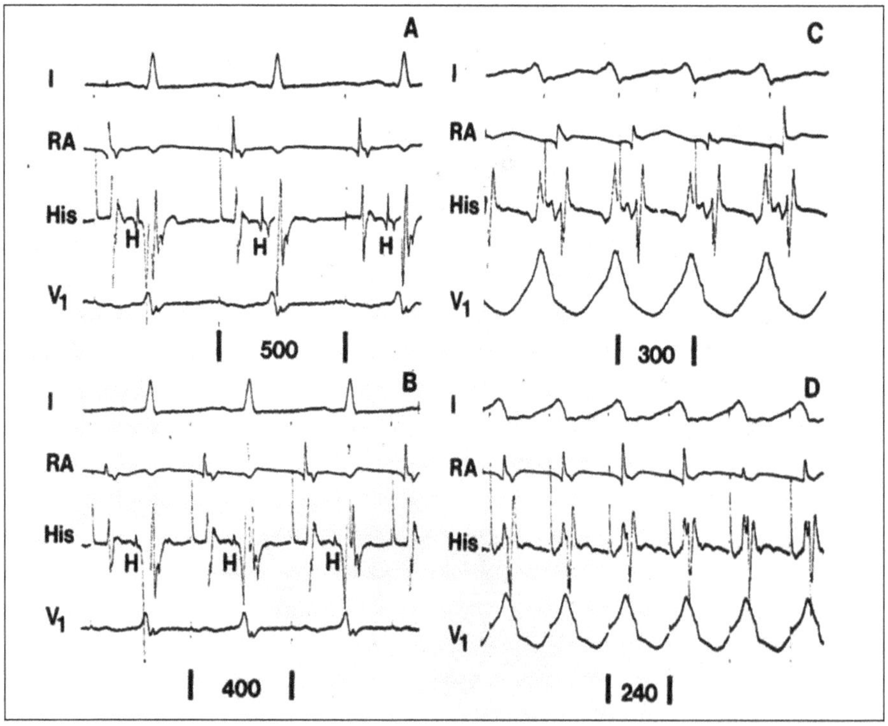

Figure 11-16 Recordings from a patient with a left lateral bypass tract during atrial pacing at different cycle lengths (labeled below V_1). ECG lead I at the **top**, V_1 at the **bottom**. RA, right atrial electrogram; His, His bundle electrogram, with H indicating the His deflection (Wellen's ECG collection).

Electrophysiological Mechanisms of Circus Movement Reentry (Tachycardia) Utilizing an A-V Bypass Tract

Supraventricular tachycardia (SVT) associated with an A-V bypass tract is caused by reentry in a circuit comprised of the normal A-V conducting system, ventricular myocardium, bypass tract, and atrial myocardium. SVT is referred to as circus movement tachycardia (CMT) because of circular impulse movement around this pathway. During orthodromic tachycardia, the most common form (Figure 11-12) the reentrant impulse travels from atria to ventricles over the normal A-V conducting system. During antedromic or preexcited tachycardia, it travels from atria to ventricles through the bypass tract (Figure 11-13).

Initiation by Atrial Premature Depolarization

In hearts with a lateral A-V bypass tract (WPW syndrome), the most common mechanism for initiation of reentrant SVT is by an atrial premature depolarization.

Figure 11-17 illustrates how reentry is initiated. During normal sinus rhythm, there is antegrade conduction (from red asterisk) to the ventricle through both pathways as shown in Panel A (blue arrow through the bypass tract (BT) and red arrow through A-V node (AVN) and His bundle). This circumstance precludes reentry because there is no excitable return pathway to the atria. Unidirectional conduction block must be established in one of the A-V conducting pathways for reentry to occur (see Figure 9-1).

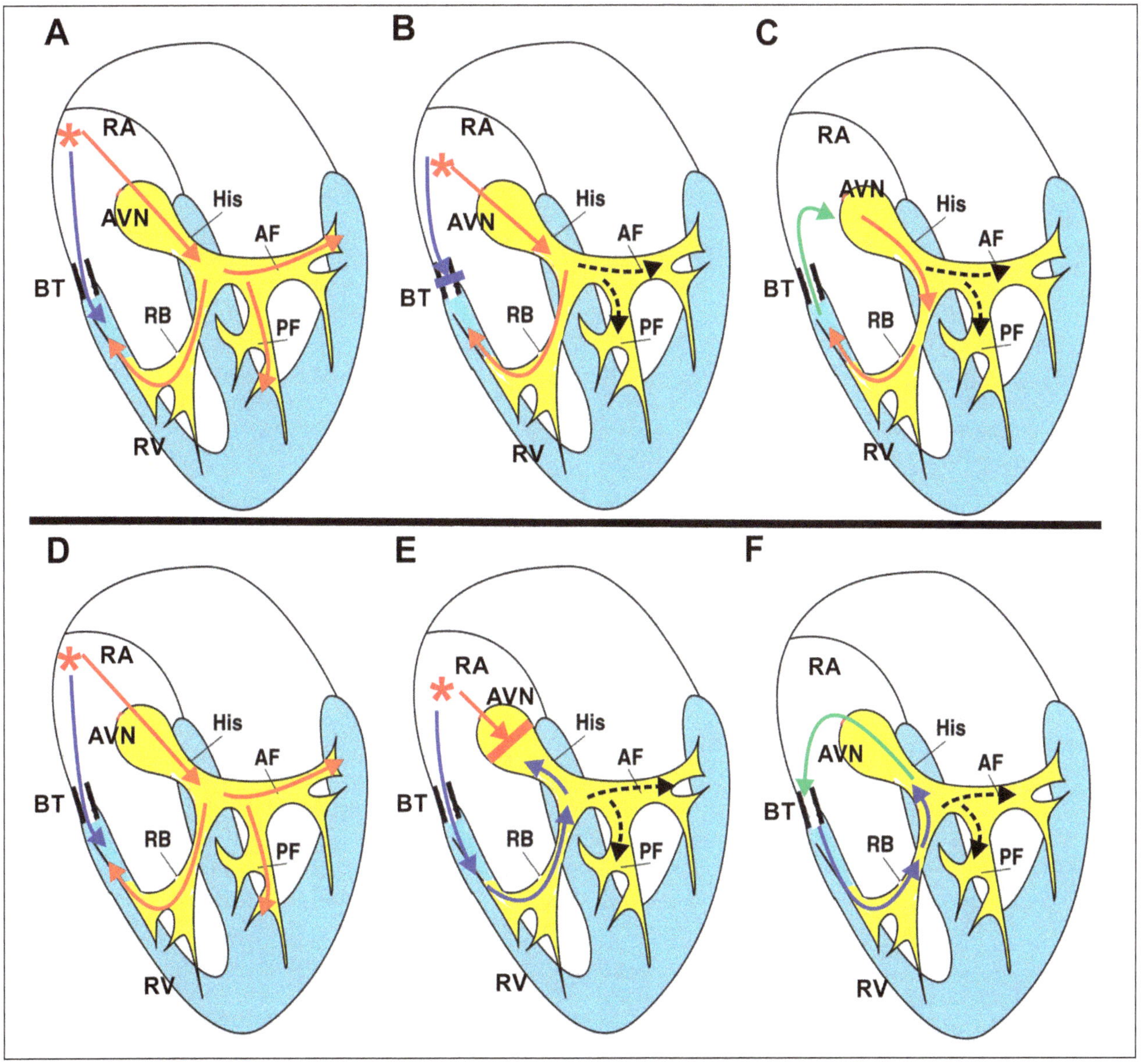

Figure 11-17 **Panels A–C:** Initiation of orthodromic circus movement, **Panels D–F:** Initiation of antidromic circus movement. Right lateral bypass tract (BT), A-V node (AVN), His bundle, right bundle (RB), anterior fascicles (AF), and posterior fascicles (PF) of the left bundle, and right ventricle (RV).

Figure 11-17, Panels B and C, diagram initiation of an orthodromic tachycardia. For this to occur, there is conduction block of an atrial premature impulse in the bypass tract in the antegrade direction (Panel B, blue arrow and horizontal bar) because in this example the effective refractory period of the bypass tract is longer than that of the normal A-V conducting system. Block can occur either at the atrial margin or in the bypass tract. Conduction of the premature impulse through the normal A-V conducting system (red arrow) should be slow enough for the bypass tract to recover excitability at its ventricular end, thus enabling retrograde propagation of the impulse that reached the ventricles from the A-V conducting system back to the atrium completing the reentrant circuit (Panel C, green arrow). The site of critical conduction delay (to allow the bypass tract to recover excitability) is most often the A-V node but can also occur in the His-Purkinje system, ventricular muscle, or a combination of these different sites. When conduction is not slow enough at long premature coupling intervals, the necessary slow conduction can occur at shorter coupled atrial premature impulses.

After returning to the atrium, the reentrant impulse can enter the normal A-V conducting system again and continue to conduct around the circuit (Panel C, red arrows) to cause circus movement tachycardia. Perpetuation of reentry requires that the refractory period of every part of the circuit be shorter than the reentrant cycle length. The wavelength of reentry changes throughout the circuit, shortening in the A-V node where conduction is slowest and lengthening in the bypass tract, ventricular conducting system, and atrial and ventricular muscle, where conduction is faster (see Figure 9-3).

Concealed Bypass Tracts

In hearts with concealed bypass tracts, circus movement reentry causing SVT follows the same process as shown in Figure 11-17, Panels A–C. Since antegrade block is already present in the bypass tract during sinus rhythm, the role of the short initiating cycle length is to cause sufficiently slow conduction through the normal conducting system to allow recovery at the atrial junction of the bypass tract during retrograde conduction, or in the bypass tract itself if there is concealed antegrade conduction of the atrial impulse into the tract.

Initiation of Antidromic Reentrant Tachycardia

Figure 11-17, Panels D–F diagrams initiation of antidromic reentrant tachycardia. Panel D again shows the pattern of activation during sinus rhythm. In a small percentage of cases, the A-V node has a longer effective refractory period than the bypass tract, causing the premature impulse to block in the A-V node (Figure 11-17, Panel E, red arrow and horizontal red bar) while antegrade conduction is maintained to the ventricles through the bypass tract (Panel E, blue arrow). This impulse can then conduct from the ventricular end of the bypass tract, retrogradely into the A-V conducting system (Panel E, blue arrow) resulting in retrograde conduction through the A-V node to the atrium (Panel F, green arrow). Propagation of the reentrant impulse is in the opposite direction, antegrade conduction is through the bypass tract, leading to a tachycardia with a wide preexcited QRS morphology (Figure 11-13). Conduction slowing and delay of the premature impulse (conducting antegrade through the bypass tract) usually occurs in ventricular muscle and the ventricular conducting system and must be sufficient to allow recovery of the A-V node and retrograde conduction through it. Concealed antegrade penetration of the premature impulse into the A-V node before it blocks may lengthen A-V nodal recovery time. When the A-V bypass tract is lateral in the left ventricle the longer conduction time back to the normal AV conducting system provides extra time for its recovery.

Circus movement tachycardia can also be initiated by premature ventricular impulses during an electrophysiological study.

Figures 11-17 illustrates only a few examples of reentrant circuits involving bypass tracts. More detailed descriptions of other possible circuits, also involving multiple bypass tracts leading to complex reentrant circuits, are described in *Josephson's Clinical Cardiac Electrophysiology*, Chapter 10.

SVT Cycle Length and Effects of Bundle Branch Block

Changes in conduction in the His-Purkinje system during circus movement reentry influence the cycle length of tachycardia since it is an important part of the reentrant circuit. The most significant effect occurs when bundle branch block develops ipsilateral to the bypass tract, illustrated in **Figure 11-18**. Panel A shows orthodromic reentry (red arrows indicate pattern of propagation) with antegrade conduction through the A-V node (AVN) and right bundle branch (RB) and retrograde conduction through a right-sided bypass tract (BT). The ECG below shows a narrow QRS in lead V_1, and a cycle length of 350 ms. The interval from ventricular (V) to atrial (P wave) activation (V-A interval in the figure) is the time it takes the circulating impulse, after it exits the His-Purkinje system, to conduct through ventricular myocardium to the bypass tract and then into the atrium. Panel B illustrates the change in the circuit that occurs if there is right bundle branch block (RBBB) (red arrow, horizontal bar). The antegrade pathway switches from the right bundle to the posterior fascicle (PF) of the left bundle, significantly prolonging the cycle length from 350 to 425 ms because of the longer reentrant circuit. This change in pathway changes the QRS to a RBBB morphology. The interval between ventricular and atrial activation (V-A) is also increased because of the increased conduction time in ventricular muscle.

Hearts with right free-wall bypass tracts have a prolongation of the cycle length and V-A interval with the development of RBBB (Figure 11-18), and those with left-sided free-wall bypass tracts show prolongation of the tachycardia cycle length and V-A interval with left bundle branch block (LBBB). On the other hand, contralateral block (LBBB in the presence of the right-sided bypass tract and RBBB in the presence of a left-sided tract) does not significantly influence tachycardia cycle length since the contralateral bundle branch is not involved in the circuit.

A-V Node Conduction Changes

Changes in conduction through the A-V node will also affect the cycle length of both orthodromic and antidromic tachycardia. In hearts with dual A-V nodal pathways (see Figure 11-3), a shift in conduction from fast to slow pathway after tachycardia starts because of block in the fast pathway due to its longer refractory period, increases tachycardia cycle length.

Atrial Fibrillation

Atrial fibrillation commonly occurs in patients with lateral A-V bypass tracts, although the reason why is uncertain. Atrial fibrillation may develop when the rapid rate of circus movement tachycardia causes multiple small functional (leading circle or rotors) reentrant atrial circuits to form (Chapter 10). It has also been hypothesized that rapid atrial tachycardia stimulates focal triggers of atrial fibrillation in the pulmonary veins (Chapter 10).

In general, the antegrade refractory period of the bypass tract correlates with the ventricular response rate during atrial fibrillation. A short antegrade refractory period of the bypass tract (less than 250 ms) is associated with rapid rates of ventricular activation during atrial fibrillation and may induce ventricular fibrillation. Even though the refractory period of the bypass tract may be longer than the A-V node at long cycle lengths, its duration decreases at the rapid rates of atrial fibrillation characteristic of ventricular muscle. Concurrently, the refractory period of the A-V node lengthens, favoring conduction through the bypass tract that causes the rapid ventricular rate. A lower risk for lethal ventricular responses during atrial fibrillation is associated with a long effective refractory period of the bypass tract.

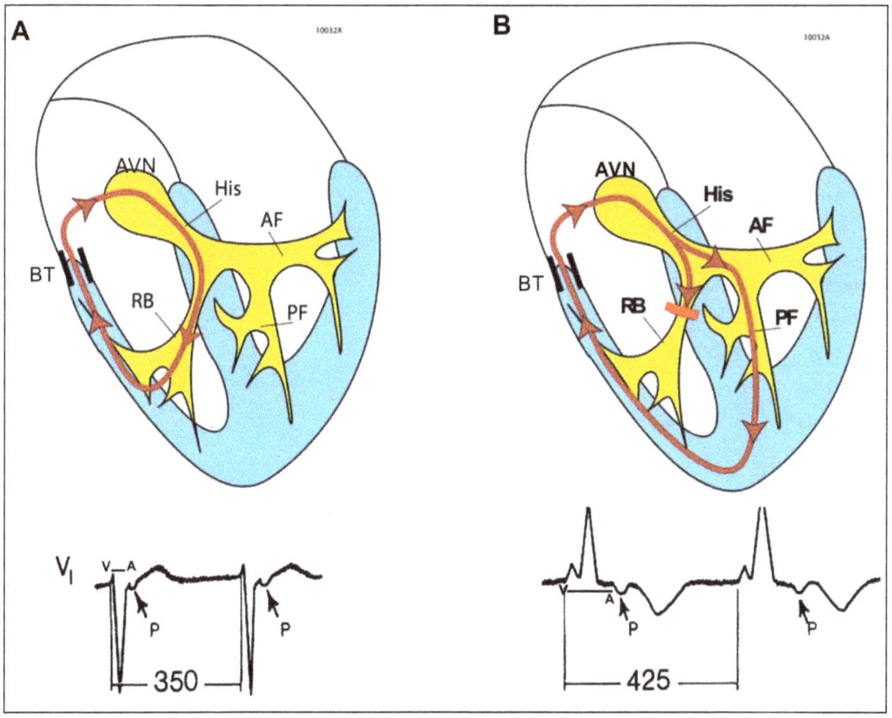

Figure 11-18 **Panel A:** Reentrant circuit (**red arrows**) involving a right-sided bypass tract causing orthodromic tachycardia. **Panel B:** Effect of RBBB. Labels are the same as Figure 11-17.

Effects of Electrical Stimulation

Initiation by Atrial Premature Stimulation

Reentry in a circuit involving the normal A-V conducting system and an A-V bypass tract can be initiated by atrial premature stimulation during programmed stimulation protocols as illustrated in Figure 11-19. The mechanism for initiation is similar to initiation by a spontaneous atrial premature impulse described in Figure 11-17. In Figure 11-19, a delta wave (d) is evident during sinus rhythm (the first impulse at the left in each panel), representing fusion activation of the ventricles both through the bypass tract and the normal A-V junctional pathway. The His bundle deflection (H) in the His bundle electrogram (HBE) comes before ventricular depolarization with an A–H = 90 ms and H–V = 30 ms, indicating activation through the normal A-V conducting system. In Panel A, a stimulated premature impulse (S, arrow below the high right atrial (HRA) recording) at a coupling interval of 380 ms produces greater preexcitation because of increased ventricular activation through the bypass tract. Increased bypass activation is attributed to greater delay of the premature impulse in the A-V node than in the bypass tract, resulting in the His bundle being activated after initial ventricular activation through the bypass tract (the QRS masks the H deflection). In Panel B, at a coupling interval of 370 ms, the premature impulse (S, arrow) blocks in the bypass tract and conducts through the normal A-V conducting system, indicated by normalization of the premature QRS and the occurrence of the His deflection (H) prior to ventricular depolarization. A-V nodal conduction delay increases (A–H = 130 ms) and His-Purkinje conduction time (H-V) is 55 ms. However, the delay in the A-V node is not sufficient to allow recovery of the bypass tract or atrial excitability and therefore retrograde activation by way of the bypass tract causing reentry does not occur (see Figure 11-17, Panel B).

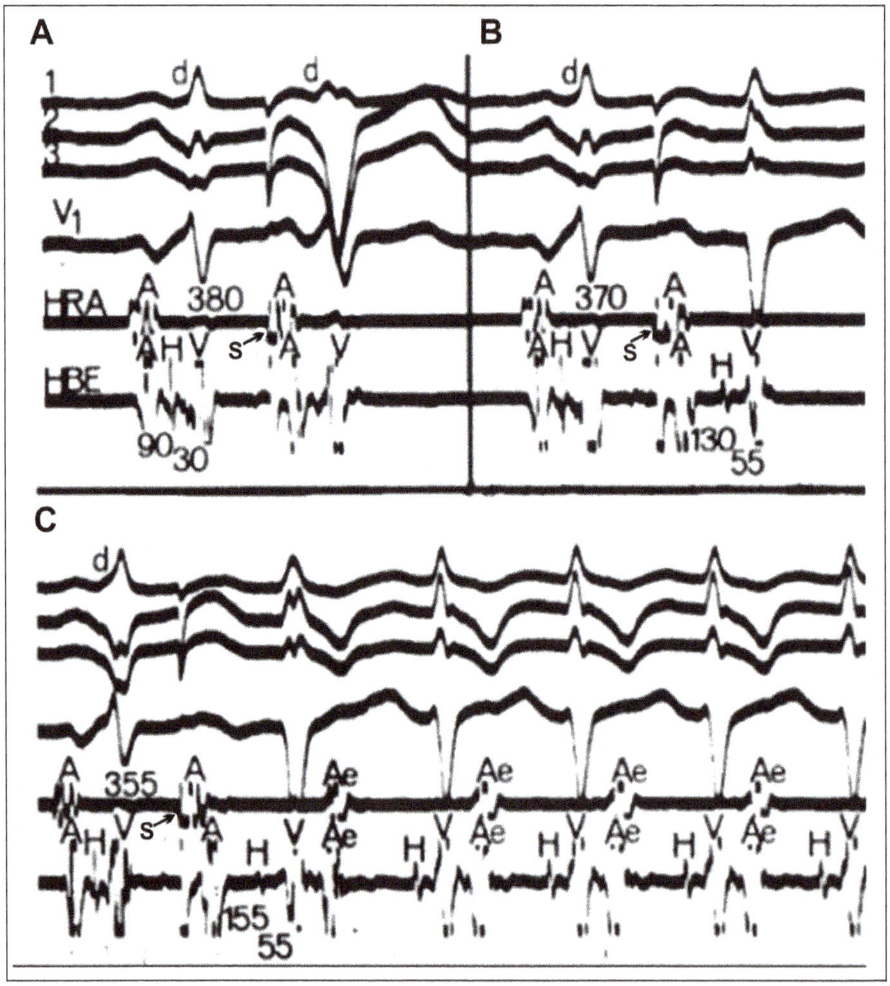

Figure 11-19 Premature atrial stimulation in a patient with a posteroseptal A-V bypass tract. ECG leads I (d indicates delta wave), II, III, and V_1, and electrograms from high right atrium (HRA) and His bundle region (HBE) (A, atrial; H, His bundle; V, ventricular).

In Figure 11-19, Panel C, orthodromic tachycardia is initiated when the premature impulse occurs at a shorter coupling interval and there is sufficient recovery of excitability in the bypass tract. In Panel C, the premature impulse occurs at a 355 ms coupling interval (S, arrow), and block occurs in the bypass tract (indicated by normal QRS in lead I). The greater conduction delay in the normal A-V conducting system (A-H increased to 155 ms) allows sufficient time for recovery of the bypass tract excitability and retrograde excitation of the atrium by the premature impulse, initiating orthodromic circus movement tachycardia. The pattern of conduction initiating the tachycardia is described in Figure 11-17, Panels B and C. Similarly, rapid atrial pacing can initiate orthodromic tachycardia when block occurs in the bypass tract and conduction through the normal A-V conducting system is sufficiently slow to allow reentry to occur. Orthodromic tachycardia can also be initiated in hearts with concealed bypass tracts by the same mechanism since there is antegrade block in the bypass tract and retrograde conduction.

Antidromic tachycardia can also be initiated by atrial premature or rapid atrial stimulation when the normal A-V conducting system effective refractory period is longer than the bypass tract refractory period, by the mechanism described in Figure 11-17, Panels E and F.

Initiation by Ventricular Premature Stimulation

Reentrant tachycardia can also be initiated by either ventricular premature stimulation or rapid ventricular pacing. Initiation of orthodromic tachycardia is diagrammed in **Figure 11-20**, Panels A–C and antidromic tachycardia in Panels D–F.

Figure 11-20, Panel A, shows right atrial (RA) activation during ventricular stimulation at the asterisk, both through the bypass tract (BT) (blue arrows) and the normal A-V conducting system (right bundle [RB], His, red arrows). In Panel B, block of a premature ventricular impulse occurs in the normal His-Purkinje system (red arrow and horizontal bar), particularly at long basic cycle lengths when the refractory period of the His-Purkinje system is long. (At long stimulus cycle lengths, repolarization time and effective refractory periods are lengthened because of cycle length dependent repolarization (see Figure 7-7).) The atrial impulse that conducted through the bypass tract (Panel B, blue arrow), then enters the normal A-V conducting system (Panel C, green arrow) and conducts antegradely to the ventricles. This pattern of circus movement then continues to cause orthodromic tachycardia. Initiation of reentry is dependent on return conduction to the ventricles through the normal A-V conducting system (Panel C, green arrows) with sufficient delay to allow the ventricles and the bypass tract to recover excitability. Retrograde block during rapid ventricular pacing can also initiate orthodromic circus movement by creating block in the A-V node rather than the His-Purkinje system. During rapid pacing the His-Purkinje refractory period shortens (Figure 7-7), but the A-V nodal refractory period lengthens and is responsible for the change in site of block.

Antidromic tachycardias can also be initiated by ventricular stimulation in hearts with an A-V bypass tract (Figure 11-20, Panels D–F). In this instance, retrograde block in the bypass tract must occur (Panel E, blue arrow and horizontal bar) and retrograde conduction proceeds only over the normal A-V conduction system (red arrow). If there is sufficient conduction delay in the His-Purkinje system or A-V node to allow bypass and ventricular recovery of excitability, antegrade conduction through the bypass tract (Panel F, green arrows) starts antidromic tachycardia.

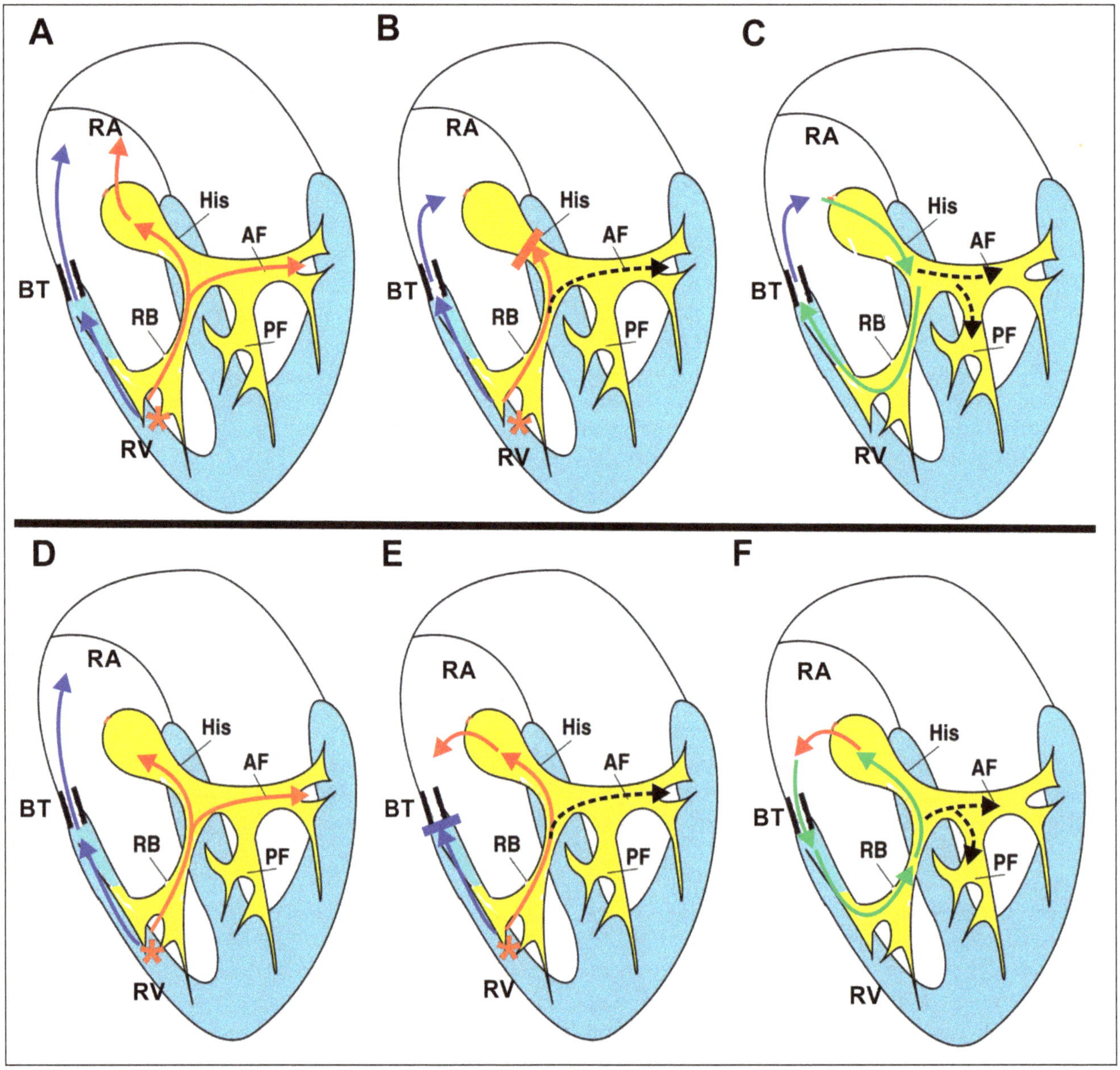

Figure 11-20 Labels are the same as Figure 11-17. **Panel A–C:** Initiation of orthodromic tachycardia by ventricular stimulation. **Panels D–F:** Initiation of antidromic tachycardia by ventricular stimulation.

Resetting, Entrainment, and Termination

Atrial- or ventricular-stimulated impulses can penetrate the large reentrant circuits that include a bypass tract and that have a large temporal and spatial excitable gap, to reset, entrain, or terminate circus movement tachycardia.

Figure 11-21 shows several patterns of activation by stimulated premature impulses during orthodromic reentry. The reentrant circuit utilizes a lateral A-V bypass tract that is diagrammed by the blue arrows in Panel A. In Panel B, an atrial premature impulse (red asterisk and arrows) collides with the reentrant impulse (blue arrow) and conducts orthodromically through the A-V node, around the circuit (red arrow). The premature impulse then would emerge from the bypass tract to depolarize the atrium retrogradely (not shown in this diagram) to reset the tachycardia. The sum of the last tachycardia cycle length and the premature cycle length is less than two tachycardia cycle lengths, indicating resetting (see Figure 9-28). However, if conduction delay of the premature impulse in the A-V node is very long, it would result in a long return cycle length, and resetting on the ECG would not be observed. During overdrive pacing and entrainment, there is continuous resetting; each stimulated impulse resets the circuit that was reset by the prior stimulated impulse (see Figure 9-29). All the features of entrainment described in detail in Chapter 9 can be demonstrated.

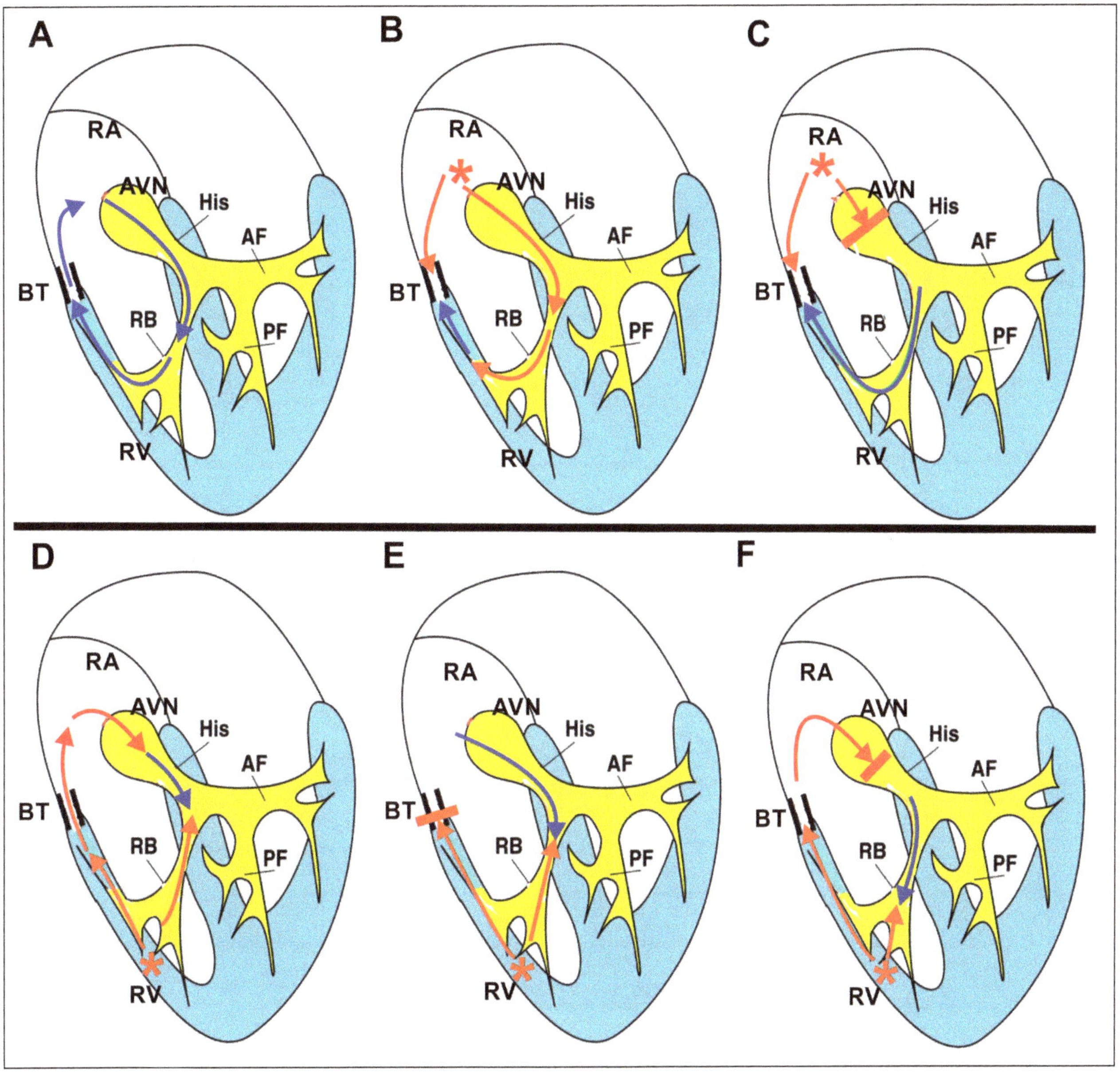

Figure 11-21 Labels on heart diagrams are the same as in Figure 11-17. Activation patterns during orthodromic tachycardia (**Panel A**), stimulated atrial premature impulses (**Panels B** and **C**), and stimulated ventricular impulses (**Panels D–F**).

Figure 11-21, Panel D, shows resetting due to ventricular stimulation (red asterisk). There is collision of the stimulated impulse (red arrow) with the orthodromic reentrant impulse (blue arrow) in the A-V conducting system and propagation of the stimulated impulse through the bypass tract (red arrow) to reset tachycardia. Entrainment occurs when overdrive pacing continuously resets the circuit with a similar pattern of activation (see Chapter 9).

Termination of circus movement reentry (Figure 11-21, Panels C, E, and F) requires block of the stimulated impulse (either premature or overdrive) in either the bypass tract or the normal A-V conducting system. The coupling interval or cycle length of stimulated impulses that terminate the tachycardia is shorter than cycle lengths of stimulated impulses that cause resetting, so that for termination, the stimulated impulses encounter the effective refractory period in a segment of the circuit. Figure 11-21, Panel C, diagrams termination by an early atrial premature impulse that blocks in the A-V node in the orthodromic direction (red arrow and horizontal bar) and collides with the reentrant impulse (blue arrow). Stimulated atrial premature impulses that terminate reentry need not block in the A-V node as shown in Panel C. They might also conduct through the node and around part of the circuit, only to block in the bypass tract.

Figure 11-21, Panels E and F, show two possible patterns of conduction of ventricular stimuli that can terminate orthodromic tachycardia. In Panel E, block of the stimulated impulse (originating at the red asterisk) occurs in the bypass tract (red arrow and horizontal bar) simultaneously with collison with the orthodromic reentrant impulse in the A-V conducting system (blue arrow). In Panel F, block occurs after the stimulated impulse conducts through the bypass tract and enters the A-V node (red arrow and horizontal bar). The stimulated impulse (red arrow) also collides with the reentrant impulse (blue arrow).

Figure 11-22 shows similar patterns of termination in a clinical study. In Panel A, a premature atrial impulse at a coupling interval of 240 ms (downward black arrow) that terminates orthodromic tachycardia using a postero septal bypass tract, blocks in the A-V node as confirmed by the lack of a His bundle depolarization (slanted red arrow and horizontal bar). In Panel B, a premature ventricular impulse (250-ms coupling, downward black arrow over the RVA electrogram) conducts to the atrium through the bypass tract (red arrow), reenters and blocks in the A-V node (blue arrow and horizontal bar).

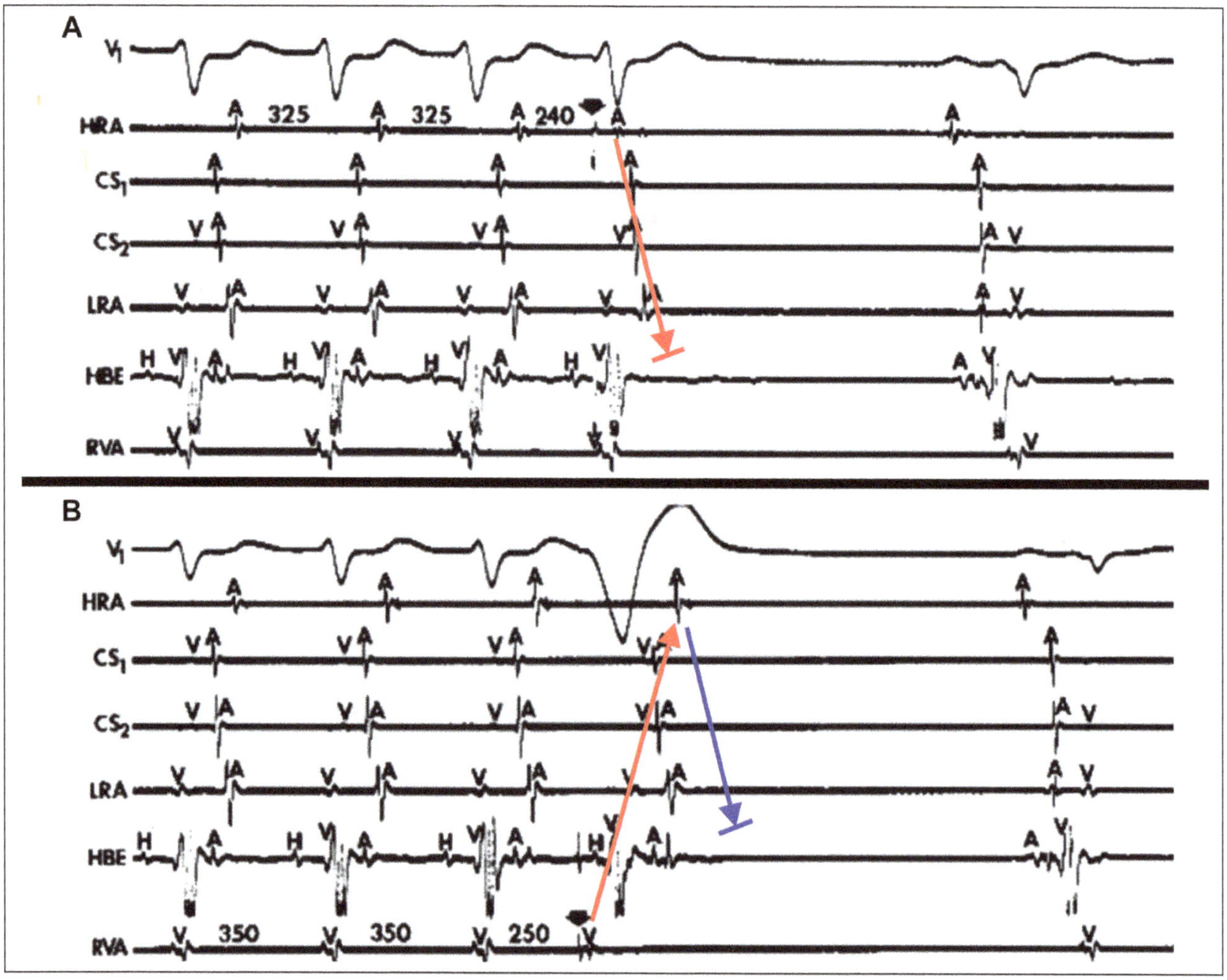

Figure 11-22 Termination of tachycardia by an atrial (**Panel A**) and a ventricular premature impulse (**Panel B**). ECG lead V_1 and electrograms from high right atrium (HRA), coronary sinus (CS), low right atrium (LRA), His bundle region (HBE); A, atrial; V, ventricular; H, His bundle), and right ventricle (RVA). (Reproduced from Josephson ME. *Josephson's Clinical Cardiac Electrophysiology: Techniques and Interpretations* (5th ed.). Philadelphia, PA: Wolters Kluwer; 2016.)

Autonomic Nervous System and Pharmacology to Distinguish Circus Movement from Automatic or DAD-Triggered Tachycardia

The reentrant mechanism causing supraventricular tachycardia utilizing a bypass tract can be differentiated from automatic and triggered mechanisms by the characteristics described above, including ECGs, His bundle electrograms, patterns of activation, and responses to electrical stimulation. The effects of autonomic mediators and blockers or selected pharmacological agents are not necessary to distinguish circus movement reentry from other arrhythmogenic mechanisms.

Autonomic mediators and blockers affect reentrant circuits formed by an A-V bypass tract and the normal A-V conducting system, mostly through their effects on conduction and refractoriness of the A-V node. Parasympathetic stimulation and parasympathomimetic drugs slow conduction through the A-V node and prolong its refractory periods without affecting the bypass tract, thereby slowing or stopping reentrant tachycardia. This selective effect can be attributed to a decrease in I_{CaL} in A-V nodal cells to reduce phase 0 depolarization but little or no effect of ACh on the I_{Na}-dependent phase 0 of ventricular muscle cells that often form the A-V bypass tract. Parasympathomimetic effects also slow supraventricular tachycardias caused by the other mechanisms, automaticity and DAD-triggered activity, and terminate triggered activity but not automaticity. The effects on automaticity and triggered activity do not correlate with slowing of A-V nodal conduction.

Sympathetic stimulation and sympathomimetc drugs have opposite actions compared to parasympathetic stimulation. The reentrant cycle length is decreased in a circuit that includes an A-V bypass tract and the normal A-V conducting system because conduction of the impulse in the A-V nodal segment of the circuit is faster due to an increase in I_{CaL}. Conduction through the bypass tract can also be accelerated and refractory periods shortened, in some but not all patients, since sympathetic stimulation can accelerate repolarization in ventricular muscle. Sympathetic stimulation during exercise may precipitate ventricular fibrillation, which can be initiated by the short cycle length of impulses activating the ventricles through the bypass tract. Bypass tracts with long refractory periods (> 300 ms) have less of a response to catecholamines decreasing the likelihood of ventricular fibrillation with exercise. Sympathetic stimulation also accelerates automatic and DAD-triggered tachycardia.

Adenosine and verapamil, which are sometimes helpful in distinguishing automaticity from triggered activity, do not identify circus movement tachycardia. Both drugs depress A-V nodal conduction to lengthen the reentrant cycle length and might terminate reentry by causing conduction block in the A-V node. Slowing without termination occurs with normal automaticity. Slowing and termination occurs with DAD-triggered SVT.

The effects of antiarrhythmic drugs that block Na^+ and/or K^+ currents are complex, since they have different effects on the A-V node and bypass tracts and may even have different effects on anterograde vs. retrograde conduction and refractoriness. Although a knowledge of these effects are important for drug therapy, they do not assist in identifying a reentrant mechanism and are not described here.

SUMMARY

Typical and Atypical AVNRT

Supraventricular tachycardias (SVT) that are caused by reentry in circuits in the normal A-V conducting pathway are called A-V nodal reentrant tachycardias (AVNRT). The basic electrophysiological characteristics of the reentrant circuit causing AVNRT can be described using a dual-pathway model consisting of two conducting pathways between the atria above and ventricles below. One pathway has slow conduction and a short refractory period (slow pathway). The other pathway has faster conduction and a longer refractory period (fast pathway). The two pathways connect with each other at the atrial and ventricular ends to form the reentrant circuit, although the exact location of the connections is still debatable. The P-R interval on the ECG during sinus rhythm is determined by conduction time in the fast pathway. Reentry that causes typical AVNRT can be initiated by an atrial premature impulse that blocks in the fast pathway due to its longer refractory period and proceeds slowly down the slow pathway. The ventricles are activated through the slow pathway that leads to a sudden prolongation ("jump") in the P-R interval. If conduction through the slow pathway is sufficiently slow, the impulse returning through the fast pathway to cause the atrial echo, can again enter the slow pathway and travel through the reentrant circuit repetitively causing typical AVNRT. Occasionally, the fast pathway has a shorter refractory period than the slow pathway. Block of the premature impulse occurs in the slow pathway and successful conduction antegrade occurs through the fast pathway and retrograde through the slow pathway. The reentrant impulse can then continue to conduct again into the fast pathway and around the circuit to cause atypical AVNRT.

Variations in conduction properties and refractory periods of cells within different regions of the A-V conducting system can provide a functional substrate for reentry without the presence of anatomically discrete pathways. An alternative model is AVNRT caused by an anatomical reentrant circuit comprised of the posterior nodal extension (PE) and the CN as the slow pathway; and then transitional AN cells that make contact with the CN that gradually turn into atrial cells as the fast pathway.

Atrial or ventricular premature stimulation or rapid pacing can initiate typical and atypical AVNRT by the same mechanism as spontaneous initiation. Premature atrial impulses can reset the reentrant circuit because this circuit has a spatial and temporal excitable gap. Premature atrial impulses can also terminate reentry causing AVNRT. Reentrant circuits causing both typical and atypical AVNRT can be entrained and terminated by overdrive pacing.

Sympathetic stimulation speeds conduction through the A-V node and shortens the cycle length of AVNRT. Parasympathetic stimulation (ACh) slows conduction and prolongs the cycle length of AVNRT and reentry can be terminated.

Adenosine and verapamil, slow A-V nodal conduction increasing the cycle length of AVNRT and can cause A-V nodal block, thus terminating the arrhythmia. They can also prevent initiation of reentry.

Preexcitation and Circus Movement Tachycardia

Reentrant SVT (called circus movement tachycardia because of the circular shape of the reentrant pathway) also occurs in patients with preexcitation syndromes. Preexcitation occurs when the atrial impulse conducts to the ventricles in a pathway in addition to the normal A-V conducting pathway called an A-V accessory pathway or bypass tract. Preexcitation results in a delta wave preceding the R wave, reflecting early ventricular myocardium activation through the bypass tract.

During orthodromic reentrant (circus movement) tachycardia that is the most common form, the reentrant impulse travels from atria to ventricles over the normal A-V conducting system and then back to the atria through the bypass tract. During antidromic or preexcited circus movement tachycardia, it travels from atria to ventricles through the bypass tract and back to the atria through the normal A-V conducting system. Initiation of an orthodromic tachycardia occurs when there is conduction block of an atrial premature impulse in the bypass tract because its effective refractory period is longer than that of the normal A-V conducting system. Slow conduction of the premature impulse through the normal A-V conducting system allows time for the bypass tract to recover excitability, enabling retrograde propagation of the impulse back to the atrium completing the reentrant circuit. Initiation of antidromic reentrant tachycardia occurs when the A-V node has a longer effective refractory period than the bypass tract causing the premature impulse to block in the A-V node while antegrade conduction is maintained to the ventricles through the bypass tract. This impulse can then conduct from the ventricular end of the bypass tract, retrogradely into the A-V conducting system.

Reentry in preexcitation can be initiated by atrial premature stimulation. The mechanism for initiation is identical to initiation by a spontaneous atrial premature impulse. Orthodromic circus movement tachycardia can also be initiated by either ventricular premature stimulation or rapid pacing. Atrial or ventricular stimulated impulses can penetrate the reentrant circuits that include a bypass tract to reset, entrain, or terminate tachycardia because the reentrant circuits have a large temporal and spatial excitable gap. Termination of circus movement reentry requires block of the stimulated impulse (either premature or overdrive stimulation) in either the bypass tract or in the normal A-V conducting system.

Parasympathetic stimulation and parasympathomimetic drugs slow conduction through the A-V node and prolong its refractory periods without affecting the bypass tract, thereby slowing or stopping reentrant tachycardia. Sympathetic stimulation and sympathomimetc drugs have opposite actions. Adenosine and verapamil both act to depress A-V nodal conduction and to lengthen the reentrant cycle length and might terminate reentry by causing conduction block in the A-V node.

SOURCES

Bardy GH, Packer DL, German LD, Gallagher JJ. Preexcited reciprocating tachycardia in patients with Wolff-Parkinson-White syndrome: Incidence, and mechanisms. *Circulation.* 1984; 377-391.

Cosio FG, Anderson RH, Kuck KH, et al. Living anatomy of the atrioventricular junction. A guide to electrophysiologic mapping. A consensus statement from the Cardiac Nomenclature Study Group,Working Group of Arrhythmias,European Society of Cardiology and the Task Force on Cardiac Nomenclature from NASPE. *Circulation.* 1999;100:e31–e37.

Durrer D, Schoo L, Schilenburg RM, Wellens HJJ. Role of premature beats in the initiation and termination of supraventricular tachycardia in the Wolff-Parkinson-White syndrome. *Circulation.* 1967;36:644–662.

Gallagher JJ, Pritchet ELC, Sealy WC et al. The preexcitation syndromes. *Progr Cardiovasc Dis.* 1978;20:285–327.

Inoue S, Becker AE. Posterior extensions of the human compact atrioventricular node: a neglected anatomic feature of potential clinical significance. *Circulation.* 1998;97:188–193.

Inoue S, Becker AE, Riccardi R, Gaita F. Interruption of the inferior extension of the compact atrioventricular node underlies successful radio frequency ablation of atrioventricular nodal reentrant tachycardia. *J Interv Card Electrophysiol.* 1999;3:273–277.

Jackman WM, Beckman KJ, McClelland JH, et al.Treatment of supraventricular tachycardia due to atrioventricular nodal reentry, by radiofrequency catheter ablation of slow-pathway conduction. *N Engl J Med.* 1992;327:313–318.

Janse MJ, van Capelle FJL, Freud GE, Durrer D. Circus movement within the AV node as a basis for supraventricular tachycardia as shown by multiple microelectrode recording in the isolated rabbit heart. *Circ Res.* 1971;28:403–414.

Josephson ME. *Josephson's Clinical Cardiac Electrophysiology: Techniques and Interpretations* (5th ed.). Philadelphia, PA: Wolters Kluwer; 2016.

Katritsis DG, Becker A. The atrioventricular nodal reentrant tachycardia circuit: A proposal. *Heart Rhythm.* 2007;4:1354–1360.

Keim S, Werner P, Jazayeri M, Akhtar M, Tchou P. Localization of the fast and slow pathways in atrioventricular nodal re-entrant tachycardia by intraoperative ice mapping. *Circulation.* 1992;86:919–925.

Kuck KH, Brugada P, Wellens HJJ. Observations on the antidromic type of circus movement tachycardia in the Wolff-Parkinson-White syndrome. *J Am Coll Cardiol.* 1983;2:1003–1010.

Lin L-J, Billette J, Khalife K, et al. Characteristics, circuit, mechanism, and ablation of reentry in the rabbit atrioventricular node. *J Cardiovasc Electrophysiol.* 1999;10:954–964.

Lin L-J, Billette J, Medkour D, et al. Properties and substrate of slow pathway exposed with a compact node targeted fast pathway ablation in rabbit atrioventricular node. *J Cardiovasc Electrophysiol.* 2001;12:479–486.

McGuire MA, Lau KC, Johnson DC, et al. Patients with two types of atrioventricular junctional (AV nodal) reentranttachycardia: Evidence that a common pathway of nodal tissue is not present above the reentrant circuit. *Circulation.* 1991;83:1232–1246.

Mendez C, Moe GK. Demonstration of a dual A-V conduction system in the isolated heart. *Circ Res.* 1966;19:378–393.

Mendez C, Moe GK. Some characteristics of transniembrane potentials of AV nodal cells during propagation of premature beats. *Circ Res.* 1966;19:993–1010.

Meijler FL, Janse MJ. Morphology and electrophysiology of the mammalian atrioventricular node. *Physiol Rev.* 1988;68:608–639.

Miller JM, Rosenthal ME, Vassalo JA, Josephson ME. Atrioventricular nodal reentrant tachycardia: Studies on upper and lower "common pathways." *Circulation.* 1987;75:930–940.

Moe GK, Preston JB, Burlington H. Physiologic evidence for a dual A-V transmission system. *Circ Res.* 1956;4:357–375.

Nikolski VP, Jones SA, Lancaster MK, et al. Cx43 and dual-pathway electrophysiology of the atrioventricular node and atrioventricular nodal reentry. *Circ Res.* 2003;92:469–475.

Otomo K, Wang Z, Lazzara R, Jackman WM. Atrioventricular nodal reentrant tachycardia: electrophysiological characteristics of four forms and implications for the reentrant circuit. In: Zipes DP, Jalife J, eds. *Cardiac Electrophysiology: From Cell to Bedside.* (3rd ed.). Philadelphia, PA: WB Saunders Co; 2000:504–521.

Plumb VJ. Catheter ablation of the accessory pathways of the Wolff-Parkinson-White syndrome and its variants. *Progr Cardiovasc Dis.* 1995;37:295–306.

Spach MS, Josephson ME. Initiating reentry: The role of nonuniform anisotropy in small circuits. *J Cardiovasc Electrophysiol.* 1994;5:182–209.

Wellens HJJ, Schuilenburg RM, Durrer D. Electrical stimulation of the heart in the study of the Wolff-Parkinson-White syndrome type A. *Circulation.* 1971;43:99–114.

Wu J, Wu J, Olgin J, et al. Mechanisms underlying the reentrant circuit of atrioventricular nodal reentrant tachycardia in isolated canine atrioventricular nodal preparation using optical mapping. *Circ Res.* 2001;88:1189–1195.

CHAPTER

12

Ventricular Reentrant Arrhythmias

LOCATION, MECHANISM, AND PROPERTIES OF REENTRY

Reentrant excitation in the ventricles occurs either in ventricular muscle, the specialized (His-Purkinje) conducting system, or a combination of the two. It is the mechanism of "sustained monomorphic ventricular tachycardia" defined as ventricular tachycardia (VT) lasting > 30 sec and characterized by a single repeating QRS pattern. Only arrhythmias that have these characteristics are described below because they best exemplify a reentrant mechanism. Although some non-sustained monomorphic and polymorphic VTs are also caused by reentry, the evidence for their mechanism is less established, owing to their short-lasting nature. Sustained monomorphic VT caused by reentry, in general, does not occur in normal hearts.

SUSTAINED MONOMORPHIC VT DUE TO CHRONIC ISCHEMIC HEART DISEASE

Panels A and B of **Figure 12-1** show sustained monomorphic VT (single repeating QRS pattern, QRS duration > 130 ms) in two different patients with ischemic heart disease, initiated by spontaneously occurring premature impulses at the arrows. The ECGs during sinus rhythm (at the left in each panel) show the presence of an old (healed) myocardial infarction anteriorly in both patients These arrhythmias occurred weeks after a coronary occlusion as compared to acutely occurring VT shortly after occlusion.

Reentrant VT in hearts with healed infarcts and/or aneurysms can be initiated by a premature ventricular impulse (similar to DAD-triggered activity) but onset of VT is not usually preceded by changes in sinus rate as it can be for automatic VT (Chapter 3) or DAD-triggered tachycardia (Chapter 6). The initiating premature impulse can originate in the same area as the VT, as indicated by the same QRS morphology (Figure 12-1, Panel A, arrow), or elsewhere, as indicated by a different QRS morphology (Figure 12-1, Panel B, arrow).

Reentrant VT does not usually exhibit a warm-up phase, and spontaneous termination is usually abrupt without gradual slowing, other features that distinguish the reentrant mechanism from DAD-triggered activity.

Chronic ischemic heart disease associated with a scar from prior infarction, often accompanied by aneurysm formation, is the most common cardiac disorder associated with sustained, reentrant monomorphic VT. The greater the wall-motion abnormalities, the higher the incidence of aneurysm formation, and the lower the ejection fraction, the more likely is the occurrence of a sustained monomorphic VT. Because of the large infarct size, aneurysms are present in nearly 85% of patients with VT associated with anteroapical infarctions and in approximately 50% of patients with VT associated with inferior infarctions. Approximately one-third of patients have their first episode of VT within the first year following myocardial infarction, which can lead to cardiac arrest by degenerating into ventricular fibrillation (VF). Subsequently, the incidence of VT occurrence increases 3% to 5% over the following 15 years, while the incidence of cardiac arrest decreases. Late occurrence of VT is more common with inferior aneurysms. The cycle length of VT occurring early after infarction (within several weeks) tends to be shorter with faster rates, and tachycardia is more poorly tolerated, than those occurring late after infarction (one year or more). This probably reflects evolving scar formation with time, which is related to longer tachycardia cycle lengths, owing to greater abnormalities of conduction.

Locating the Origin of Sustained Monomorphic VT

12-Lead ECG

The site of VT origin, which indicates the myocardium that is activated earliest by the reentrant impulse after it exits from the circuit, can sometimes be deduced from the 12-lead ECG. However, locating the origin from the ECG postinfarction is less precise than for VTs in patients without structural heart disease because of the effects of the large infarcts and regions of fibrosis and scarring on the QRS. The larger the infarct, the less predictive are ECG patterns for specific sites of origin, with about only one-half of tachycardia morphologies predictive of a specific site of origin.

Electrophysiological Foundations of Cardiac Arrhythmias: A Bridge Between Basic Mechanisms and Clinical Electrophysiology, Second Edition.
© 2020 Andrew L. Wit, Penelope A. Boyden, Mark E. Josephson, Hein J. Wellens. Cardiotext Publishing, ISBN: 978-1-942909-42-2.

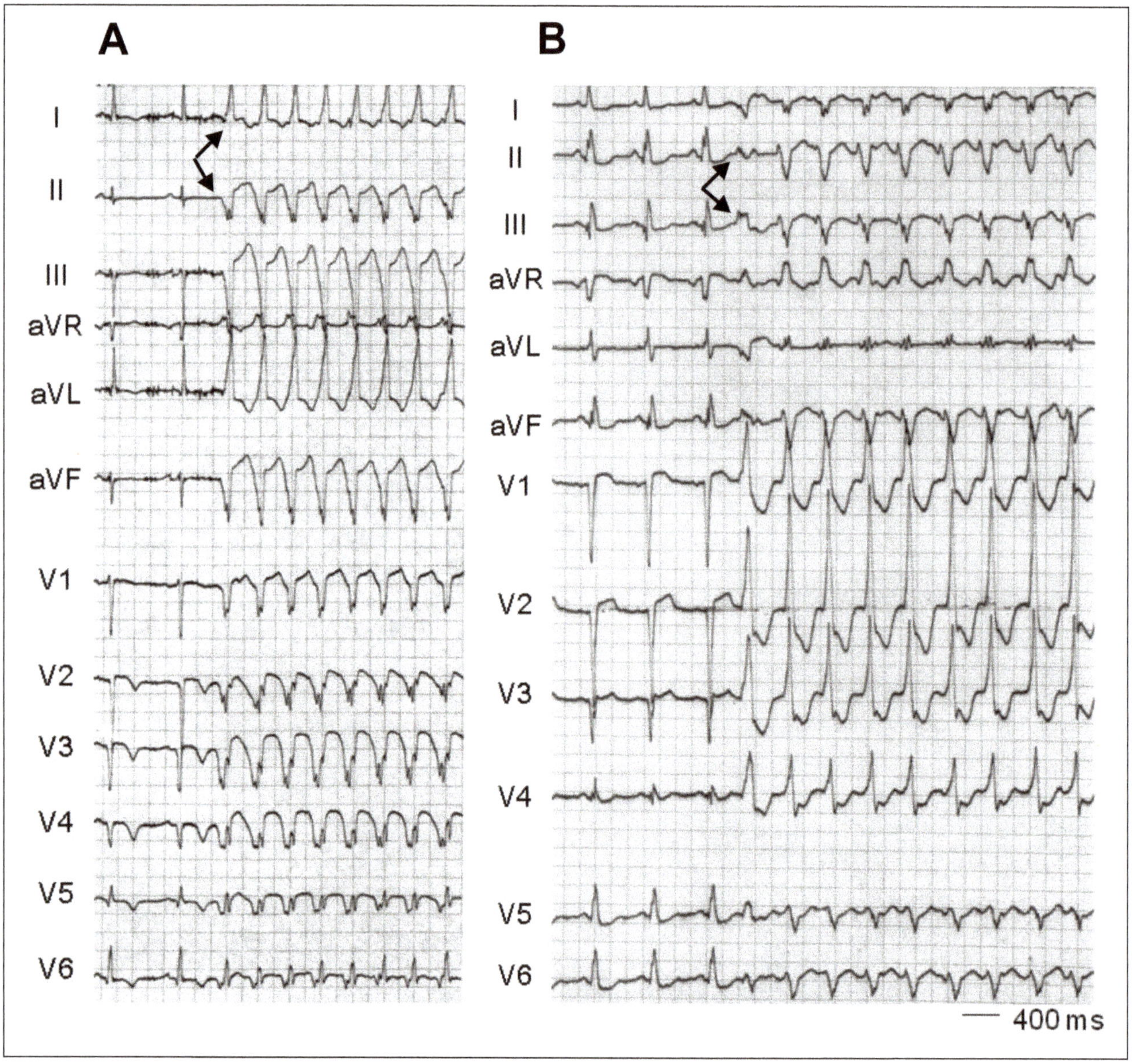

Figure 12-1 A 12-lead ECG showing spontaneous initiation of VT (**arrows**) in healed anterior myocardial infarction by premature ventricular impulses in two patients (**Panels A** and **B**) (Wellens' ECG collection).

The following is a general summary:

- The presence of Q wave in leads I, V_1, V_2, and V_6 in VTs with RBBB or left bundle branch block (LBBB) morphology indicate an origin near the apex but not inferobasal parts of the heart.
- R waves in leads I, V_1–V_6 are specific for VTs with a posterior origin.
- An inferior QRS axis in the frontal plane suggests a VT with a basal origin, and a superior frontal QRS axis, an inferior origin.

(For a more detailed description, consult *Josephson's Clinical Cardiac Electrophysiology*; Chapter 11).

Activation Mapping

Activation mapping utilizing recordings of local electrograms from multiple sites (described in Chapter 2) during VT can locate the site of VT origin, which is the exit from the circuit where the ventricles are first activated. The circuit itself can sometimes also be located. The "site of origin" of VT is the earliest recorded electrogram relative to the onset of the QRS. The earliest electrogram is arbitrarily designated as the one closest to mid-diastole to distinguish it from late electrograms occurring after the QRS. VT origin is invariably in a region of dense scar in or adjacent to an aneurysm. The earliest electrogram is often abnormal and fractionated

(Figure 9-12) and can show discrete systolic and diastolic components. These electrogram features reflect the characteristics of the substrate in which reentry occurs, nonuniform anisotropic myocardium (see Figure 9-11). Since reentry involves continuous electrical activity as the reentrant impulse propagates around the circuit, electrograms may be found throughout the diastolic and systolic intervals when recording directly from the circuit (unlike those with a focal origin of impulse initiation caused by automaticity or DAD-triggered activity).

Sites of VT origin. A subendocardial or septal origin of VT occurs in more than 80% of cases. Patients with left ventricular aneurysms usually have a subendocardial site of origin, within 2–5 mm of the subendocardial surface. Tachycardias associated with blotchy, nontransmural infarctions with or without aneurysms may have subendocardial, intramural, or subepicardial sites of origin.

Figure 12-2 shows subendocardial electrograms in a patient with chronic ischemic heart disease and a ventricular aneurysm on the posterior left ventricular wall, during VT with a subendocardial origin (diagram at the left shows location of recording sites). The earliest site of activation is at site LV 8 on the border of the aneurysm where a discrete mid-diastolic potential (arrow) occurs that is –153 ms before the QRS (see dotted vertical line from surface ECG). This electrogram also has a later, larger amplitude component coincident with the onset of the QRS. Presystolic activity also occurs at adjacent sites LV 6 (–112 ms) and LV 5 (–82 ms), suggesting activation of a pathway from LV 8 to LV 6 and LV 5 during diastole (diagram at the left, wide curved arrow). These electrograms all have multiple components, are fractionated and are characteristic of electrograms recorded from chronic ischemic regions (see below). The other LV sites away from the aneurysm (LV 9, LV 10) have more discrete electrogram deflections as expected from normal regions and occur after the onset of the QRS.

When mid-diastolic electrograms or presystolic activity at least 50 ms before the QRS do not occur in endocardial maps, it is likely that the origin of VT is intramural or subepicardial or that these regions are part of a reentrant circuit that also includes the subendocardium. Presystolic electrograms with the same fractionated characteristics are recorded on the epicardial surface when the circuit is located epicardially.

Mid-diastolic electrograms that are the site of VT origin have a stable time relationship between the electrogram and onset of the QRS during VT with a constant cycle length. If the time relationship changes, for example during a change in VT cycle length, or if the electrogram only appears sporadically, it is likely not representative of VT origin but may be from a region of slow activation that is not an integral part of the reentrant circuit.

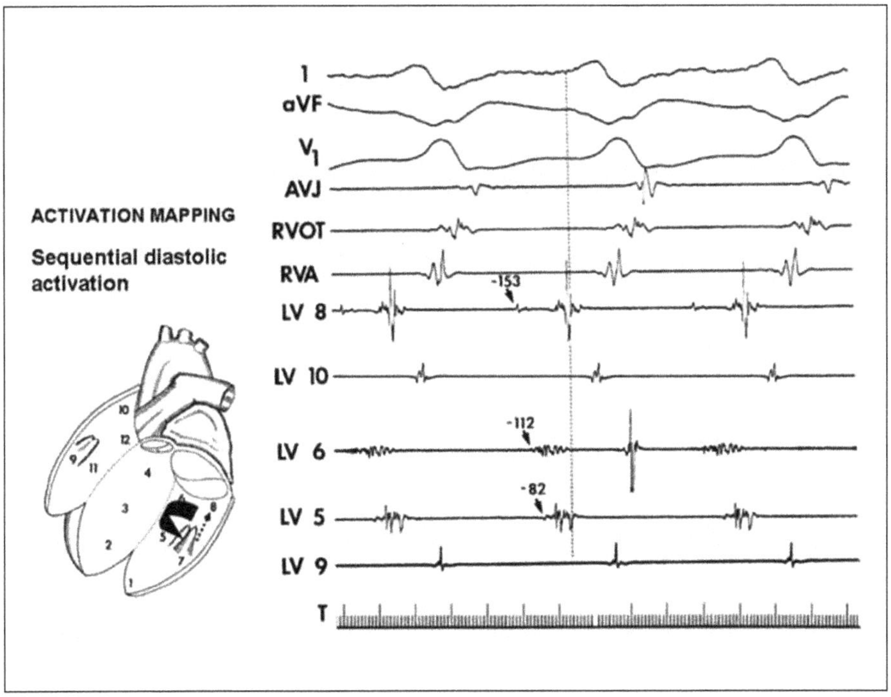

Figure 12-2 Endocardial catheter activation map showing subendocardial site of origin of sustained monomorphic VT. Leads I, aVF, and V_1 are shown with electrograms from the A-V junction (AVJ), right ventricular outflow tract (RVOT), right ventricular apex (RVA), and several left ventricular (LV) sites. The recording sites 1–12 are depicted in the drawing at the left. Time scale (T) = 100 ms subdivided into 10-ms intervals. (Reproduced from Josephson ME. *Josephson's Clinical Cardiac Electrophysiology: Techniques and Interpretations* (5th ed.). Philadelphia, PA: Wolters Kluwer; 2016.)

When the reentrant circuit is located in the subendocardium, there is little correlation between earliest epicardial breakthrough and epicardial activation with circuit location. Epicardial breakthrough usually occurs after the onset of the QRS. The conduction pathway from a subendocardial circuit to the epicardium is not direct and may involve slow, tortuous pathways through or around scarred regions, delaying arrival of activation at the epicardium, which is at a distance from the circuit. When tachycardias arise in the septum, epicardial breakthrough usually begins paraseptally, superiorly, or inferiorly and after the onset of the QRS irrespective of where on the septum the tachycardia originates. Earliest activation on the epicardium usually occurs with inferior infarctions and the absence of an aneurysm when the circuit is partly or completely located epicardially. When this occurs, the subendocardium is activated late through intramural conduction pathways.

Relationship to His Bundle Electrogram

Usually, reentrant circuits causing VT are entirely in ventricular myocardium and do not involve the His-Purkinje conducting system as part of the circuit. Even though the reentrant circuit does not directly involve the His-Purkinje conducting system, it may be activated retrogradely after ventricular depolarization has already begun. During retrograde conduction to the His bundle from the site of origin of VT, the His deflection usually starts after the QRS onset, rarely before. When after, there may be no detectable His bundle deflection (H) when it is obscured by the large ventricular deflection. His deflection can also occur in the terminal part of the QRS, or follow the QRS with a long V-H interval. When before, the H-V interval is shorter than the supraventricular H-V interval. Also, changes in VT cycle length resulting from spontaneous or induced changes in conduction in the reentrant circuit can change the relationship between the His bundle deflection and ventricular depolarization, showing that the origin is not in the His bundle (see description of bundle branch reentry later in this chapter). Engagement of the His-Purkinje system early allows for more rapid activation of the myocardium, which in turn results in a narrower QRS during VT.

Activation Patterns of Reentrant Circuits

The reentrant circuits that cause VT may form as early as two weeks after coronary occlusion. Despite the continuing changes expected in the substrate as the infarcts heal and fibrosis occurs, reentrant circuits that develop during the first three weeks can persist with fairly stable electrophysiological properties for many months in some patients (VT with same QRS and cycle length) or can undergo changes in other patients (shorter cycle lengths and/or QRS at three weeks compared to months later). In some patients, VT does not first appear for months or even years, likely reflecting time-dependent changes in structure of the infarct and ischemic regions that are necessary for formation of circuits.

Circus Movement Pattern

The reentrant circuits that cause VT can have different sizes and shapes. **Figure 12-3** shows a left ventricular endocardial activation map of a reentrant circuit, causing an incessant monomorphic VT in a patient with a large ventricular aneurysm secondary to an old inferior infarction. The inexcitable region of the aneurysm lacking viable muscle is indicated by the grey region, surrounded by surviving muscle (colored isochrones). The border of the aneurysm is indicated by tan circles (pointed out by the white arrows).

According to the color code of activation times at the upper right of Figure 12-3 (earliest activation is the red area followed by orange, yellow, and green), the reentrant impulse circles around the viable margin of the aneurysm from left to right (curved solid black arrow indicates the segment of the circuit that is mapped on the anterior surface of the image). The remainder of the circuit that is in the back of the image that is not seen, has light blue, dark blue, and purple isochrones and is indicated by the dashed arrows. This reentrant pattern around the aneurysm is the circus (circular) movement pattern (solid and dashed arrows) explained in Figure 9-1 (not to be confused with circus movement tachycardia associated with an accessory pathway in Chapter 11) and the aneurysm (gray area) is the central inexcitable obstacle.

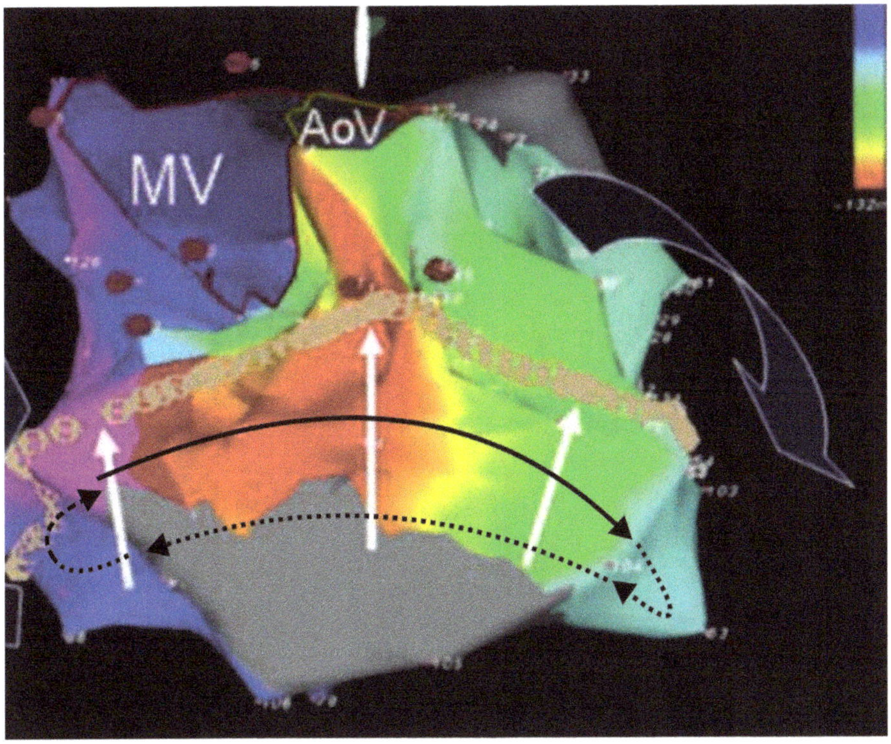

Figure 12-3 Electroanatomical activation map of a macroreentrant circuit around a ventricular aneurysm. AoV, aortic valve; MV, mitral valve. (Reproduced from Josephson ME. *Josephson's Clinical Cardiac Electrophysiology: Techniques and Interpretations* (5th ed.). Philadelphia, PA: Wolters Kluwer; 2016.)

The different widths of the isochrones show that conduction velocity changes in different regions of the circuit, which changes the wavelength (see Figure 9-3). Very slow conduction is indicated by narrow isochrones (red and yellow), while more rapid conduction is indicated by broader isochrones (green and orange). The cause for the slow and nonuniform conduction in the substrate of chronic ischemia is described in the next section on electrophysiological mechanisms.

Most of the circuits of the kind shown in Figure 12-3 are isolated from surrounding myocardium by fibrous tissue. Exit of reentrant impulses from the circuit to activate the ventricles are then through discrete exit pathways that connect the circuit to the surrounding myocardium. There may be multiple connections but one pathway usually predominates leading to the stable QRS morphology of monomorphic VT. The other discrete connections may serve as entrance pathways that allow stimulated impulses to enter the circuit.

Figure-Eight Pattern

Another pattern of reentry is shown in **Figure 12-4**, which is an endocardial activation map from a patient with an inferoposterior infarction in whom VT arose from the basal septum. Earliest activation in the period of time shown occurs in the dark red area. The reentrant impulse moves in a narrow band (upwards; red, orange isochrones). This single wavefront then splits into two, moving left and right (yellow, green isochrones). Both wavefronts move downwards, back to the origin (green, blue, purple isochrones, curved arrows), completing two reentrant circuits. Activation is the "figure-eight" pattern described in **Figure 9-17**.

In Figure 12-4, the single wavefront moving upward (vertical arrow, red, orange isochrones) is in the central common pathway for both the right and left circuits, also called the isthmus of the circuit. Each reentrant wavefront revolves around a line of block (large arrows), the exact extent of which is difficult to estimate (dashed black lines). The cause of block may be an anatomical obstacle formed by fibrosis. The exit site from the circuit appears to be from the isthmus, at the asterisk. Subendocardial figure-eight reentrant circuits appear to have a circuit area probably in excess of 4 cm^2. Central common pathways that are activated during diastole and act as diastolic exit pathways are about 1–3 cm long and a few millimeters to 1 cm wide. However, the actual circuit may be smaller if part of the lines of block are actually functional barriers (not anatomical) as also shown in Figure 12-4 (small arrows). In this case, there may be slow propagation across functional barriers, transverse to myocardial fiber orientation (small arrows), referred to as "pseudo block" because there seems to be block in the activation maps. This pattern of activation results in a smaller circuit than the large arrows indicate. If this was the case, ablation lesions at the exit site of the isthmus (asterisk), would not be effective in stopping the tachycardia.

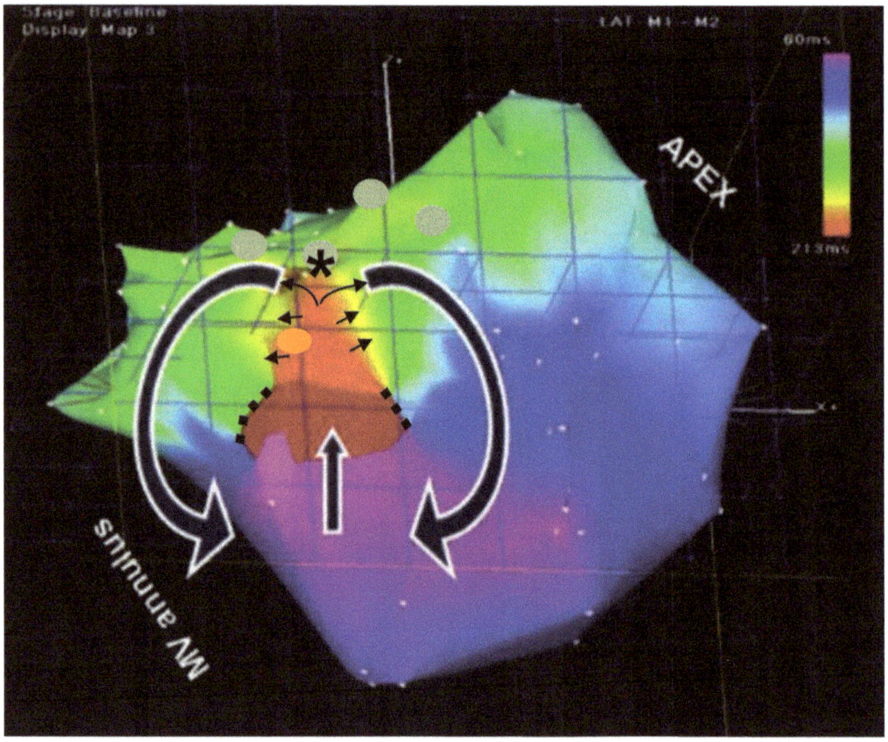

Figure 12-4 Activation map showing a figure-eight pattern, displayed in the posterolateral view at site of VT origin in the basal septum. Color scale is shown at the upper right. (Reproduced from Josephson ME. *Josephson's Clinical Cardiac Electrophysiology: Techniques and Interpretations* (5th ed.). Philadelphia, PA: Wolters Kluwer; 2016.)

Conduction velocity and wavelengths change in different regions of the circuit as shown by the changing width of the isochrones. The causes of these changes are described below in the section on electrophysiological mechanisms.

When the barriers around which the two reentrant wavefronts circulate are structural (formed by fibrosis) the impulse can exit the circuit from the isthmus (at the asterisk in Figure 12-4) that connects to surrounding myocardium. Fibrous tissue of the scar bounds the two loops, likely providing obstacles that prevent exit from other locations around the circuit. High-density activation maps with many recording electrodes covering a small region may be necessary to see the figure-eight activation pattern. In low-density activation maps, when the circuit is small, the pattern of endocardial activation may appear to be focal with centrifugal spread from that site.

Interrelationship of Substrate Structure and Electrophysiological Mechanisms of Reentry

Formation and Structure of Infarct Border Zones

Reentrant circuits form to cause VT at locations where myocardial cells survive in and around an infarcted region. Over the ensuing hours after an acute proximal coronary artery occlusion, cell death progresses as a "wavefront of necrosis" from the region of most intense ischemia (usually subendocardial) toward both the endocardial and epicardial surfaces, as well as laterally. Expansion of the infarct can continue over days to many weeks. Viable myocardial and Purkinje cells often remain on the subendocardial surface because of continued perfusion from the ventricular cavity, possibly by retrograde flow through venous channels. Some intramural and subepicardial muscle may survive in the necrosing region because of collateral blood flow. The extent and location of collateralization determines the amount and location of the surviving muscle. The necrotic myocardium is then replaced by fibrous tissue over the following weeks and months, while the muscle that survives becomes trapped in the infarct scar forming the arrhythmogenic infarct border zones. Surviving Purkinje and myocardial cells trapped in the scar in the subendocardium form the subendocardial border zone even in regions of transmural infarction, aneurysms, or adjacent to aneurysms where many of the reentrant circuits are located. Muscle cells in the subepicardium form the subepicardial border zone, also where reentrant circuits are sometimes located. In some hearts, bundles of myocardium also traverse the scar connecting subendocardial and subepicardial border zones and also form part of reentrant circuits that may involve both border zones or which may be intramural.

Figure 12-5 shows the microscopic structure of the subendocardium (subendocardial border zone) in a region where VT originated adjacent to an aneurysm.

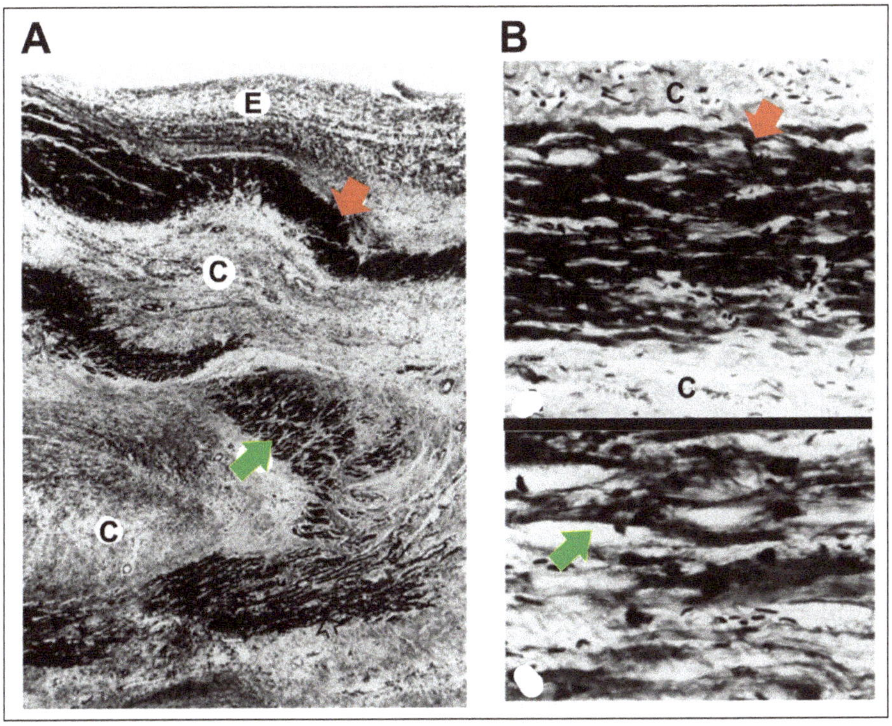

Figure 12-5 Subendocardial resection from a patient with sustained monomorphic VT. **Panel A:** Original magnification ×94. **Panel B** shows additional magnification of myocardial cells at the **red arrows** and **green arrows** in **Panel A**. **Panel B:** Upper section (magnification ×240) and lower section (magnification ×360).

Resection of this region during surgery abolished VT. Panel A shows a thickened endocardial surface (E) and dense connective tissue (C) within which are embedded bundles of myocardial cells that are widely separated from one another (red and green arrows). In some bundles the myocardial cells are relatively compact (Panel A, red arrow and Panel B top, red arrow at higher magnification) and in some bundles the cells are separated by connective tissue (Panel A, green arrow and Panel B bottom, green arrow at higher magnification). The trapped subendocardial muscle may be separated from surviving intramural muscle (if present) by the extensive subendocardial scar, or there may be connections with surviving muscle bundles that are transmural and follow a zig-zag course through the scar. These transmural bundles may also connect with surviving muscle in the subepicardium that form an epicardial border zone. Muscle bundles around the lateral aspects of the infarcted region may also protrude into the scarred region as lateral border zones. The surviving muscle bundles form anatomical reentrant circuits around inexcitable regions of fibrosis, either within the aneurysm (Figure 12-3) or smaller subendocardial regions (Figure 12-4).

Electrophysiology of Infarct Border Zones

Although resting potentials are partially depolarized and action potential phase 0 are reduced by the initial ischemic event, after several weeks (when sustained monomorphic VT usually occurs), the action potentials in the surviving muscle in infarct border zones, for the most part, have nearly normal resting potentials and phase 0 depolarization. In **Figure 12-6**, a representative ventricular muscle action potential that appears normal is shown at the upper right. The action potential was recorded from a surviving cell in the epicardial border zone of a 2-month-old experimental canine infarct. The recording is from a region with very slow conduction as indicated by the narrow spacing of the isochrones in the activation map below. Also shown in the upper left of Figure 12-6 is a fractionated bipolar electrogram recorded from this region that is characteristic of slow conduction in muscle bundles trapped in scar tissue (see Figure 9-12). Reduction of inward depolarizing (I_{Na}) current is not a major factor in causing the slow conduction and unidirectional block necessary for reentry. The conditions for reentry are established by the structure of the surviving muscle bundles trapped in the scar. In addition to forming anatomical circuits, their separation by fibrous tissue disrupts gap junction connections particularly in the transverse direction, resulting in slowed transverse conduction and nonuniform anisotropy (Figure 9-11). Reduction in the quantity of gap junctions caused by ischemia contributes to both slow longitudinal and slow transverse conduction. Interconnections between small and larger fiber bundles cause slow conduction and block through the mechanism of impedance mismatch described in Figure 9-16.

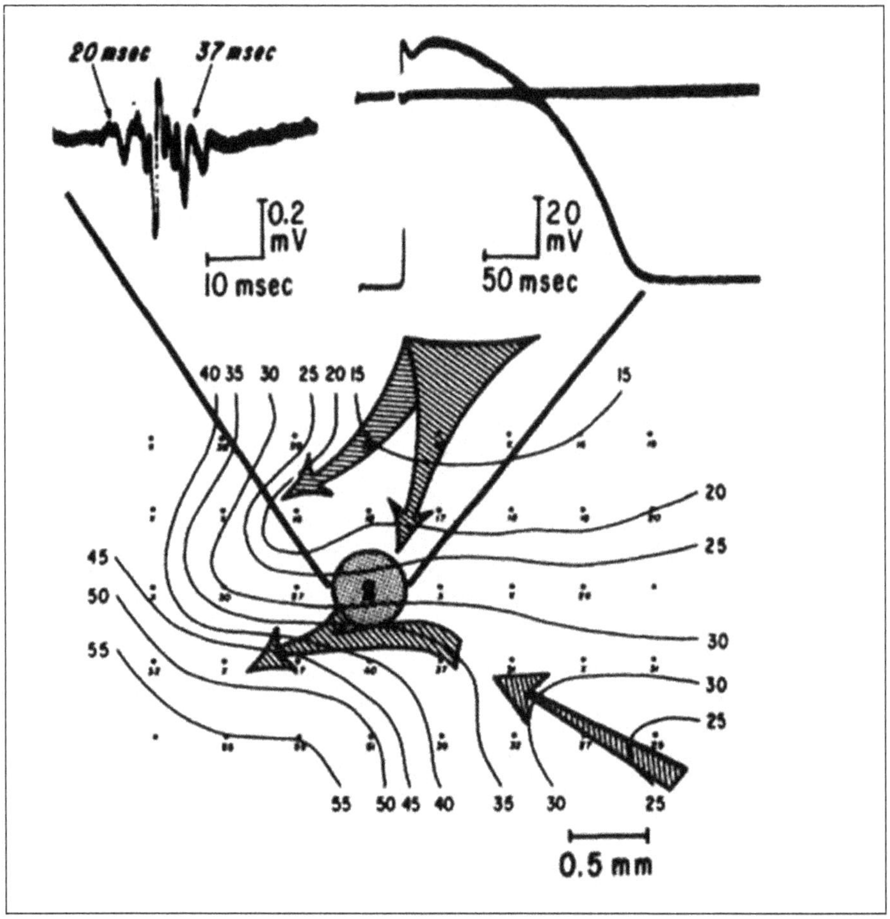

Figure 12-6 Action potential recorded from a surviving ventricular muscle cell in epicardial border zone of a two-month-old canine infarct is at the **top right**. Activation map of the region is shown **below with dots** indicating each point at which an action potential was recorded, with isochrones at 5-ms intervals. The direction of propagation is shown by arrows. Location and size of a bipolar electrode is indicated by the **stippled circle** and the fractionated electrogram recorded from this electrode is shown **above at the left**. The distance scale is shown below.

The effects of these structural features on reentry are shown in the circuits in Figure 12-3 and Figure 12-4. In Figure 12-3, the changes in the width of the isochrones as the impulse traverses the circuit around the aneurysm reflect changes in conduction velocity, more rapid in the wide isochrones of the orange and green regions and very slow in the narrow isochrones of the yellow and dark red regions. The changes in conduction velocity may be caused by changes in orientation of the muscle with faster conduction in the longitudinal direction and slower conduction in the transverse direction (Figure 9-11). It may also be caused by changes in the size of the muscle bundles with conduction slowing where small bundles connect to larger bundles (Figure 9-16). In the figure-eight reentrant circuit shown in Figure 12-4, slow transverse conduction is evident in the yellow isochrone, between the orange and green isochrones (small arrows). The lines of conduction block (dashed lines) may also be a result of gap junction uncoupling. In addition, wavefront curvature where the impulse moves from the central isthmus into the outer pathways (small curved arrows above at the asterisk) contributes to conduction slowing. Convex curvature occurs where impulses conduct from a narrow pathway (the isthmus) into a wider pathway as explained in Figure 9-13.

The wavelength of the reentrant impulse and the spatial excitable gap change in different parts of the circuit. The wavelength is short and the gap widens when the impulse is in regions of slow conduction and the wavelength is long and the gap shortens when the impulse is in regions of more rapid conduction (see Figure 9-3).

Characteristics of Bipolar Electrograms

Abnormal conduction caused by the structural features of the infarcted region that result in reentry can be detected in the characteristics of bipolar electrograms recorded during sinus rhythm. These electrograms are abnormal and show low amplitudes, multiple components, and prolonged duration, and frequently occur after the end of the QRS indicating delayed activation of the infarcted region.

Figure 12-7 shows these general features of abnormal electrograms recorded with a bipolar catheter electrode from the subendocardial border zone of a patient with a healed myocardial infarction.

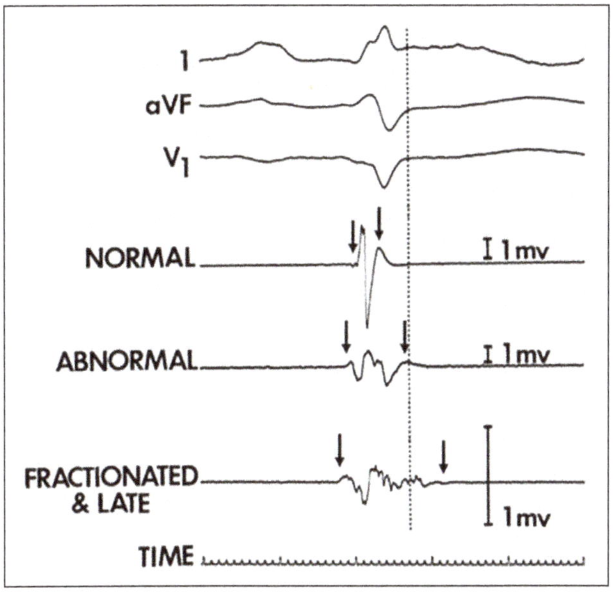

Figure 12-7 ECG leads I, aVF, and V_1 at the top. Below electrograms recorded with a bipolar catheter. Voltage calibrations are at the **right**. Note the difference between the calibrations for abnormal, fractionated, and normal electrograms. **Arrow** indicates duration of electrogram at each recording site. (Reproduced from Cassidy DM, et al. Endocardial catheter mapping in patients in sinus rhythm: Relationship to underlying heart disease and ventricular arrhythmias. *Circulation*. 1986;73:645–652.)

The actual quantitative values of electrogram characteristics depend on the size of the electrodes and the distance between bipoles that determine the area of myocardium from which electrical activity is being recorded. The mapping catheter used to construct the electroanatomic maps in Figure 12-3 and Figure 12-4 had a tip electrode 4 mm in length and a ring electrode 2 mm in length, with an interelectrode distance of 2 mm on a 7- to 8-Fr diameter catheter. With this size, normal electrogram amplitude is equal or greater than 1.5 mV (Figure 12-7, Normal) reflecting little or no scar, a rapid depolarization (phase 0) of the underlying myocardial cells and rapid conduction. At the border of the scar (Figure 12-7, Abnormal) where connective tissue interdigitates with muscle, the amplitude is 0.5–1.5 mV. The presence of dense scar is indicated when amplitude is equal or less than 0.5 mV (Figure 12-7, Fractionated and Late). An electrogram with an amplitude of 0.1 mV or less suggests that the scar is 90% transmural with only small bundles of surviving muscle fibers. The amplitude of the signal is dependent on several factors: The insulating properties of the connective tissue forming the scar, the distance the electrodes are from the viable muscle bundles because of scar thickness, the density of the muscle bundles trapped in the scar generating the electrical signal and the conduction velocity of the impulse in those bundles. A large scar, small bundles, and slow conduction can all cause low-amplitude electrograms. Therefore, there can be a great deal of variability in electrogram amplitude, particularly when the scar is less than 90% transmural. Abnormal electrograms with low amplitudes can also be fractionated with multiple components and long durations (Figure 12-7, fractionated and late, long duration indicated by downward black arrows). Long duration is caused by slow conduction in poorly coupled cells. The fractionation is a result of the "zig-zag" and asynchronous pattern of propagation in nonuniform anisotropic myocardium (Figure 9-11). These electrograms may occur late, that is, after the end of the QRS because of the prolonged activation time caused by the slow conduction. Patients with sustained monomorphic VT have a greater number of sites demonstrating these abnormal electrograms compared to patients with coronary artery disease and no VT or nonsustained VT.

The relationship between sites of abnormal electrograms and origin of VT can be demonstrated by recording electrograms at numerous sites during sinus rhythm; a procedure known as "substrate mapping." The location of abnormal electrograms often correlates with the site of origin of VT.

Electrogram characteristics within scarred tissue. Within the connective tissue scarred region, pathways of conduction that form reentrant circuits can also be located on the basis of electrogram characteristics during sinus rhythm. **Figure 12-8** shows a sinus rhythm (substrate) voltage map obtained with an electrode catheter, in such a region where VT originated. This substrate map focuses on electrogram amplitude and not earliest activation.

The entire region within the dark blue boundaries (white arrow at left) is characterized by electrograms with a low-voltage amplitude of less than 0.5 mV. Within this region conducting "channels" are formed by bundles of muscle cells that give rise to electrograms, with amplitudes of between 0.1 and 0.3 mV indicated in green, that course through and around very low voltage regions (red, < 0.1 mV) comprised mostly of fibrotic tissue. A hypothetical figure-eight reentrant circuit based on the electrogram amplitudes, but not mapped during VT, is shown by the curved black arrows. The two loops (1 and 2) course around anatomical obstacles formed in the red region and an isthmus is formed by the green region and dashed white line that is part of both reentrant circuits. That this channel is the isthmus was proven by successful abolition of VT by ablation lesions placed at the sites indicated by the small brown circles.

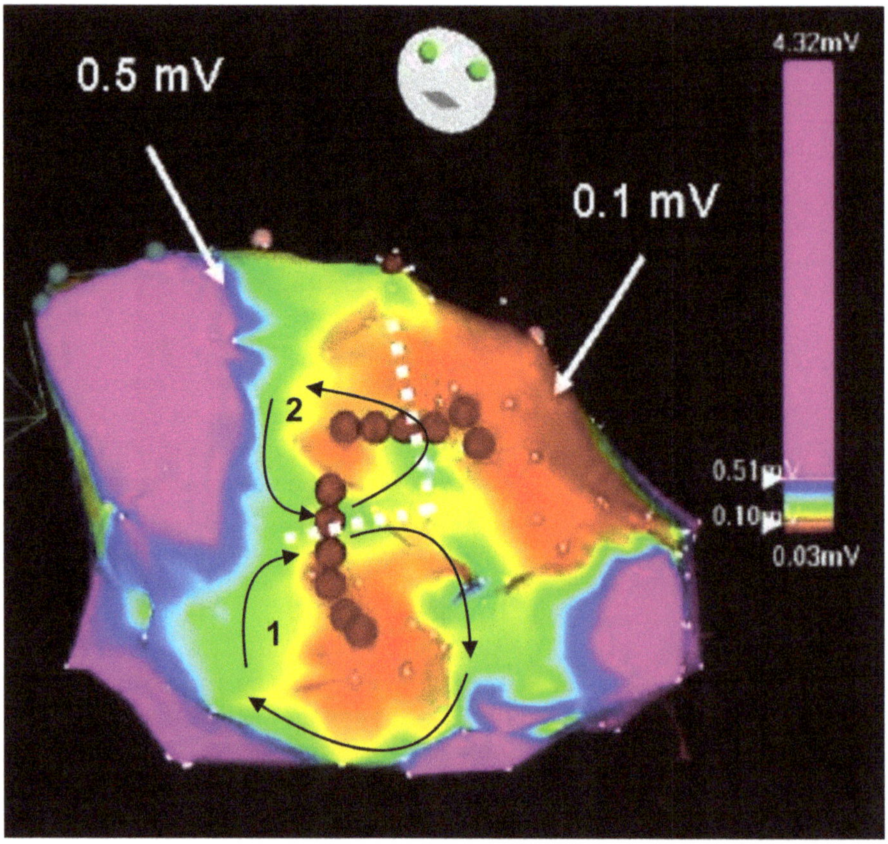

Figure 12-8 The endocardial surface of the left ventricle is shown. Amplitude of electrograms are plotted with color coding at the right.

Further evidence that these channels are conducting pathways in the reentrant circuit can sometimes be obtained from pacing during sinus rhythm (pace maps), within the region where the circuits form. When the isthmus of a figure-eight circuit with fibrous tissue boundaries is stimulated, the paced impulse is forced to exit the circuit through the same pathway as the reentrant impulse giving rise to the same QRS morphology as during VT.

Electrogram characteristics during VT. Not only do electrogram characteristics during sinus rhythm indicate sites of origin of reentrant VT, electrogram characteristics during VT can also show the location of the reentrant circuit. As described in Figure 12-2, electrograms at sites of origin of VT have long duration, low amplitude, and fractionated activity that likely represent the exit route of the impulse from the reentrant circuit. When electrodes are positioned directly on a small reentrant circuit, electrical activity can be detected throughout the tachycardia cycle length as the wavefront transits around the circuit. These electrograms are referred to as having "continuous electrical activity."

Continuous electrical activity during VT is found at sites that demonstrate abnormal electrograms during sinus rhythm. **Figure 12-9** shows ECGs and electrograms recorded during sinus rhythm (NSR, left) and during VT (right) in a patient with a posteroseptal aneurysm. During sinus rhythm, the electrogram recorded at the distal LV septum post infarct (d) has multiple components (fractionated), low amplitude and long duration (180 ms) and extends beyond the end of the QRS. During VT, at this same site, continuous electrical activity is present as the wavefront travels around the complete reentrant circuit. This activity is not detected on the ECG because of the relatively small extracellular signal recorded from a small pathway. Continuous activity ceases when VT terminates.

Failure to record continuous activity during VT suggests that the circuit may be larger than the recording area of the catheter and/or that the entire circuit is not located in the region where the electrodes are positioned. For example, endocardial electrodes will not detect continuous activity if part (or all) of the circuit has an intramural or epicardial location.

Additional comments. All abnormal and fractionated electrograms recorded either during sinus rhythm or VT do not represent sites of VT origin. Such activity may represent recording artifacts such as during electrode movement, or electrical activity in regions of the infarct with the similar structural characteristics as the site of origin but unrelated to the genesis and maintenance of the tachycardia. Mid-diastolic electrograms can also be recorded from "dead end" pathways that are connected to the reentrant circuit but are not part of the reentrant pathway.

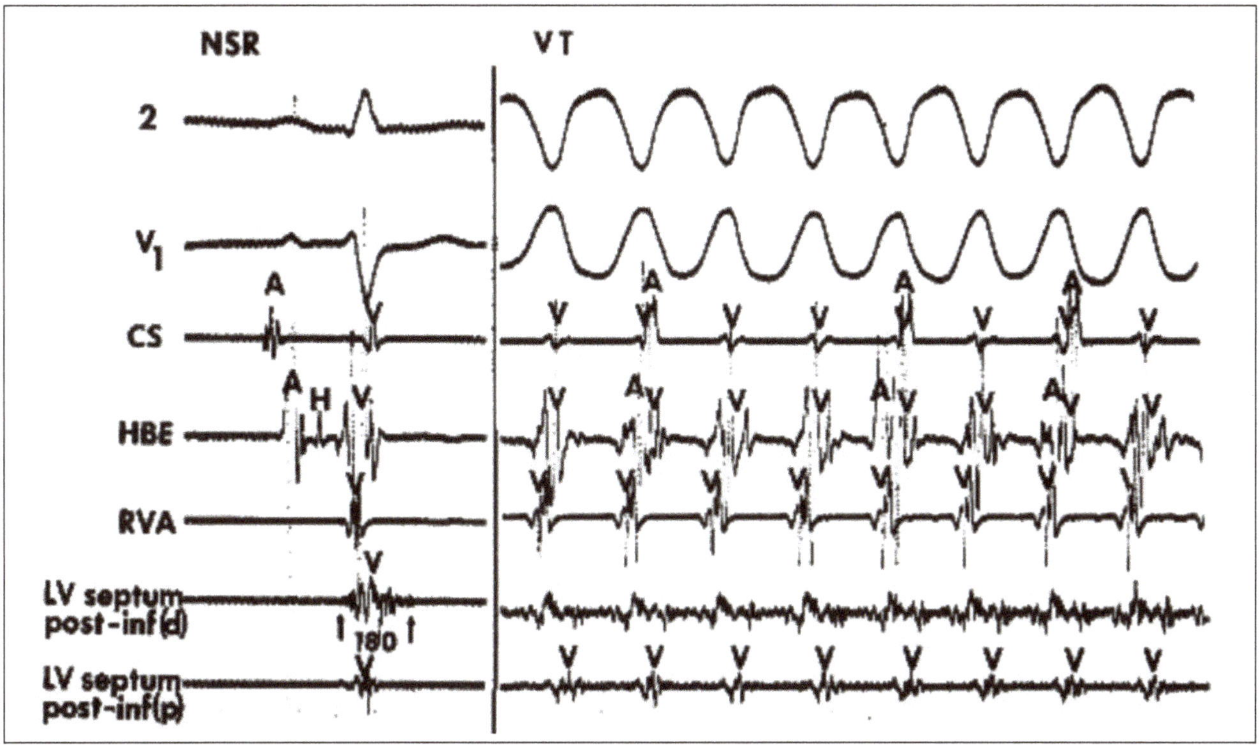

Figure 12-9 ECG leads II and V_1 along with electrograms from coronary sinus (CS), His bundle (HBE), right ventricular apex (RVA), posterior inferior left ventricle (LV) septum from distal (d), and proximal (p) pair of electrodes on the same catheter. Normal sinus rhythm (NSR) is at the **left**, VT at the **right**. A, atrial; V, ventricular; H, His bundle electrogram. (Reproduced from Josephson ME, et al. Continuous local electrical activity. A mechanism of recurrent ventricular tachycardia. *Circulation*. 1978;57:659–665.)

Effects of Electrical Stimulation

Programmed electrical stimulation can start sustained reentrant monomorphic VT in most patients with spontaneously occurring VT, with the induced arrhythmia having identical ECG characteristics as the spontaneous one. Initiation by stimulation is a property of reentry (Chapter 9).

Initiation by Programmed Premature Stimulation

As described in the model of anatomical reentry shown in Figure 9-25, reentry can be initiated by premature stimulation because it establishes the necessary conditions of slow conduction and unidirectional conduction block. **Figure 12-10** illustrates initiation of reentrant VT by premature stimulation in a patient with recurrent sustained monomorphic VT and an old inferoposterior myocardial infarction.

In each panel of Figure 12-10, from left to right, the first two complexes are the last of 8 paced impulses at the right ventricular apex (RVA) at a basic cycle length of 600 (S1) followed by a single prematurely stimulated impulse (S2) (labeled above the RVA recording). The coupling intervals of the premature impulses (S2) are 300 ms (Panel A), 290 ms (Panel B), and 280 ms (Panel C). In Panel C, VT is initiated at the large arrow above ECG lead II (2). The bottom electrogram (LV-An) recorded from the subendocardial region of the aneurysm related to the infarct shows fractionated activity during basic pacing (V_1). The duration of the electrogram and number of fractionated components increases for premature impulses after V_2 (small upward pointing arrow in panels A and B below the LV-An recording,), until at the 280 ms coupling interval (Panel C), the electrical activity spans the diastolic interval coincident with the initiation of VT indicating sufficiently slow conduction to start reentry.

Inverse relationship of coupling intervals. As premature coupling intervals decrease, the premature impulses conduct more slowly around an anatomical circuit resulting in an increase in the time between entry into the circuit and exit from the circuit (Figure 9-25). **Figure 12-11** illustrates this inverse relationship during the initiation of VT in a clinical electrophysiological study. In each panel the first two impulses at the left are at the end of a period of pacing from the right ventricular apex (RVA) at a basic cycle length of 700 ms. The third impulse is a premature impulse with the coupling interval indicated by the horizontal black bar.

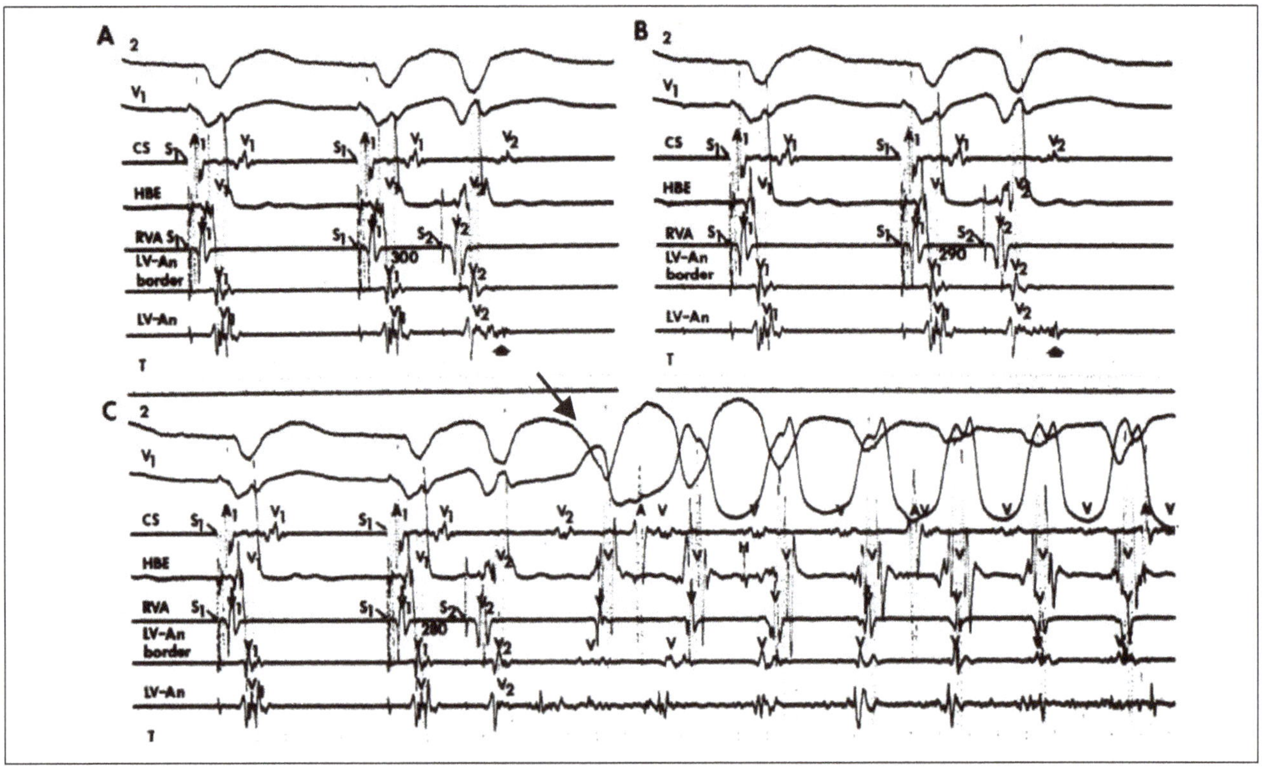

Figure 12-10 Initiation of VT with premature electrical stimulation. ECG leads II and V_1 and electrograms from coronary sinus (CS), His Bundle (HBE), right ventricular apex (RVA), border of left ventricular aneurysm (LV-An border), and left ventricular aneurysm (LV-An). Labels of electrograms, A1 and V_1 = atrial and ventricular electrograms during basic drive; V_2 = ventricular electrograms of premature impulse; S1 = basic drive stimulus; S2 = premature stimulus. (Reproduced from Josephson ME, et al. Continuous local electrical activity. A mechanism of recurrent ventricular tachycardia. *Circulation.* 1978;57:659–665.)

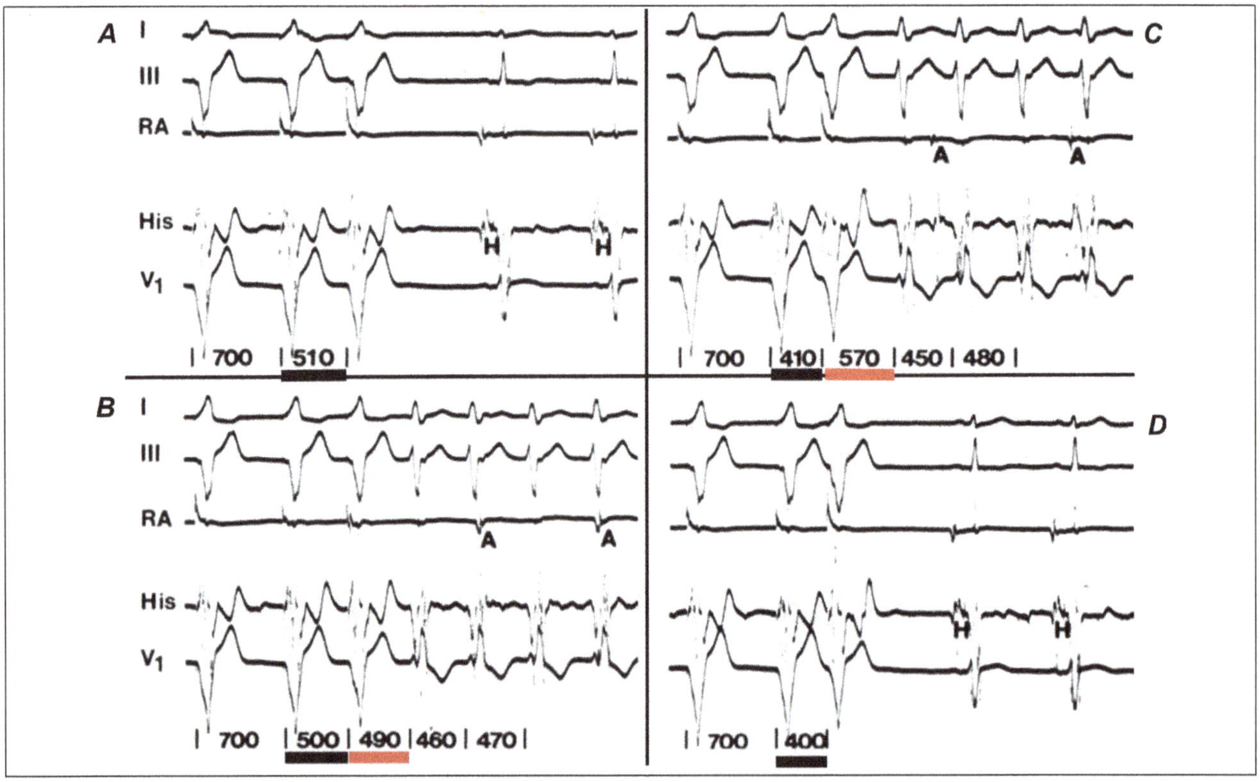

Figure 12-11 ECG leads I, III, V_1, right atrial (RA), and His bundle (His) electrograms in each panel showing an inverse relationship during initiation of VT (Wellens' ECG collection).

In Figure 12-11, Panel A, a premature impulse at a coupling interval of 510 ms does not induce reentry. In Panel B, a premature impulse with a coupling interval of 500 ms (thick black bar) initiates VT and the coupling interval to the first tachycardia impulse is 490 ms (thick red bar). In Panel C a premature impulse with a coupling interval of 410 ms (thick black bar) induces VT with the coupling interval to the first tachycardia impulse of 570 ms (thick red bar). In Panel D, at a shorter coupling interval of 400 ms (thick black bar) VT is not induced. All single premature impulses in the coupling interval range 500 to 410 ms initiated VT indicating in this patient a wide tachycardia initiating zone. In Panels B and C, there is an inverse relationship between the stimulated premature impulse coupling interval and the first impulse of tachycardia. Failure to induce VT at the shortest coupling interval in Panel D is attributed to block of the premature impulse in the circuit and defines the inner boundary of the window of vulnerability (the range of coupling intervals that initiate reentry) (see Chapter 9). This inverse relationship when comparing Panels B and C is in contrast to the direct relationship for the coupling intervals during initiation of triggered rhythms due to DADs (Figure 5-6).

Initiation by Overdrive Pacing

VT can also be initiated by overdrive pacing at a critical cycle length that causes unidirectional conduction block and slow conduction as explained in Figure 9-23. Although overdrive also can initiate DAD-triggered activity (Figure 5-4), the necessary changes in conduction required for reentry are not involved in initiation of triggered activity. Overdrive pacing is not as effective in initiating reentrant VT as programmed premature stimulation. During overdrive at short cycle lengths, repolarization and refractoriness may shorten in ventricular muscle with normal action potentials that occur in arrhythmogenic border zones (see Figure 7-6). The decrease in refractory period can prevent the necessary amount of slow conduction and/or block for initiation of reentry. In contrast, DAD-triggered activity is more easily induced by overdrive than premature stimulation, since overdrive results in more Ca^{2+} entry into triggerable cells than one or several premature stimuli (Table 5-1).

Resetting and Termination

The effects of premature stimulation on reentry causing sustained monomorphic VT conform with the description of the anatomical model of reentry in Figure 9-27. In **Figure 12-12**, Panels A and B show the resetting response for a circuit with a fully excitable gap. Panels C and D show the response of a different circuit characteristic of a partially excitable gap.

Figure 12-12, Panel A shows the effects of single premature stimuli applied to the right ventricular apex (indicated by "S" on the RVA recording) on a VT with a cycle length of 380 ms. The return cycle in response to premature coupling intervals of 350 ms (A1), 310 ms (A2), and 250 ms (A3) is constant at 400 ms (labeled above the RVA recording). Tachycardia is reset in each case since the sum of the premature and return cycle lengths are less than twice the tachycardia cycle length. The graph in Panel B shows the constant return cycle (RC) over the range of premature coupling intervals (PCI, filled circles), a flat response. This characteristic indicates conduction of the premature impulses in the completely excitable gap of the circuit (described in Figure 9-27). At shorter coupling intervals, premature impulses fail to enter and reset the circuit, possibly because they encounter refractory myocardium outside the circuit. Resetting with double premature stimuli (Panel B, unfilled circles) enables premature impulses with shorter coupling intervals to enter the circuit, since application of the first premature stimulus shortens the refractory period of intervening myocardium, enabling the second premature impulse to more easily access the circuit. The constant 400 ms coupling to the return tachycardia impulse is extended to even shorter coupling intervals (unfilled circles).

In Panel C, in a different patient, only double premature stimuli (indicated by S, and S below the RVA recording) were utilized to characterize the resetting response of a different VT with a cycle length of 315 ms. The first premature stimulus that is set at a constant 300 ms facilitates the ability of the second one to reach and penetrate the circuit by shortening the refractory period of myocardium between the stimulation site and the circuit. The coupling interval of the second premature impulse is decreased from 295 ms (Panel C1) to 270 ms (Panel C2), and 240 ms (Panel C3). The second premature impulse is the one that enters and resets the circuit. The return cycle increases from 350 ms (Panel C1) to 355 ms (Panel C2) to 380 ms (Panel C3). The graph in Panel D shows the inverse relationship between the return cycle and premature coupling interval between the second and first stimulus (S-S CI). This characteristic is a result of slowing of conduction of the premature impulse in the partially excitable gap of the reentrant circuit, as the coupling interval decreases (Figure 9-27). There is no large, fully excitable gap since there is no flat segment of the response curve.

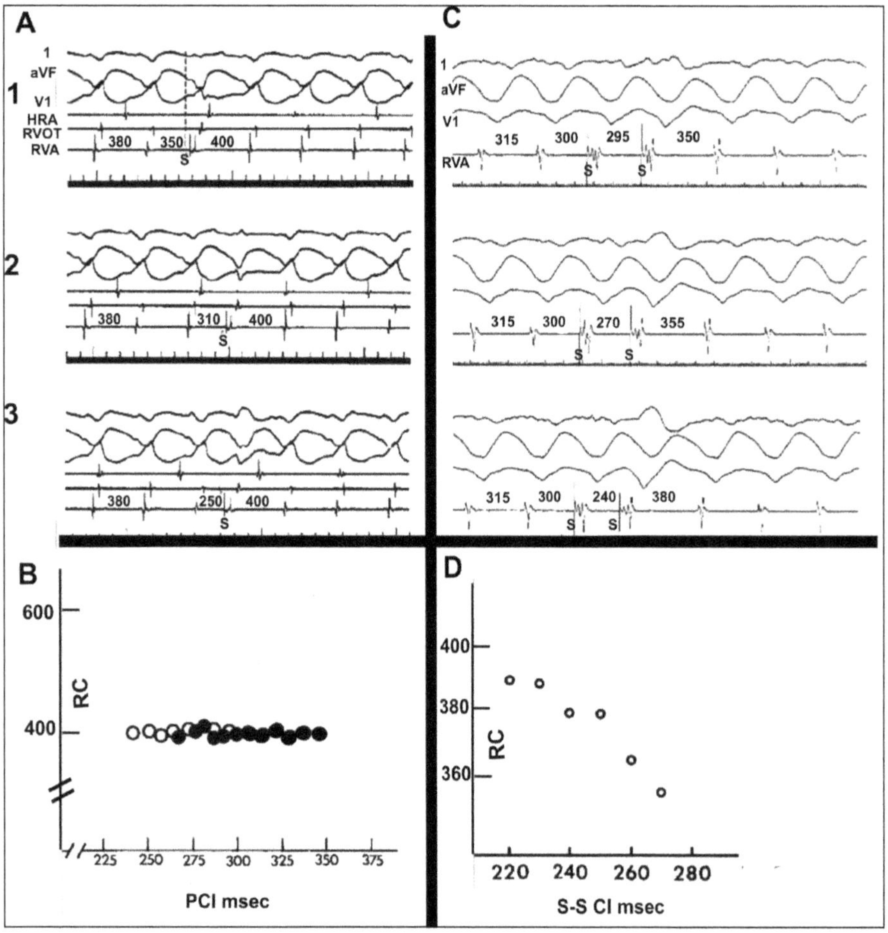

Figure 12-12 Resetting response patterns in two different patients. ECG leads I, aVF, V_1, and electrograms from high right atrium (HRA), right ventricular outflow tract (RVOT), and right ventricular apex (RVA).

Termination. The VT in Figure 12-12 (Panels A and B) was terminated at a coupling interval of 230 ms (not shown in the figure). The length of the horizontal response line shows the duration of the fully excitable gap. However, it is possible that an ascending part of the curve that shows a small partially excitable gap just prior to the coupling interval that caused block and termination, was missed since premature stimuli were not applied at small enough decrements. Reentrant circuits with fully excitable gaps also have partially excitable gaps that can be very small. In Panel D tachycardia was terminated at premature coupling intervals less than 220 ms, also indicating the inner boundary of the partially excitable gap. Other circuits can have a mixed response consisting of flat and ascending segments enabling measurement of the fully and partially excitable gap (see Figure 9-28).

Figure 12-13 shows an example of termination of another sustained VT (cycle length 410 ms) by a single stimulated premature impulse. A premature stimulus delivered to the right ventricular apex (RVA) at a coupling interval of 230 ms (at the arrow) terminates tachycardia.

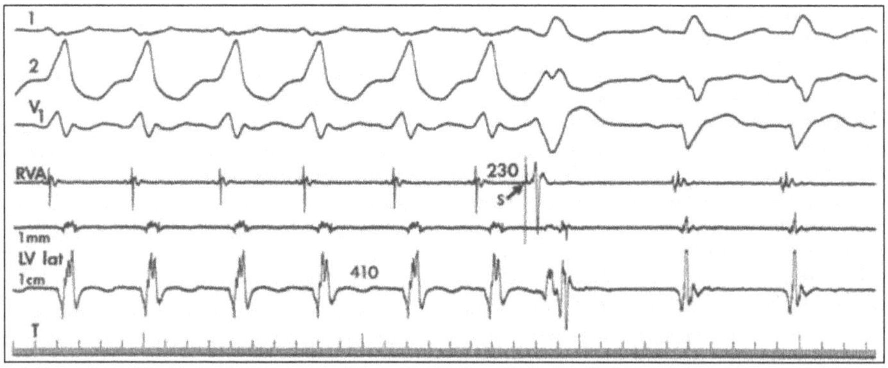

Figure 12-13 Termination of VT by a premature stimulus (**arrow**). ECG leads 1, 2, and V_1, and electrograms recorded from right ventricular apex (RVA) and lateral left ventricle (LV lat). (Reproduced from Josephson ME. *Josephson's Clinical Cardiac Electrophysiology: Techniques and Interpretations* (5th ed.). Philadelphia, PA: Wolters Kluwer; 2016.)

Overdrive and Entrainment

As described in Chapter 9, transient entrainment is continuous resetting of a reset circuit by overdrive pacing (Figure 9-29). Entrainment of VT with a left apical origin is illustrated in **Figure 12-14**. Panel A shows the ECG and electrograms during VT (cycle length 380 ms). The left ventricular (LV) electrogram recording site is at the exit from the circuit; the LV electrogram comes before the onset of the QRS (vertical dashed line) and is fractionated, characteristics of the site of VT origin. The electrogram at the right ventricular apex (RVA) is at the stimulus site and during overdrive pacing provides a rough estimate of the time the stimulated impulse enters the circuit (discounting conduction time from stimulus site to the circuit). Panel B shows the QRS morphology during pacing from the right ventricular (RVA) site during sinus rhythm.

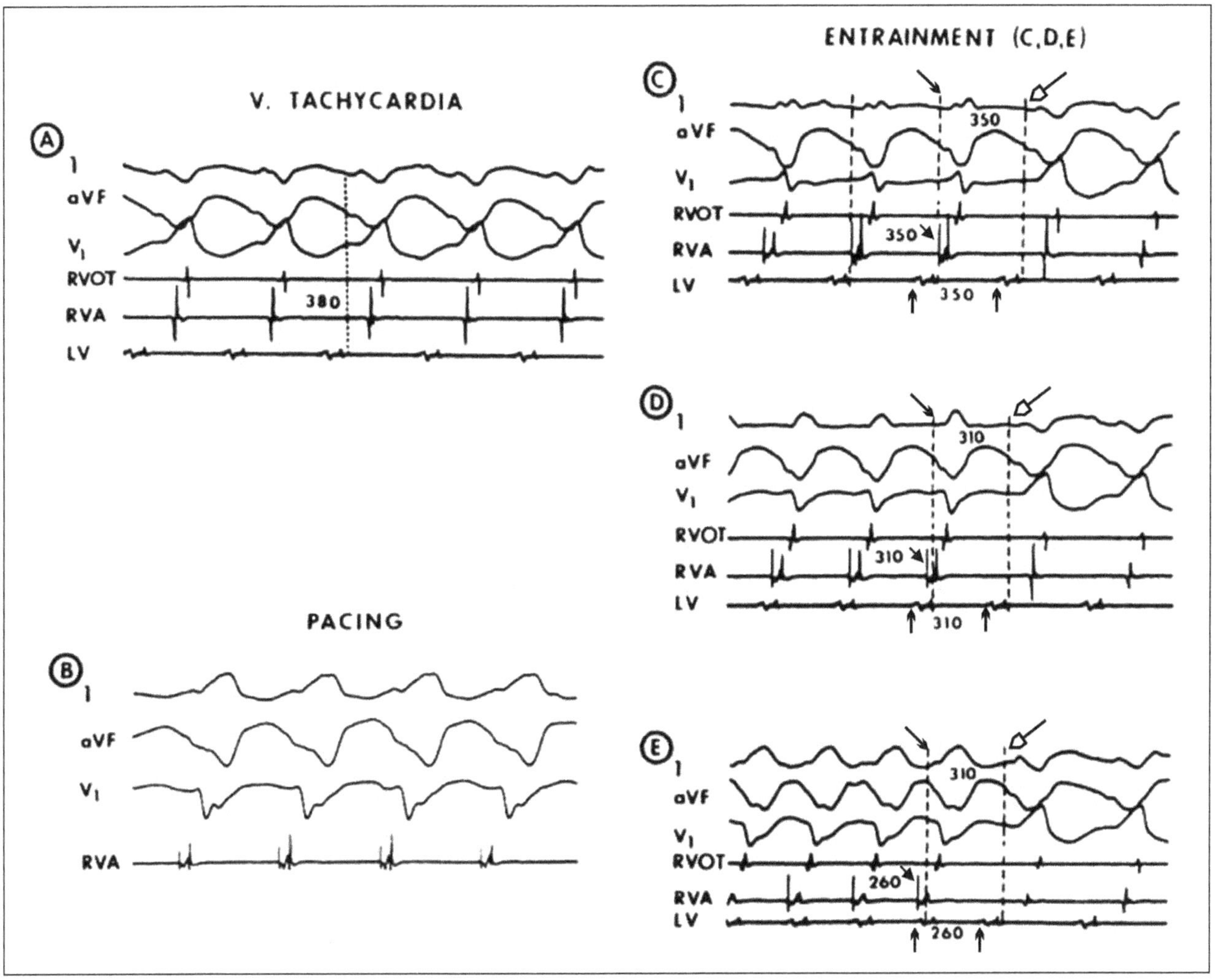

Figure 12-14 Entrainment of VT. Each panel shows three surface electrocardiographic leads (I, aVF, and V_1), along with intracardiac recordings from the right ventricular apex (RVA, pacing site) and from the left ventricle at the site of origin of tachycardia (LV). **Panel A:** Recordings during VT. **Panel B:** Pacing during sinus rhythm. **Panels C, D,** and **E** pacing during VT. (Reproduced from Josephson ME. *Josephson's Clinical Cardiac Electrophysiology: Techniques and Interpretations* (5th ed.). Philadelphia, PA: Wolters Kluwer; 2016.)

In Figure 12-14, Panels C, D, and E show entrainment of the VT from this RVA site. The first three QRS complexes of each panel are the last of a period of overdrive pacing at cycle lengths of 350 ms (Panel C), 310 ms (Panel D), and 260 ms (Panel E). The following features of entrainment are illustrated.

1. The surface electrocardiogram and all intracardiac recordings are accelerated to the pacing rate.
2. There is immediate resumption of the original VT on cessation of pacing (last paced impulse shown by black arrows above lead I and RVA). The last paced impulse travels around the circuit to cause the first impulse with a QRS morphology characteristic of the VT (unfilled arrow above lead I) (as diagrammed in Figure 9-32).
3. Fusion is evident. The QRS morphology during pacing in Panels C and D is intermediate between that of the VT (Panel A) and pacing during sinus rhythm (Panel B) (fixed fusion) and increasingly resembles the paced QRS at shorter pacing cycle lengths (progressive fusion) (as diagrammed in Figure 9-31 and 9-32).
4. In Panel E, the QRS is the same as the paced QRS although the circuit is still entrained. Entrainment can still be identified since activation at the stimulus site (RVA, downward arrow) occurs simultaneously with the LV electrogram (LV, upward arrow), which precedes the QRS and does not change its morphology indicating that it is activated orthodromically. Even at the fastest pacing cycle length during which the QRS resembles a fully paced QRS (Panel E), local fusion still occurs, the stimulus impulse occurs simultaneously with the beginning of the orthodromically activated LV electrogram.
5. Following the last stimulated impulse in Panels C, D, and E, the return cycle from the last paced complex to the first VT complex, measured at the orthodromically activated exit site from the circuit (vertical arrows below LV electrogram) is the same as the pacing cycle length (also see Figure 9-29).
6. The interval from the last RVA electrogram (vertical dashed line) to the onset of the QRS caused by the orthodromic impulse from the circuit (dashed vertical line and unfilled arrow) is a measurement of conduction of the stimulated impulse through the circuit plus normal myocardium that is seen as the onset of the QRS. Therefore, measurements of the first cycle length of VT on the QRS can be longer than measurements at the exit from the circuit because of the additional conduction delay (Panel E).

Termination at short pacing cycles. A characteristic of entrainment is termination of the tachycardia at a short pacing cycle with reversion of the ECG to that characteristic of the pacing site (diagrammed in Figure 9-30). This feature is illustrated in **Figure 12-15**. Panel A shows VT at a cycle length of 380 ms. The fractionated left ventricular electrogram (LV) is recorded at the site of origin, the initial component occurs prior to the onset of the QRS (arrows).

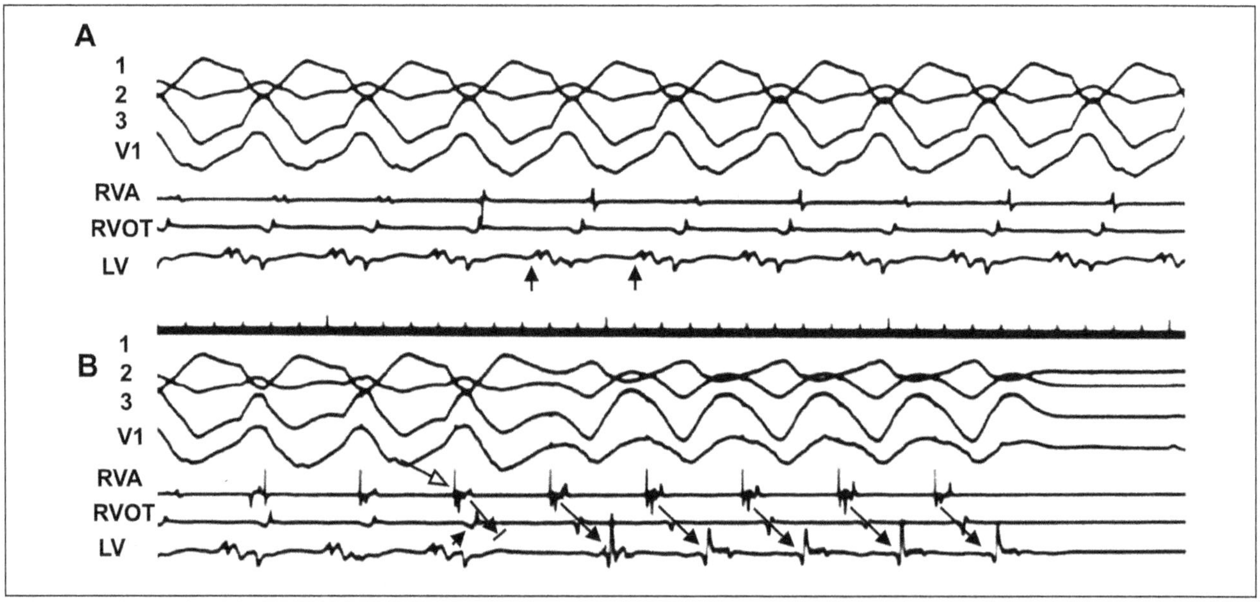

Figure 12-15 Termination of VT by overdrive pacing. ECG leads I, II, III, and V_1, and electrograms recorded from right ventricular apex (RVA), right ventricular outflow tract (RVOT), and left ventricular site of VT origin (LV) are shown in each panel. (Reproduced from Josephson ME. *Josephson's Clinical Cardiac Electrophysiology: Techniques and Interpretations* (5th ed.). Philadelphia, PA: Wolters Kluwer; 2016.)

In Figure 12-15, overdrive pacing begins in Panel B. The first stimulus does not capture the ventricles. Following the third overdrive stimulus (unfilled arrowhead on RVA), block occurs in the orthodromic direction (arrow pointing to LV). The subsequent stimulated impulses conduct antidromically to the presystolic electrogram with a shorter activation time (slanted black arrows), also indicated by the change in LV electrogram morphology. A change in QRS morphology shows that the ventricles are no longer activated by an orthodromic impulse from the circuit. When overdrive is stopped at the far right, VT is not present.

Concealed entrainment. Figure 9-33 describes the mechanism for concealed entrainment (also referred to as exact entrainment) when pacing occurs inside the circuit and the paced impulses exit through the same pathway as the intrinsic reentrant impulses so that the paced QRS is exactly the same as the QRS of the VT. Exact entrainment of VT is illustrated in **Figure 12-16**. The 12-lead ECG during VT is shown in Panel A and entrainment of the VT from a stimulus site in a protected isthmus of the circuit is in Panel B. The QRS complex in all 12 leads during entrainment (Panel B) is identical to the VT (Panel A) with comparable notching and amplitudes. Stimulation sites at which exact entrainment occurs are channels of surviving myocardium in the scar that form a protected isthmus (Figure 12-8).

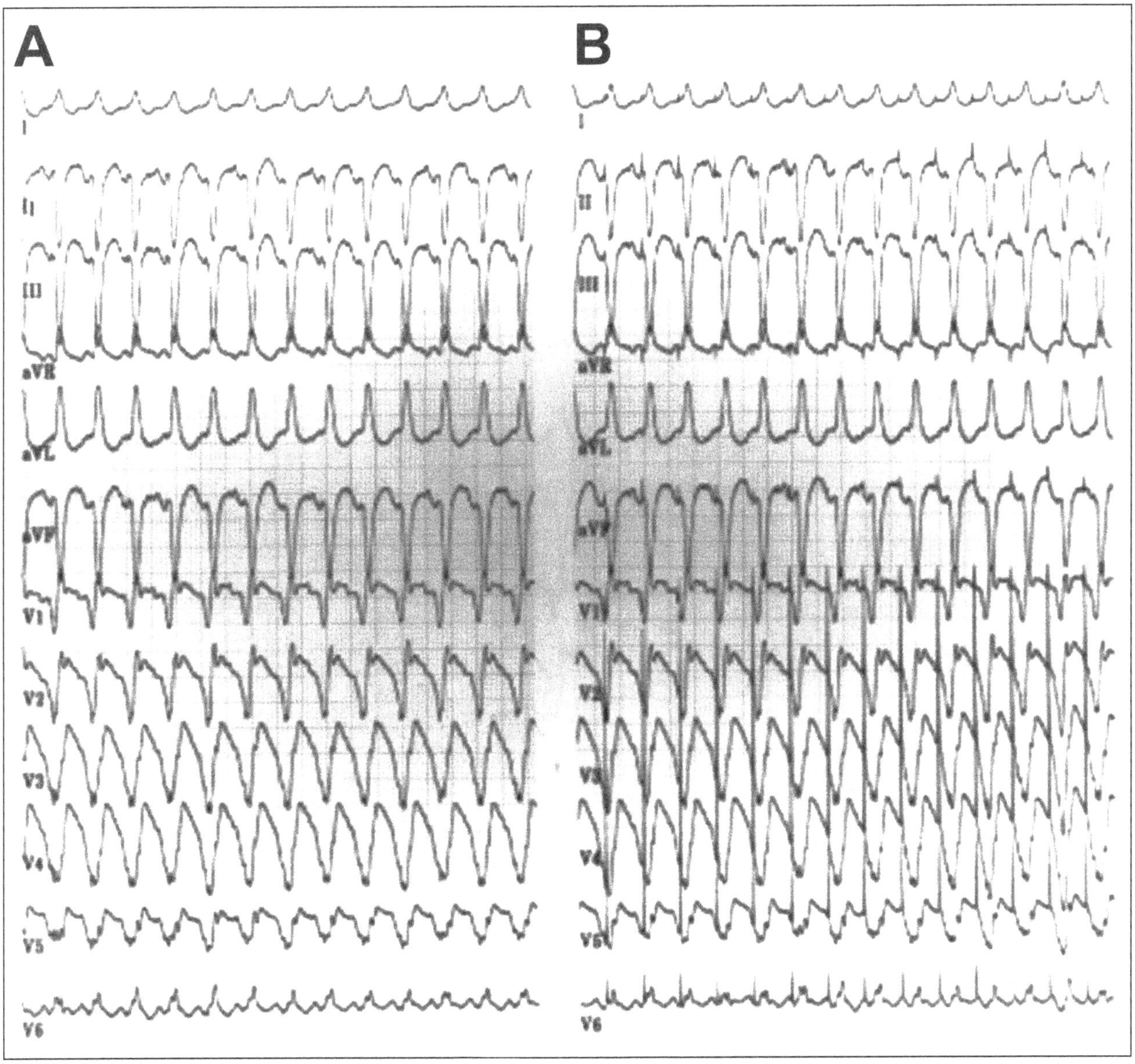

Figure 12-16 Exact (concealed) entrainment. **Panel A** shows the 12-lead ECG during VT. **Panel B** shows entrainment from a stimulus site in the protected isthmus of the VT circuit. (Reproduced from Josephson ME. *Josephson's Clinical Cardiac Electrophysiology: Techniques and Interpretations* (5th ed.). Philadelphia, PA: Wolters Kluwer; 2016.)

Autonomic Nervous System (ANS) and Drugs

Information pertaining to the effects of the ANS, drugs that act on the ANS (agonists and antagonists), and other types of drugs that are helpful in identifying the arrhythmogenic mechanisms of automaticity and triggered activity, is described in Chapters 1, 3, 5, and 6. The effects of these agents are of limited usefulness in identifying a reentrant mechanism as a cause of sustained monomorphic VT related to infarct scarring.

In general, β_1-adrenergic stimulation (from sympathetic activity or administration of β-adrenergic agonists) has little effect on electrophysiological properties of the substrate of healed infarction. While β_1-adrenergic stimulation usually accelerates repolarization of ventricular muscle, it does not influence reentrant circuits significantly that have a fully excitable gap. Also, conduction is little affected in myocardial cells with well-polarized membrane potentials in the reentrant VT substrate (Figure 12-6). Therefore, tachycardia cycle length is usually not affected, in contrast to the shortening of the cycle length of triggered and automatic tachycardia.

Spontaneous onset of reentrant VT is not necessarily related to sympathetic stimulation; there is often no increase in sinus rate prior to occurrence of VT. There is often an acceleration of rate prior to onset of DAD-triggered activity. Occasionally, isoproterenol may facilitate initiation of VT by programmed stimulation by shortening the refractory period at the site of stimulation, enabling stimulation with shorter coupled premature impulses that may be necessary to cause sufficiently slowed conduction or block to initiate reentry. β_1-receptor blockers do not prevent reentry. Isoproterenol facilitates induction of DAD-triggered activity and β-receptor blockers prevent this arrhythmogenic mechanism. Also, parasympathetic activation does not alter the electrophysiological properties of the reentrant substrate nor alter VT initiation or cycle length. The lack of a parasympathetic effect distinguishes reentrant VT related to prior infarction from some DAD-triggered VTs that can be terminated by parasympathetic stimulation. The lack of effects of adenosine and verapamil on reentrant VT related to healed infarction because they do not affect the muscle action potentials in the reentrant circuit, also distinguishes it from DAD-triggered tachycardia which is terminated by these drugs (see Chapters 5 and 6).

The response to antiarrhythmic drugs (other than verapamil described in the preceding paragraph) does not, in general, help distinguish reentrant VT from the other arrhythmogenic mechanisms and so is not described in detail here. Class IA antiarrhythmic drugs such as procainamide facilitate initiation of VT by programmed premature stimulation. This effect would not be expected of the other arrhythmogenic mechanisms and so can be used to confirm that reentry is the mechanism. This effect is likely caused by facilitating the occurrence of unidirectional block and/or slow conduction in a potential reentrant circuit related to the Class IA action to decrease I_{Na}, sometimes evident by prolongation of the duration of electrograms recorded from the circuit. Drugs such as procainamide that slow conduction in the reentrant circuit by reducing I_{Na} will prolong VT cycle length. Slowing conduction shortens the wavelength and lengthens the excitable gap. If tachycardia terminates, it likely does so because of conduction block due to insufficient axial current that results from the decreased I_{Na} and not because of effects on the excitable gap. These drugs are also expected to prolong the cycle length of arrhythmias caused by other mechanisms so changes in VT cycle length does not distinguish among mechanisms (Chapters 1 and 5). A more detailed description of antiarrhythmic drug effects on infarct scar-related VT can be found in *Josephson's Clinical Cardiac Electrophysiology*, Chapter 11.

Reentry Associated With Nonischemic Cardiomyopathy

SUSTAINED MONOMORPHIC VT

The nonischemic cardiomyopathies include dilated cardiomyopathy (DCM), hypertrophic cardiomyopathy (HCM), and arrhythmogenic right ventricular cardiomyopathy (ARVC)—the latter has been more recently referred to as arrhythmogenic cardiomyopathy since it can also involve the left ventricle. They are also characterized by sustained monomorphic VT that occurs less frequently than in ischemic heart disease. Nevertheless, when it occurs, it is usually caused by reentry in ventricular muscle that has pathological abnormalities. The ventricular conducting system is sometimes involved in the reentrant circuit.

Origin of Sustained Monomorphic VT

In contrast to the frequent subendocardial origin of infarct-related sustained monomorphic VTs, the VTs associated with nonischemic cardiomyopathies can arise in reentrant circuits located almost anywhere in the endocardium, midmyocardium, or epicardium of the left and right ventricles because of the widespread myocardial structural changes that can form reentrant circuits (see below). VT origin associated with the different cardiomyopathies differs since the location of the structural changes are different. It is estimated that reentrant circuits causing up to 50% of VTs in DCM occur either intramurally or epicardially as compared to about 10% for infarct-related VTs. A small percentage of VTs are also caused by reentry using the bundle branches of the conducting system as the reentrant circuit. The origin of reentrant tachycardia in HCM has not been located although it is likely in the septum where the most severe structural changes occur. In ARVC many of the circuits are on the endocardium of the right ventricle, a major site of structural abnormalities, although a left ventricular site of origin has been documented in patients who have left ventricular structural changes.

The basic ECG features that locate the origin of VT are the same as described previously for ischemic VT. **Figure 12-17** shows monomorphic sustained VT in a patient with dilated nonischemic cardiomyopathy (DCM). Panel A shows VT with a superior QRS axis in the frontal plane. The initial positivity in lead I suggests an origin at the midlevel between the septum and apical border of the posterior papillary muscle. Q-S complexes from V_3 to V_6 indicate an inferoapical origin in the left ventricle that may be epicardial. During sinus rhythm (Panel B), LBBB with low QRS voltage in the extremity leads indicate marked cardiac enlargement.

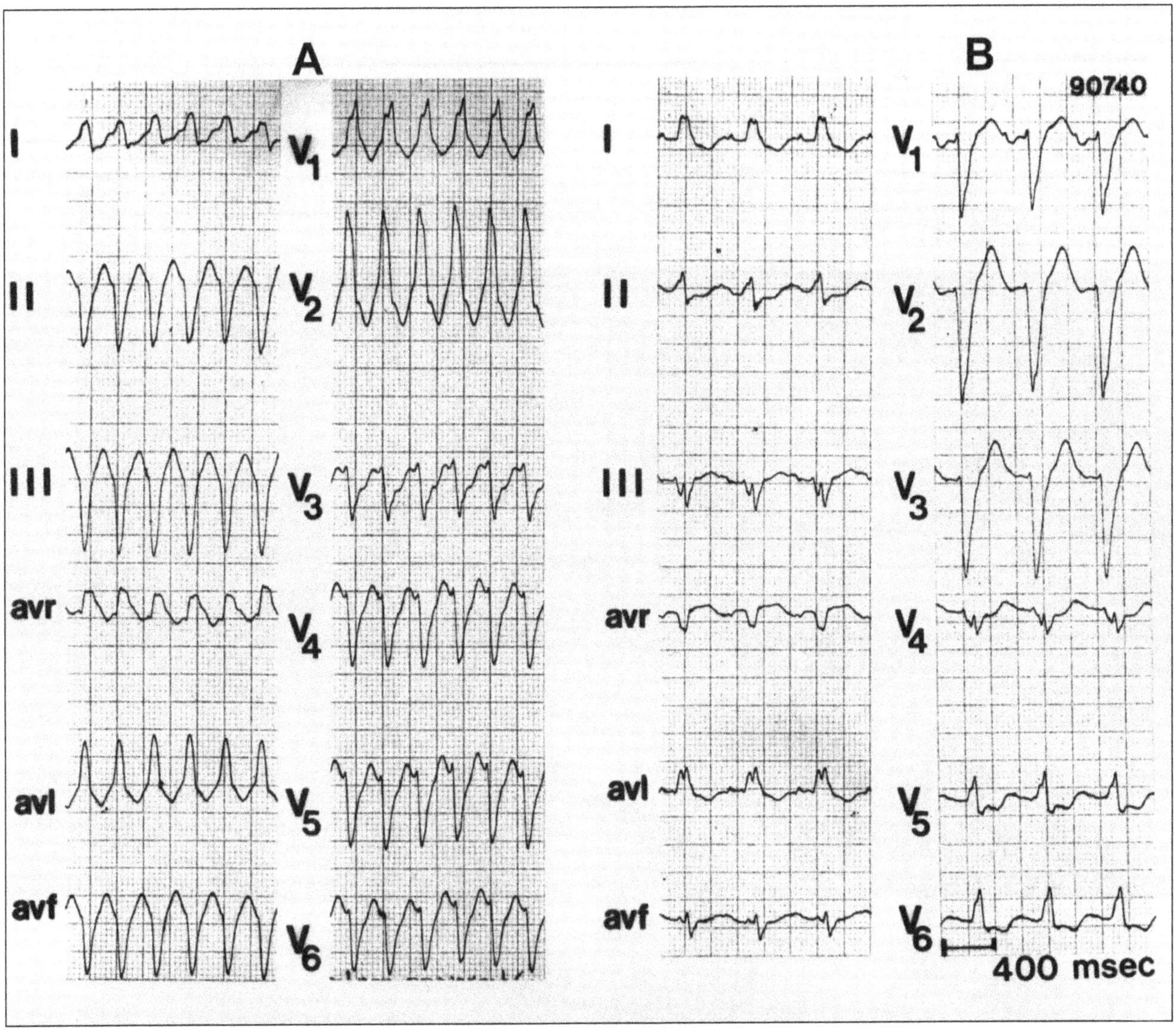

Figure 12-17 A 12-lead ECG during VT (**Panel A**) and sinus rhythm (**Panel B**) from a patient with dilated nonischemic cardiomyopathy (Wellens' ECG collection).

Activation Mapping and Patterns of Reentrant Circuits

Activation mapping, as described for Figure 12-2, can also be utilized to locate the site of origin. However, when the circuit has an intramural or epicardial location, earliest endocardial activity as determined by the usual procedure of catheter mapping is usually not mid-diastolic but occurs closer to the onset of the subsequent QRS. Epicardial mapping using special techniques show that the site of origin of an epicardial reentrant circuit is activated much earlier than the earliest endocardial site and can be mid-diastolic. Intramural mapping is not feasible in clinical studies. When a circuit is intramural, the earliest site activated on the endocardium is later than the actual earliest activated site intramurally, reflecting conduction time from the circuit to the endocardium.

In DCM, reentrant circuits are located either in the subendocardium or subepicardium, or involve both regions depending on the location of the structural changes that form the circuits. **Figure 12-18**, Panels B and D show how the activation pattern of an epicardial reentrant circuit appears on both the epicardial and endocardial surfaces. (Panels A and C show electrogram voltage maps during sinus rhythm that are described later in the section on structure and electrophysiology.)

In Figure 12-18, Panel B, shows an epicardial activation map of a figure-eight reentrant pattern (see Figure 9-17) as pointed out by the arrows (activation is from red → yellow → green → blue → magenta).

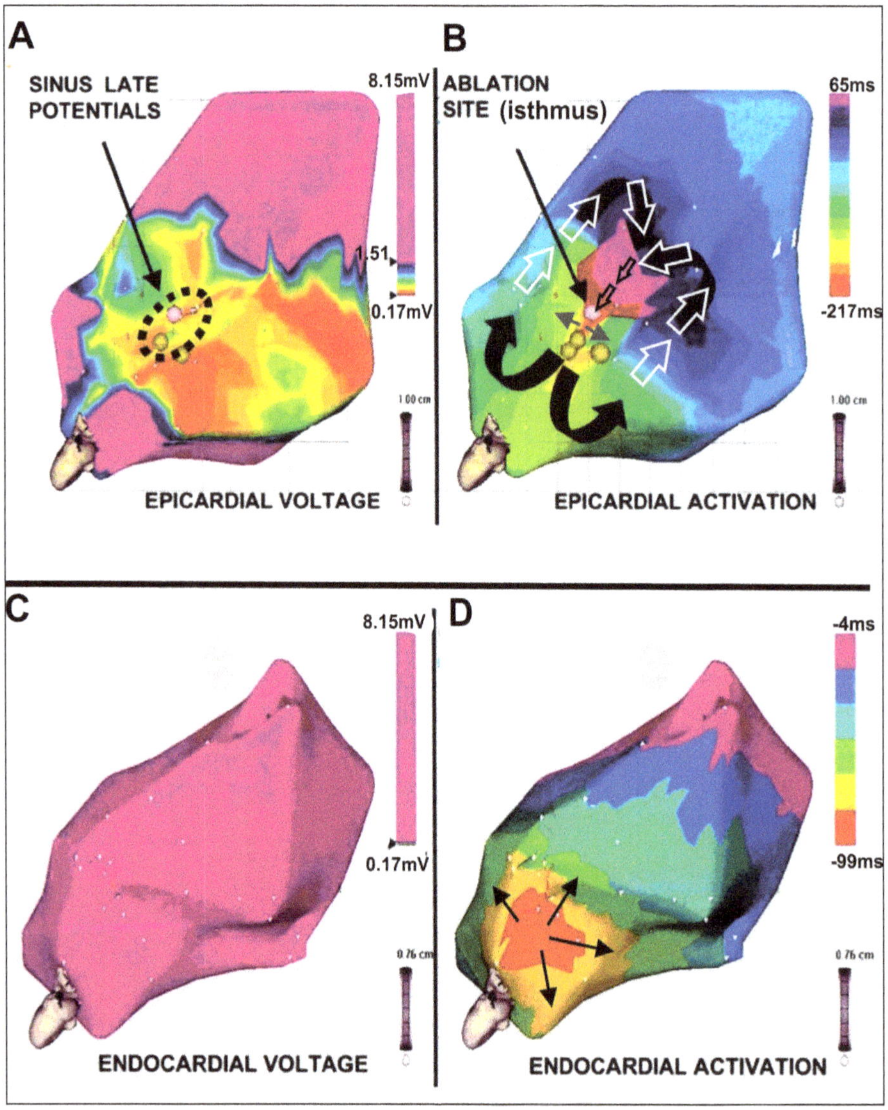

Figure 12-18 **Panel A:** Electrogram amplitudes (**color scale at the right**) plotted on posterior oblique view of the left ventricle during sinus rhythm. **Panel B:** Epicardial activation map during VT. Color code is activation times. **Panel C:** Endocardial sinus rhythm voltage map (**color scale at the right**), of the left ventricle in the left posterior oblique view. **Panel D:** Activation map of the endocardial surface during VT. **Color code at right** indicates activation times. (Reproduced with permission from Swarup V, et al. Ablation of epicardial macroreentrant ventricular tachycardia associated with idiopathic nonischemic dilated cardiomyopathy by a percutaneous transthoracic approach. *J Cardiovasc Electrophysiol.* 2002;13:1164–1168.)

There are two reentrant circuits (larger white arrows) with a narrow central common pathway or isthmus indicated by the small black unfilled arrows. The latest activated region (magenta) adjacent to the earliest (red) in the central common pathway is characteristic of reentrant circuits. Exit from the circuit is from the end of the isthmus in dark red, 217 ms before the onset of the QRS (–217 on the color code at the right) (large curved black arrows). The map shows slow activation in regions with closely spaced isochrones and more rapid activation in regions with widely spaced isochrones likely related to the amount of structural damage in different regions of the circuit. The site in the isthmus where ablation stopped reentry is indicated by the long black arrow.

Panel D shows a map of endocardial activation during the same VT. When the reentrant circuit is epicardial, the earliest endocardial activation site represents the site at which the impulse from the circuit first reaches the endocardium but not its origin. The earliest activation in red (–99 ms before the onset of the QRS, color code at the right) represents the endocardial breakthrough of the impulse conducting from the epicardial circuit and appears to be focal. From this site, there is radial activation (arrows). In this case, epicardial ablation in the narrow isthmus (labeled in Panel B), rather than endocardial ablation, terminates VT.

Interrelationship of Substrate Structure and Electrophysiological Mechanisms of Reentry

Structure of the Arrhythmogenic Substrate

Table 12-1 summarizes the structural changes in nonischemic cardiomyopathies and compares them to the changes that underlie reentrant VT in ischemic heart disease and healed infarcts that were described in the first part of this chapter. The electrical basis for arrhythmias in the nonischemic cardiomyopathies may be due to the underlying substrate specific to the disease.

Fibrosis is a prominent feature in all, leading to separation of muscle bundles, disruption of gap junction connections, formation of muscle bundles of different sizes, and changes in orientation of muscle bundles. Myocytes may also be hypertrophied. In DCM, these structural changes are widespread throughout the left and right ventricles, resulting in formation of reentrant circuits in subendocardial, mid-myocardial, subepicardial regions (Figure 12-18), or reentrant circuits that encompass several different regions of the ventricular wall. In DCM, mutations in lamin A/C (LMNA) have been noted in some patients and lead to aberrant cell Ca^{2+} handling, which may be related to the structural changes. In HCM, cellular hypertrophy is accompanied by genetic based myofibrillar disarray. Septal myocardium shows the most disorganized architecture with adjacent hypertrophied cardiac muscle cells arranged perpendicularly and obliquely. This site (the septum) would seem to have the most propensity to develop reentrant circuits. In ARVC, ankyrinB and desmosomal gene mutations have been identified. There is loss of electrical coupling between cells that can lead to cell death and scarring. The right ventricle is mostly involved with myocardial replacement by fibrous and fatty tissue, or just fatty tissue, leading to formation of reentrant circuits mostly in the subepicardium or subendocardium. However, when pathological changes occur in the left ventricle, circuits may locate here as well.

Table 12-1 Components of the Arrhythmogenic Substrate in Ischemic and Nonischemic Structural Heart Disease

Structural Heart Disease	Fibrosis	Separation of Muscle Bundles, Changes in Bundle Size and Orientation	Gap Junction Disruption and Remodeling	Nonuniform Anisotropy	Ion Channel Remodeling
Ischemic cardiomyopathy					
Coronary artery disease/myocardial infarction	++++	++++	++++	++++	++++
Nonischemic cardiomyopathy					
Dilated cardiomyopathy	++++	++++	++++	++++	??
Hypertrophic cardiomyopathy	++++	++++	++++	++++	++
Arrhythmogenic cardiomyopathy	++++	++++	++++	++++	++++

+ = presence of property indicated in left column. ?? = likely that ion channel remodeling changes action potential characteristics but detailed quantification is not available.

Relationship of Structural Changes to Electrophysiology

The structural changes in Table 12-1, have similar electrophysiological consequences that were described for healed, scarred infarcted hearts. The combination of fibrosis and gap junction remodeling is a cause of nonuniform anisotropy, which is involved in the slow conduction that enables reentry to occur. Interconnections of large and small diameter myocardial bundles results in regions of impedance mismatch and wavefront curvature, also contributing to the slow conduction and block crucial for occurrence of reentry.

Low-amplitude bipolar electrograms. The structural features of the nonischemic cardiomyopathies listed in Table 12-1 that cause the abnormalities in conduction that result in reentry, can be detected by the characteristics of bipolar electrograms recorded during both sinus rhythm and VT. During sinus rhythm, abnormal electrograms that have multiple components, low amplitudes, and prolonged durations (similar to those shown for ischemic cardiomyopathy in Figure 12-7) are characteristic of regions where reentrant circuits form.

In Figure 12-18, Panel A, epicardial electrogram amplitudes during sinus rhythm are plotted on a reconstruction of the posterior oblique view of the left ventricle for the same region where the reentrant circuit in Panel B was located. This voltage map shows a large region of abnormal, low-amplitude electrograms, < 0.5 mV (red, yellow, green, blue area; purple area is normal) in the epicardium during sinus rhythm. A region activated after the end of the QRS (late potentials) enclosed by the dashed oval, coincides with the location of the isthmus of the epicardial reentrant circuit (note the similarity to the voltage map for an ischemic site of VT origin, Figure 12-8). Structural changes in regions not associated with reentrant circuits, can also cause abnormal electrograms. In contrast, patients with DCM often have normal, large-amplitude endocardial electrograms during sinus rhythm when the reentrant circuit is epicardial or intramural as shown by the sinus rhythm voltage map in Figure 12-18, Panel C.

Electrograms during VT. Similar to VT associated with infarction (Figure 12-2), in nonischemic cardiomyopathies, electrograms recorded at the location of the reentrant circuit during VT can be mid-diastolic, fractionated, and sometimes continuous throughout diastole (continuous activity). Figure 12-19 shows electrograms from the epicardial surface of the left ventricle in a patient with DCM, recorded with an electrode catheter inserted into the pericardial space with a subxyphoid approach. The epicardial electrograms during sinus rhythm (left panel, ABL 3-4, and ABL 1-2) have a low amplitude (voltage calibration is absent), long duration, and are fractionated, with components occurring after the QRS (arrowheads in left panel indicate late potentials). Electrogram fractionation and duration increase during VT in the right panel so that it is almost continuous activity, with the earliest component of the electrogram in ABL-1-2 occurring in mid-diastole; both features are expected to occur at the site of origin of reentrant VT, similar to ischemic VT.

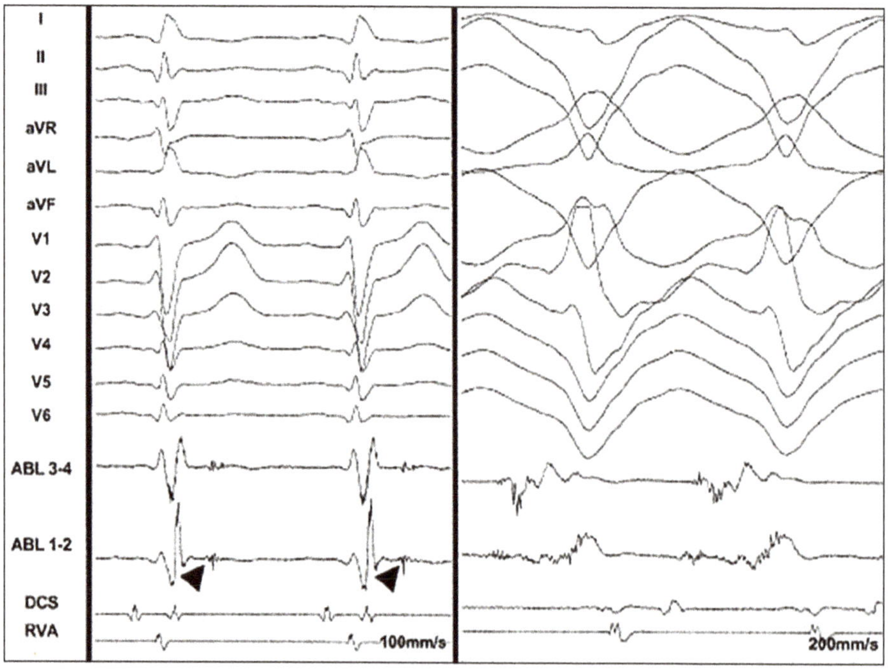

Figure 12-19 A 12-lead surface ECG and electrograms recorded from epicardium of left ventricle during sinus rhythm (**left**) and VT (**right**) in a patient with DCM. Electrogram recording location: epicardial ablation catheter (ABL 3-4, ABL 1-2), distal coronary sinus (DCS), and endocardial right ventricular apex (RVA). **Arrows at left** point to isolated late potentials during sinus rhythm. (Reproduced from Swarup V, Morton JB, Arruda M, Wilbur DJ. Ablation of epicardial macroreentrant ventricular tachycardia associated with idiopathic nonischemic dilated cardiomyopathy by a percutaneous transthoracic approach. *J Cardiovasc Electrophysiol.* 2002;13:1164–1168.)

Mid-diastolic, long-duration, fractionated electrograms should also occur at intramural sites during VT when the circuit is located in that region. Although documented in experimental animal studies by inserting electrodes intramurally, intramural mapping is not feasible in clinical studies.

Effects of Electrical Stimulation

The effects of electrical stimulation in patients with sustained monomorphic VT no matter the underlying disease conform to the expected effects of stimulation on reentrant circuits. The concepts described in detail for sustained monomorphic VT in ischemic heart disease apply to nonischemic cardiomyopathies and will only be briefly summarized here.

In most patients with sustained monomorphic VT, the same tachycardia can be initiated either by overdrive pacing or programmed premature stimulation that establish the necessary conditions of slow conduction and unidirectional conduction block. **Figure 12-20** illustrates VT initiated by overdrive pacing in a patient with hypertrophic cardiomyopathy. The first three QRS complexes at the left are the last of a period of atrial pacing at a cycle length of 400 ms (indicated by S on the HRA recording), and are followed by VT with a LBBB morphology that is similar to spontaneous VT in this patient.

VT can also be induced by programmed premature stimulation with either single or multiple stimuli. As with induction of VT in ischemic heart disease, a critical pacing or premature cycle length is necessary to initiate VT. The anatomical model of induction of reentry in Figure 9-23 and Figure 9-25 explains the mechanisms for initiation. An inverse relationship occurs between the initiating cycle length and the first cycle length of tachycardia similar to the relationship shown for VT in ischemic disease in Figure 12-11.

Once VT is initiated it can also be reset, and entrained by premature or overdrive stimulation. Termination occurs at a critical stimulus cycle length. Characteristics of the excitable gap have not been determined. The features of entrainment described in Chapter 9, occur demonstrating that VT is caused by reentry. Exact entrainment can occur from the site where the reentrant circuit is located. For example, when the circuit is on the epicardial surface, exact entrainment can only occur with epicardial stimulation.

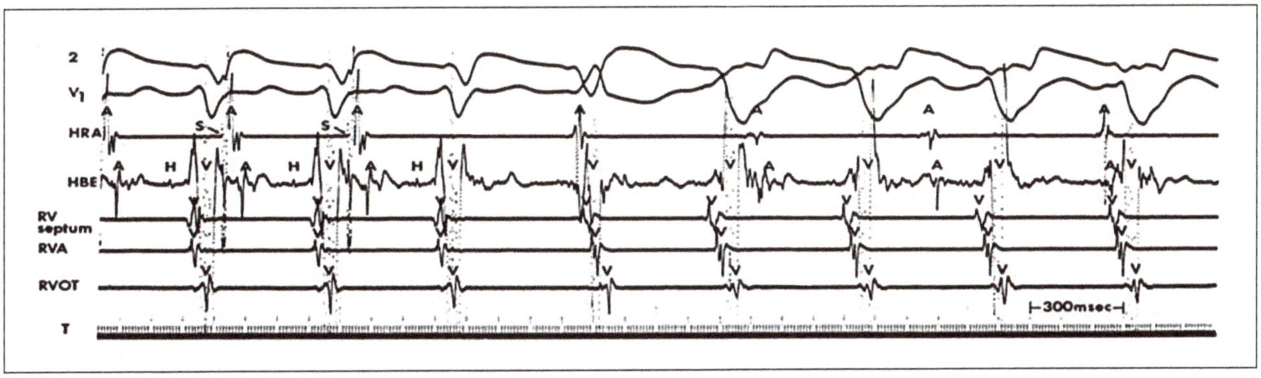

Figure 12-20 Initiation of VT by atrial pacing in a patient with hypertrophic cardiomyopathy. ECG leads II, and V_1, and electrograms from high right atrium (HRA), His bundle region (HBE), right ventricular (RV) septum, right ventricular apex (RVA), and right ventricular outflow tract (RVOT). (Reproduced from Josephson ME. *Josephson's Clinical Cardiac Electrophysiology: Techniques and Interpretations* (5th ed.). Philadelphia, PA: Wolters Kluwer; 2016.)

Reentry in the Ventricular Conducting System

BUNDLE BRANCH REENTRANT VT

ECG Characteristics

The ECG in **Figure 12-21** shows a sustained monomorphic VT at the left with a RBBB pattern, caused by bundle branch reentry. Tachycardia was terminated by two stimulated ventricular premature impulses (arrows) and after three conducted sinus beats, spontaneously reoccurred. During tachycardia the QRS is similar to the QRS during sinus rhythm, which is typical for bundle branch reentrant VT. This classification of reentry utilizes an anatomic reentrant circuit formed by the distal end of the His bundle and the left and right bundle branches described in Figure 12-22.

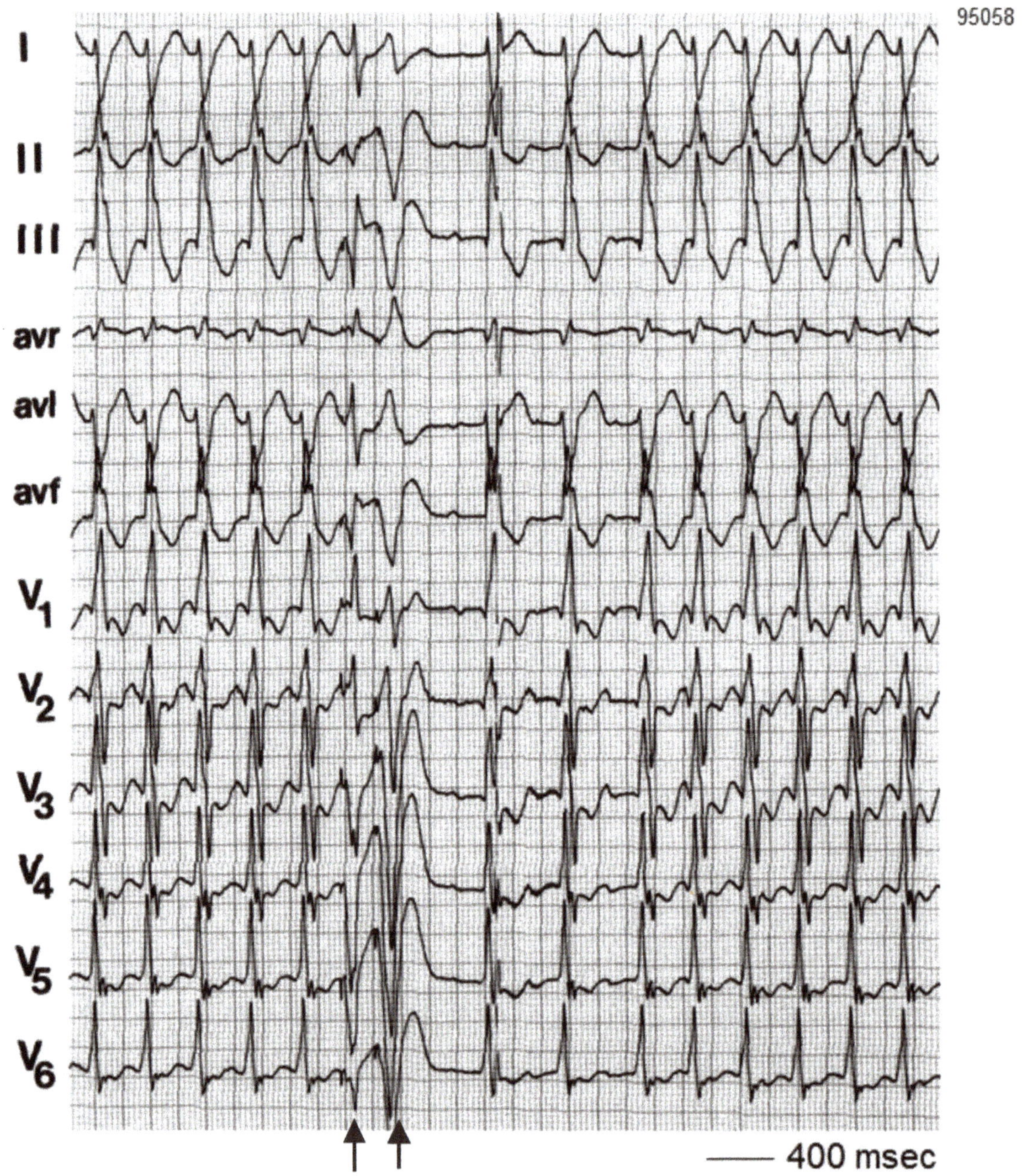

Figure 12-21 A 12-lead ECG of ventricular tachycardia caused by bundle branch reentry (Wellens' ECG collection).

Bundle branch reentry causes less than 10% of all sustained monomorphic VTs. It is most often associated with a large post infarct anteroseptal scar or a nonischemic dilated cardiomyopathy, but sometimes occurs in patients with myotonic dystrophy or with aortic valvular heart disease. In some patients it may have a genetic component, a mutation in the *LMNA* gene that encodes lamin proteins or a loss in function mutation in the Na^+ channel gene, *SCN5A*. VT can have a LBBB or RBBB pattern.

Bundle branch reentry can cause VT in patients with a healed myocardial infarction resulting from proximal occlusion of the left anterior descending coronary artery before the first septal branch that results in damage to the superior part of the inter ventricular septum with scar formation. Those patients with septal infarcts with bundle branch reentrant tachycardia, usually have a RBBB pattern with or without fascicular block during VT. Bundle branch reentry can only be diagnosed with certainty by using intracardiac electrogram recordings from both the right and left conducting system (see next section on origin and Figure 12-22). This necessary proof in septal infarction must still be obtained. RBBB during bundle branch reentry must also be distinguished from interfascicular reentry, which may have identical ECG characteristics but involves a circuit comprised of the anterior and posterior fascicles of the LBB. Interfascicular reentry is described later in this chapter. Analysis of the timing of both RBB and LBB electrograms in relation to the His bundle electrogram (HBE) in sinus rhythm and during VT are required to distinguish between bundle branch reentry with RBBB and interfascicular reentry.

Patients with tachycardia caused by bundle branch reentry have evidence of conduction system disease as indicated by sinus rhythm ECG patterns showing intraventricular conduction delays, incomplete/complete anterograde LBBB, or incomplete/complete anterograde RBBB. Physiological complete bundle branch block is actually not present even though ECG criteria for anterograde block might be met, since the reentrant impulse must be able to conduct through the bundle branches that form the reentrant circuit.

Origin of Bundle Branch Reentrant VT

In sustained monomorphic VT caused by bundle branch reentry, the anatomic circuit consists of the bundle branches, septal ventricular myocardium and distal part of the His bundle that connects the bundle branches (diagrammed and explained in Figure 12-22). Parts of the circuit have abnormal conducting properties caused by disease, necessary for sustained reentry, as evidenced by a bundle branch block pattern and long H-V interval in the His bundle electrogram during sinus rhythm. Initiation of bundle branch reentry requires the transient occurrence of complete block in one of the bundles that is unidirectional (see the model for initiation of reentry in Figure 9-1 and Figure 9-14). That block may occur spontaneously during sinus rhythm or after a decrease in supraventricular or ventricular cycle length, often in the form of an atrial or ventricular premature impulse. The bundle branch in which unidirectional block occurs can be either the right or left bundle. The blocked bundle branch determines the antegrade pathway from the circuit to activation of ventricular muscle and thus whether the VT has a LBBB or RBBB pattern.

Reentrant Bundle Branch VT with a LBBB Pattern

In **Figure 12-22**, Panel A, conduction slowing in the LBB during sinus rhythm as it might occur in nonischemic dilated cardiomyopathy is diagrammed by the dashed yellow arrows, with normal antegrade conduction in the RBB, indicated by the solid yellow arrow. Therefore, initial ventricular activation is via the RBB and the QRS has a LBBB morphology. Panel B shows the initiation of the most common form of reentrant tachycardia with a LBBB pattern in this pathology, after a premature ventricular impulse caused by any mechanism, originating near the asterisk. The initiating impulse blocks retrogradely in the RBB (green arrow with horizontal black line) with slowing of retrograde conduction characteristic of a premature impulse, through the LBB (dashed yellow arrow). The time course of repolarization (phases 2 and 3) and refractory periods of Purkinje cells in the right bundle are normally longer than in the left, leading to the more prevalent conduction block in the right bundle, of ventricular premature impulses that initiate reentry (Figure 2-22, Panel B).

In Figure 12-22, Panel B, the retrograde impulse in the LBB (yellow dashed arrow) then enters the RBB through the connecting distal His bundle (HB) (curved dashed yellow arrow) and propagates antegradely in the RBB (dashed yellow arrow continues). If conduction is sufficiently slow for it to arrive at the site at which the premature impulse initially blocked, after it has recovered excitability, the impulse will conduct through the RBB (beginning at the asterisk in Figure 12-22, Panel C), from which it activates the ventricles. The reentrant impulse then crosses back to the LBB through septal myocardium (dashed green arrow), and again conducts retrogradely through the LBB, continuing to propagate through the reentrant circuit with this pattern. Maintenance of reentry is enabled by slowed conduction in one or both of the bundle branches at the decreased cycle length (Figure 12-22, Panel C). (Panel D showing the RBBB pattern is described later).

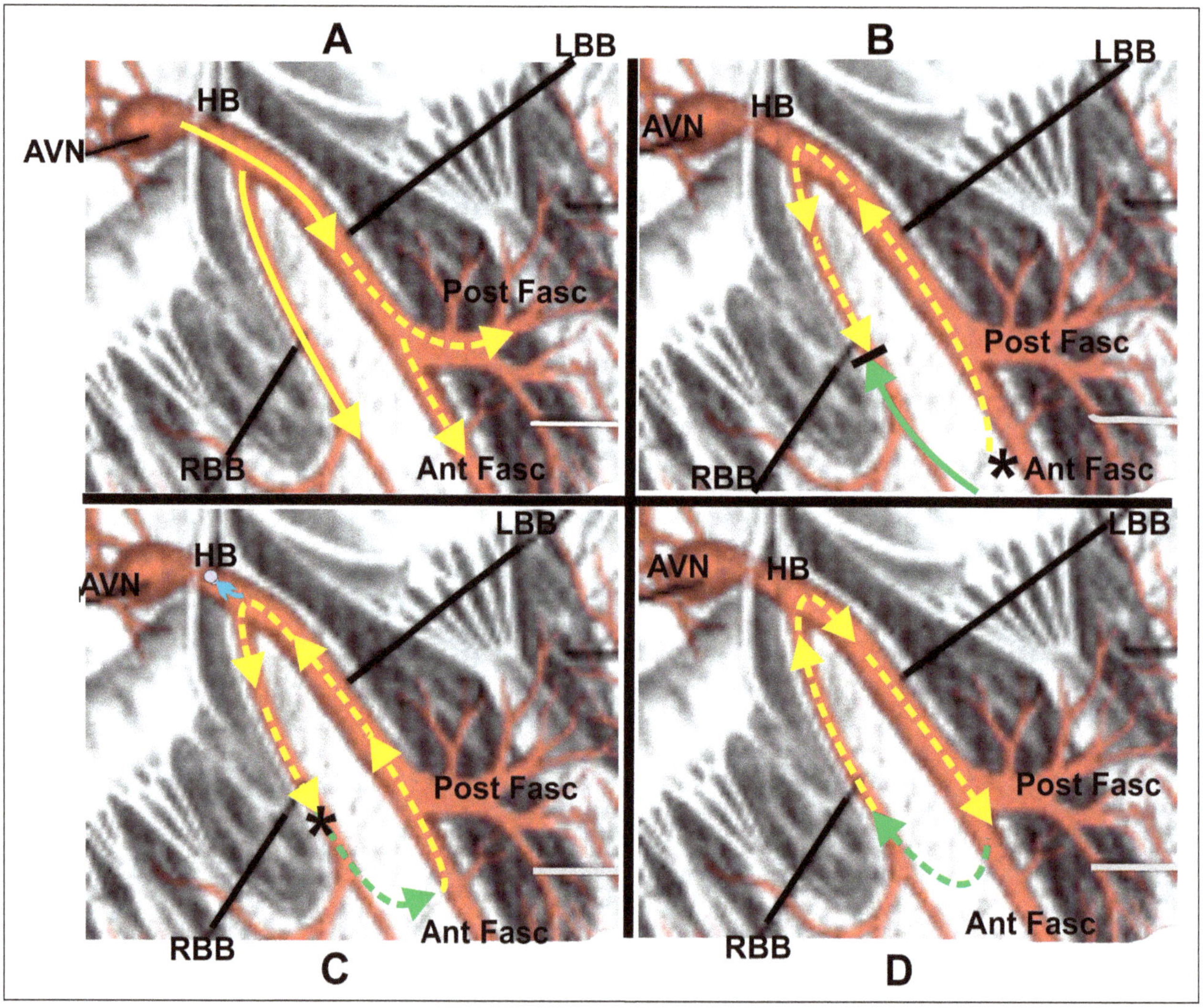

Figure 12-22 Each panel shows the A-V node (AVN), His bundle (HB), right bundle branch (RBB), left bundle branch (LBB), posterior fascicle (Post Fasc), and anterior fascicle (Ant Fasc).

The sequence of activation in the circuit in Figure 12-22 Panels B and C is shown in **Figure 12-23** in a patient with dilated cardiomyopathy and a VT with a LBBB pattern. The electrograms and arrows point out the sequence of activation from the left Purkinje system–LBB (dLPF) retrograde to → His bundle (H) → antegrade to right bundle branch (RBB) → to ventricular muscle (VM) and then back into the left Purkinje system.

His bundle activation in bundle branch reentry. In Figure 12-23, a His bundle electrogram is shown during tachycardia. Usually the His bundle is retrogradely activated due to retrograde activation of its distal end connecting the bundle branches (Figure 2-22, Panel C, blue arrow). Antegrade His bundle activation may occur when there is a marked distance between the origin of the bundle branches; when the anterogradely conducting bundle branch originates much lower from the His bundle than the retrogradely conducting bundle branch. In both situations (retrograde or antegrade His bundle activation), the His bundle deflection (H) is in between two QRS complexes during bundle branch reentrant VT (Figure 12-23). This pattern is unlike VT caused by myocardial reentry where the His bundle deflection is often obscured by the ventricular electrogram since the His bundle is usually not part of the circuit.

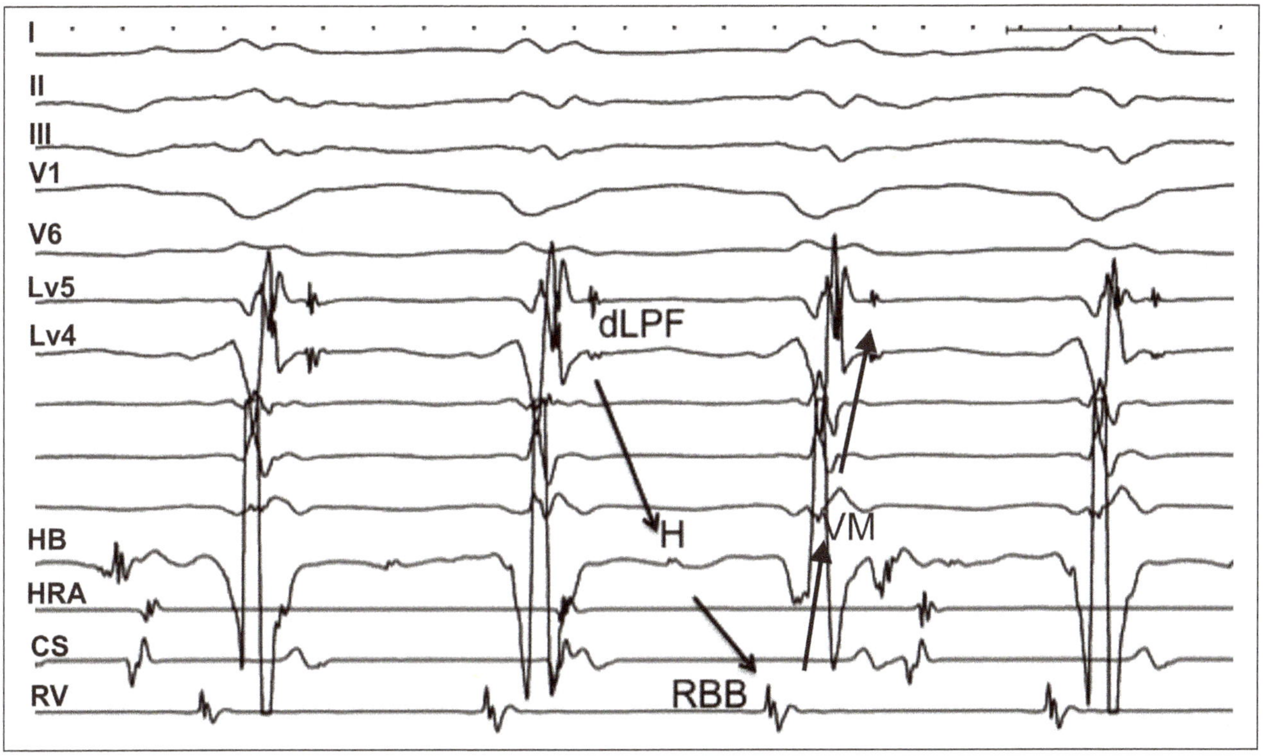

Figure 12-23 ECG leads I, II, III, V_1, and V_6, and bipolar electrograms recorded from distal left bundle branch (Lv5, Lv4; labeled dLPF, distal left Purkinje electrogram), His bundle (HB and H, His bundle deflection); VM, septal ventricular muscle; HRA, high right atrium; CS, coronary sinus; RV, right ventricle; RBB, right bundle branch electrogram.

During VT caused by bundle branch reentry, the interval from the His bundle electrogram to the VT QRS depends on anterograde or retrograde His bundle activation. The H-V interval will be similar to that interval during sinus rhythm when part of the His bundle is incorporated into the tachycardia circuit. It will be shorter, when only the distal end of the His bundle connecting the bundle branches is part of the circuit, and almost the entire His bundle is retrogradely activated (see Figure 12-22, Panel C, blue arrow).

Bundle Branch Reentry with a RBBB Pattern

If the ventricular premature impulse that initiates VT blocks in the LBB rather than the RBB (not shown), for reasons described below, the antegrade pathway for ventricular activation would be through the left bundle and a VT with a RBBB pattern would occur (Figure 12-22, Panel D).

Supraventricular Initiation

Supraventricular impulses can also initiate bundle branch reentry. A diagram of the activation pattern is shown in **Figure 12-24**. In this example, there is slowing of conduction through the right bundle branch during sinus rhythm (Panel A) indicated by the dashed yellow arrow. Propagation through the left bundle is more rapid (blue arrows) resulting in initial ventricular activation through the left bundle giving rise to an incomplete RBBB QRS pattern.

In Figure 12-24, Panel B diagrams complete (unidirectional) block in the RBB (dashed yellow arrow and horizontal line at the asterisk) that initiates reentry, as might occur after a decrease in atrial cycle length (premature impulse or period of supraventricular tachycardia). The impulse from the LBB can then cross through the septum and invade the RBB retrogradely (Figure 12-24, Panel B, curved blue arrow), propagating through the region where initial block occurred (asterisk) to complete the reentrant circuit (dashed blue arrow in Figure 12-25, Panel C). The sequence of activation in the circuit during tachycardia is then as follows: RBB → distal end of the HB → LBB → septal VM → RBB, and the VT has a RBBB QRS morphology. Most of the His bundle is activated retrogradely.

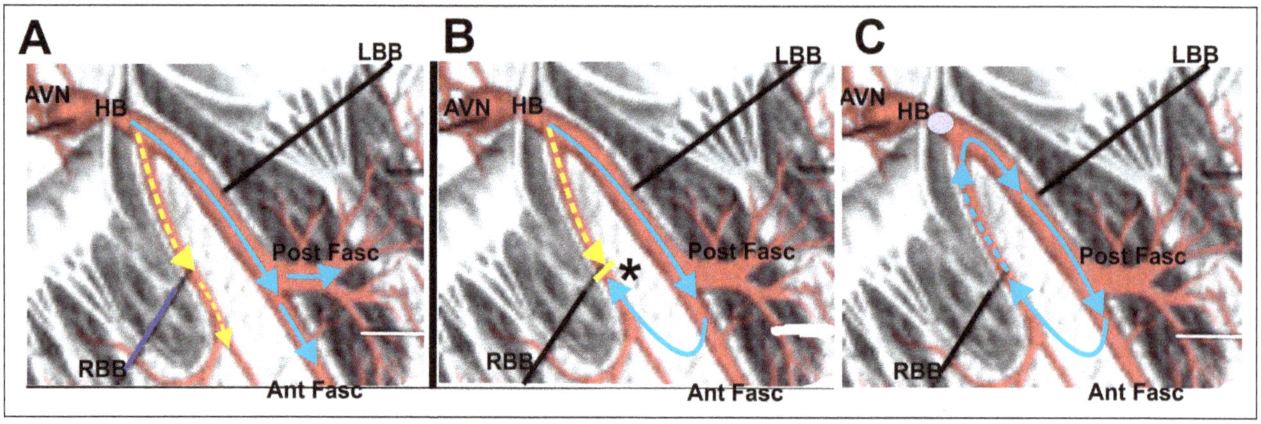

Figure 12-24 Initiation of bundle branch reentry by a supraventricular impulse. AVN, A-V node; Ant Fasc, anterior fascicle; HB, His bundle; LBB, left bundle branch; Post Fasc; posterior fascicle; RBB, right bundle branch.

Electrophysiological Mechanisms

The necessary depression of conduction in either the RBB or LBB that enables reentry to become sustained, no matter what the underlying pathology, is likely caused by depressed (less negative) Purkinje cell resting membrane potentials that reduces phase 0 I_{Na} (see Figure 4-5) resulting from conducting system disease. Stretch from chamber dilation in patients with dilated cardiomyopathy may also contribute.

Action potentials with low membrane potentials have postrepolarization refractoriness that lasts longer than complete repolarization (Figure 9-7). At a decreased basic or premature cycle length, postrepolarization refractory periods get longer, a response similar to the A-V node, rather than shortening, which is the normal response of Purkinje cells. This property may occasionally cause initial block of a premature impulse in the LBB if it is more diseased than the RBB, instead of the usual block in the RBB. Slowing of conduction in the muscle forming the transseptal part of the reentrant circuit may also occur in patients with dilated cardiomyopathy and in patients with a large anteroseptal scar because of the myocardial structural changes.

Effects of Electrical Stimulation

Initiation

In the normal heart, bundle branch reentrant impulses can be initiated by ventricular premature stimulation but reentry is rarely sustained and terminates after one or two reentrant impulses (called the V_3 phenomenon; V_1 is the basic stimulated impulse, V_2 is the premature stimulated impulse and V_3 is the reentrant impulse). Block of the premature impulse occurs retrogradely in the RBB because of its longer refractory periods. However, rapid conduction through the normal conducting system in a reentrant pattern (e.g., retrograde through the LBB to the distal His bundle and antegrade through the RBB), without the additional conduction delay caused by disease, usually results in block in the LBB during the second or third excursion through the circuit. In the normal conducting system, the decrease in the basic cycle during overdrive is not expected to initiate bundle branch reentry because refractory periods decrease due to accelerated repolarization (Figure 7-6), preventing conduction block.

In patients with spontaneously occurring bundle branch reentrant VT, the same VT can be initiated by overdrive pacing or premature stimulation at critically short cycle lengths from either the atria or ventricles because of the additional slowing of conduction in one of the bundle branches associated with conduction system disease (evidenced by the bundle branch block pattern during sinus rhythm). The mechanism for initiation by stimulation is the same as for spontaneous initiation described in Figure 12-22 and Figure 12-24.

Figure 12-25 shows initiation of bundle branch tachycardia with a RBB pattern by an atrial premature stimulus. During atrial pacing (A-A = 550 ms at the left) a RBBB pattern is present with an H-V interval of 120 ms. The ladder diagram below indicates ventricular activation via slow conduction through the LBB (squiggly blue line).

An atrial premature impulse (A-A = 460 ms) blocks in the RBB (red line and horizontal bar), conducts slowly through the LBB to the ventricles (squiggly blue line), transeptally (horizontal blue bar), and retrogradely in the RBB (red arrow) to the distal His bundle from which it returns to the ventricles through the LBB (squiggly blue line initiating bundle branch reentrant tachycardia. Note the retrograde conduction through the His bundle resulting in an H-V interval of 60 ms that is shorter than the antegrade H-V during atrial pacing. A caveat is that the timing of both RBB and LBB electrograms in relation to the His bundle electrogram (HBE) is required to definitively distinguish between bundle branch reentry with RBBB and interfascicular reentry. In bundle branch reentrant tachycardia with RBBB there is anterograde activation of the LBB and retrograde activation of the RBB. In contrast with interfascicular reentry there is retrograde activation of the LBB and anterograde RBB activation (see below).

If the initial block occurs in the LBB during initiation of VT by a supraventricular impulse instead of the RBB, the sequence of activation of the circuit would be the opposite, resulting in antegrade activation of the ventricles through the RBB and VT with a LBB pattern (not shown).

Rapid overdrive stimulation can also initiate VT when there are depressed action potentials in one of the bundle branches, leading to slow conduction and block because of the lengthening of postrepolarization refractoriness described above (also see Figure 9-7).

Resetting, Entrainment, and Termination

Reentrant impulses causing bundle branch reentrant tachycardia have a wavelength that shortens when the impulse is in regions where conduction is depressed and lengthens when the impulse is in regions of more rapid conduction (see Figure 9-3). The average wavelength is short enough to leave a large fully excitable gap, enabling ventricular premature impulses to penetrate and reset the circuit by the mechanism diagrammed in **Figure 12-26**. Panel A shows a reentrant pattern of activation during bundle branch reentrant VT. In Panel B, still during VT, a stimulated ventricular premature impulse (black arrows originating at the asterisk) conducts in the RBB segment of the circuit to collide with the orthodromic reentrant impulse (dashed yellow arrows) and also propagates orthodromically (with respect to the pattern of reentry) in the LBB. In Panel C, the stimulated impulse propagating in the LBB, continues to the His bundle (dashed black arrow is a continuation of Panel B) and then into the right bundle and ventricular muscle (dashed black arrows), resetting the circuit. Reentry continues as indicated by the dashed yellow arrow in Panel C.

Return cycles remain constant over a range of premature coupling intervals giving a flat response pattern (see Figure 9-28), because the premature impulses conduct at the same velocity through the completely excitable gap over a wide range of coupling intervals. Figure 12-26, Panel D diagrams termination of reentry with a short coupled premature impulse (black arrows). The stimulated impulse blocks in the circuit in the LBB because it is refractory (black arrow and horizontal black bar), while colliding with the orthodromic reentrant impulse (dashed yellow arrow) in the RBB.

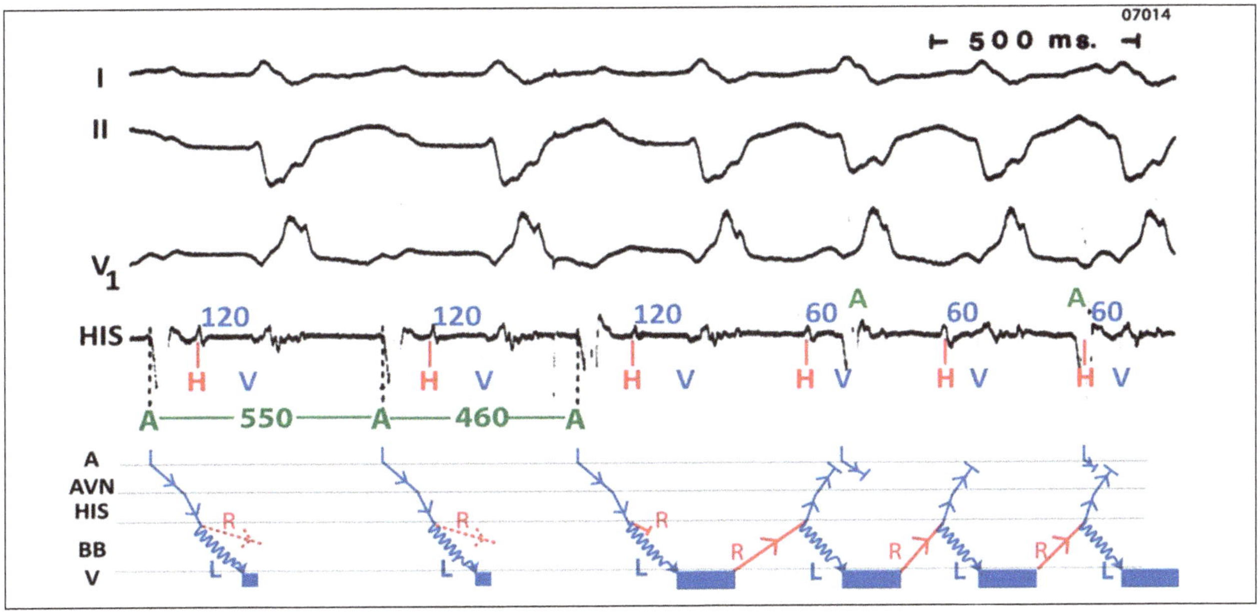

Figure 12-25 Initiation of bundle branch tachycardia by a stimulated atrial premature impulse in a patient with an anteroseptal scar. From **top to bottom** are ECG leads I, II, and V_1, and His bundle recording (H, His; V, ventricle depolarization). H-V intervals in **blue** above His recording, atrial cycle lengths in **green** below His recording. Ladder diagram below shows sequence of activation (A, atria; AVN, AV node; His, BB, bundle branches; V, ventricular septum) (Wellens' ECG collection).

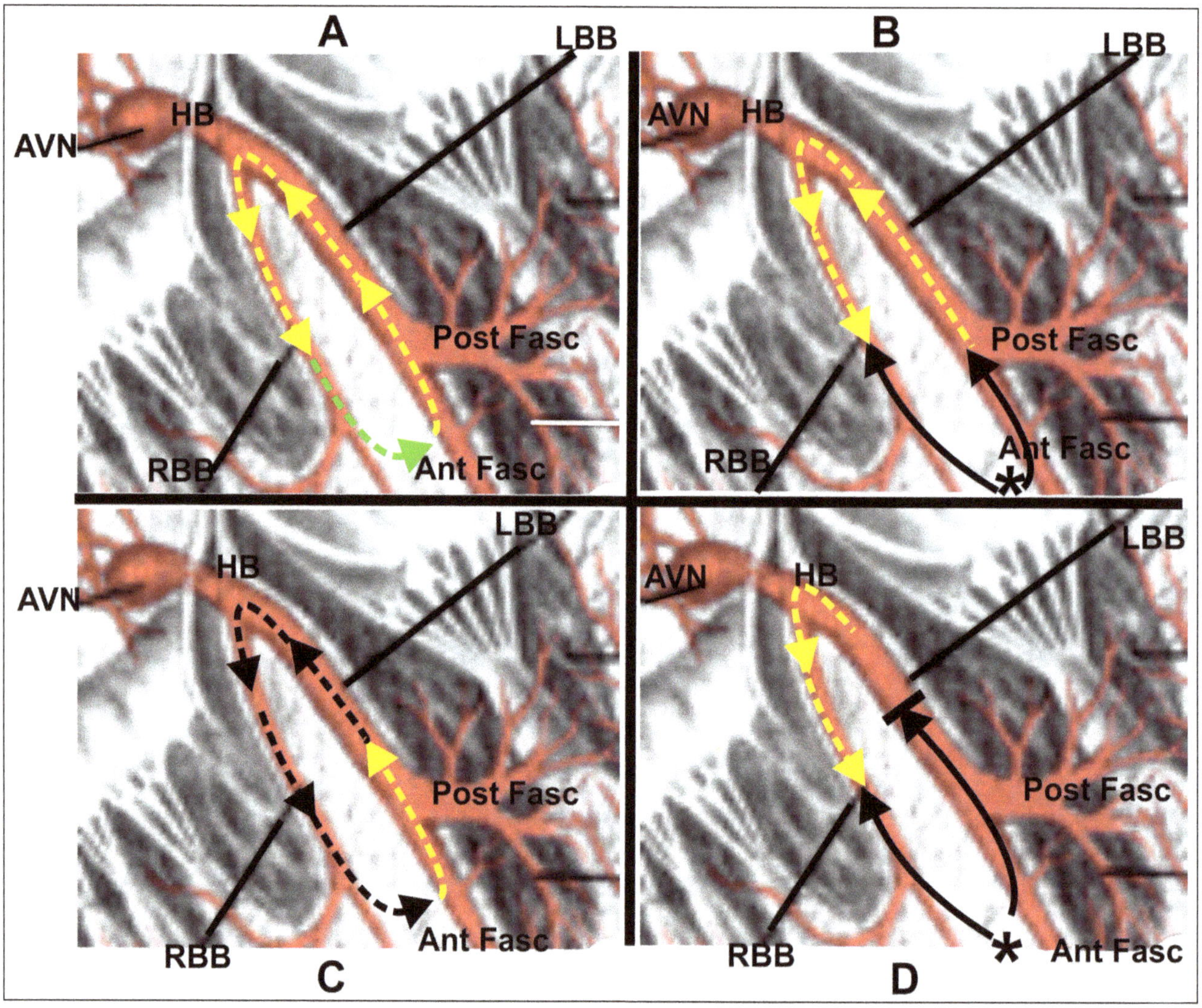

Figure 12-26 **Panel A** diagrams reentry with a LBB pattern. **Panel B** and **C** show conduction of a stimulated impulse during entrainment. **Panel D** shows termination of reentry.

Entrainment. Bundle branch reentry can be entrained, a characteristic of reentrant circuits with an excitable gap. Figure 12-26, Panels B and C, also illustrate the activation pattern for each paced impulse during entrainment with ventricular stimulation: collision of the antidromic paced impulse (black arrow) with the orthodromic reentrant impulse in the RBB (dashed yellow arrow) and propagation of the paced impulse orthodromically through the circuit (black arrow), resetting it (Panel C). All the characteristics of entrainment described in Figures 9-29, Figure 9-30, and Figure 9-31 can be demonstrated, including cycle length–dependent fixed and progressive fusion and termination of reentry at a critically short pacing cycle length.

If there is no retrograde conduction to the His bundle during bundle branch reentrant tachycardia, atrial stimulated impulses can reset and entrain bundle branch reentrant tachycardia. Exact or concealed entrainment of a bundle branch reentrant circuit can occur during atrial overdrive pacing, since paced impulses enter the circuit from the atrial pacing site via the His bundle, comparable to directly pacing the His bundle part of the circuit. Concealed entrainment of a bundle branch reentrant tachycardia is shown in **Figure 12-27**.

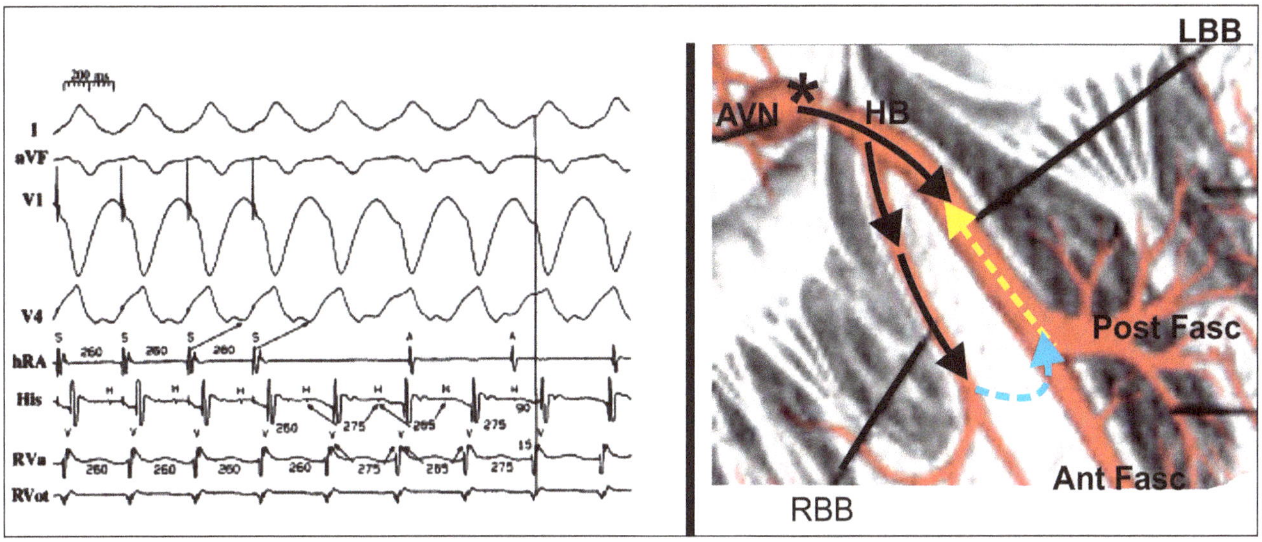

Figure 12-27 **Left Panel:** ECG leads I, aVF, V_1, and V_4, and bipolar electrograms from high right atrium (hRA, S = stimulus artifact); His bundle (H = His bundle electrogram); right ventricular apex (RVa, V = ventricular electrograms); and right ventricular outflow tract (RVot). Numbers on hRA recording are pacing cycle length, numbers on His and RVa recordings are H and V cycle lengths. (Reproduced from Merino JL, et al. Transient entrainment of bundle-branch reentry by atrial and ventricular stimulation. *Circulation*. 1999;100:1784–1790. **Right Panel:** Diagram of pattern of impulse propagation during exact entrainment with atrial stimulation. AVN, A-V node; Ant Fasc, anterior fascicle; HB, His bundle; LBB, left bundle branch; Post Fasc, posterior fascicle; RBB, right bundle branch.

Figure 12-27 (left panel) shows the last four paced impulses during atrial overdrive pacing of bundle branch reentrant tachycardia at a cycle length of 260 ms (S on hRA recording indicates paced impulses). On the His and right ventricular (RVa) electrograms that show orthodromic activation (the H-V interval of 90 ms during pacing is same as during tachycardia), the interval from the last paced impulse to the first tachycardia impulse is the same as the pacing cycle length (260 ms) followed by resumption of the VT cycle length (arrows, 275 ms). The QRS morphology of tachycardia is the same as during entrainment.

Concealed entrainment occurs because the atrial paced impulse enters the circuit from the His bundle (Figure 12-27, right panel, asterisk and black arrows) as would occur if the pacing site were located in this segment of the reentrant circuit. Collision of the paced impulse (black arrow) with the reentrant impulse (yellow arrow) occurs in the LBB, with orthodromic activation of the circuit down the RBB (black arrow) and across the septum to the LBB (dashed blue arrow). No part of the ventricles is directly activated by the paced impulse accounting for the lack of fusion and a QRS during pacing identical to the QRS during tachycardia.

INTERFASCICULAR TACHYCARDIA

VT caused by interfascicular reentry (**Figure 12-28**), where the anterior and posterior fascicles of the LBB comprise the circuit, most commonly occurs in patients with anterior infarction, and either anterior or posterior hemiblock. RBBB is complete and bidirectional, so true bundle branch reentry cannot occur.

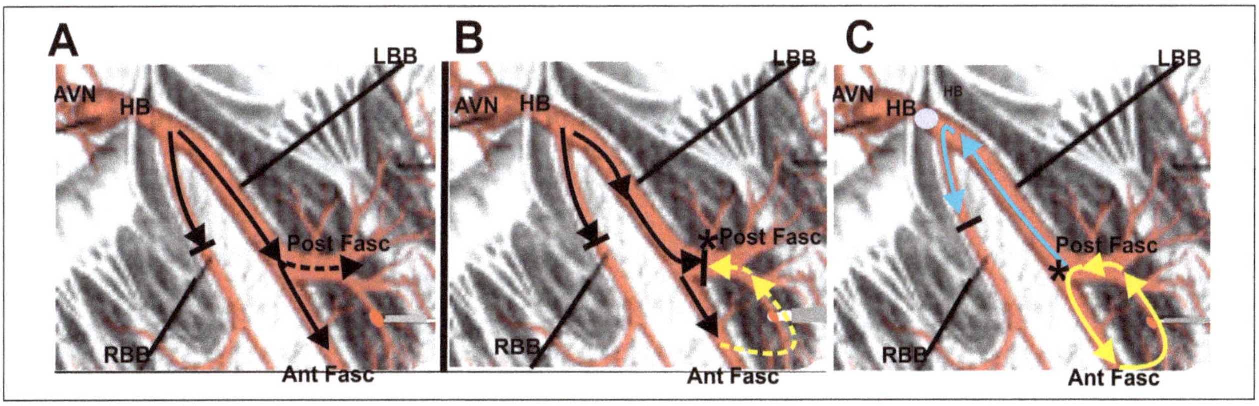

Figure 12-28 Abbreviations are same as in Figure 12-29. **Panel A:** Activation during sinus rhythm with RBBB. **Panel B:** Activation during an atrial premature impulse. **Panel C:** Reentry involving anterior and posterior fascicles (**yellow arrows**).

In Figure 12-28, Panel A diagrams RBBB (indicated by the end of the curved black arrow at the horizontal line) and slowed conduction in the posterior fascicle indicated by the dashed arrow. Initiation of interfascicular reentry occurs when an atrial or ventricular premature impulse or an increase in heart rate causes transient block in the slowly conducting posterior fascicle (Panel B, black arrow and black line, at the asterisk). The impulse conducts over the anterior fascicle, and retrogradely enters the blocked posterior fascicle (Panel B, yellow dashed arrows). Conduction back through the region of initial block (Panel C, yellow arrow at the asterisk) leads to reentry.

The left bundle branch and His bundle are activated retrogradely (blue arrow in Panel C) as the reentrant impulse activates ventricular muscle antegradely (yellow arrow).

Other Reentrant Arrhythmias

Reentry is the cause of other ventricular arrhythmias. The list below is not all-inclusive. Only brief summaries are provided.

VERAPAMIL-SENSITIVE VENTRICULAR TACHYCARDIA

A type of reentrant idiopathic VT arising in the left ventricle is distinguished by its "verapamil sensitivity"; that is, it is terminated by verapamil, unlike the reentrant tachycardias described above. This tachycardia is characterized by a RBBB, and a superior frontal axis QRS morphology. Earliest ventricular activation occurs either at the level of the posterior third (left superior axis) or apical third (right superior axis) of the septum. Tachycardias characteristically have relatively narrow QRS complexes and rapid initial forces unrelated to hypertrophy. Electrophysiological characteristics of this VT that indicate a reentrant mechanism are the following:

1. VT can be induced and terminated by programmed stimulation.
2. During initiation, there is an inverse relationship between the initiating premature coupling interval and the first complex of the tachycardia.
3. Entrainment and resetting with fusion are possible from multiple sites in the right ventricle and from the atrium.

The substrate of the reentrant circuit is not well characterized. The circuit is likely to be very small since exact entrainment is difficult to accomplish. Electrograms at or near the site of origin in sinus rhythm are usually normal although in some patients isolated diastolic potentials may occur that are characteristic of a region of slow conduction. The exact location and components of the reentrant circuit causing VT is not certain. The involvement of the Purkinje system in the circuit is controversial. Purkinje fiber potentials may precede or follow the onset of the QRS during VT making involvement of the septal Purkinje system questionable. In addition, atrial pacing can depolarize the septal Purkinje system without affecting the tachycardia. Therefore, it is likely that the septal Purkinje system is activated by the reentrant impulse after it leaves the circuit rather than being part of the circuit.

A distinguishing feature of the reentrant circuit is that verapamil blocks conduction in the antegrade pathway (prior to the diastolic electrogram) to stop VT. It is likely that this segment has partially depolarized membrane potentials in the range of approximately −65 to −75 mV which inactivates most of the inward I_{Na} and leaves the verapamil-sensitive I_{CaL} responsible for phase 0 (Figure 4-5 and Figure 4-6). (Remember that verapamil also terminates VT caused by DAD-triggered activity (Chapter 6 and Figure 6-22).

VENTRICULAR PREMATURE DEPOLARIZATIONS CAUSED BY REENTRY

Ventricular premature depolarizations (VPDs) caused by reentry, occur either in ventricular muscle or the distal Purkinje system. They are usually associated with myocardial disease that causes partial depolarization of the membrane potential and regions of slow conduction and block (**Figure 9-4**) and can arise from either anatomical or functional reentrant circuits.

POLYMORPHIC VENTRICULAR TACHYCARDIA/ VENTRICULAR FIBRILLATION

Polymorphic VT that terminates spontaneously or progresses to VF can be caused by reentry. Reentrant circuits that cause polymorphic VT in hearts with ischemic and nonischemic cardiomyopathies likely share some properties with the circuits that cause monomorphic VT, such as nonuniform conduction (anisotropy), slowing and block. Polymorphic VT can be induced by rapid pacing or by multiple premature stimuli. Because of the nonsustained nature, other effects of electrical stimulation characteristic of reentry cannot be evaluated. Activation maps in animal models have shown stable reentrant circuits with multiple exit routes that are constantly changing, or multiple reentrant circuits in different regions. In patients with chronic ischemic heart disease and healed infarcts, polymorphic VT can sometimes be converted to sustained monomorphic VT with an antiarrhythmic drug that slows conduction, such as procainamide. This feature suggests a relationship exists between the reentrant circuit causing polymorphic VT and monomorphic VT and that shortening the wavelength leads to a stable reentrant circuit. Polymorphic VT can also be induced in normal hearts, where it cannot be converted to sustained monomorphic VT by procainamide because of the lack of a structurally defined reentrant circuit. The mechanism in normal hearts may involve functional circuits, similar to VF (see below).

Why polymorphic VT is sometimes self-terminating and sometimes goes on to VF is not well understood. When VF occurs, an accelerated phase of VT precedes VF with progressive conduction delay until fractionation and irregular activity evident in local electrograms occurs throughout the ventricles.

Ventricular Fibrillation (VF)

VF is likely to be caused by reentry. There are several different theoretical explanations. It may be caused by multiple small reentrant circuits that are either anatomical or functional, with exiting impulses activating different regions of the ventricles. Functional circuits (rotors or leading circle) are small enough so that many can exist at one time and can migrate (meander) through the ventricles. Functional circuits can form, dissolve, and then reform depending on the spatial dispersion of repolarization and refractoriness, giving rise to multiple nonstationary wavefronts. Alternatively, there may be only a few small reentrant circuits with emanation of impulses to surrounding myocardium at rapid rates, leading to "fibrillatory conduction" of wavefronts (see **Figure 10-20**. This term basically means that at the short cycles, impulses encounter partially and completely refractory myocardium, causing them to block or conduct slowly in circuitous patterns dictated by the heterogeneity of refractoriness, giving rise to fibrillatory patterns of activation. That VF more readily occurs in diseased rather than normal hearts may reflect the increased heterogeneity of conduction and refractory properties that result from structural changes. Increased heterogeneity may also be caused by genetic alterations. In patients with idiopathic VF, DPP6 which is an important subunit of the transient outward K^+ current, can be mutated causing a gain in function and accelerated repolarization of Purkinje cells.

The polymorphic VT with periodic changes in QRS complexes known as torsades de pointes is associated with genetic and acquired long QT syndrome (Chapter 8, Figure 8-1 and Figure 8-3). Although onset of the arrhythmia is attributed to early afterdepolarizations (EADs), perpetuation beyond the initial impulses may result from reentry. Although attributed to heterogeneities in repolarization (see Chapter 7), questions remain concerning the mechanism for reentry and the reason for the periodic changes in ventricular activation reflected in changes in QRS axis, since mapping data has not been obtained in clinical studies.

ACUTE ISCHEMIC ARRHYTHMIAS

The acute phase of ischemia refers to events occurring within the first 2 to 4 hours after sudden onset of coronary occlusion. Information on the mechanisms of arrhythmias at this time comes from experimental animal studies. The loss of K^+ and subsequent Ca^{2+} overload that occur within minutes because of changes in permeability characteristics of the sarcolemma lead to partial membrane potential depolarization, decreased action-potential amplitude and velocity of phase 0 depolarization, and increased postrepolarization refractoriness. Increased myocardial resistivity results from collapse of the vascular bed and osmotic cell swelling, reducing extracellular space. All these factors cause a precipitous slowing and heterogeneity of conduction and block and the formation of reentrant circuits around regions of inexcitability, which results in polymorphic arrhythmias.

A marked decrease in gap junction conductance occurs after around 15 minutes of ischemia. Potassium loss from cells and accumulation in extracellular space is associated with development of intracellular acidosis that closes gap junction channels. The decrease in pH renders gap junctions more sensitive to effects of increasing intracellular calcium, which results in decreasing gap junction conductance. Accumulation of lysophosphoglycerides, arachidonic acid, and other metabolic substances also reduce gap junctional conductance. Gap junction uncoupling is greater intramurally than in border zone regions, where some recovery of the severely depressed transmembrane potentials may occur. This recovery leads to the eventual formation of surviving myocardium that form the border zones where reentrant circuits that cause chronic arrhythmias are located (see Figure 12-5). As a consequence of these changes, conduction velocity in intramural regions falls steeply and inhomogeneously, creating an environment suitable for reentry.

SUMMARY

Reentry in Ventricular Muscle

Reentrant circuits underlying sustained monomorphic VT are comprised of ventricular muscle both in chronic ischemic heart disease and in nonischemic cardiomyopathies. In ischemic disease, a subendocardial or septal origin of VT is most common. In hearts with healed myocardial infarcts, reentrant circuits form to cause VT at locations where myocardial cells survive in and around the infarcted region. Reentrant circuits are often associated with ventricular aneurysms. In ischemic heart disease subepicardial, intramural, and subendocardial myocardium can survive both within an aneurysm and in scarred regions bordering aneurysms. Separation of muscle bundles by fibrous tissue disrupts gap junction connections, particularly in the transverse direction, resulting in slowed transverse conduction and nonuniform anisotropy. Interconnections of small and large fiber bundles also cause slow conduction and block through the mechanism of impedance mismatch. These mechanisms also apply to muscle bundles in DCM that are embedded in scarred ventricle. In the case of DCM, reentrant circuits form in damaged and fibrotic regions.

During sinus rhythm, the site of origin of VT can be located by electrical mapping (substrate mapping). It is characterized by electrograms that occur closest to middiastole, which is invariably in a region of dense scar, in or adjacent to an aneurysm. In substrate mapping, the earliest electrograms near the site of origin are abnormal, with low amplitudes, and fractionated, often with discrete systolic and diastolic components. These abnormal electrograms also have a long duration caused by slow conduction in poorly coupled cells. The fractionation is a result of the "zig-zag" and asynchronous pattern of propagation in nonuniform anisotropic myocardium.

During VT, electrograms occur throughout the diastolic and systolic intervals (continuous electrical activity) when recording directly from the circuit. Whereas these electrogram features are found mostly in the subendocardium in ischemic disease, in DCM, they are often on the epicardial surface where reentrant circuits can occur.

Overdrive pacing and programmed premature stimulation can initiate VT in most patients with spontaneously occurring sustained VT in either ischemic or nonischemic cardiomyopathy, with the induced arrhythmia having identical ECG characteristics as the spontaneous one. The duration and number of fractionated components of electrograms increases as the cycle length is reduced reflecting slowing of conduction and conduction block necessary for reentry. Initiation of VT is characterized by an inverse relationship between the premature coupling interval and the coupling interval between premature impulse and the first tachycardia impulse, a specific feature of reentry. Reentry can be reset and terminated by premature stimulation during VT because the circuits have excitable gaps. Circuits can also be entrained by overdrive pacing.

Information pertaining to the effects of the autonomic nervous system (ANS), drugs that act on the ANS (agonists and antagonists), and other types of drugs that are helpful in identifying automaticity and triggered activity (adenosine and verapamil) is not necessary for identifying a reentrant mechanism. However, the lack of significant effects of most of these agents on reentry can distinguish reentry from automaticity and triggered activity.

Reentry in the Ventricular Conducting System

Sustained monomorphic VT can be caused by bundle branch reentry, where an anatomic reentrant circuit is formed by the LBB and RBB, the distal His bundle that connects them and ventricular muscle. It is associated with a postinfarct scar or nonischemic dilated cardiomyopathy. Parts of the circuit have abnormal conducting properties (caused by disease) as evidenced by a bundle branch block pattern and long H-V interval during sinus rhythm. Initiation of bundle branch reentry requires the transient occurrence of complete block in one of the bundle branches that is unidirectional. This may occur spontaneously during sinus rhythm or after a decrease in supraventricular or ventricular cycle length. The specific blocked bundle branch determines whether the VT has a LBBB or RBBB pattern. The depression of conduction that enables reentry to become sustained is likely caused by conducting system disease. VT can also be caused by interfascicular reentry where the anterior and posterior fascicles of the LBB comprise the circuit, most commonly in patients with anterior infarction, and either anterior or posterior hemi block. RBBB in this instance is complete and bidirectional, so true bundle branch reentry cannot occur.

In patients with spontaneously occurring bundle branch or interfascicular reentrant VT, the same VT can be initiated by overdrive pacing or premature stimulation at critically short cycle lengths. The circuits have a large fully excitable gap, enabling atrial or ventricular premature or overdrive impulses to penetrate the circuits, resulting in resetting, entrainment, and termination.

Other Reentrant Arrhythmias

Verapamil-sensitive tachycardia arises in the left ventricle and can be terminated by verapamil (unlike other forms of reentrant VT). Verapamil blocks conduction in the antegrade pathway to stop VT.

Polymorphic VT that terminates spontaneously or progresses to VF can be caused by reentry. Reentrant circuits likely share some properties with the circuits that cause monomorphic VT, such as nonuniform anisotropy. VF is also likely to be caused by multiple small reentrant circuits. Ventricular arrhythmias that occur during the acute phase of ischemia, within the first 2 to 4 hours after sudden onset of coronary occlusion, are caused by reentry caused by slow conduction and block in ischemic myocardial cells with low resting potentials and reduced phase 0 depolarization.

SOURCES

Akar FG, Spragg DD, Tunin RS, et al. Mechanisms underlying conduction slowing and arrhythmogenesis in nonischemic dilated cardiomyopathy. *Circ Res.* 2004;95;717–725.

Almendral J, Caulier-Cisterna R, Rojo-Alvarez R. Resetting and entrainment of reentrant arrhythmias: Part I: Concepts, recognition, and protocol for evaluation: Surface ECG versus intracardiac recordings. *Pacing Clin Electrophysiol.* 2013;36: 508–532.

Almendral J. Resetting and entrainment of reentrant arrhythmias: Part II: Informative content and practical use of these responses. *Pacing Clin Electrophysiol.* 2013;36:641–661.

Bolick DR, Hackel DB, Reimer KA, et al. Quantitative analysis of myocardial infarct structure in patients with ventricular tachycardia. *Circulation.* 1986;74:1266–1279.

Carmeliet E. Cardiac ionic currents and acute ischemia from channels to arrhythmias. *Physiol Rev.* 1999;79:917–1017.

Caceres J, Jazayeri M, McKinnie J, et al. Sustained bundle branch reentry as a mechanism of clinical tachycardia. *Circulation.* 1989;79:256–270).

Fenoglio JJ Jr, Pham TD, Harken AH, et al. Recurrent sustained ventricular tachycardia: Structure and ultrastructure of subendocardial regions in which tachycardia originates. *Circulation.* 1983;68:518–533.

Hsia HH, Marchlinski FE. Characterization of the electroanatomic substrate for monomorphic ventricular tachycardia in patients with nonischemic cardiomyopathy. *J Pacing Clin Electrophysiol.* 2002;25:1114–1127.

Janse MJ, Wit AL. Electrophysiological mechanisms of ventricular arrhythmias resulting from myocardial ischemia and infarction. *Physiol Rev.* 1989;69:1049–1169.

Josephson ME, Almendral J, Callans DJ. Resetting and entrainment of reentrant ventricular tachycardia associated with myocardial infarction. *Heart Rhythm.* 2014;11:1239–1249.

Marchlinski FE, Zado E, Dixit S, et al. Electroanatomic substrate and outcome of catheter ablative therapy for ventricular tachycardia in setting of right ventricular cardiomyopathy. *Circulation.* 2004;110:2293–2298.

Markowitz SM, Lerman BB. Mechanisms of focal ventricular tachycardia in humans. *Heart Rhythm.* 2009;6:S81–S85.

Poll DS, Marchlinski FE, Buxton AE, et al. Sustained ventricular tachycardia in patients with idiopathic dilated cardiomyopathy: Electrophysiologic testing and lack of response to antiarrhythmic drug therapy. *Circulation.* 1984;70:451–456.

Richardson AW, Callans DJ, Josephson ME. Electrophysiology of postinfarction ventricular tachycardia: A paradigm of stable reentry. *J Cardiovasc Electrophysiol.* 1999;10:1288–1292.

Saffitz JE. Arrhythmogenic cardiomyopathy and abnormalities of cell-to-cell coupling. *Heart Rhythm.* 2009;6:S62–S65.

Soejima K, Stevenson WG, Sapp JL, et al. Endocardial and epicardial radiofrequency ablation of ventricular tachycardia associated with dilated cardiomyopathy. The importance of low-voltage scars. *J Am Coll Cardiol.* 2004;43:1834–1842.

Tchou P, Jazayeri M, Denker S, et al. Transcatheter electrical ablation of right bundle branch. A method of treating macroreentrant ventricular tachycardia attributed to bundle branch reentry. *Circulation.* 1988;78:246–257.

Tomaselli GF, Zipes DP. What causes sudden death in heart failure? *Circ Res.* 2004;95:754–763.

Index

Page references followed by "*f*" denote figures; those followed by "*t*" denote tables

B

C

D

E

F

G

H

I

P

Q

R

S

W

www.ingramcontent.com/pod-product-compliance
Lightning Source LLC
Chambersburg PA
CBHW050238220326
41598CB00047B/7437
9781942909422